Video Contents

Dear Yo —

Thank you for your professionalism, expertise, friendship, and loyalty over nearly ten years.

You are a special person.

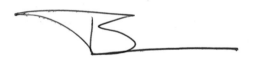

Surgical Management
of Spinal Deformities

Surgical Management
of Spinal Deformities

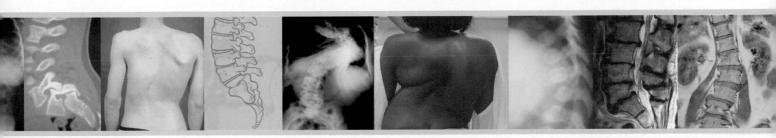

Thomas J. Errico, MD
Associate Professor of Orthopaedic Surgery
Associate Professor of Neurosurgery
New York University School of Medicine
Attending Physician
Tisch Hospital–New York University Langone Medical Center
Bellevue Hospital–New York University Langone Medical Center
Manhattan Veterans Administration Hospital
Orthopedic Institute, New York University Hospital for Joint Diseases
New York, New York

Baron S. Lonner, MD
Clinical Associate Professor of Orthopaedic Surgery
New York University School of Medicine
Director, Spinal Deformity Center
New York University Hospital for Joint Diseases
New York, New York

Andrew W. Moulton, MD
Assistant Professor of Orthopedic Surgery
Coordinator of Spine Surgery Education
New York Medical College
Attending Physician
Westchester Medical Center
Valhalla, New York

SAUNDERS

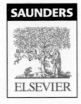

ELSEVIER

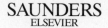

1600 John F. Kennedy Boulevard
Suite 1800
Philadelphia, PA 19103-2899

SURGICAL MANAGEMENT OF SPINAL DEFORMITIES   ISBN: 978-1-4160-3372-1
Copyright © 2009 by Saunders, an imprint of Elsevier Inc.

Notice

Knowledge and best practice in this field are constantly changing. As new research and experience broaden our knowledge, changes in practice, treatment and drug therapy may become necessary or appropriate. Readers are advised to check the most current information provided (i) on procedures featured or (ii) by the manufacturer of each product to be administered, to verify the recommended dose or formula, the method and duration of administration, and contraindications. It is the responsibility of the practitioner, relying on their own experience and knowledge of the patient, to make diagnoses, to determine dosages and the best treatment for each individual patient, and to take all appropriate safety precautions. To the fullest extent of the law, neither the Publisher nor the Editors assume any liability for any injury and/or damage to persons or property arising out or related to any use of the material contained in this book.

The Publisher

Library of Congress Cataloging-in-Publication Data

Surgical management of spinal deformities / [edited by] Thomas J. Errico, Baron S. Lonner, Andrew W. Moulton.—1st ed.
    p. ; cm.
  Includes bibliographical references.
  ISBN 978-1-4160-3372-1
  1. Spine—Abnormalities—Surgery. I. Errico, Thomas J. II. Lonner, Baron S. III. Moulton, Andrew W.
  [DNLM: 1. Musculoskeletal Diseases—surgery. 2. Orthopedic Procedures—methods. 3. Musculoskeletal Abnormalities—surgery. WE 190 S9605 2009]
  RD768.S76 2009
  617.5'6059—dc22

2008012084

Acquisitions Editor: Daniel Pepper
Developmental Editor: Ann Ruzycka Anderson
Design Direction: Ellen Zanolle
Marketing Manager: Catalina Nolte

Printed in China

Last digit is the print number: 9 8 7 6 5 4 3 2 1

I would like to dedicate this text to my parents, Joseph and Nancy Errico; my in-laws, Frank and Santina Chillemi; and my beloved niece Leigh Grieco Cascarilla, all of whom passed on during the preparation of this book. Most important, I would like to thank my wife and children, who helped "keep me grounded" during the difficult times we shared together.

Thomas J. Errico

To my sons, Noah and Jadon, who have been a source of inspiration to me.

Baron S. Lonner

To Carmen, Geraldine, and Ella, whose love and support have allowed me to pursue this work.

Andrew W. Moulton

Contributors

Sheila Conway Adams, MD
Assistant Professor
Department of Orthopaedics
University of Miami School of Medicine
Miami, Florida
Pediatric Neoplasms of the Spine

Daniel Alfonso, MD
Chief Orthopaedic Surgery Resident
Department of Orthopaedic Surgery
New York University Hospital for Joint Diseases
New York, New York
Congenital Scoliosis

M. Darryl Antonacci, MD
Clinical Assistant Professor of Orthopaedic Surgery
Mount Sinai School of Medicine
Attending
Lenox Hill Hospital
New York, New York
Consultant
Shriners Hospital for Children
Philadelphia, Pennsylvania
Spinal Cord Injury

Vincent Arlet, MD
Professor of Orthopaedic Medicine
University of Virginia School of Medicine
Professor of Orthopaedic Surgery
Professor of Neurological Surgery
University of Virginia
Charlottesville, Virginia
Myelomeningocele Spinal Deformities

Ritika Arora, MD
Lenox Hill Radiology and Medical Imaging Associates
New York, New York
Radiologic Imaging of Spinal Deformities

Joshua D. Auerbach, MD
Fellow
Adult and Pediatric Spinal Reconstructive Surgery
Washington University School of Medicine
St. Louis, Missouri
Pediatric Infections of the Spine

Carlos A. Bagley, MD
Assistant Professor
Duke University School of Medicine
Durham, North Carolina
Adult Neoplasia

Randal R. Betz, MD
Shriners Hospital for Children
Philadelphia, Pennsylvania
Infantile and Juvenile Idiopathic Scoliosis

Oheneba Boachie-Adjci, MD
Professor of Medicine
Weill Medical College of Cornell University
Chief of Scoliosis Service
Hospital for Special Surgery
Attending Orthopaedic Surgeon
New York Presbyterian Hospital
New York, New York
Revision Deformity Surgery

David A. Bomback, MD
Attending Orthopedic Spine Surgeon
Danbury Hospital
Connecticut Neck and Back Specialists
Danbury, Connecticut
Revision Deformity Surgery

Elliot R. Carlisle, MD
Encino-Tarzana Regional Medical Center
Orthopedic Consultants Medical Group
Encino, California
Sherman Oaks Hospital
Sherman Oaks, California
Bone Graft and Fusion Enhancement

Gilbert Chan, MD
Visiting Orthopedic Surgeon
Veterans Memorial Medical Center
Quezon City, Philippines
Spinal Deformity in Skeletal Dysplasia

Alvin H. Crawford, MD
Professor of Orthopaedic Surgery and Pediatrics
University of Cincinnati College of Medicine
Director, Pediatric Orthopaedic Fellowhip
Director of Spine Center
Cincinnati Children's Hospital Medical Center
Cincinnati, Ohio
Neurofibromatosis

Bernard K. Crawford, MD
Assistant Professor of Surgery
New York University School of Medicine
New York University
Director, General Thoracic Surgery
Tisch Hospital–New York University Langone
   Medical Center
New York, New York
Thoracic Exposures for Spinal Deformity Surgery

Matthew E. Cunningham, MD, PhD
Instructor
Orthopaedic Surgery
New York Presbyterian Hospital
Instructor
Clinician-Scientist Track
Research Division
Hospital for Special Surgery
Weill Medical College
New York Presbyterian Hospital
Cornell Medical Center
Assistant Attending
Orthopaedic Surgery
New York Presbyterian Hospital
Weill-Cornell Medical Center
Hospital for Special Surgery
New York, New York
Revision Deformity Surgery

John P. Dormans, MD
Professor of Orthopaedic Surgery
Children's Hospital of Philadelphia
University of Pennsylvania School of Medicine
Chief of Pediatric Orthopaedic Surgery
University of Pennsylvania
Philadelphia, Pennsylvania
*Pediatric Infections of the Spine; Pediatric Neoplasms
   of the Spine*

Thomas J. Errico, MD
Associate Professor of Orthopaedic Surgery
Associate Professor of Neurosurgery
New York University School of Medicine
Attending Physician
Tisch Hospital–New York University Langone
   Medical Center
Bellevue Hospital–New York University Langone
   Medical Center
Manhattan Veterans Administration Hospital
Orthopedic Institute, New York University Hospital
   for Joint Diseases
New York, New York
*Introduction to Spinal Deformity; Scheuermann's Kyphosis;
   Cerebral Palsy and Other Neuromuscular Disorders in
   Children; Isthmic and Dysplastic Spondylolisthesis; Adult
   Idiopathic Scoliosis and Degenerative Scoliosis;
   Degenerative Spondylolisthesis*

Jean-Pierre Farcy, MD
Clinical Professor of Orthopedic Surgery
New York University
Attending Orthopedic Surgeon
New York University Hospital for Joint Diseases
New York, New York
Complications in Spinal Deformity Surgery

David S. Feldman, MD
Associate Professor of Orthopedic Surgery
New York University School of Medicine
New York University Hospital for Joint Diseases
Chief, Pediatric Orthopedic Surgery
New York University Hospital for Joint Diseases
New York, New York
Congenital Scoliosis

Jeffrey S. Fischgrund, MD
Fellowship Doctor, Spine Surgery
William Beaumont Hospital–Royal Oak
Royal Oak, Michigan
Bone Graft and Fusion Enhancement

Ziya L. Gokaslan, MD, FACS
Donlin M. Long Professor
Professor of Neurosurgery
Oncology and Orthopaedic Surgery Vice-Chair
Director of Spine Program
Department of Neurosurgery
Johns Hopkins University School of Medicine
Baltimore, Maryland
Adult Neoplasia

Thomas R. Haher, MD
Professor
Department of Orthopaedic Surgery
New York Medical College
Valhalla, New York
Department of Orthopaedic Surgery
Community General Hospital
Syracuse, New York
Biomechanics of Spinal Instrumentation

John P. Kostuik, MD FRCS(C)
Chief of Spinal Surgery (Retired)
Johns Hopkins University
Baltimore, Maryland
Adult Idiopathic Scoliosis and Degenerative Scoliosis

Renata La Rocca Vieira, MD
Research Fellow
New York University Hospital for Joint Diseases
New York, New York
Radiologic Imaging of Spinal Deformities

Willam Lavelle, MD
Fellow, Spine Surgery
Cleveland Clinic Foundation
Cleveland, Ohio
Scheuermann's Kyphosis

Lawrence G. Lenke, MD
The Jerome J. Gilden Professor of Orthopaedic
    Surgery
Professor of Neurological Surgery
Department of Orthopaedic Surgery
Washington University School of Medicine
Co-Chief, Adult/Pediatric Scoliosis and
    Reconstructive Spinal Surgery
Department of Orthopaedic Surgery
Barnes-Jewish Hospital
Department of Orthopaedic Surgery
St. Louis Children's Hospital
Chief, Spinal Surgery
Department of Orthopaedic Surgery
Shriners Hospital for Children–St. Louis Unit
St. Louis, Missouri
Adolescent Idiopathic Scoliosis

Baron S. Lonner, MD
Clinical Associate Professor of Orthopaedic Surgery
New York University School of Medicine
Director, Spinal Deformity Center
New York University Hospital for Joint Diseases
New York, New York
*Spinal Deformity in the Clinical Setting; Congenital
    Scoliosis; Isthmic and Dysplastic Spondylolisthesis;
    Inflammatory Arthropathies*

William G. Mackenzie, MD
Assistant Professor
Jefferson Medical College of Thomas Jefferson
    University
Philadelphia, Pennsylvania
Chairman
Department of Orthopedic Surgery
Nemours/duPont Hospital for Children
Wilmington, Delaware
Spinal Deformity in Skeletal Dysplasia

Jeffrey A. Morgan, MD
Clinical Instructor
Cardiothoracic Surgery
Columbia Presbyterian Medical Center
New York, New York
Thoracic Exposures for Spinal Deformity Surgery

Andrew W. Moulton, MD
Assistant Professor of Orthopedic Surgery
Coordinator of Spine Surgery Education
New York Medical College
Attending Physician
Westchester Medical Center
Valhalla, New York
Clinically Relevant Spinal Anatomy

Bart E. Muhs, MD, PhD
Co-Director, Endovascular Program
Assistant Professor of Vascular Surgery
Section of Vascular Surgery
Yale University School of Medicine
Yale–New Haven Hospital
New Haven, Connecticut
*A Modified Anterior Muscle-Sparing Retroperitoneal
    Approach to the Lumbar Spine: Technique and
    Outcomes*

Matthew M. Nalbandian, MD
Clinical Assistant Professor of Surgery and
    Orthopedics
New York University School of Medicine
New York, New York
*A Modified Anterior Muscle-Sparing Retroperitoneal
    Approach to the Lumbar Spine: Technique and
    Outcomes*

Peter O. Newton, MD
Associate Clinical Professor
Department of Orthopedic Surgery
University of California, San Diego
Director of Scoliosis Service and Orthopedic Research
Rady Children's Hospital
San Diego, California
Future Developments in Spinal Deformity Surgery

Roy M. Nuzzo, MD, FAAOS, FAAP
Associate Professor of Orthopedics
New York University Medical School
New York, New York
Associate Professor of Orthopedics
Seton Hall Graduate School of Medical Education
Paterson, New Jersey
Medical Director, Orthopedics
Childrens Neuromuscular Center
Atlantic Health System
Overlook Hospital
Summit, New Jersey
*Cerebral Palsy and Other Neuromuscular Disorders
    in Children*

Jean Ouellet, MD
Assistant Professor of Spine Surgery
Chief, Scoliosis and Spine Group
McGill University Health Centre
Clinical Director of Scoliosis and Spine Surgery
Montreal Shriners Hospital
Montreal Children's Hospital
Montreal, Quebec, Canada
Myelomeningocele Spinal Deformities

Matías G. Petracchi, MD
Spine Fellow
Department of Orthopaedic Surgery
Maimonides Medical Center
Brooklyn, New York
Complications in Spinal Deformity Surgery

Anthony Petrizzo, DO
Assistant Professor of Orthopaedic Surgery
New York University
New York, New York
Section Head of Pediatric Scoliosis and Spinal
  Deformities
Schneider Children's Hospital
New Hyde Park, New York
Introduction to Spinal Deformity

Martin Quirno, MD
Orthopaedic Resident
Department of Orthopaedic Surgery
New York University Hospital for Joint Diseases
New York, New York
Degenerative Spondylolisthesis

Afshin E. Razi, MD
Clinical Assistant Professor
Department of Orthopaedic Surgery
New York University Langone Medical Center
New York, New York
Congenital Scoliosis

Andrew D. Rosenberg, MD
Professor of Anesthesiology and Orthopedic Surgery
Department of Anesthesiology
Executive Vice Chair
New York University School of Medicine
Chair, Department of Anesthesiology
New York University Hospital for Joint Diseases
Department of Anesthesiology
New York, New York
*Anesthesia for Spine Surgery and Management of Blood
  Loss*

Amer F. Samdani, MD
Shriners Hospital for Children
Philadelphia, Pennsylvania
Infantile and Juvenile Idiopathic Scoliosis

Aaron K. Schachter, MD
Orthopaedic Surgeon
Orthopedic Health LLC
Milford Hospital
Milford, Connecticut
Congenital Scoliosis

Frank Schwab, MD
Associate Professor
New York University School of Medicine
Chief of Spinal Deformity
New York University Hospital for Joint Diseases
New York, New York
Complications in Spinal Deformity Surgery

Mark E. Schweitzer, MD
Professor and Chair of Radiology
University of Ottawa
Ottawa, Ontario, Canada
Radiologic Imaging of Spinal Deformities

Suken A. Shah, MD
Co-Director, Spine and Scoliosis Service
Attending Pediatric Orthopaedic Surgeon
Alfred I. duPont Hospital for Children
Wilmington, Delaware
Assistant Professor of Orthopaedic Surgery
Thomas Jefferson University
Philadelphia, Pennsylvania
Operative Treatment of Neuromuscular Spinal Deformity

Alok D. Sharan, MD
Chief, Orthopedic Spine Service
Montefiore Medical Center
Bronx, New York
Scheuermann's Kyphosis

Fernando E. Silva, MD
Director of Spine Surgery
Hillcrest Health Systems
Waco, Texas
Adolescent Idiopathic Scoliosis

Harvey Smith, MD
Fellow, Spine Surgery
Department of Orthopaedic Surgery
Thomas Jefferson University
Philadelphia, Pennsylvania
Operative Treatment of Neuromuscular Spinal Deformity

Edward W. Song, MD
Spinal Reconstructive Surgeon
The Center for Spainal Disorders
Phoenix, Arizona
Isthmic and Dysplastic Spondylolisthesis

George J. Spessot, MD
Clinical Associate Professor
Department of Anesthesiology
New York University School of Medicine
Attending Anesthesiologist
Department of Anesthesiology
New York University Hospital for Joint Diseases
    Orthopaedic Institute
New York, New York
*Anesthesia for Spine Surgery and Management of Blood
    Loss*

Jeffrey M. Spivak, MD
Assistant Professor
Department of Orthopaedic Surgery
New York University School of Medcine
Director, New York University Hospital for Joint
    Diseases Spine Center
Department of Orthopaedic Surgery
New York University Hospital for Joint Diseases
New York, New York
Inflammatory Arthropathies

Paul D. Sponseller, MD
Professor
Johns Hopkins University School of Medicine
Baltimore, Maryland
Spinal Surgery in Connective Tissue Disorders

Eeric Truumees, MD
Adjunct Faculty
Bioengineering Center
Wayne State University
Detroit, Michigan
Orthopaedic Director
Gehring Biomechanics Laboratory
Attending Spine Surgeon
William Beaumont Hospital
Royal Oak, Michigan
Osteoporosis

Antonio Valdevit, MSc
Senior Lecturer
Biomechanics and Biomaterials
The Stevens Institute of Technology
Hoboken, New Jersey
Biomechanics of Spinal Instrumentation

Diane Von Stein, MD
Clinical Assistant Professor
Nationwide Children's Hospital
Ohio State University
Columbus, Ohio
Neurofibromatosis

David S. Weiss, PhD
Department of Orthopedics
Lenox Hill Hospital
New York, New York
Intraoperative Monitoring
North Shore–LIJ Hospital
Glen Cove, New York
Neuromonitoring for Scoliosis Surgery

Christopher Zarro, MD
Spine Surgeon
Spine Care and Rehabilitation
Roseland, New Jersey
Inflammatory Arthropathies

Joseph M. Zavatsky, MD
Ochsner Medical Center
Spine Center
New Orleans, Louisiana
Inflammatory Arthropathies

Preface

This book was undertaken in light of recognition that the "specialty" of spinal deformity has continued to evolve and develop rapidly over the past decade. In the middle of the previous century, interest in spinal deformity had a pediatric focus. By the 1960s, it was clear that surgical treatment was possible into adulthood. Today, we have developed surgical treatments even for the geriatric population, although not without greater inherent risks and problems. Historically, most of the focus was on coronal plane deformities. Over time, it became evident that equal, if not greater, emphasis must be placed on sagittal plane deformities. Early on, we strived to understand the biomechanics of spinal problems and spinal instrumentation; however, important biomechanical principles also must be understood in the context of the overall "harmony" of the spine in both planes. Even monosegmental procedures have a long-term, if not short-term, effect on overall spinal harmony. One can no longer say, "I am purely a 'degenerative' surgeon and the scope of this text is beyond the needs of my practice and my patients."

Increasingly, both orthopedic and neurologic surgeons know that they need to understand the overall global principles of spinal deformity. This text represents an attempt to put together these evolving topics in a text in which individual disease states are covered comprehensively. In this book, we cover not only the primary processes such as scoliosis, kyphosis, spondylolisthesis, and so on, but also the short- and long-term complications of previous attempts at surgical corrections of these problems. With the knowledge that a picture is worth a thousand words, great effort has been made to accompany selected chapters with videos of surgical techniques described in the chapters. A more complete "transfer of knowledge" can be obtained through careful study of both formats together. The text creates the underlying knowledge base that allows the videos to enlighten the student further.

A text such as this is a living work that evolves over time. It is said that textbooks are outdated by the time they are published. Without doubt, there is some truth to this statement, but every surgeon who continues to develop his or her skills is also a work in progress. The basic principles and tenets of this textbook will stand over time, even though surgical techniques continually evolve. Using this text as part of a surgeon's evolution will hopefully yield rewards for surgeons and patients alike.

Acknowledgments

This book would not have been possible without the assistance of Nicole Martingano Reinhart, Alex Lee, Rose McAndrew, and Frank Martucci.

Thomas J. Errico

I would like to acknowledge my family for their support and encouragement during my work on this book. The advice and guidance of my wife, Melissa, over the years has been invaluable—she has not heard that enough from me. A special note of gratitude goes to my parents, who have provided the blueprint. Without their dedication and direction, I would not have written this book.

I would like to acknowledge and thank my colleagues at NYU Hospital for Joint Diseases for their insightfulness and camaraderie. Special recognition goes to Tom Errico, MD, my chief and co-editor of this book, who is an exceptional chief.

Finally, I would like to acknowledge my teachers, especially Stanley Hoppenfeld, MD; Oheneba Boachie-Adjei, MD; and Patrick F. O'Leary, MD, for providing me with the framework for my career and academic interests.

Baron S. Lonner

I would like to acknowledge Tom Errico, Baron Lonner, and Thomas Haher, whose enthusiasm for spinal deformity care has inspired me.

Andrew W. Moulton

Contents

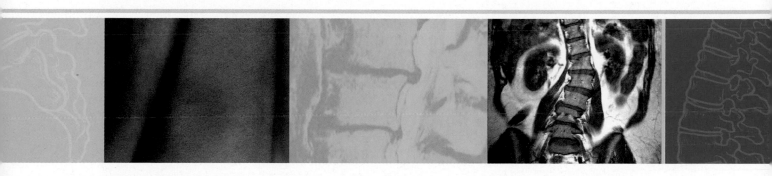

General Introduction/Principles

CHAPTER I

Introduction to Spinal Deformity

THOMAS J. ERRICO *and* ANTHONY PETRIZZO

Historically as well as scientifically, references to spinal deformity date back to antiquity. The Andry tree has become the symbol of our surgical specialty, and the definition of the orthopedic discipline has evolved from the concept of spinal deformity. The treatment of spinal deformity has evolved over the past four centuries from nonoperative modalities, such as traction, casting, and bracing, to spinal fusions, reduction of deformity, and adjunctive use of spinal instrumentation. During this evolution, we have amassed research on the natural history of several common spinal deformities and the effects of intervention. We have also developed an appreciation of the consequences of untreated deformity progressing and creating instability, symptomatic imbalance, spinal stenosis in the concavity of the curves, or lateral spondylolisthesis. With spinal deformity, the musculoskeletal system can lose its deformity compensation capacity by the juxta-articular regions, which can be spinal or extraspinal segments.

Paramount to treating spinal deformity, there needs to be a clear understanding of normal sagittal and coronal parameters to appreciate the magnitude of the deformity and its potential for disability. The normal three-dimensional parameters ensure a balance of the spine in the sagittal and coronal planes and promote efficiency in balance and motion. Spinal deformity can potentially affect the coronal and sagittal planes by creating a multiplane deformity with progression, causing symptomatic imbalance. The normal spine is without curves in the coronal plane. The sagittal alignment is more complicated. It has four normal curves. There is a fixed sacral kyphosis and a primary thoracic kyphosis, which are apparent at birth. Cervical lordosis develops when the infant can maintain an upright head posture. The next curve, which typically develops once a child starts to walk, is the lumbar lordosis. Lumbar lordosis is often absent in nonambulators. Between each of the sagittal curves is a transition zone, where alignment is neutral relative to the vertical sagittal axis of the body. The inflection point in a spinal region is the segment that changes from lordotic to kyphotic or vice versa. Each

of these curves is designed to efficiently transfer the weight of the body and distribute it down through the pelvis. Abnormalities of normal alignment can occur at any segment, as well as at extraspinal locations. These alterations can affect regional as well as global alignment of the spine.

The treatment of spinal deformity requires not only a thorough understanding of the underlying disease processes but also, equally important, an appreciation of spinal mechanics and balance. Once those tasks are understood, it becomes possible to define and treat a deformity. After the deformity has been recognized, a comprehensive understanding of the natural history of the disease process is required to educate the patient and predict the implications. With a complete understanding of the natural history, we can evaluate the risks, benefits, and goals of conservative or operative treatment.

There is also an increased awareness of the importance of prospective outcomes studies, which have been validated. Such studies evaluate the quality of life for both general health and specific disease with attention to pain, function, and satisfaction with the intervention. Our depth of knowledge of spinal deformity has advanced significantly in the last decade as a result of long-term and outcomes-based research. There now exists an advancing middle-aged population of patients who were treated with older methods of posterior spinal fusion and instrumentation. This population can be compared to control groups in regard to long-term and adjacent-level effects. Additionally, it can be determined whether the intervention has changed the natural history of the disease process or the quality of life for those who are affected. Third-party payers evaluating cost effectiveness and threatening pay-for-performance issues will require documentation of treatment and validated outcomes. Furthermore, the technology to process all this information and to communicate and combine the data through multiple centers provides the scientific community exponential access to information.

CLINICAL PRESENTATION

Patients with deformity often present to the orthopedic specialist from referral sources. Patients with idiopathic scoliosis are typically referred by pediatricians or by school screening programs after some degree of asymmetry has been noted. These patients are often free of symptoms with the exception of occasional parathoracic spasm. Older teenagers or adults can present with deformity that was previously thought not to be important or was not noticed. Older adults can present with indirect complaints such as that they are "getting shorter" or their "clothes fit them differently." Adult scoliosis patients experience fatigue symptoms, especially if they have a trunk shift or decompensation in the coronal plane.

Patients with a Scheuermann's kyphosis may also experience back pain in the apex of the curve. This muscle fatigue is often more symptomatic when the apex of the curve is in the thoracolumbar area.

Patients with local segmental deformity present with more subjective complaints than structural complaints. Isthmic or degenerative spondylolisthesis presents with low back pain. Symptoms of neurogenic claudication, which is secondary to nerve root compression, can present later.

DEFORMITY ANALYSIS

Evaluation

To appreciate a spinal deformity, a careful history and physical examination are critical. Parameters such as the characteristics of the pain and duration of symptoms are an important part of the subjective assessment. Neurologic assessments for deficits are imperative objective findings. Family history, rate of progression, and goals of treatment are also important considerations.

Radiographs should be obtained from a standing 36-inch posteroanterior (PA) and lateral radiographs. New digital imaging techniques allow for adequately large views of the entire spine. Patients should stand in their normal posture. This is important in the lateral radiograph, in which the upper limbs are often flexed to be cleared out of the radiograph view, inadvertently flexing or extending the spine. Full-length radiographs permit calculation of the frontal and sagittal plane and the global offset of the plumb line. By using the Cobb technique, thoracic kyphosis, lumbar lordosis, and thoracolumbar junctional measurements can be obtained. An important consideration is the overall sagittal balance. This is determined by dropping a plumb line from the center of the odontoid or seventh cervical vertebra and measuring the distance from the anterior aspect of the S2 body to this line (Fig. 1-1). This line is perpendicular to the horizon and measured on full-length lateral radiographs. Normally, this plumb line should be within 2 cm anterior or posterior (according to the Scoliosis Research Society) to the sacrum. In addition, this plumb line should continue and bisect the femoral heads

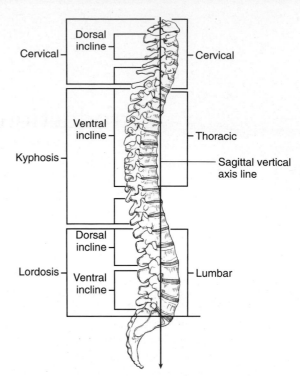

Figure 1-1. Sagittal plumb line.

and continue down through the malleoli of the ankles. Advanced degenerative changes in the diarthrodial joints can magnify spinal symptomatology and should be taken into consideration during the spinal examination.

The PA films should allow a wide enough field to allow for evaluation of the iliac crest apophysis and rib physis to aid in the determination of bone maturity in children.

If specific pathology, such as a nonunion in a postoperative patient is suspected, other radiographs might be needed, including dynamic studies to assess junctional stability. If neurologic symptoms are present, computed tomography, magnetic resonance imaging, and/or myelography might also be needed.

Cervical Region

C1, C2, and C7 are atypical vertebrae with respect to morphology and function, whereas C3 through C6 are commonly described as typical cervical vertebrae. The atlanto-occipital joint (O-C1) acts as a pivot for the flexion/extension motion of the cranium, with 13 degrees average flexion/extension and 8 degrees lateral bending, thus allowing only a few degrees of axial rotation. The atlanto-axial complex (C1-2) has a total axial rotation of approximately 80 to 90 degrees, coupled with a flexion/extension of approximately 10 degrees and minor lateral bending. The prominent motion of the subaxial cervical spine is flexion/extension with some segmental rotation, the latter being facilitated through the alignment of the apophyseal joints and the presence of uncinate processes. The C5-6 interspace is generally found to have the greatest range of flexion/extension motion of the subaxial spine. Flexion/

extension motion decreases as one progresses toward the cervicothoracic junction, which includes an inflection point typically at C7-T1, where it changes from lordosis to kyphosis. It is important in imaging cervical pathology to be able to visualize this region. The cervical lordotic curve normally ranges from 25 to 50 degrees with an apex at C4. The C7 vertebra is atypical and morphologically takes on the appearance of a thoracic vertebra. It has the only transverse process in the cervical spine that does not contain a foramen transversarium to transmit the vertebral artery. It also has a prominent spinous process (vertebra prominens), which is a useful palpable landmark intraoperatively in identifying operative vertebral levels. Its pedicle morphology better accommodates pedicle screws as opposed to positioning them through its lateral mass.

As cervical degenerative changes advance, the intervertebral discs desiccate, causing the space to narrow. Posterior facet joints hypertrophy, causing a loss of cervical lordosis or kyphosis. These degenerative changes can also cause significant narrowing in the anterior-posterior diameter and spinal cord compression. In this situation, patients will present with signs of myelopathy on examination.

Thoracic Region

The thoracic spine anatomically refers to the named vertebral levels from T1 to T12. This region is usually kyphotic, with its apex around T7. The caudal aspect of the kyphosis typically decreases in sagittal angulation until the relatively neutral thoracolumbar junction, which has a relatively straight inflection point. Patients with adolescent idiopathic scoliosis and a thoracic structural curve are hypokyphotic often less than 20 degrees.

Multiple studies of thoracic measurements show a large degree of variability in thoracic kyphosis. Normal thoracic kyphosis usually ranges from 20 to 50 degrees in adults. There is a large variation in this measurement, which occurs for many reasons. Foremost, the shoulders obscure upper thoracic anatomy and create discrepancies in measurement. To avoid this discrepancy, many radiographic studies include only T4 to T12. However the upper thoracic spine is also kyphotic, and including all kyphotic segments would increase the overall number. Also, while the thoracic spine ends at T12, it is not uncommon for the upper lumbar vertebrae to still be in the kyphotic segment of the thoracic curve and not yet reach its inflection point.

Hyperkyphosis can also be a presenting complaint in children and adults. Thoracic radiographs should be closely inspected for the presence of anterior wedging of three adjacent thoracic vertebrae, greater than 5 degrees. Thoracic wedging in three contiguous segments can be a cause of hyperkyphosis. Wedging in addition to Schmorl's nodes, which are irregularities in the vertebral endplates, might suggest Scheuermann's kyphosis. These curves are typically more rigid than a postural kyphosis is. Scheuermann's changes have also been described in the thoracolumbar and lumbar spine.

Lumbar Region

The normal lumbar lordosis is between 40 and 70 degrees with an apex located at the L3-4 interspace. A large discrepancy in the lumbar spine also exists, based on which levels are included in the measurement. This measurement is going to be significantly less than the lordotic L5-S1 if the caudal aspect of vertebrae measurement stops at L5.

The lumbosacral junction is an inflection point for the lordotic segment of the lumbar spine to the kyphotic sacrum. With an isthmic spondylolisthesis, the cephalad vertebral body (usually L5) translates forward and caudal, creating a worsening kyphotic defect. This local kyphosis is measured by the angle created between a line along the inferior aspect of L5 and a line along the superior border of S1. This is also referred to as the *slip angle* and can be used to quantify progression.

Lumbosacral-Pelvic Relationships

One of the most critical relationships in the human spine that sets parameters for sagittal balance is the lumbosacral pelvis. Recent studies report that sagittal plane balance is mediated by the following independent factors: sacral slope, pelvic tilt, pelvic incidence, and lumbar lordosis (Fig. 1-2). Sacral slope is the angle between the superior border of S1 and a line parallel to the horizon. The pelvic tilt is the angle between a line perpendicular to the horizon

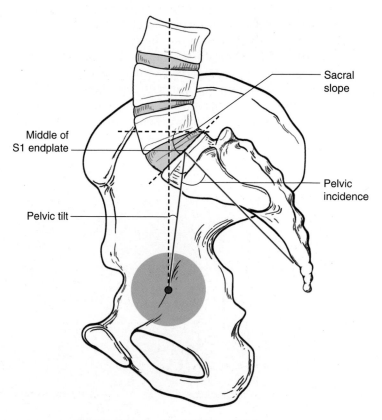

Pelvic incidence = Sacral slope + Pelvic tilt

Figure 1-2. Pelvic tilt and incidence.

and a line joining the middle of the superior sacral end plate.

Pelvic Incidence

Pelvic incidence (PI), or pelvisacral angle, is defined as the angle between a line perpendicular to the sacral plate at its midpoint and a line connecting the same point to the center of the bicoxofemoral axis. This number is fixed and some believe it is the angle on which all other spinal curves are based. Pelvic incidence has been receiving acceptance as being an important anatomic parameter for determining sagittal balance and with higher numbers leading to increased lordosis. Higher numbers are also seen with isthmic spondylolisthesis.

It has become increasingly important to develop an understanding of the reciprocal relations of lumbosacral-pelvic interrelations and their implications on global balance. There is a growing body of evidence suggesting that the sacral pelvic correlations are established primarily and the spinal segments adjust to maintain balance. Computer integrated digital software and further studies will undoubtedly better elucidate these interrelationships.

Spinal-Femoral Angles

When a spinal deformity is recognized, it is important to assess whether the spine is balanced. If the spine is balanced, the patient can still be globally decompensated, especially in the setting of hip or knee contractures. It is important to examine the lower extremities or the angle of the femurs with respect to the spine.

This angle is clinically relevant in two patient populations: previously fused patients with progressive sagittal imbalance and nonambulators with dislocated or fixed hip contractors. Contractures occur in the elderly population with the progression of arthritis and scarring of the anterior hip capsule. These patients with prior sagittal imbalance lose the ability of their hips to compensate for sagittal imbalance. The second population is quadriplegics, a population in which the patients are nonambulators, are confined to a wheelchair, and have hip contractures or subluxations.

INTERPRETING DEFORMITY

Cartesian Coordinates

In describing deformity, the relative position of translation, rotation, or change in relation to another point can be described in many ways. One useful standardized method is based on the Cartesian coordinate system. The Cervical Spine Research Society and the Scoliosis Research Society has standardized coordinates to represent translational motion along the x-, y-, or z-axis. When a free-body diagram is utilized with the sacrum as the reference point, the x-axis lies in the sagittal plane and projects anterior, the y-axis lies in the coronal plane and projects to the left, and the z-axis projects out the head in a cephalad direction. This uses a three-dimensional figure that relates positive and negative changes on the basis of Fleming's right-hand rule (Fig. 1-3). Positive vectors are described in relation to the way the digits of the right hand are pointing. This can be described to represent local, regional spinal, or global curves and clinically is most useful in comparing one vertebral level to another and not regional or global curves.

Coupled Motion

Subtle secondary motion, or coupled motion, of the spine occurs in response to the primary motion. The coupled pattern occurs with motion in the axial, sagittal, or coronal plane; that is, the direction of axial rotation in the subaxial spine is such that the spinous processes rotate into the convexity of the spine on side bending. Coupled motion is

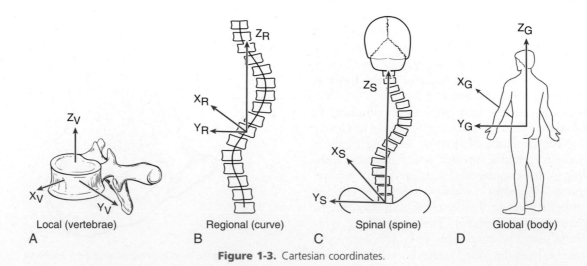

Figure 1-3. Cartesian coordinates.

A Local (vertebrae)   B Regional (curve)   C Spinal (spine)   D Global (body)

a part of the physiologic bending patterns of the spine. It can also be exemplified in pathologic states. For example, scoliosis may be indirectly inferred by performing a forward bending Adams test on clinical examination, in which the clinician looks not only at the scoliosis but also at the amount of vertebral and rib rotation.

Scoliosis deformity is evident in the axial and coronal planes and is often flat or hypokyphotic in the sagittal plane. The end vertebrae are maximally tilted in the coronal plane. The apical vertebrae are often maximally rotated but neutral in the coronal plane.

Coronal Zones of Stability

In evaluating a scoliotic deformity, it is important to assess which curves should be included to balance the spine. The first principle of correction is that the deformity must be appreciated in all three dimensions. PA radiographs should be inspected for the end vertebrae and apical vertebrae. A coronal plumb line should be established to determine which levels are involved in the deformity, and this should be addressed during surgery. Harrington suggested that the caudal level of fusion should be defined by parallel lines that are drawn through the lumbosacral facets. This zone is referred to as the *stable zone of Harrington* (Fig. 1-4). King

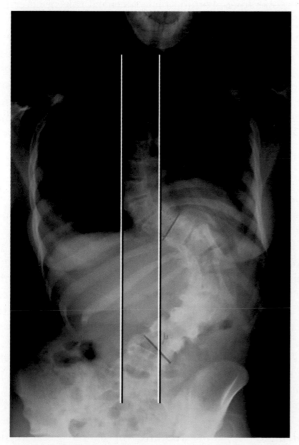

Figure 1-4. Stable zone of Harrington.

and colleagues provided a more specific region termed the *center vertical sacral line*.

Center Vertical Sacral Line

The center vertical sacral line is a single line that is drawn through the center of the sacrum and perpendicular to the iliac crests. The vertebra that is bisected by this line is referred to as the *stable vertebra*. However, it is important to note that in preoperatively planning the fusion levels, one cannot only rely on a PA film. It is important that the lateral radiograph also demonstrates the end vertebra to be stable in the sagittal plane.

Preoperative radiographs should include bending films that differentiate structural curves from compensatory curves. Structural curves remain rigid despite efforts to bend the curve straight. A satisfactory bending film will include either bending over a bolster, a push-prone film, or a bend with head tilted and arms on the convex side over the midline. This bending potential, or flexibility index, should be confirmed on physical examination.

Classification Systems

King, Moe, and coworkers published a classification system with the intent of stratifying a subgroup of adolescents with thoracic idiopathic scoliosis that can have a selective thoracic fusion and potentially avoid a fusion to the caudalmost lumbar segments. In this landmark retrospective study of 405 patients, the authors outlined several important parameters that correlated with a satisfactory result in their study population. First was that the caudalmost segment of the fusion has to be centered over the sacrum and be neutral from a rotation standpoint. The authors also stressed the importance of bending films to determine the degree of correction expected.

The benefit of this study was that it allowed surgeons to selectively choose a thoracic-only fusion and select a subset of patients who would benefit from this thoracic fusion. It also reported on 2-year clinical follow-up of these patients and established how the patients fared postoperatively on the basis of the curve type. Some shortcomings of the study were that isolated thoracolumbar, lumbar, and triple thoracic curves were excluded. Also sagittal balance was not addressed, and all patients underwent posterior spine fusion with Harrington instrumentation, which is not currently used as a primary fixation method. Subsequent articles examined the interobserver and intraobserver reliability, using the classification of King and colleagues. Using posterior anterior and lateral radiographs as well as left and right forced side bending radiographs made with the patient supine, some studies cite poor intraobserver and interobserver reliability of this classification.

Lenke and colleagues proposed an expanded version of this classification system in an attempt to include all curve types as well as to categorize the curve in two dimensions:

TABLE 1-1. Lenke Classification of Curve Types

| Curve Type | Description | Characteristic Curve Patterns* | | | Structural Region of Each Curve Type |
		Proximal Thoracic	Main Thoracic	Thoracolumbar/ Lumbar	
1	Main thoracic	Nonstructural	Structural (major)	Nonstructural	Main thoracic
2	Double thoracic	Structural	Structural (major)	Nonstructural	Proximal thoracic, main thoracic
3	Double major	Nonstructural	Structural (major)	Structural	Main thoracic, thoracolumbar/lumbar
4	Triple major	Structural	Structural (major†)	Structural (major†)	Proximal thoracic, main thoracic, thoracolumbar/lumbar
5	Thoracolumbar/lumbar	Nonstructural	Nonstructural	Structural (major)	Thoracolumbar/lumbar
6	Thoracolumbar/lumbar–main thoracic	Nonstructural	Structural	Structural (major)	Thoracolumbar/lumbar, main thoracic

*A structural proximal thoracic curve has a Cobb angle of ≥25 degrees on side-bending radiographs and/or kyphosis between the second and fifth thoracic levels of at least +20 degrees. A structural main thoracic curve has a Cobb angle of ≥25 degrees on side-bending radiographs and/or kyphosis between the tenth thoracic level and the second lumbar level of at least +20 degrees. A structural thoracolumbar/lumbar curve has a Cobb angle of ≥25 degrees on side-bending radiographs and/or kyphosis between the tenth thoracic level and the second lumbar level of at least +20 degrees.
†Either the main thoracic or the thoracolumbar/lumbar curve can be the major curve.
From Lenke LG, Betz RR, Harms J, et al: Adolescent idiopathic scoliosis: A new classification to determine extent of spinal arthrodesis. J Bone Joint Surg Am 2001;83:1169–1181.

coronal orientation and sagittal plane. Lenke and colleagues' classification is divided into six major groups with two additional modifiers to account for sagittal thoracic and lumbar modifier (Table 1-1). This classification system was evaluated for reproducibility and interobserver reliability first by the five deformity surgeon members of the Scoliosis Research Society who had developed the classification system, followed by seven randomly selected surgeons, also members of the Scoliosis Research Society community.

Lenke and colleagues defined several goals for this classification system. First, it had to include all types of curves in adolescent idiopathic scoliosis. It had to provide a two-dimensional assessment to add the surgical curves as well. It had to recommend selective fusions and avoid fusing nonstructural regions. Finally, they recommended that it be practical, easy to understand, and usable by surgeons and their trainees.

TREATMENT PRINCIPLES

Adolescent Scoliosis

Treatment principles for scoliosis include spinal fusion to prevent curve progression, achieving global spinal balance in the coronal and sagittal planes, and preserving caudal mobile disc spaces if possible. There are three classic ways to categorize surgical treatment of scoliosis. The first is the traditional posterior approach with instrumentation and fusion. The second is anterior with stand-alone anterior instrumentation and fusion techniques. The third is reserved for special situations in which both anterior and posterior techniques are used in the same patient in either staged or same-day surgeries. Traditionally, anterior surgeries have been reserved for three indications: (1) when

there are larger, stiffer curves; (2) in an attempt to save all-important distal mobile disc spaces; and (3) in skeletally immature children (Risser I or II) to prevent crankshaft or continued spinal growth around a solid posterior fusion. The recent popularization of entire pedicle screw constructs has started to redefine the specific indications for all three of these surgical categories.

Preoperative planning plays a crucial role in determining which levels of the spine will be included in the fusion construct. This is determined by preoperative radiographs and, more important, the physical examination. Visual inspection of the scoliosis helps us to determine our cephalad as well as caudal levels. It also gives us an indication of the flexibility of the spine. Observation of the shoulder height gives an indication of the flexibility of the upper thoracic curve. A right thoracic curve should have an elevated right shoulder. If, on inspection, the left shoulder is elevated, that should alert the clinician to a structural proximal thoracic curve, which should be included in the fusion. Incorporation of the proximal thoracic region will often carry the fusion up to T1 as compared to T4 for a symmetric or right elevated shoulder.

Trunk shift or a lateral deviation of the head from the midline on a PA film indicates a coronal decompensation. This is often seen when the thoracolumbar and lumbar curves are larger than the thoracic curves. These curves are often the most cosmetically unpleasant to the patient. Flexibility is also important here to restore the head over the plumb line.

Determining the caudal end of the fusion construct is complex and based on several parameters. Ideally, the caudal end should be a stable vertebra with respect to rotation and coronal tilt. Traditionally, this level is the caudalmost level that fell within the stable zone of Harrington or, more recently, the center sacral vertical line. With pedicle screw fixation and current instrumentation systems, we are able to manipulate the caudal end of the construct to potentially derotate the spine to neutral and horizontalize the distal level, potentially saving caudal levels from a fusion. Preoperative assessments such as the bending films that show reversal of the typical trapezoidal shape of the last disc space suggest that the caudal level can be repositioned to neutral. Intraoperative postreduction radiographs should be obtained to confirm. The impetus for saving distal levels is reinforced by recent studies that show a high likelihood of degenerative changes caudal to the fusion when there is one or two remaining disc spaces.

Sagittal parameters also play an important role in determining fusion vertebral levels. It is fair to say that any abnormal segment should be corrected and included in the fusion. Patients who are hyperkyphotic in the upper thoracic spine should be included in the curve independent of the Cobb measurement on PA films (see the Case Presentation later in the chapter). Also, the caudal segment must be neutral in the sagittal plane. Any thoracolumbar kyphosis greater than 20 degrees should be included in the fusion independent of its Cobb angle.

Neuromuscular Scoliosis

The important considerations of treating neuromuscular scoliosis are the activities of daily living and surgical goals.

For non–wheelchair-independent ambulators, you want to use the same balancing principles and avoid fusing to the pelvis. For wheelchair-independent ambulators the goals of treatment involve preventing curve progression and creating a balanced pelvis for proper seating. It is important to consider that the fusion will not impede any of their self functions including propelling a wheelchair or bending for self-catheterization. Nonambulating patients with neuromuscular curves should focus on balancing the spine and, importantly, reducing the pelvic obliquity. This often requires fusion to the pelvis.

It is important to consider the specific type of neuromuscular condition that is causing the scoliosis. Treatment of spastic neuromuscular curves will require more rigid fixation and often fusion to the pelvis compared to nonspastic neuromuscular scoliosis, in which the goals are to avoid exposure into the chest cavity and which often requires fewer fixation points.

Sagittal Plane Deformity

Iatrogenic flat-back syndrome is a postural disorder and a recognized complication following spine surgery; it most often occurs in the treatment of pediatric or adult scoliosis. For example, with distraction-type instrumentation such as Harrington rods, the posterior distraction force decreases the segmental and regional thoracolumbar and lumbar lordosis, resulting in sagittal imbalance (Fig. 1-5). Iatrogenic

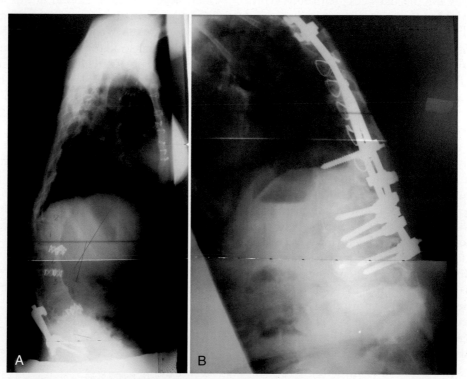

Figure 1-5. A and **B,** Sagittal standing roentgenograms in flat-back deformity syndrome.

flat-back syndrome can also occur after surgery in adults for nonscoliotic degenerative processes or instability-related pathology. Loss of sagittal balance may be secondary to pseudarthrosis within a fusion or below a previous fusion level. The degree of imbalance depends on several factors, including the alignment of the thoracic kyphosis and the thoracolumbar junction, the flexibility of any mobile distal lumbar discs, and the flexibility of the hip joints. The resultant loss of lordosis results in forward inclination of the trunk, back pain, and an inability to stand erect without flexing the knees.

The physical difficulty of maintaining an erect posture for patients with flat-back syndrome places select muscle groups under a constant strain and results in pain and fatigue in the otherwise unaffected areas of the spine (i.e., the thighs and the buttocks). The sagittal malalignment of the flat back places high demands on the muscles, ligaments, and discs of the vertebral column. Minimal disturbances in sagittal alignment are usually compensated for by muscle action to maintain a level gaze (horizontal visual field). However, increasing loss of normal lumbar lordosis leads to a decreased paraspinal lever arm; therefore, significant forces and energy expenditures are required to maintain an erect posture. The progressive decompensation in alignment can be theorized as a gradual process of failure of muscle mechanics (dynamic stabilizers) to maintain posture, followed by a gradual failure of the ligaments and capsular structures (rigid stabilizers). A progression of the deformity is associated with persistent pain and limited function for the patient.

Treatment options for the flat-back deformity evolve around obtaining global balance in the sagittal plane as well as the coronal plane. Paramount to performing this deformity correction is a complete physical and radiologic evaluation and obtaining a preoperative plan.

In most cases of flat-back deformity, the mainstay of treatment involves vertebral wedge osteotomies stabilized with rigid fixation. Osteotomy technique is best guided with the surgeon's experience, the degree of correction, and the location of the deformity. Single osteotomies may be used in relatively mild deformities when the principle deformity is in the middle to lower lumbar spine. When the spinal fusion must be extended to the level of the lower lumbar spine or sacrum, the use of distraction instrumentation must be avoided to prevent recurrent deformity. Conventional wisdom among spinal deformity surgeons is that multiple osteotomies are preferred to ensure better total correction with less chance of neurologic injury. A combined anterior-posterior approach is recommended with a sagittal plane imbalance of more than 4 cm, when the lumbosacral curve is rigid and a source of pain, or when the patient has been previously fused and remains imbalanced. The goals of treatment are to enable the patient to resume a more erect posture, decreasing the strain of adjacent cephalad and caudal muscle groups; to restore horizontal visual field; to relieve compression of abdominal

viscera; and to improve diaphragmatic respiration as well as overall cosmesis.

EVALUATING THE IMPACT OF DEFORMITY

Outcomes research applied to treating spinal disorders is generated to address a plethora of important issues. Treatment of spinal deformity is diverse, costly, and often extensive. A multitude of outcomes are measured to evaluate this spectrum of disease, including monetary cost, length of hospitalization, complications, and perioperative morbidity. In recent years, there has been a shift in research and evaluative bodies to apply evidence-based medicine techniques and outcomes as a foundation for clinical decision making.

The standard history and physical examination provide objective findings that support subjective complaints to develop an overall assessment of the spinal disorder. This "standard" examination often does not assess the impact of the deformity on the patient's quality of life. Functional scales can potentially be useful to measure the impact of disease on the performance of common daily activities. Defining a standard evaluation for functional disability is difficult, because functional activity can be influenced by many factors independent of symptoms and signs, such as age, psychological ability to cope with disease, and the demands of professional activity. They can also vary according to cultural regions and practices. Several validated instruments for evaluating back dysfunction are widely available and are listed in Box 1-1.

The MOS 36-Item Short Form Health Survey (SF-36), developed for the Medical Outcomes Study, is an example of a traditional scale for functional assessment. This questionnaire has obtained an overall usefulness in the general reporting of musculoskeletal ailments; however, it does not report on specific deformity or disability because it is a generic questionnaire that evaluates general health quality of life.

Within the last 10 years, the Scoliosis Research Society introduced a deformity-specific questionnaire based on patients with adolescent idiopathic scoliosis and questions relative to the perception and limitations of their deformity as well as the social impact and limitations caused by the spinal deformity. This SRS-30 was thoroughly ana-

---

BOX 1-1 Standard Instruments for Evaluating Spinal Deformity

MOS 36-Item Short Form Health Survey (SF-36)
SRS-22
SRS-24
SRS-30
Patient-Specific Functional Scale
EQ-5D

lyzed for reproducibility and consistency. It was modified and reanalyzed, and its most current validated version is the SRS-22. Questions are divided into five domains: function/activity, pain, self image/appearance, mental health, and satisfaction with management. This current SRS-22 has high internal consistency and reproducibility and has been validated in a patient population with adolescent idiopathic scoliosis. There are current studies that suggest that SRS-22 is an effective tool to assess adult scoliosis as well.

EQ-5D is a generic measure of health-related quality of life in which health status is defined in terms of five dimensions: mobility, self-care, usual activities, pain/discomfort, and anxiety/depression. Each dimension has three qualifying levels of response roughly corresponding to "no problems," "some difficulties/problems," and "extreme difficulties."

Information generated by the five-dimensional descriptive system and EQ VAS is increasingly being used to generate population reference data (population norms). These norms can be used as reference data to compare profiles for patients with specific conditions and to assess the burden of disease.

CONCLUSION

The rapid evaluation of spinal technology is allowing surgeons to raise the bar with regard to surgical correction, stabilization, and ability to obtain a solid fusion. Within this expansion, the science of spine care is equally expanding and forcing spine physicians to keep pace with technology. As scientists, we have been improving classification systems that allow us to standardize a disease, communicate this information, and report the benefits of this technology. We have also been reporting well-designed prospective long-term studies.

With the expansion of the aging population and a trend toward profound financial implications, patients will continue to push for more acceptable treatments, insurance carriers will demand validation of the costs, surgeons will focus on utilizing outcome studies, and ultimately, patients will benefit from all these interventions.

Illustrative Case Presentation

CASE 1. An Adolescent Girl Status Post Posterior Hook-Rod Instrumentation for Adolescent Idiopathic Scoliosis Who Developed Proximal Junctional Kyphosis

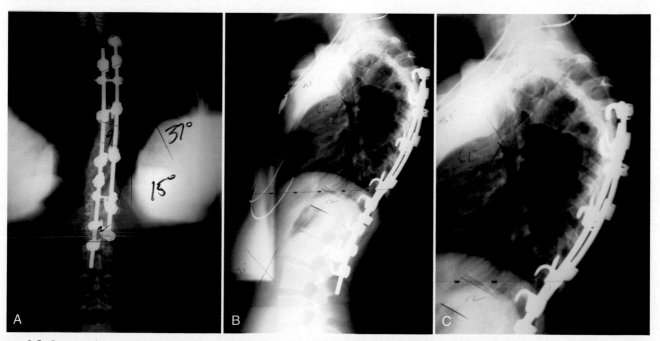

Figure 1-6. Preoperative posteroanterior (**A**) and lateral (**B** and **C**) radiographs of the spine in an adolescent girl status post posterior hook-rod instrumentation for adolescent idiopathic scoliosis who developed proximal junctional kyphosis.

Continued

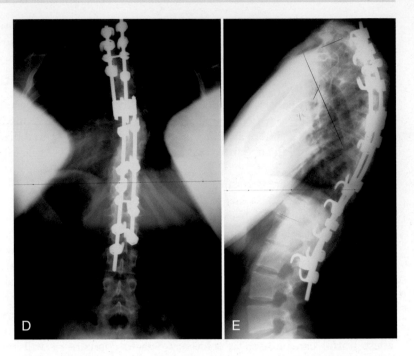

Figure 1-6, cont'd. Postoperative revision posteroanterior (**D**) and lateral (**E**) radiographs following extension of the fusion proximally.

REFERENCES

Boachie-Adjei O, Girardi FP, Hall J: Posterior lumbar decancellation osteotomy. In Margulies JY, Aebi M, Farcy JC (eds): Revision Spine Surgery. St. Louis: Mosby, 1999, pp 568–575.

Booth KC, Bridwell KH, Lenke LG, et al: Complications and predictive factors for the successful treatment of flatback deformity. Spine 1999;24:1712–1720.

Bradford DS, Tribus CB: Current concepts and management of patients with fixed decompensated spinal deformity. Clin Orthop Rel Res 1994;306:64–72.

Farcy JPC, Schwab FJ: Management of flatback and related kyphotic decompensation syndromes. Spine 1997;22:2452–2457.

Kostuik JP, Maurais GR, Richardson WJ, Okajima Y: Combined single stage anterior and posterior osteotomy for correction of iatrogenic lumbar kyphosis. Spine 1988;13:257–266.

LaGrone MO: Flat-back syndrome: Avoidance and treatment. Semin Spine Surg 1998;10:328–338.

Lenke LG, Betz RR, Harms J, et al: Adolescent idiopathic scoliosis: A new classification to determine extent of spinal arthrodesis. J Bone Joint Surg Am 2001;83:1169–1181.

Lowery GL, Bhat AL, Pennisi AE: Pedicle subtraction osteotomy and lumbar extension osteotomy for iatrogenic flatback. In Margulies JY, Aebi M, Farcy JC (eds): Revision Spine Surgery. St. Louis: Mosby, 1999, pp 576–588.

Noun Z, Lapresle L, Missenard G: Posterior lumbar osteotomy for flat back in adults. J Spinal Disord 2001;4:311–316.

Voos K, Adjei OB, Rawlings BA: Multiple vertebral osteotomies in the treatment of rigid adult spine deformities. Spine 2001;26:526–522.

Ware JE Jr, Sherbourne CD: The MOS 36-item short-form health survey (SF-36). Med Care 1992;30:473–483.

Wu SS, Hwa SY, Lin LC, et al: Management of rigid post-traumatic kyphosis. Spine 1996;21:2260–2267.

SUGGESTED READINGS

Asher MA, Burton DC: The surgical evaluation and analysis of the deformed spine. In Spine: State of the Art Reviews, vol 14, no 1. Philadelphia: Hanley and Belfus, 2000.

Provides a systematic approach to interpreting and describing spinal deformity as well as an overview of scoliosis curve classification.

Asher M , Lai SM, Burton D, et al: The reliability and concurrent validity of the Scoliosis Research Society-22 Patient Questionnaire for Idiopathic Scoliosis. Spine 28;1;63–69.

This study demonstrates the reliability, reproducibility, and internal consistency of the SRS-22.

Bigos S, Bowyer O, Braen G, et al: Acute low back problems in adults. Clinical Practice Guideline No. 14. AHCPR Publication No. 95–0642. Rockville, MD: Agency for Health Care Policy and Research, Public Health Service, U.S. Department of Health and Human Services. December 1994.

Applies evidence-based medicine to provide an overview of common causes and interventions for back pain.

King HA, Moe JH, Bradford DS, Winter RB: The selection of fusion levels in thoracic idiopathic scoliosis. J Bone Joint Surg 1983;65A: 1302–1313.

This classic article stratified a subgroup of adolescents with thoracic idiopathic scoliosis that can have a selective thoracic fusion and potentially avoid a fusion to the caudalmost lumbar segments. It also set parameters that correlated with a satisfactory result.

Vialle R, Levassor N, Rillardon L, et al: Radiographic analysis of the sagittal alignment and balance of the spine in asymptomatic subjects. J Bone Joint Surg 2005;87A:260–267.

This is a comprehensive radiographic study of 300 asymptomatic volunteers. It obtained mean values for lumbar lordosis, sacral slope, pelvic tilt, pelvic incidence, and sagittal offset.

CHAPTER 2

Clinically Relevant Spinal Anatomy

Andrew W. Moulton

THE OCCIPUT

The occiput forms the posterior-inferior wall of the calvarium. It is the bony protection for the cerebellum and posterior fossa (Fig. 2-1). The foramen magnum passes through the base of the occipital bone. The anterior border and posterior border of the foramen are called the basion and opisthion, respectively. The two occipital condyles are lateral to the foramen magnum and articulate with the atlas. The occipital condyles are located along the anterior one third of the lateral margin of the foramen magnum. The joint surfaces are elliptical and biconvex. The hypoglossal canal passes through the occipital condyles anterolaterally. The hypoglossal nerve (twelfth cranial nerve) runs within this canal and supplies the muscles of the tongue.

The two most important landmarks on the occiput are the inion, or external occipital protuberance, and the superior nuchal line (Fig. 2-2). The inion is the thickest portion of the occiput, ranging from 11 to 17 mm in depth. The occiput is usually thicker than 8 mm within 2 cm lateral to the inion. The external occipital crest runs caudally from the inion to the foramen magnum, and its thickness can range from 5 to 15 mm.

Transverse occipital landmarks include the supreme, superior, and inferior nuchal lines. The most clinically important is the superior nuchal line. The thickness of the occiput decreases as one moves distally from the superior nuchal line to the foramen magnum. The superior nuchal line runs laterally from the inion. Instrumentation placed cephalad to the superior nuchal line may be too superficial and can result in erosion of the scalp. The superior nuchal line is a landmark not only for bony thickness but also for the internal dural sinuses, a potential surgical hazard if the inner cortex is breached.

Instrumentation of the Occiput

Optimal fixation in the occiput may be seen as the "T" that is formed by the confluence of the superior nuchal line transversely and the external occipital crest vertically.

Sublaminar wires and hooks may be placed unicortically but might not provide as rigid fixation as screws, particularly with osteoporotic bone. Unicortical screw fixation is similar in effectiveness to bicortical fixation (and minimizes potential perforation of the venous plexus). Eight-millimeter screws can safely be placed 2 cm lateral to the midline at the level of the inion, 1 cm from the midline at 1 cm below the inion, and 0.5 cm from the midline at 2 cm below the inion.

THE ATLAS

The first cervical vertebra, or atlas, articulates with the occiput rostrally and the axis caudally. It consists of two articulating lateral masses that are connected anteriorly and posteriorly by neural arches (Fig. 2-3). The lateral masses are also connected coronally by the transverse atlantal ligament. The superior articulation with the occiput is biconcave and provides flexion and extension. The inferior articulating surface of the atlas articulates with the rostral joint surfaces of the axis in a noncongruent manner. This allows for a wider rotational range of motion but a greater potential for instability. The atlas has been described as acting as an intercalated segment, in that its movements are a reaction to the motion of the occiput versus the axis and lower cervical spine (Fig. 2-4), for example, its rotating and translating with lateral bending of the occipitocervical spine.

THE AXIS

The second cervical vertebra, or axis, has a very large and prominent spinous process (Fig. 2-5). This serves as a landmark for localization in performing surgery on the upper posterior cervical spine. Unlike the atlas, the axis has a vertebral body, which articulates with the third cervical vertebra. The dens is the rostral projection from the vertebral body of the axis and represents the remnant of the atlas body. The dens articulates with the anterior arch of the atlas. The stability of this articulation is maintained by the transverse atlantal ligament posterior to the dens (Fig.

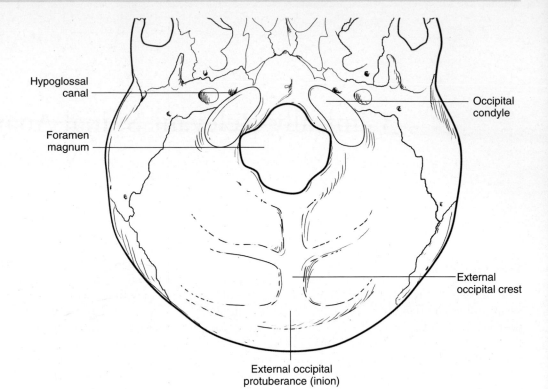

Figure 2-1. Inferior view of the occiput.

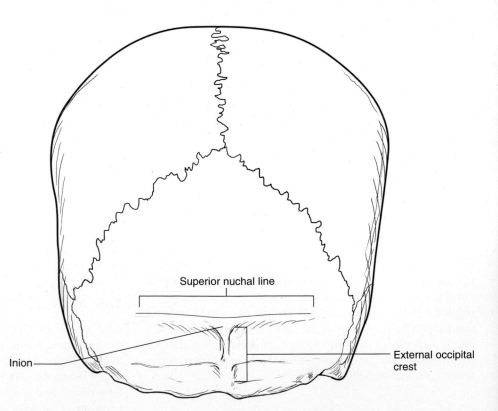

Figure 2-2. Posterior view of the occiput.

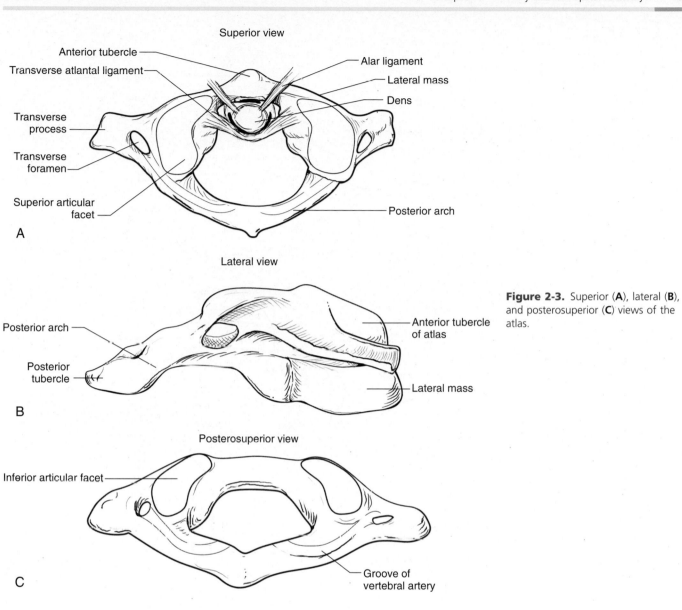

Superior view

Anterior tubercle

Transverse atlantal ligament

Transverse process

Transverse foramen

Superior articular facet

A

Alar ligament

Lateral mass

Dens

Posterior arch

Lateral view

Posterior arch

Posterior tubercle

B

Anterior tubercle of atlas

Lateral mass

Posterosuperior view

Inferior articular facet

C

Groove of vertebral artery

Figure 2-3. Superior (**A**), lateral (**B**), and posterosuperior (**C**) views of the atlas.

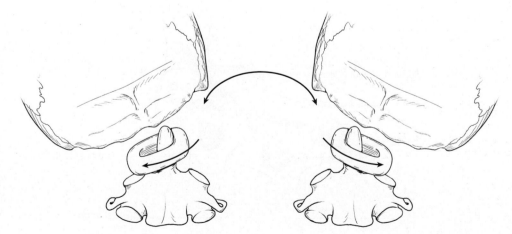

Figure 2-4. Lateral flexion/extension of the occipital-atlantoaxial articulation.

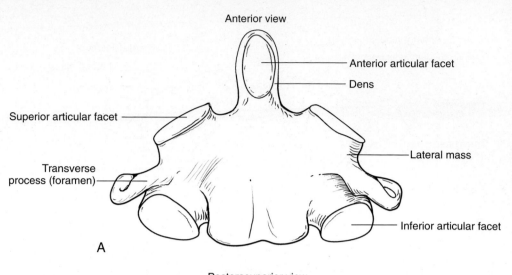

Anterior view

Anterior articular facet

Dens

Superior articular facet

Lateral mass

Transverse process (foramen)

Inferior articular facet

A

Figure 2-5. Anterior (**A**), posterosuperior (**B**), and lateral (**C**) views of the axis.

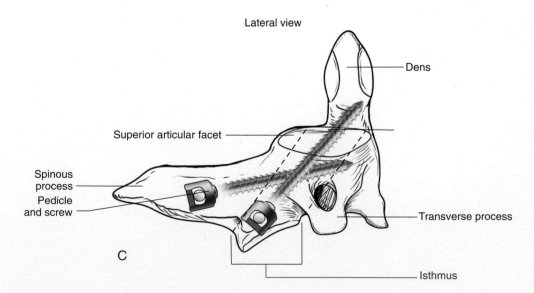

Posterosuperior view

Dens

Posterior articular facet

Superior articular facet

Pedicle

Transverse process (foramen)

Isthmus (pars)

Pedicle

Spinous process

B

Lateral view

Dens

Superior articular facet

Spinous process

Pedicle and screw

Transverse process

Isthmus

C

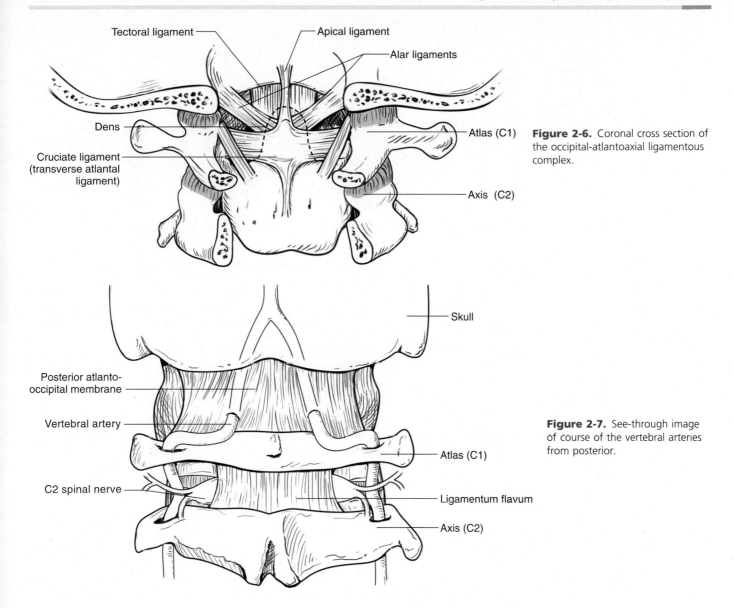

Figure 2-6. Coronal cross section of the occipital-atlantoaxial ligamentous complex.

Figure 2-7. See-through image of course of the vertebral arteries from posterior.

2-6). The alar and apical ligaments connect the tip of the dens to the occiput and are important secondary stabilizers of the atlantoaxial-occipital articulation. The vertebral arteries arise from the transverse foramen of the axis laterally, coursing medially around the posterior aspect of the lateral masses to lie along the rostral surface of the ring of the atlas and progress posteriorly to within 8 mm of the midline before turning superiorly (Fig. 2-7). Computed tomography (CT) angiography may prove helpful in planning instrumentation around the upper cervical spine.

Instrumentation of the Atlantoaxial Level

The importance of selective fusion at the occipitocervical junction must be kept in mind in that more than half of flexion of the cervical spine happens at the atlanto-occipital joint, whereas more than half of rotation of the cervical spine occurs at the atlantoaxial articulation. Atlanto-occipital fixation is almost nonviable, owing to the large momen-

tum of the head in comparison to the atlas as well as the relative bony instability of the C1-2 articulation. For isolated dens fractures, healing can be obtained with direct screw fixation, but this requires minimal displacement and comminution.

Various approaches have been taken to atlantoaxial fixation. The Gallie technique consists of passing sublaminar wires rostrally beneath the lamina of C1, or atlas, and then around the spinous process of C2 with the addition of a clothespin-shaped bone graft (Fig. 2-8). The bilateral wires add more resistance to rotation. The Brooks technique consists of sublaminar wires beneath the lamina of the atlas and axis with two cortical bone graft struts (Fig. 2-9). Hooks may be used over the arch of C1 and under the lamina of C2 to create a "claw." A clamp has specifically been designed for this purpose (Fig. 2-10).

Recently, screw fixation has become more popular. Magerl has described a transarticular technique. The screw traverses the isthmus of the axis and enters the posterior

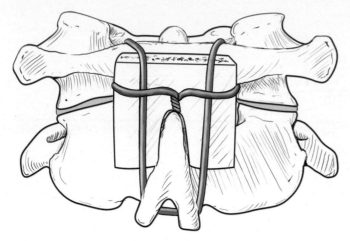

Figure 2-8. Posterior view of the Gallie fixation of C1-2.

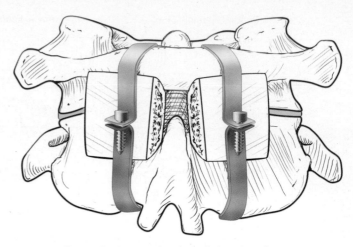

Figure 2-10. Posterior view of clamping of C1-2.

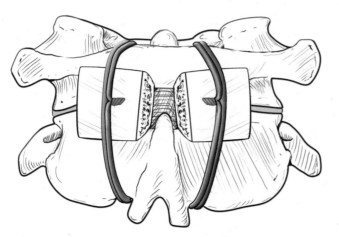

Figure 2-9. Posterior view of the Brooks technique.

aspect of the atlantoaxial joint on its way to the lateral mass of the atlas. There are various contraindications to the transarticular screw, mostly focusing on the course of the vertebral artery (Fig. 2-11). The vertebral artery passes in a groove through the axis before entering the transverse foramina of the atlas. If the depth of the groove exceeds 5 mm, the remaining height of the lateral mass and pedicle width of C2 may be less than 2 mm. This would make it impossible to pass a 3.5-mm screw safely. Also, if the isthmus of the axis is less than 5 mm in height or width, the chance of penetration into the vertebral artery by a 3.5-mm transarticular screw increases. To be aware of these anatomic variations, it is necessary that preoperative CT scans with sagittal and coronal or three-dimensional reconstructions be done prior to transarticular screw placement (Fig. 2-12). An additional complication of the transarticular screw is hypoglossal nerve injury. The twelfth cranial nerve courses anterior to the lateral tip of the C1 lateral mass. If the screws are too long or the lateral mass is overdrilled, injury to this nerve can occur, resulting in motor paresis of the tongue.

Atlantoaxial stabilization can also be accomplished by connecting lateral mass screws from C1 to pedicle screws in C2 (Fig. 2-13). This has the advantage of allowing reduction of the atlas on the axis after individual instrumentation of each and locking them in place with connecting bars. The pedicle lies posterior and medial to the transverse foramen. The pedicle projection is 5 mm caudal to the superior laminar edge and 7 mm lateral to the lateral border of the spinal canal. The pedicle axis is directed 30 degrees medial to the sagittal plane and 20 degrees rostral to the axial plane. The inferior pedicle width is approximately 3 mm less than the width of the superior pedicle. Therefore, to avoid vertebral artery injury and to maintain adequate purchase in the C2 pedicle, the screw should be directed to the superior medial portion of the pedicle.

Another option that might be underutilized for C1-2 instrumentation is the C2 intralaminar screw, having a safer trajectory and similar pullout strength (Fig. 2-14).

THE SUBAXIAL SPINE (C3 to C7)

Posterior Anatomy

The vertebrae from C3 to C7 are relatively uniform, the major differences being the increasing size of their bodies and spinous processes at each adjacent caudal level (Fig. 2-15). The spinous processes are typically bifid except for C7, which is the longest and is commonly used as a landmark for posterior dissection of the cervical spine. The vertebral body is kidney shaped with the concavity facing posteriorly. The vertebrae of the subaxial spine contain lateral masses. The lateral mass is the bony junction between the superior and inferior articular surfaces. The lamina joins the lateral mass medially, and this junction is seen as a shallow groove. The posterior projection of the lateral mass is defined by this groove, the lateral margin of the lateral mass and the posterior aspect of the facet joint above and below. This groove also roughly represents the

Magerl technique

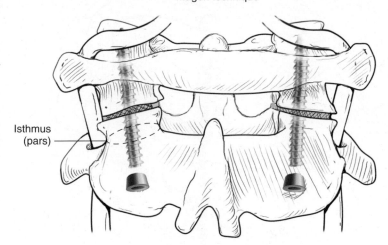

Isthmus
(pars)

A

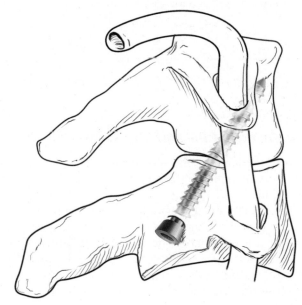

B

Figure 2-11. Posterior (**A**) and lateral (**B**) views of the transarticular Magerl screw with vertebral artery overlay.

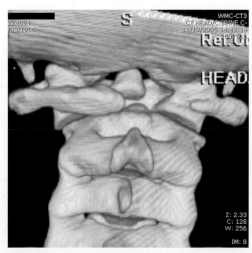

Figure 2-12. Posterolateral view of three-dimensional CT of a patient with a congenital anomaly of the odontoid and atlas.

posterior projection of the medial border of the vertebral artery. The artery's lateral border projects to the middle of the lateral mass (slightly medial to it from C3 to C5 and lateral to it at C6). The vertebral artery runs anterior to the nerve in the transverse foramen. The distance from the posterior midpoint of the lateral mass to the transverse foramen ranges from 9 to 12 mm. Immediately anterior to the lateral mass is the nerve root within the neural foramen. The spinal roots exit the cervical foramen above the respective pedicle and lie anterior to the superior articular process. The nerve branches into dorsal and ventral rami. The distance between the dorsal rami and the anterior lateral corner of the superior facet ranges from 5 to 7 mm. The ventral rami lie 1 to 2 mm anterior to the ventral cortex of the lateral mass. Therefore, the surgeon must take care not to place screws anterior to the tip of the superior articular process to avoid injuring the dorsal rami

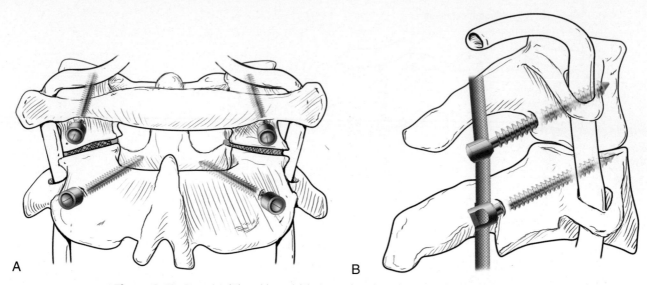

Figure 2-13. Posterior (**A**) and lateral (**B**) views of C1 lateral mass and C2 pedicle screws.

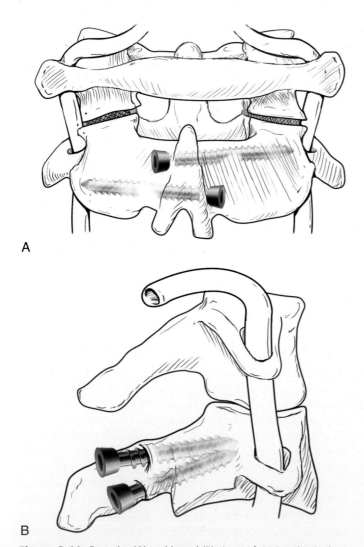

Figure 2-14. Posterior (**A**) and lateral (**B**) views of C2 intralaminal screws.

or directly anterior to the lateral mass to avoid the ventral rami (Fig. 2-16).

Instrumentation of the Posterior Subaxial Spine

Posteriorly, the laminae provide excellent fixation for sublaminar wires or hooks. Sublaminar wires have potentially large canal intrusion when passed, but they have low volumetric displacement and provide segmental fixation. Hook constructs achieve segmental fixation as well but also result in canal intrusion and large volumetric displacement (Fig. 2-17). Lateral mass screws result in adequate fixation, but care must be taken in their trajectory. The distance from the posterior midpoint of the lateral mass to the transverse foramen ranges from 9 to 12 mm. The lateral border of the artery lies 6 degrees lateral to the midpoint of the lateral mass at C6. Therefore, lateral mass screws are started 1 mm medial to the midpoint of the lateral mass and are directed at least 10 degrees lateral to the sagittal plane. To avoid the nerve root, the trajectory should parallel the facet joint with a rostral inclination. Practically, this can be accomplished by laying the drill guide shaft against the spinous process. This will help to ensure the required lateral angulation and anterosuperior trajectory, carrying the tip of the screw between the exiting nerve roots and lateral to the vertebral artery.

The lateral masses of C7 are too small to place screws. Pedicle screws are a better choice and provide better fixation. The posterior projection of the axis of the pedicle of C7 is 1 mm inferior to the middle of the transverse process and 2 mm medial to the lateral border of the lateral mass. The pedicles are angulated posterior superior to anterior inferior about 25 degrees and directed approximately 35 degrees medially. From C3 to C6, the pedicles may be

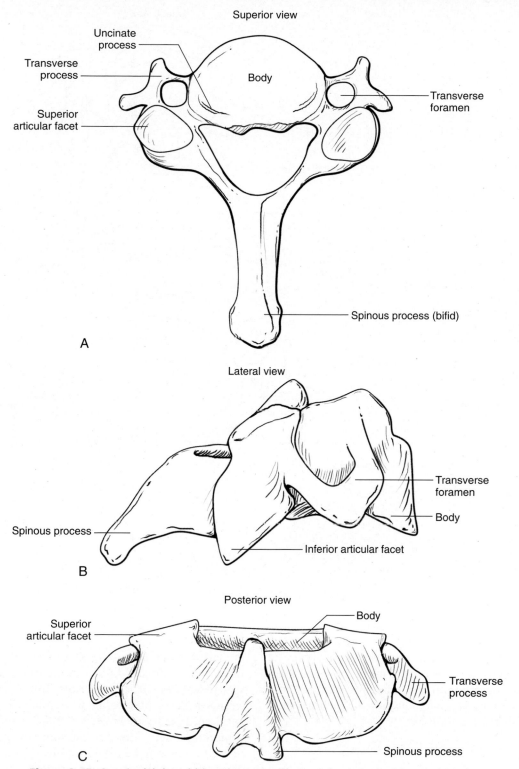

Figure 2-15. Superior (**A**), lateral (**B**), and posterior (**C**) views of typical subaxial cervical vertebra.

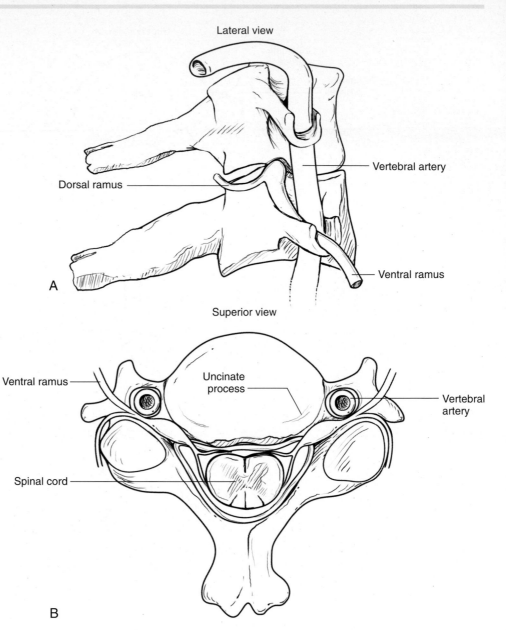

Figure 2-16. See-through lateral (**A**) and superior (**B**) views of subaxial vertebra with nerves and artery projection from posterior.

small and sclerotic, with little room for error. There is no space between the pedicle and the nerve root superiorly or between the pedicle and the dura medially. Specific radiographic planning is prudent at these levels because of the variability of their anatomy.

Anterior Anatomy

When approaching from anterior, many surgeons prefer to use the left side to avoid trauma to the recurrent laryngeal nerve, which descends within the carotid sheath and then a branch of the vagus nerve. On the left, it passes under the aortic arch before coursing deep within the tracheoesophageal groove back up to the larynx. On the right side, it loops around the subclavian artery and returns to

the larynx diagonally in a more variable path (Fig. 2-18). It may be injured while ligating the inferior thyroidal artery, with which it often runs. Injury to the recurrent laryngeal nerve may result in dysphagia, dysphonia, and vocal cord paralysis. However, these symptoms are more commonly due to the direct trauma of the self-retaining retractor and may be minimized by decreasing the length of or amount of pressure or by repositioning the endotracheal tube cuff (it should be inflated and deflated after the retractors are positioned).

The vertebral artery arises from the subclavian artery on the right and the brachiocephalic artery on the left. It enters the transverse foramen of C6 and ascends through the cervical vertebrae. The mean distance from the medial edge of the longus colli to the medial edge of the vertebral artery is approximately 10 mm.

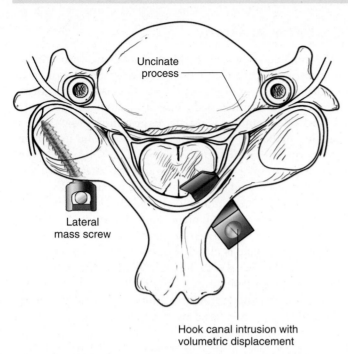

Figure 2-17. Lateral sagittal image of wire and hook canal intrusion and volumetric displacement.

The longus colli muscle lies on the anterior aspect of the atlas and transverse processes of C3 to C6. The sympathetic trunk lies in the loose areolar tissue anterior to the longus colli muscles approximately 10 mm lateral to their medial border. Therefore, dissection of the anterior cervical vertebrae must be carried out through the midline, retracting the longus colli laterally, being careful not to section the muscle. Injury to the cephalad sympathetic trunk may result in Horner's syndrome (ipsilateral ptosis, meiosis, anhydrosis, and enophthalmos).

Upon discectomy, it can be seen that the superior surface of the vertebral body is nearly flat and the inferior

surface is concave. The average depth of the end plate at the midline is 14 mm. The characteristic uncovertebral joints are important landmarks for lateral dissection. Approximately 3 to 4 mm lateral to the uncovertebral joint is the vertebral artery. These joints are also in direct proximity to the exiting nerve roots.

Instrumentation of the Anterior Subaxial Spine

The vertebral bodies provide good screw fixation anteriorly. Because of the kidney shape of the vertebral body, screws that are placed in a converging orientation tend to be shorter than those placed in a diverging orientation. However, diverging screws could result in screw penetration into the neuroforamen or the transverse foramen, resulting in either nerve root or vertebral artery injury. Converging screws meet in the softer central cancellous bone. Therefore, diverging screws might be preferred in certain situations, such as in multilevel corpectomies in patients with severe osteoporosis.

THE THORACIC SPINE

The thoracic region is the longest segment of the axial skeleton, consisting of 12 vertebrae (Fig. 2-19). The first 10 thoracic vertebrae and their corresponding ribs articulate with the sternum to form the rib cage. The T1 vertebral body has characteristics similar to those of the cervical vertebrae, such as the uncinate processes. The T11 and T12 vertebrae represent a transition between the thoracic and lumbar spines. T2 to T8 represent the typical thoracic vertebral anatomy.

Anterior Anatomy

The vertebral bodies are heart shaped with a deeper anterior posterior dimension than medial lateral dimension

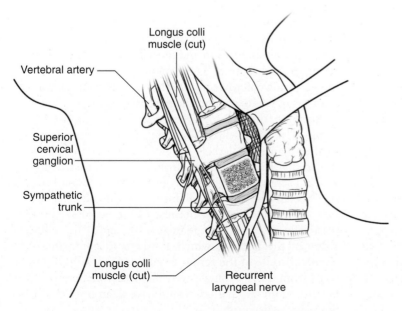

Figure 2-18. Anterior view of C3 to C7 with recurrent laryngeal nerve, longus coli, vertebral artery, sympathetic trunk, and corpectomy.

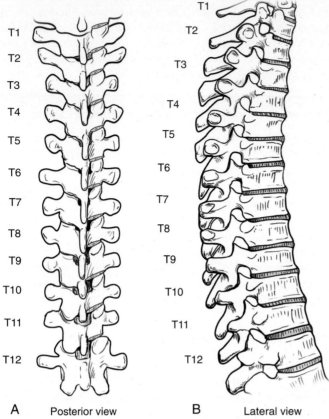

Figure 2-19. Posterior (**A**) and lateral (**B**) views of the thoracic spine.

Posterior Anatomy

The thoracic pedicles are elliptical in shape with a larger rostral-caudal dimension than transverse dimension. The medial cortex is significantly thicker than the lateral cortex. The average thoracic pedicle width is approximately 6 to 8 mm. The diameter is usually largest in the low thoracic region, smallest in the midthoracic region, and intermediate in the proximal thoracic spine. The transverse plane angulation of the pedicle at T4 is approximately 15 degrees medially and gradually becomes more parallel to the sagittal plane as the vertebrae move caudally. The pedicles are inclined in the sagittal plane approximately 22 degrees from posterior superior to anterior inferior. The medial wall of the pedicle is closely bounded by the exiting nerve roots and the thecal sac. The rib head and its costovertebral joint and ligamentous complex lie lateral, protecting the major vascular structures. Superiorly and inferiorly, the pedicles are bordered by their neuroforamen and the nerve roots within them.

Thoracic facet joints are similar from T1 to T11. The articular surfaces are flattened and are oriented primarily in the coronal plane. The orientation of these facet joints allows for mainly lateral bending. The transverse processes arise from the pedicles and laminae at their bases and extend posterolaterally. The laminae of the thoracic spine are in close proximity to each other, and the overlap of the facet joints gives the effect of shingles on a roof.

Instrumentation of the Posterior Thoracic Spine

The transverse processes, laminae, and spinous processes have been incorporated into points of fixation using various techniques with hooks and wires. The size, shape, and strength of the transverse processes below T8 are variable and usually are not amenable to hook fixation. Laminar hooks in a supralaminar and infralaminar position, as well as pedicle hooks, have been extensively used. However, both hooks and sublaminar wires encroach on the spinal canal. Hook-type fixation is also limited in that it provides only semiconstrained fixation and must be paired with a hook in the opposite direction. These methods also limit fixation to the posterior column only, leaving the anterior and middle columns to rotate around the posterior fixation.

Recently, thoracic pedicle screws have been used more commonly. Most thoracic pedicles will accommodate a smaller-diameter pedicle screw, but some studies have shown that the pedicles might be too small to accept even a 4-mm screw. It has been suggested that a screw 110% of the size of the outside diameter of the pedicle can be inserted intrapedicularly because of the pedicle's ability to plastically deform. This may also be due to the elliptical shape of the pedicle, which allows it to conform to the circular profile of the screw. In addition, measured dimensions from a CT scan showed the actual pedicle width to be 1 to 2 mm larger than would have been predicted from the plain radiograph.

(Fig. 2-20). The bodies gradually increase in size from rostral to caudal. The pressure of the aorta flattens the surface of the left side of the vertebral bodies. There may be a dominant segmental arterial supply to the anterior spinal artery known as the *artery of Adamkiewicz*. It is more often on the left than the right, and 90% of the time it originates between T8 and L1.

Instrumentation of the Anterior Thoracic Spine

The thoracic spine may be instrumented anteriorly with vertebral body screws connected with plates or rods. The screws are positioned laterally to avoid injury to the great vessels anteriorly and the contralateral foramen or spinal canal posteriorly (Fig. 2-21). They are directed perpendicular to the vertebral body and kept within the coronal plane. The starting point should not be posterior to the midbody to avoid the canal. Because the body is primarily cancellous, bicortical purchase might be necessary and will increase pullout strength by 40%. Staples also somewhat improve screw fixation but compromise the segmental vessels. Juxta-end-plate position of the screw will provide increased purchase due to increased bone mineral density in this area. Augmentation with methylmethacrylate cement can be particularly helpful in osteoporotic bone, almost doubling pullout strength.

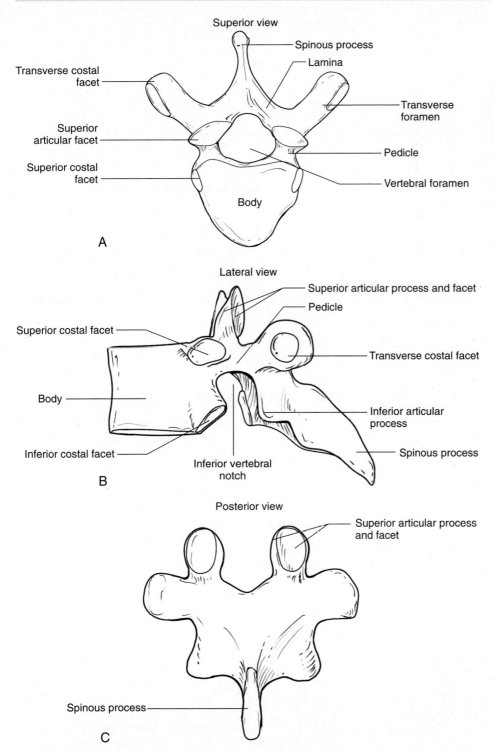

Superior view

Spinous process

Lamina

Transverse costal facet

Superior articular facet

Superior costal facet

Transverse foramen

Pedicle

Vertebral foramen

Body

A

Lateral view

Superior articular process and facet

Pedicle

Superior costal facet

Transverse costal facet

Body

Inferior articular process

Inferior costal facet

Spinous process

Inferior vertebral notch

B

Posterior view

Superior articular process and facet

Spinous process

C

Figure 2-20. Superior (**A**), lateral (**B**), and posterior (**C**) views of thoracic vertebra.

Accuracy for the starting point for thoracic pedicle screws is imperative. The center of the posterior projection of the pedicle lies adjacent to the superior edge of the transverse process and 2 mm medial to the lateral edge of the lamina. This varies critically from rostral to caudal (Fig. 2-22). The pedicle trajectories fall within an anatomic box bounded by the midline of the facet medially, the lateral facet edge laterally, the base of the facet rostrally, and the superior third of the base of the transverse process caudally. Within this box they follow a pattern, being "low and outside" at T1, progressing to "high and inside" at T8

and back to low and outside at T12. This will serve as the entry portal for the "anatomic" approach to the pedicle. The "straightforward" approach allows use of uniaxial or fixed screws and has a slightly different starting point and trajectory (Fig. 2-23), their relative trend being to start lower and aim less caudally.

Angulation of the pedicle in the transverse plane is greatest at T1 at approximately 30 degrees. The transverse angulation decreases going caudally in the thoracic spine and reaches approximately 0 degrees at T12. Angulation in the sagittal plane is approximately 20 to 22 degrees

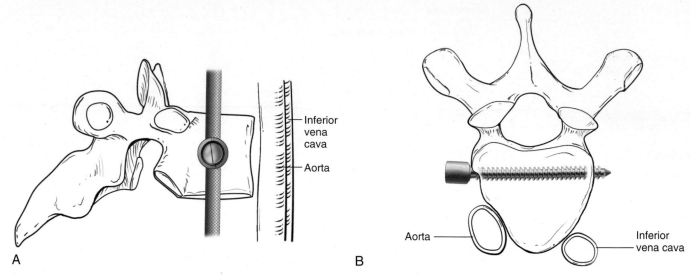

Figure 2-21. Lateral view of hook and wire fixation demonstrating single-column fixation (**A**) and superior view of thoracic vertebral body screw trajectory (**B**).

posterior superior to anterior inferior at T1, also moving toward zero by T12.

Screws may also be placed in a lateral, "extrapedicular" fashion to engage the transverse process, the lateral aspect of the pedicle, and the medial aspect of the rib, ending in the vertebral body (Fig. 2-24). This "in-out-in" screw trajectory provides 75% of the pullout strength of intrapedicular screws. Other studies show that extrapedicular screws could be stronger than some intrapedicular models. Since there is no epidural space between the dura and the medial edge of the pedicle, this method may allow for less chance of spinal cord injury. Clinically, the surgeon will feel resistance as the probe passes through the transverse process and then a sudden giving way as the probe passes lateral to the pedicle. Resistance will then be felt again as the probe enters the lateral aspect of the vertebral body. Lateral pedicle penetration is somewhat protected by the rib head, unless the screw tip is excessively long, anterior and lateral on the left side, in which case the aorta may be

in danger. Care must be taken with severe or dysplastic deformities, in particular the "windswept" pedicle.

THE LUMBAR SPINE

There are five lumbar vertebrae, similar in configuration but increasing in size from rostral to caudal. The lumbar spine is lordotic in alignment with the L4-5 and more so the L5–sacral discs, accounting for the majority of this along with a lesser amount of vertebral body wedging.

Anterior Anatomy

Lumbar vertebral bodies are kidney shaped with the anterior posterior diameter smaller than the transverse diameter (Fig. 2-25). The body has a concave shape posteriorly, and the anterior body height is greater than the posterior body height, contributing to the overall lordosis of the lumbar spine. The size of the vertebral bodies increases as we move

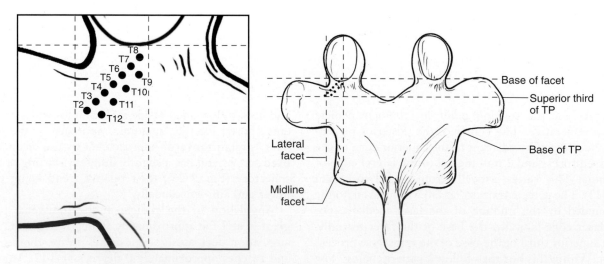

Figure 2-22. Posterior view of thoracic vertebra with projected pedicle and landmarks.

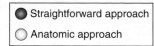

● Straightforward approach
○ Anatomic approach

Posterior view

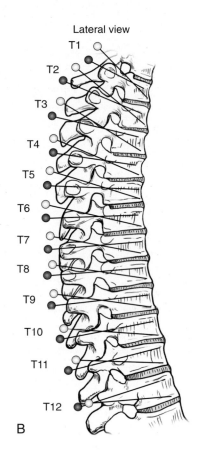

Lateral view

Level	Cephalad-Caudad Starting Point	Medial-Lateral Starting Point
T1	Midpoint TP	Junction: TP-lamina
T2	Midpoint TP	Junction: TP-lamina
T3	Midpoint TP	Junction: TP-lamina
T4	Junction: Proximal third–midpoint TP	Junction: TP-lamina
T5	Proximal third TP	Junction: TP-lamina
T6	Junction: Proximal edge–proximal third TP	Junction: TP-lamina-facet
T7	Proximal TP	Midpoint facet
T8	Proximal TP	Midpoint facet
T9	Proximal TP	Midpoint facet
T10	Junction: Proximal edge–proximal third TP	Junction: TP-lamina-facet
T11	Proximal third TP	Just medial to lateral pars
T12	Midpoint TP	At the level of lateral pars

A

B

Figure 2-23. Lenke's schematic.

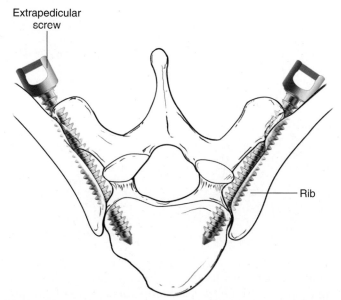

Figure 2-24. Superior view of thoracic vertebra and rib head with extrapedicular screw.

caudally in the lumbar spine. Owing to the concavity of the vertebral bodies circumferentially, the width is slightly larger at the end plate level than at the middle of the body. The ring apophyses of the superior and inferior end plates have a 2- to 3-mm elevation at the perimeter. During anterior disc excision, this is an important landmark, as it is seen just before takedown of the annulus fibrosus.

Instrumentation of the Anterior Lumbar Spine

Anterior fixation of the lumbar spine is similar to that of the thoracic spine. The screws should be placed laterally and directed in the coronal plane. The same dangers and precautions that were discussed in regard to the thoracic spine can be applied to the lumbar spine. An awareness of the vascular and visceral anatomy around the lumbar spine is essential to instrumentation at these levels (Fig. 2-26). The bifurcation of the aorta into the common iliac arteries and the confluence of the common iliac veins into the inferior vena cava occur just cephalad to the L4-5 disc space. The surgeon must be aware of the medial extent of left common iliac vein during the anterior approach to the lower lumbar spine, as it may appear as a thin veil when it is compressed. The great vessels must be mobilized to instrument the lumbar spine. This might require identifying and ligating the middle sacral and segmental vessels. Particular attention should be paid to ligating the left iliolumbar vein when attempting to retract the vena cava and left common iliac vein medially to expose the L4-5 disc.

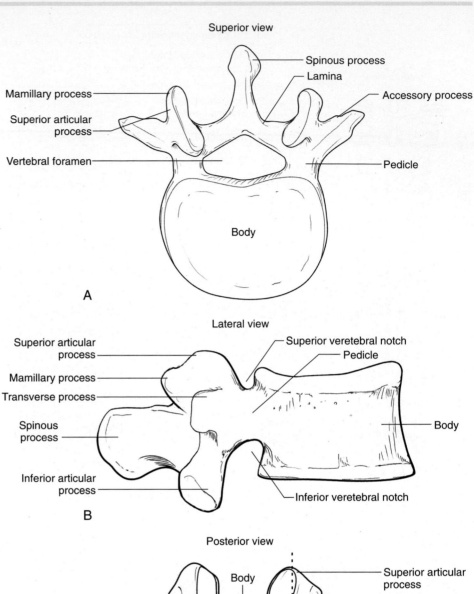

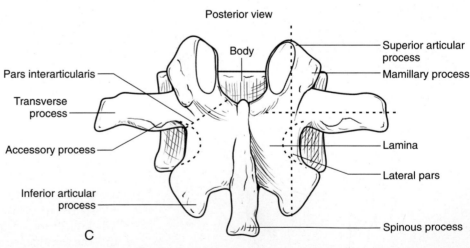

Figure 2-25. Superior (**A**), lateral (**B**), and posterior (**C**) views of a lumbar vertebra.

The ureter is also vulnerable, as it is mobilized medially with the viscera. Injury to the presacral sympathetic plexus can result in retrograde ejaculation. The plexus is located anterior to the sacrum and lower lumbar spine. Blunt dissection sweeping from the midline laterally with minimal electrocautery could decrease the incidence of this. Although this condition is most commonly temporary, male patients should be warned of the possibility.

Unilateral damage to the plexus can lead to increased appearance of the basal parasympathetic tone of the vasculature, the operative side being flush and the other leg feeling relatively cooler to the touch. This might be misconstrued postoperatively as a vascular injury or venous thrombosis.

Methods to increase the anterior body screw pullout strength are the same as those for the thoracic vertebra:

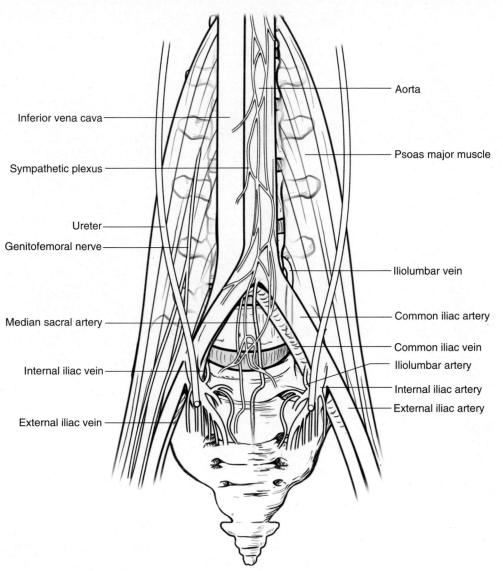

Inferior vena cava

Sympathetic plexus

Ureter

Genitofemoral nerve

Median sacral artery

Internal iliac vein

External iliac vein

Aorta

Psoas major muscle

Iliolumbar vein

Common iliac artery

Common iliac vein

Iliolumbar artery

Internal iliac artery

External iliac artery

Figure 2-26. Anterior anatomy of the lumbar spine.

juxta–end-plate position of the screw, bicortical purchase, and cement augmentation.

Posterior Anatomy

The lumbar pedicles tend to be short and medially inclined. The transverse diameter of the pedicles ranges from 8 to 18 mm. The height of the lumbar pedicle is approximately 15 mm on average. The lumbar pedicle axis is directed approximately 7 degrees medially at L1 and increases at each lumbar level to approximately 18 degrees at L5. The projection of the lumbar pedicle may be found by using the following landmarks (Fig. 2-27). The midline of the transverse process corresponds to the middle of the pedicle. The pedicle axis projects 2 to 4 mm superior from L1 to L3, is at the midline at L4, and is approximately 1.5 mm inferior to the midline at L5. The zygapophyseal joint line gives the most medial aspect of the pedicle, and the lateral aspect of the superior articular facet gives its lateral border. The pedicle's posterior projection may also be defined by

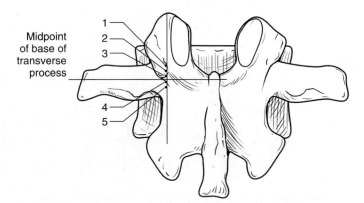

Midpoint
of base of
transverse
process

1
2
3

4
5

Figure 2-27. Posterior view of a lumbar vertebra with projection of pedicle and landmarks.

a confluence of the lamina, the transverse process, and the inferior aspect of the superior facet. The lumbar pedicle, on average, is 5 mm from the superior adjacent nerve root, 1.5 mm from the inferior adjacent nerve root, and 1.5 mm from the lateral dural edge.

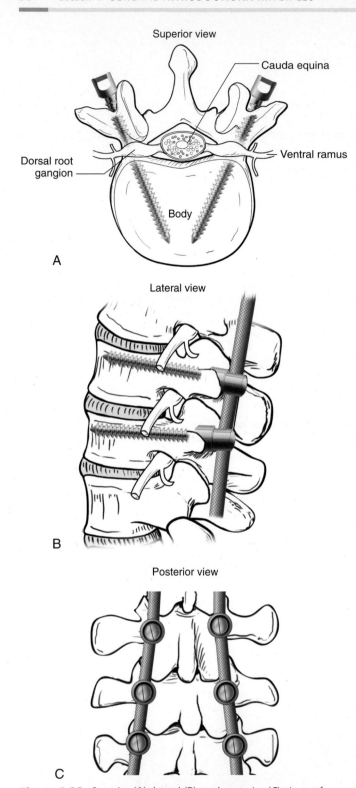

Figure 2-28. Superior (**A**), lateral (**B**), and posterior (**C**) views of lumbar vertebrae instrumented with translaminar screws, hooks, and wires.

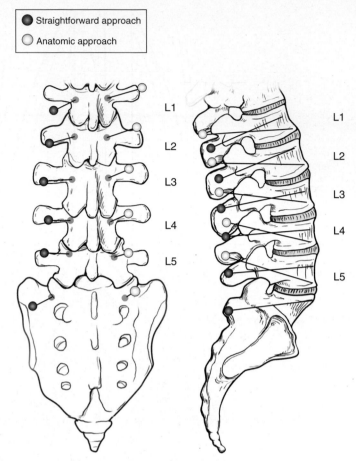

Figure 2-29. Schematic for the lumbar spine similar to Lenke's schematic for the thoracic spine.

Instrumentation of the Posterior Lumbar Spine

The mean thickness of the lamina has been found to be approximately 4 mm. The lamina thickness increases toward the inferior aspect and will allow for the insertion of a 4.5-mm screw for translaminar fixation. Anatomic danger to the insertion of translaminar screws is to the cauda equina at the laminar portion of the path and the exiting nerve root in its foraminal portion. As with the thoracic spine, the lumbar lamina can be instrumented with supralaminar or infralaminar hooks or sublaminar wires. The surgeon must be aware of the insertion of the ligamentum flavum and be sure to develop a plane between the ligamentum and the lamina prior to the insertion of laminar hooks. Care must be taken to insert sublaminar wires midline, in the median raphe of the ligamentum flavum.

Pedicle screws are the most commonly used instrumentation technique for the lumbar spine (Fig. 2-28). Magerl has proposed the starting point as the lateral edge of the superior facet at the level of the midline of the transverse process. Medial angulation of the screw depends on the level of instrumentation. From T12 down, one should aim 5 degrees medially for each level so that the L5 level corresponds to approximately 30 degrees medial angulation (Fig. 2-29).

THE SACRUM

The sacrum consists of five fused vertebrae in kyphotic alignment (Fig. 2-30). The dorsal surface of the sacrum is

Lateral view

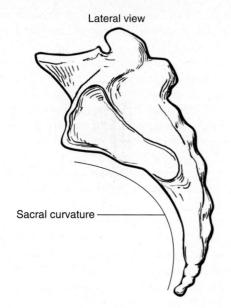

Sacral curvature

A

Anterior view

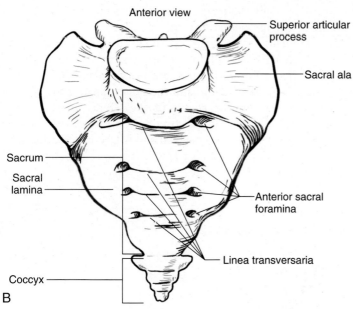

Superior articular process

Sacral ala

Sacrum

Sacral lamina

Anterior sacral foramina

Linea transversaria

Coccyx

B

Figure 2-30. Lateral (**A**), anterior (**B**), and posterior (**C**) views of the sacrum.

Posterior view

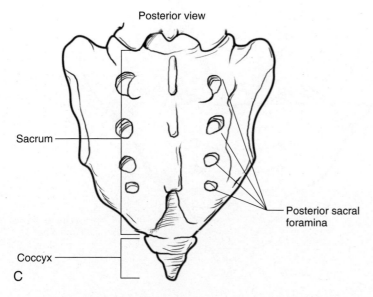

Sacrum

Posterior sacral foramina

Coccyx

C

convex. The sacral laminae unite posteriorly in the middle and form the median sacral crest. The posterior sacral foramina are located lateral to the sacral laminae. The posterior rami exit from these posterior sacral foramina along with the vasculature. There are similar sacral foramina anteriorly. Each sacral vertebra is separated from the adjacent vertebrae by a transverse line known as the linea transversaria anteriorly. The superior aspect of the sacrum is made of the S1 vertebral body, the alae, the posterior arch, and the S1 superior facets. The sacral alae are actually lateral masses that represent the fusion of the vestigial costal elements and transverse processes. The superior aspect of the alae is at the level of the S1 body posteriorly, but anteriorly, the alae are 11 mm lower than the promontory. The promontory is the anterior border of the superior aspect of S1. The angle between the anterior body of L5 and S1 is 140 degrees. This angle is easily palpable and is a useful landmark during anterior surgery. The S1 pedicles are trapezoid in shape. They are bound medially by the spinal canal, laterally by the SI joints, superiorly by the sacral alae, and inferiorly by the first sacral foramina. The S1 pedicles are the widest in the spine, at approximately 20 mm, and are 25 to 30 mm in height. The anteroposterior dimension of the pedicles can be as short as 12 mm.

Instrumentation of the Sacrum

The most effective pedicle fixation of S1 comes from converging screws into the cortex of the apex of the sacral promontory (Fig. 2-31). Another option is the alar screw, which should be directed 30 to 45 degrees laterally to avoid neurovascular injury. Fixation into the far cortex again significantly improves pullout strength. The base of the facet joint serves as the starting point for both of these. S2 pedicle screws are most appropriately oriented 20 degrees laterally. Specific implants have been devised to take advantage of combinations of the above fixation points (Chopin Block and Tacoma Plate).

In performing surgery at the L5-S1 level, various structures are at risk. The posterior structures that are at risk are the cauda equina when medially angled screws enter the canal. Anteriorly, the common iliac vessels are at risk when the anterior cortex is breached. At the level of the promontory, a "safe zone" has been identified that allows for placement of bicortical sacral screws. The safe zone is medial to the left common iliac vein and the right common iliac artery and is 50 mm wide and 30 mm high above the promontory. The bicortical screws that do not exit the safe zone not only will injure the iliac vessels but might also injure the lumbosacral trunk.

The Dunn-McCarthy "S" rod fits over the sacral ala and is particularly useful for boney deficits of the posterior elements or ilium as found in myelodysplasias (Fig. 2-32). These rods pass behind and then over the ala and buttress against the anterior cortex of the lateral masses. Their greatest strength is in resisting flexion forces, and they are less stable to rotation. Jackson and McManus use an intrasacral placement of the rods themselves, attached to S1 screws (Fig. 2-33). The rods are placed into the sacral

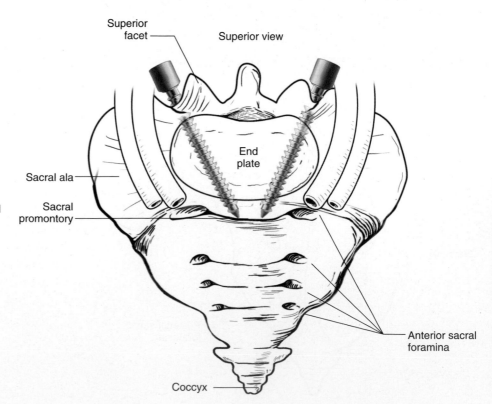

Figure 2-31. Transverse section of the sacrum showing the trajectory of screws and pelvic neurovascular structures.

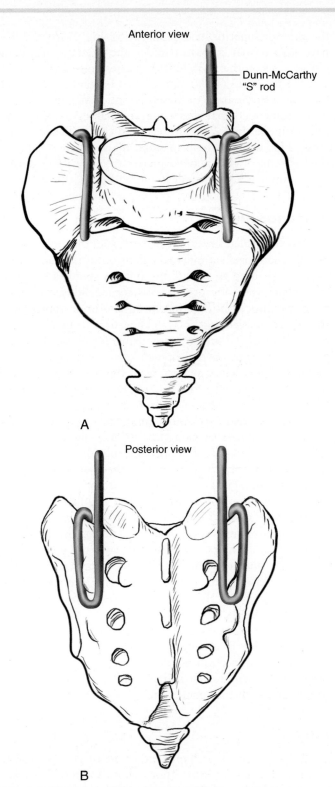

Anterior view

Dunn-McCarthy "S" rod

A

Posterior view

B

Figure 2-32. Anterior (**A**) and posterior (**B**) views of the Dunn-McCarthy "S" rod.

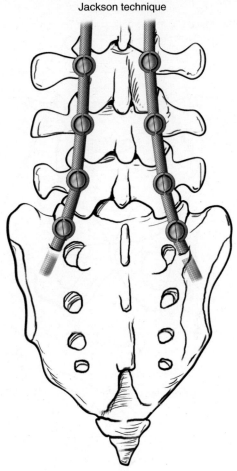

Jackson technique

Figure 2-33. Oblique view of the Jackson technique.

Iliac fixation is the most powerful anchor to the lumbo-pelvic level. This may be done with a Galveston rod or an iliac post or screw. The starting point is the posterosuperior iliac spine, and the device is directed toward the anteroinferior iliac spine, within 2 cm of the greater sciatic notch (Fig. 2-34). The wedge created by the inner and outer tables of the greater sciatic notch gives very good purchase for the screw. Penetration of the greater sciatic notch risks injury to the superior gluteal artery.

AUTOGENOUS GRAFT

The iliac crest is commonly used as a bone graft donor site, and even with the introduction of various alternatives such as allograft and bone morphogenetic proteins, autogenous bone grafting remains the gold standard for spinal fusion. Cancellous bone may be harvested through a trapdoor in the crest. Unicortical grafts may be taken from the lateral table of the posterior ilium, and tricortical graft may be taken from the midilium. The rib may be readily available during anterior thoracic exposures. The fibula is an effective structural graft but requires a remote incision. Each has its own specific anatomic considerations.

lateral masses immediately below and S1 screws, lateral to the S1-2 foramen. There is a large margin for error, as the average distance between the lateral cortex of the S1 foramen and the sacroiliac joint is 28 mm.

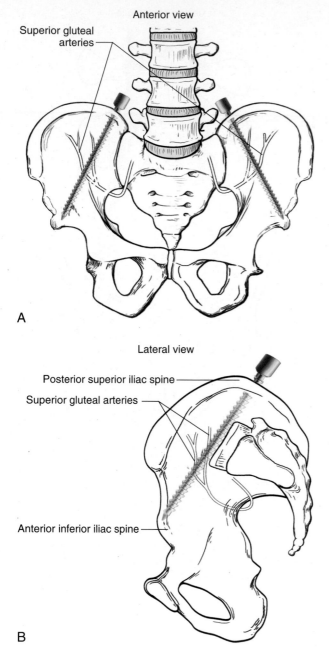

Anterior view

Superior gluteal arteries

A

Lateral view

Posterior superior iliac spine

Superior gluteal arteries

Anterior inferior iliac spine

B

Figure 2-34. See-through anterior (**A**) and lateral (**B**) views of the pelvis with iliac screws.

Anterior Ilium

A trapdoor may be created from which cancellous bone may be harvested, or a tricortical structural graft may be taken with a saw or osteotome (Fig. 2-35). Care should be taken to approximate the fascia in closing.

The main anatomic consideration in this approach is the lateral femoral cutaneous nerve (LFCN). Injury to this nerve may lead to meralgia paresthetica, a dysesthesia in the anterolateral thigh. It is essential to understand its course to avoid injury. The LFCN runs along the lateral border of the psoas, crosses the ilium, and heads toward the anterior superior iliac spine (ASIS) (Fig. 2-36). Studies have shown that it passes under the inguinal ligament (58%), runs on the ASIS (29%), crosses posteriorly within 2 cm of the ASIS (11%), and crosses beyond 2 cm 2% of the time. On the basis of these anatomic considerations, it is recommended that dissection and harvest of the crest remain more than 2 cm posterior to the ASIS along the crest. This will also help to avoid injury to the origin of the sartorius. Care to avoid penetrating the inner cortex will minimize risk to the deep circumflex iliac artery.

Posterior Ilium

The posterior iliac crest may be harvested through a separate incision, or a suprafascial extension of the same incision can be used to expose the lumbar spine. The outer table may be taken to provide corticocancellous graft. The main anatomic consideration in the posterior approach is the cluneal nerves (Fig. 2-37). They arise from the posterior rami of L1-L3 and are responsible for sensation of the gluteal area. The medial branch of the superior cluneal nerve may be as close as 8 cm from the posterior superior iliac spine. Therefore, it is recommended that the dissection not be extended more than 8 cm anterolateral to the posterior superior iliac spine. Injury to these nerves can result in numbness or painful neuromas. Temporary dysesthesias are not uncommon, probably due to traction; they usually resolve in 3 months. If they persist, cortisone injections or surgical excision of a neuroma might be necessary. The donor site itself may be painful in 12% of patients 6 months after the procedure.

Injury to the superior gluteal artery during this approach has also been described. The artery leaves the pelvis superior to the piriformis muscle directly in contact with the greater sciatic notch. The artery can be lacerated by an osteotome or saw if the graft is harvested too deeply. The artery can also be injured by a retractor placed in the notch. If injured, it may retract into the pelvis, leading to a life-threatening situation. To avoid this, it is recommended that dissection not be carried out inferior to the insertion of the gluteus maximus and that retractors should not be placed in the sciatic notch.

Rib

The ribs can provide significant autograft and be readily available during anterior approaches. Vulnerable structures include the pulmonary pleura and intercostal neurovascular bundle. The key is to perform a careful subperiosteal dissection. Pleural violation can result in pneumothorax and might require chest tube placement. It should be checked for with an intraoperative Valsalva maneuver and postoperative chest radiograph. Intercostal neurovascular bundle injury will lead to bandlike dysesthesias and bleeding, potentially in the intrathoracic region. Injection of long-acting anesthetic into the costovertebral junction just

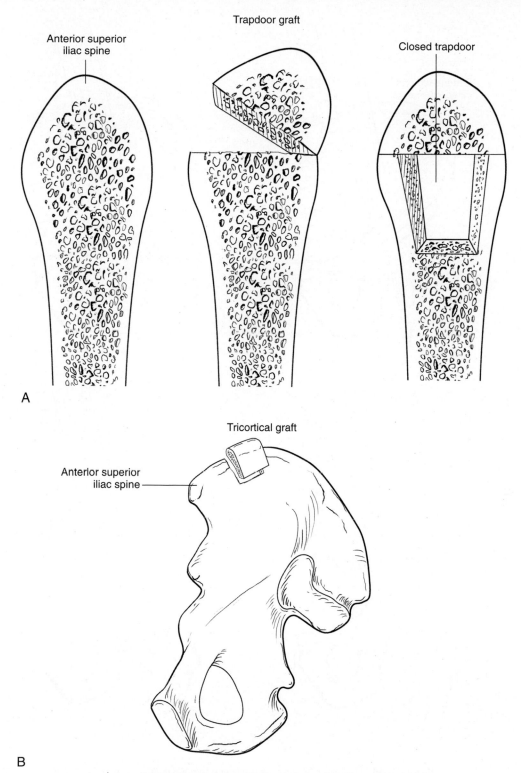

Figure 2-35. Trapdoor (**A**) and tricortical (**B**) grafts.

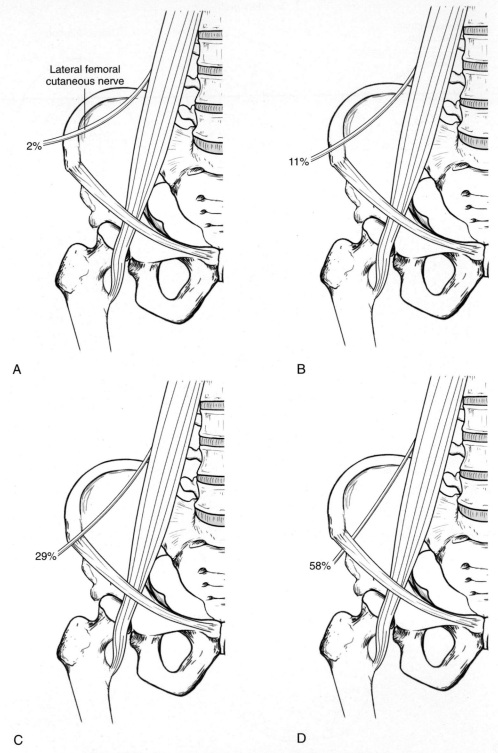

Figure 2-36. Possible trajectories of the lateral femoral cutaneous nerve.

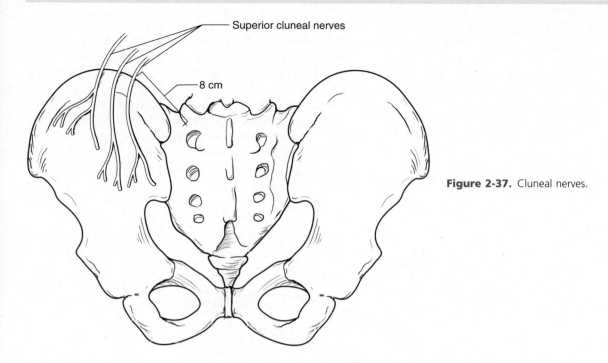

Figure 2-37. Cluneal nerves.

prior to closure can reduce postoperative ventilatory compromise and pain.

Fibula

The fibula provides an excellent structural graft of potentially long dimension. The ankle syndesmosis extends 10 cm above to the joint line and must be preserved. Proximally, the common peroneal nerve runs over the neck of the fibula within the peroneus longus muscle. The exposure should be from the posterior intermuscular septum, starting at the border between the distal and middle thirds of the shaft (Fig. 2-38). Subperiosteal dissection is essential to avoid injury to the peroneal muscles on the anterolateral surface, the extensor digitorum longus anteriorly, the tibialis posterior anteromedially, the flexor hallucis longus posteromedially, and the soleus posteriorly. The neurovascular bundle containing the deep peroneal nerve and the anterior tibial artery and vein lies anteromedial to the fibula within the interosseous membrane. The tibial nerve and peroneal artery and vein also lie medial and somewhat posterior to the fibula.

Vascularized Bone Grafts

Virtually all of the above-mentioned grafts can be taken with a vascular pedicle. This increases operative time and

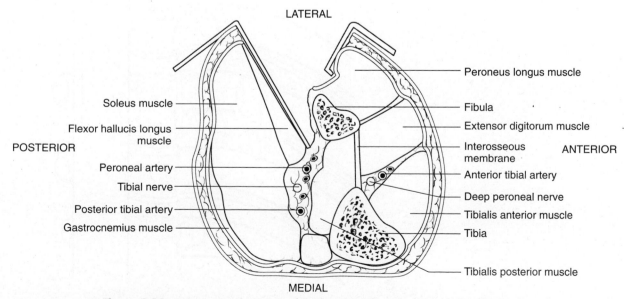

Figure 2-38. Cross-sectional anatomy of the leg with trajectory of approach to the fibula.

risks to local anatomy. However, Hayashi and colleagues have found it to be a particularly useful technique in the face of infection. It greatly increased the rate and success of graft incorporation by providing an immediate continuous blood supply, minimizing late weakening and fatigue failure of the structural graft (Fig. 2-39).

LIGAMENTS

The spinal ligaments provide spinal stability in conjunction with the musculature during physiologic loading and protect the spinal cord from injury. The anatomy is essential to understand, as these ligaments are encountered during surgical approaches, are seen on magnetic resonance imaging scans, and may themselves impinge on the spinal cord.

There are seven common spinal ligaments, as follows: anterior longitudinal ligament, posterior longitudinal ligament, intertransverse ligament, capsular ligaments, ligamentum flavum, interspinous ligaments, and supraspinous ligaments (Fig. 2-40). Those of major clinical significance will be discussed below.

Figure 2-39. Rib autograft with vascular pedicle. Corpectomy site (**A**) and structural graft placement (**B**).

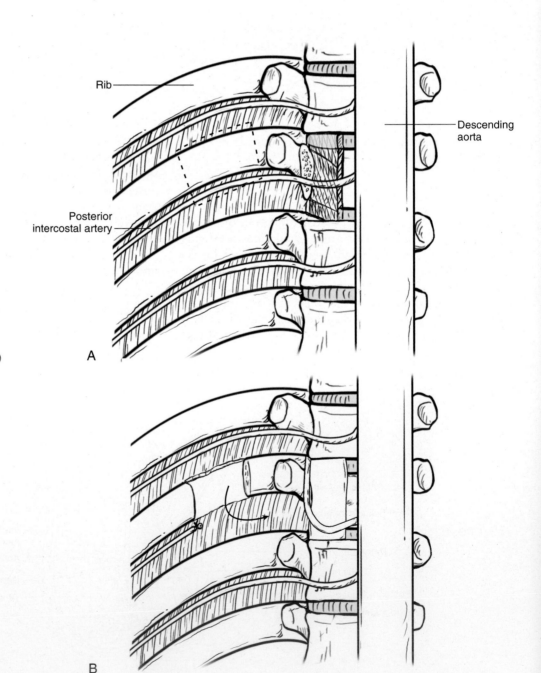

The anterior longitudinal ligament is a band of dense fibrous tissue that runs from the occiput to the sacrum on the ventral surface of the spine. It is loosely attached to the disc annulus and adheres to the edges of the vertebral bodies. The posterior longitudinal ligament arises from the basion and terminates at the coccyx over the posterior aspect of the vertebral bodies. It is wider and thinner over the intervertebral disk than over the vertebral body. In the cervical spine, the posterior longitudinal ligament has two layers. The deep layer sends fibers to the annulus. The ligamentum flavum is a thick elastic fibrous band that is found between each spinal segment from C2 to the sacrum.

Sagittal cross-sectional view

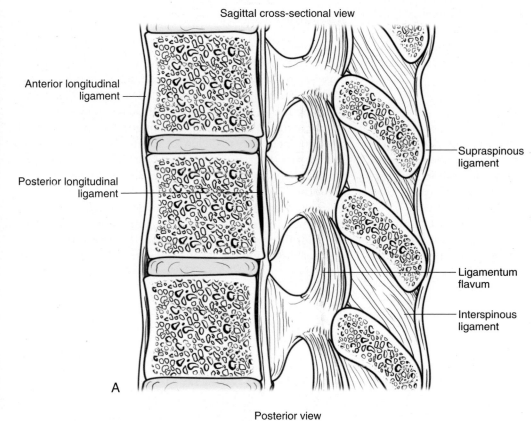

Anterior longitudinal ligament

Posterior longitudinal ligament

Supraspinous ligament

Ligamentum flavum

Interspinous ligament

A

Figure 2-40. Sagittal cross-sectional (**A**) and posterior (**B**) views of ligaments.

Posterior view

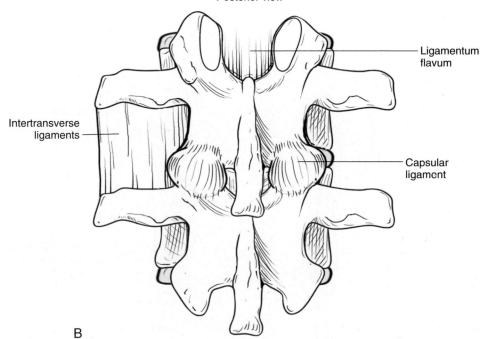

Ligamentum flavum

Intertransverse ligaments

Capsular ligament

B

It runs from the anterior surface of the rostral lamina to the superior edge of the lamina below. It extends laterally to the facet joint and is divided into two ligaments midline by the median raphe.

MUSCLES

Clinically, the spinal musculature blends together and is commonly dissected as a unit during the surgical approach. The spinal musculature therefore forms a functional unit of intrinsic (paravertebral) and extrinsic (hamstrings, abdominals, etc.) muscles. They aid in spinal stability, motion, and balance. The spinal muscles can be divided into posterior and anterior musculature.

Posterior

The superficial posterior musculature includes the trapezius, latissmus dorsi, and serratus posterior. They aid movement and stability of the shoulder girdle and respiration. They are innervated by the proximal spinal cord (Fig. 2-41).

The deeper intrinsic muscles have a segmental innervation and are supplied by the posterior rami of the spinal nerves. These muscles can be divided into three groups based on the direction of the muscle fibers (Fig. 2-42).

The first group, the spinotransversalis group (splenius muscles), runs from the midline to the transverse processes. The second group (erector spinae) runs longitudinally between the transverse processes and ribs or the spinous processes. The third group, the transversospinalis group (semispinalis, multifidus, and rotators), runs cephalad and medially from the transverse processes to the spinous processes.

Anterior

The anterior musculature of the spine can be found in the cervical and lumbar regions. In the cervical region, the muscles are the anterior and lateral rectus capitus, longus colli, longus capitus, and three scalene muscles (Fig. 2-43). The longus colli extends from the third and fourth thoracic vertebrae to the atlas. In approaching the anterior cervical spine, it is necessary to divide the longus colli in the midline and dissect laterally subperiosteally. This will help to protect the sympathetic chain, damage to which can lead to Horner's syndrome.

In the lumbar region, the muscles are the quadratus lumborum, iliacus, and psoas major and minor (Fig. 2-44). An anterior approach to the upper lumbar spine might require dissection of the psoas and the crus of the diaphragm.

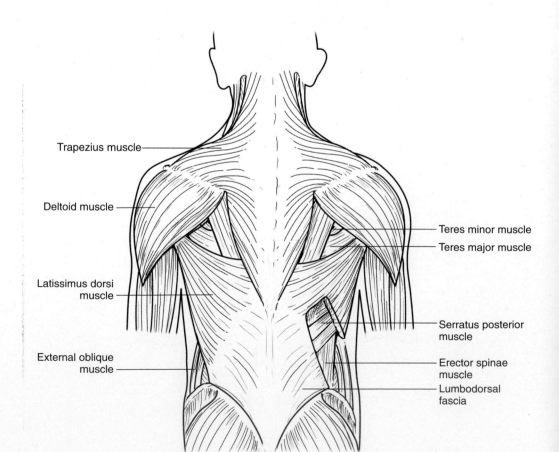

Figure 2-41. Posterior view of superficial musculature.

Trapezius muscle

Deltoid muscle

Latissimus dorsi muscle

External oblique muscle

Teres minor muscle

Teres major muscle

Serratus posterior muscle

Erector spinae muscle

Lumbodorsal fascia

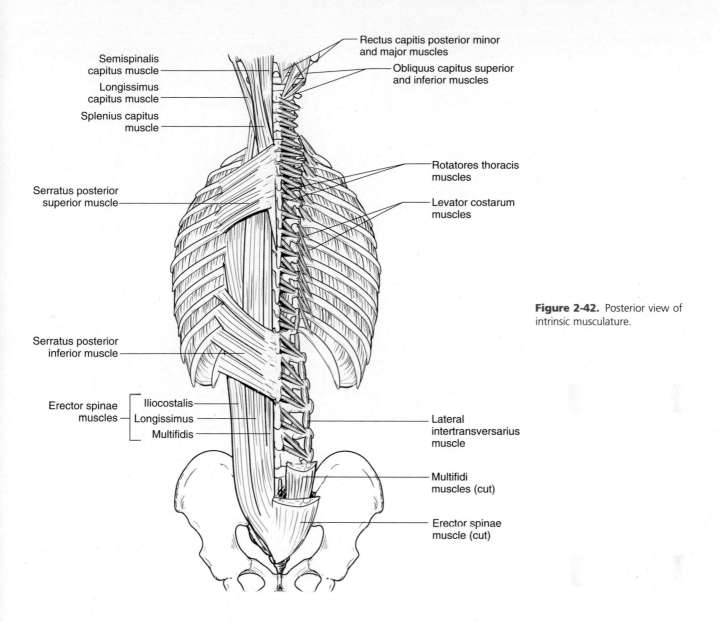

Semispinalis
capitus muscle

Longissimus
capitus muscle

Splenius capitus
muscle

Serratus posterior
superior muscle

Serratus posterior
inferior muscle

Erector spinae
muscles

Iliocostalis

Longissimus

Multifidis

Rectus capitis posterior minor
and major muscles

Obliquus capitus superior
and inferior muscles

Rotatores thoracis
muscles

Levator costarum
muscles

Lateral
intertransversarius
muscle

Multifidi
muscles (cut)

Erector spinae
muscle (cut)

Figure 2-42. Posterior view of
intrinsic musculature.

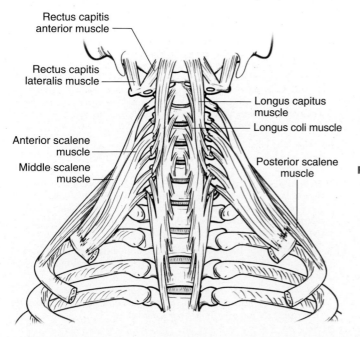

Rectus capitis
anterior muscle

Rectus capitis
lateralis muscle

Anterior scalene
muscle

Middle scalene
muscle

Longus capitus
muscle

Longus coli muscle

Posterior scalene
muscle

Figure 2-43. Anterior view of cervical musculature.

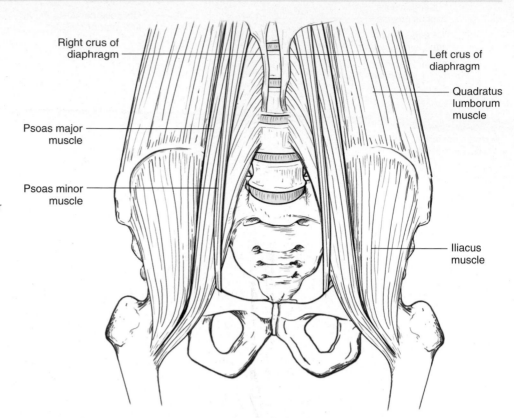

Figure 2-44. Anterior view of lumbar musculature.

REFERENCES

Dawson EG, Lotysch III M, Urist MR: Intertransverse process lumbar arthrodesis with autogenous bone graft. Clin Orthop 1981;154: 90–96.

DeWald RL, Arlet V, Carl A, O'Brien MF: Spinal Deformities: The Comprehensive Text. New York: Thieme Medical Publishers, 2003, pp 2–45.

Ebraheim NA, Xu R, Challagren E, Heck B: Location of the sacral pedicle, foramina and ala on the lateral aspect of the sacrum: A radiographic study. Orthopedics 1998;23:971–974.

Esses SI, Botsford DJ, Huler RJ, Rausching W: Surgical anatomy of the sacrum: A guide for rational screw fixation. Spine 1991;16: S283–S288.

Hayashi A, Maruyama Y, Okajima Y, Motegi M: Vascularized iliac bone graft based on a pedicle of upper lumbar vessels for anterior fusion of the thoracolumbar spine. Br J Plast Surg 1994;47:425–430.

Jackson RP, McManus AC: The iliac buttress: A computed tomographic study of sacral anatomy. Spine 1993;18:1318–1328.

Koshino T, Murakami G, Morishita K, et al: Does the Adamkiewicz artery originate from the larger segmental arteries? J Thorac Cardiovasc Surg 1999;117:898–905.

McCarthy RE, Dunn H, McCullough FL: Luque fixation to the sacral ala using the Dunn-McCarthy modification. Spine 1989;14; 281–283.

O'Brien M, Lenke L, Mardjetko S, et al: Pedicle morphology in thoracic adolescent idiopathic scoliosis: Is pedicle fixation an anatomically viable technique? Spine 2000;25:2285–2293.

Puschak TJ, Vaccaro AR, Rauschning W, Taliwal RV: Relevant surgical anatomy of the cervical, thoracic, and lumbar spine. In Vaccaro AR, Betz RR, Zeitman SM (eds): Principles and Practice of Spine Surgery, 3rd ed. St. Louis: Mosby, 2003, pp 15–33.

Suk S, Lee C, Kim W, et al: Segmental pedicle screw fixation in the treatment of thoracic idiopathic scoliosis. Spine 1995;20: 1399–405.

Suk S, Lee JH: A study of the diameter and change of the vertebral pedicle after screw insertion. Presented at the 3rd Intermeeting SIROT, Boston, Massachusetts, October 1994.

Xu R, Ebraheim NA, Yeasting RA, et al: Morphometric evaluation of the first sacral vertebra and the projection of its pedicle on the posterior aspect of the sacrum. Spine 1995;20:936–940.

Zindrick MR, Wiltse LL, Doornik A, et al: Analysis of the morphometric characteristics of the thoracic and lumbar pedicles. Spine 1987;12: 160–166.

Zipnick RI, Merola AA, Gorup J: Occipital morphology: An anatomic guide to internal fixation. Spine 1996;21:1719–1724.

SUGGESTED READINGS

Berry JL, Moran JM, Berg WS, Steffee AD: A morphometric study of human lumbar and selected thoracic vertebrae. Spine 1987;12: 392–367.

Twenty-seven dimensions were measured from thoracic (T2, T7, T12) and lumbar (L1–L5) vertebrae using prepared spinal columns from 30 skeletons. Maximum and minimum pedicle dimensions indicated that the pedicles are less symmetric cephalad than they are caudal. Vertebral body height increases caudally except posteriorly, where, after an initial increase, it decreases in the lower lumbar region. Major and minor body diameters and the major spinal canal diameter slightly increase caudally, whereas minor spinal canal diameter exhibits little or no change.

Ebraheim NA, Jabaly G, Xu R, Yeasting RA: Anatomic relations of the thoracic pedicle to the adjacent neural structures. Spine 1997;22: 1553–1556.

This study analyzed anatomic parameters between the thoracic pedicles and the spinal nerve roots. Measurements were taken from the pedicle to the nerve root superiorly and inferiorly as well as between the pedicles. Also, the superoinferior diameter of the nerve root and the frontal angle of the nerve root were measured.

Ebraheim NA, Lu J, Biyani A, et al: An anatomic study of the thickness of the occipital bone: Implications for occipitocervical instrumentation. Spine 1996;21:1725–1729.

The authors measured the thickness and quality of occipital bone regions to determine screw placement during occipitocervical fusion and described the projection of the posterior dural venous sinuses.

Ebraheim NA, Lu J, Haman SP, Yeasting RA: Anatomic basis of the anterior surgery of the cervical spine: Relationships between uncus-artery-root complex and vertebral artery injury. Surg Radiol Anat 1998;20:389–392.

Twenty-eight cadavers were dissected to determine the location and relationships of the fibroligamentous tissues to the uncinate process, vertebral artery, and nerve roots from the C3 to C6 levels. The vertebral artery and nerve root are encased by a fibroligamentous band at the level of the intertransverse space. This fibroligamentous band is attached to the lateral aspect of the uncinate process and uncovertebral joint, which combines the vertebral artery, nerve root, and uncinate process to form a complex or unit.

Ebraheim NA, Rollins JR Jr, Xu R, Yeasting RA: Projection of the lumbar pedicle and its morphometric analysis. Spine 1996;21: 1296–1300.

This study defined the projection point of the lumbar pedicle on its posterior aspect and its relation to a reliable landmark and reported pedicle dimensions based on 50 lumbar spines.

Ebraheim NA, Xu R, Ahmad M, Heck B: The quantitative anatomy of the vertebral artery groove of the atlas and its relation to the posterior-atlantoaxial approach. Spine 1998;23:320–323.

An evaluation of the vertebral artery groove of the atlas vertebra using dry bony vertebrae. The anatomic evaluation focused on the vertebral artery groove and its relation to the midline. The results of this study suggest that dissection on the posterior aspect of the posterior ring should remain within 12 mm lateral to the midline, and dissection on the superior aspect of the posterior ring should remain within 8 mm of the midline.

Ebraheim NA, Xu R, Ahmad M, Yeasting RA: Projection of the thoracic pedicle and its morphometric analysis. Spine 1997;22:233–238.

This study defined the projection point of the thoracic pedicles on their posterior aspect and its relation to a reliable landmark. It also reported pedicle dimensions based on 43 thoracic spines. Anatomic evaluation focused on the determination of the projection point of the thoracic pedicle axis on its posterior aspect and the anatomic relationship of this point to the lateral edge of the superior facet and the midline of the transverse process.

Ebraheim NA, Xu R, Yeasting RA: The location of the vertebral artery foramen and its relation to posterior lateral mass screw fixation. Spine 1996;21:1291–1295.

This study evaluated the anatomic relationship between the vertebral artery foramen and the posterior midpoint of the cervical lateral mass using cervical spine specimens. Forty-three cervical spines from C3 to C6 were directly evaluated for this study. The vertical distances from the posterior midpoint of the lateral mass to the vertebral artery foramens at C3–C6 averaged from 9.3 to 12.2 mm.

Karaikovic EE, Kunakornsawat S, Daubs MD, et al: Surgical anatomy of the cervical pedicles: Landmarks for posterior cervical pedicle entrance locations. J Spinal Disord 2000;13:63–72.

The posterior entrance to the cervical pedicle is described using quantitative and descriptive parameters. Fifty-three spines (C2 to C7) were evaluated by using a digital caliper and by visual inspection using bony landmarks. The location of the pedicle entrance was unique at each cervical level. Their distribution followed the cervical spinal cord enlargement. These landmarks should assist with safe placement of pedicle screws.

O'Brien MF, Lenke LG, Mardjetko S, et al: Pedicle morphology in thoracic adolescent idiopathic scoliosis: Is pedicle fixation an anatomically viable technique? Spine 2000;25:2285–2293.

A radiographic study of thoracic pedicle anatomy in a group of adolescent idiopathic scoliosis (AIS) patients. On the basis of the data identified in this group of adolescent patients, it is reasonable to consider pedicle screw insertion at most levels and pedicle-rib fixation at all levels of the thoracic spine during the treatment of thoracic AIS.

Weinstein JN, Rydevik BL, Rauschning W: Anatomic and technical considerations of pedicle screw fixation. Clin Orthop 1992;84: 34–36.

Pedicle screw systems provide significant and, in many cases, improved and previously unattainable spinal fixation. However, pedicle screw systems represent difficult surgical techniques involving several potential problems and complications. Only by detailed knowledge of the anatomy of the spine, with a clear understanding of the pedicle screw systems implementation, can the risks of complications be minimized.

CHAPTER 3

Radiologic Imaging of Spinal Deformities

Renata La Rocca Vieira, Ritika Arora, *and* Mark E. Schweitzer

The normal thoracolumbar spine is relatively straight in the sagittal plane and has a double curve in the coronal plane. As is shown in Figure 3-1, the thoracic spine is convex posteriorly (kyphosis) and the lumbar spine is convex anteriorly (lordosis). Normally, there should be no lateral curvature of the spine. Any change in the configuration of these curves will result in what has been termed *spinal deformity* (kyphosis, lordosis, and scoliosis), the imaging of which is the focus of this chapter.

Anomalies of the spine are varied and frequent. This chapter focuses on the important structural abnormalities of the spine, especially scoliosis. Listhesis, kyphosis, and lordosis will also be discussed.

SCOLIOSIS

Scoliosis refers to a lateral spinal curvature in the coronal plane (Fig. 3-2). This coronal orientation differentiates it from *kyphosis*, a posterior curvature of the spine in the sagittal plane, and *lordosis*, an anterior curvature of the spine also in the sagittal plane.

Epidemiology

Scoliosis occurs relatively frequently in the general population. The absolute frequency depends on the magnitude of the curve being described. A scoliosis greater than 25 degrees has been reported in about 1.5 of 1000 people in the United States.

The majority of cases are idiopathic and have an onset during childhood. When a curve magnitude of greater than 10 degrees is used as the criterion for the diagnosis of idiopathic scoliosis, reported prevalence rates range from 1.9% to 3%. There is an overall female predominance, which increases even further for patients with larger curves. For mild curves (11 to 20 degrees), the female-to-male ratio is 1.4:1; but for moderate to severe curves (greater than 20 degrees), this ratio is more than 4:1.

More than 90% of the adolescent idiopathic curves that occur in the thoracic region have curve apices that are to the right. In fact, left thoracic curves are considered atypical, and there is a 20% incidence of spinal cord abnormalities, such as tumor, syringomyelia, hydromyelia, and tethered cord, in children who have a left thoracic curve. In contrast, left curves in the lumbar spine region are common in adults and children and are not associated with an increased risk of spinal cord abnormality.

Most curves can be treated nonoperatively if they are detected before they become too severe. Therefore, scoliosis screening is done in schools across the United States and in several other countries.

Classification

Clinical Classification

Clinically, there are two major types of scoliotic curves: structural and nonstructural. Nonstructural (functional) curves are mild, nonprogressive, and correctable by ipsilateral bending. It may be postural or compensatory and there is no evidence of rotational deformity. Structural scoliosis has vertebral morphologic deformities, which include various focal dysplasias such as wedging as well as rotation.

Etiologic Classification

On the basis of its etiology, a scoliosis may be idiopathic (80%), congenital (10%), or associated with an important miscellaneous group, including developmental, neuromuscular, and tumoral causes (Fig. 3-3). These are presented in Box 3-1, which is based on the nomenclature of the Scoliosis Research Society that was developed in 1969 and later modified in 1970 and 1973.

Idiopathic Scoliosis. Although the majority of scoliosis cases are idiopathic, a conscientious approach with judicious use of imaging is a necessary prerequisite to exclude occult causes of scoliosis. The scoliosis should be considered idiopathic only after other causes have been excluded.

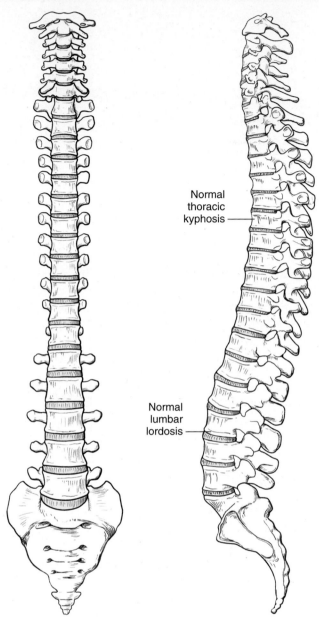

Figure 3-1. Normal spine demonstrating the normal thoracic kyphosis and lumbar lordosis.

Normal thoracic kyphosis

Normal lumbar lordosis

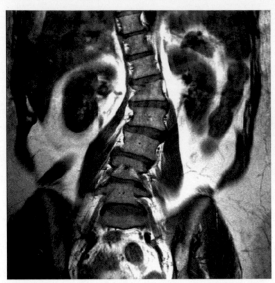

Figure 3-2. Degenerative scoliosis. Coronal T1-weighted image of the lumbar spine demonstrates levoconvex scoliosis and multilevel disc degenerative changes.

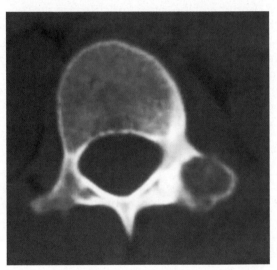

Figure 3-3. Osteoblastoma. Axial CT image of the lumbar vertebra demonstrates a lytic lesion in the right pedicle with surrounding sclerosis. Tumors in this region may result in scoliosis.

Idiopathic scoliosis is subdivided into three groups based on the age of onset: infantile (appears between birth and age 3 years), juvenile (between 3 and 10 years of age), and adolescent (after the age of 10 and before skeletal maturity).

The terms *early onset* and *late onset* are now being used to differentiate the onset of scoliosis before and after the age of 5 years. The distinction is based on the risk of cardiopulmonary complications. Progressive early-onset deformities can lead to cardiopulmonary compromise later in life, whereas late-onset idiopathic scoliosis does not.

Infantile scoliosis has a striking geographic distribution. It is relatively common in the United Kingdom but considered rare in the United States. Resolution of the spinal curvature occurs in 74% of cases; however, scoliotic curves greater than 50 degrees usually progress. Associated plagiocephaly has been noted in 86% of cases. Since the cranial flattening and scoliosis both develop in the first 6 months of life, they are thought to result from plastic deformation of bone in infants who were wrapped too tightly.

Juvenile scoliosis is recognized between the ages of 4 and 10 years. About 13% of all cases of scoliosis are discovered in this age period, but because many of the abnormal curvatures that are found later in life must have had their inception at a young age, the establishment of juvenile scoliosis as a separate category is of doubtful validity. Boys are affected predominantly when the diagnosis is made before the age of 6 years. Juvenile scoliosis usually progresses with growth.

BOX 3-1 Etiologic Classification of Scoliosis

Idiopathic

Early-onset
Late-onset
Adult

Congenital

Osteogenic (vertebral anomaly)
   Anomalous formation
      Wedge vertebra
      Hemivertebra
   Anomalous segmentation
      Unilateral bar
      Fused ribs
      Fused vertebra
Neuropathic (spinal dysraphism)
   Tethered cord
   Chiari malformations
   Syringomyelia
   Diastematomyelia
   Meningocele/myelomeningocele

Neuromuscular

Neuropathic
Upper motor neuron

Neuromuscular—cont'd

Spinocerebellar degeneration
Cerebral palsy
Lower motor neuron
Poliomyelitis
Myopathic
Congenital hypotonia
Duchenne muscular dystrophy

Developmental Syndromes

Skeletal dysostosis (e.g.,
   neurofibromatosis)
Skeletal dysplasias (e.g., osteogenesis
   imperfecta)

Tumor Associated

Vertebral
Osteoblastoma
Osteoid osteoma
   Intraspinal
      Intramedullary (e.g.,
        astrocytoma)
      Extramedullary (e.g.,
        neurofibroma)

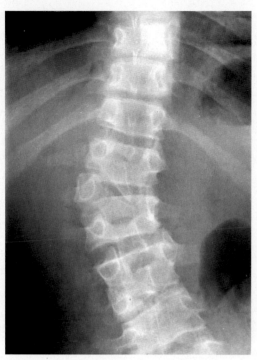

Figure 3-4. Hemivertebra. Anteroposterior view of the thoracolumbar transition. There is a dextroconvex curvature of the spine. There is a right-side, partially fused hemivertebra between the L1 and L2 vertebral bodies.

Adolescent scoliosis is the most common type of idiopathic scoliosis in the United States and is found more frequently in girls. Although idiopathic scoliosis by itself is thought to be asymptomatic, 23% of such patients seek medical attention for back pain caused by associated conditions.

Congenital Scoliosis. Congenital malformation of the vertebrae (Fig. 3-4) can produce unbalanced growth of the spine with the development of early childhood scoliosis, which can range in severity from asymptomatic mild curves to life-threatening severe curves that require early surgical treatment in infancy. The term *congenital scoliosis* is, unfortunately, a misleading one. It implies that there is always abnormal spinal curvature at birth. However, only the vertebral malformations are present at birth in all patients, whereas the scoliosis might or might not subsequently develop.

The incidence of congenital scoliosis is unknown, but it is certainly rarer than idiopathic scoliosis. If multiple vertebral anomalies are present, the risk of similar anomalies in either siblings or children of the patient is between 10% and 15%.

Congenital scoliosis may be classified into three groups, according to MacEwen: those that result from a failure in vertebral formation, which may be partial or complete; those that are caused by a failure in vertebral segmentation, which may be asymmetric and unilateral or symmetric and bilateral; and those that result from a combination of the first two. Neural anomalies such as syringomyelia, diastematomyelia, tethered cord, and lipoma may also be present.

Progression of congenital scoliosis is seen in about 75% of patients. The poorest prognosis occurs with a unilateral bar in association with a contralateral hemivertebra. Associated rib anomalies are common. Investigators have shown an association between congenital scoliosis and genitourinary tract abnormalities (unilateral renal agenesis, horseshoe kidneys, renal ectopia). For this reason, examination of the genitourinary tract is indicated in all patients with congenital anomalies of the spine.

Miscellaneous Scoliosis. Secondary forms of scoliosis with an underlying specific etiology may also develop, such as those secondary to trauma, neuromuscular disorders, infection, tumors (see Fig. 3-3), neurofibromatosis (Fig. 3-5), or degenerative disease (see Fig. 3-2). These types are particularly common and important in adults, especially the elderly.

Imaging

Plain radiography is still the first examination that is required for the initial diagnosis of scoliosis and evaluation of the degree of curve. This is measured by the Cobb angle. Underlying vertebral anomalies can also be identified.

Until the introduction of magnetic resonance imaging (MRI), myelography and computed tomography (CT), with or without intrathecal contrast medium, were used to detect suspected intraspinal disease. Now MRI has become

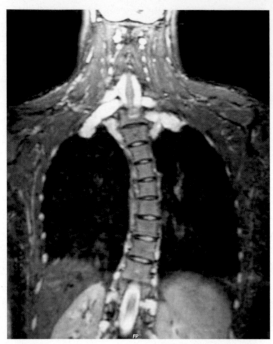

Figures 3-5. Neurofibromatosis. Coronal T2-weighted MR image of the thoracic spine demonstrates a levoconvex scoliosis and multiple neurogenic tumors in the cervical-thoracic spine transition characterized by increased T2 signal intensity.

the imaging modality of choice for the further workup, when necessary, of scoliosis. The main disadvantages of MRI include, most important, cost, as well as the frequent need for sedation or general anesthesia in younger patients and the occasional difficulty in imaging patients who are claustrophobic. The major use of MRI is to detect abnormalities of the neuroaxis prior to treatment of scoliosis, particularly with instrumentation that lengthens the spine, which can have serious neurologic consequences.

Because of the high concomitant incidence of renal disease, evaluation of the genitourinary tract in patients with congenital scoliosis is often indicated. It is accomplished by screening sonography followed by other urographic techniques when indicated.

Radiography

Once a spine deformity has been confirmed clinically, plain radiographs are usually performed. Conventional radiography has three roles. First, it will confirm the diagnosis and occasionally suggest the etiology, such as a hemivertebra, of a clinically diagnosed scoliosis. Second, the subsequent monitoring of the child depends largely on the radiographs. This is because evaluation of the severity of the scoliosis, and particularly the degree of progression over time, cannot be assessed adequately using only clinical methods. Third, the radiographs provide a method of assessing skeletal maturity.

The radiologist has to ensure that the radiographs are of optimal quality. This initial radiographic examination is

the best opportunity to identify congenital abnormalities. The minimum required views are a frontal and a lateral assessment of the whole of the thoracic and lumbar spine, with the patient standing erect, using a long cassette film or with digital techniques, in a process known as *stitching*. On the frontal view, the vertebrae from C7 to the sacrum and iliac crest are included, while the lateral plain radiograph should reveal the reduction of the normal thoracic kyphosis that is characteristic of idiopathic scoliosis. The sacrum needs to be included on the lateral view, as does the cervical spine to exclude a Klippel-Feil deformity, which can herald congenital or cord abnormalities. The posteroanterior projection is preferred on follow-up radiographs because it reduces the radiation dose to the thyroid and breast. Various sponges are utilized so that the X-ray beam penetration is uniform.

The frontal plain radiograph should include enough of the pelvis to show the iliac crests in their full lateral extent in order to visualize the developing apophysis (Risser index) (Fig. 3-6). This index is a function of the ossification of the iliac apophysis, which radiographically commences laterally, extending medially to cap the entire crest and eventually fusing to the underlying ilium. Grading according to this system divides this ossification excursion into four temporally related segments. Ossification of the lateral one fourth of the apophysis is Risser 1, of one half is Risser 2, and of three fourths is Risser 3. The complete excursion of the ossification before fusion is Risser 4. Risser 5 denotes fusion of the iliac apophysis to the adjacent ilium. Complete excursion (Risser 1 to 4) of the ossification takes approximately 1 year, while fusion of the completely ossified apophysis to the ilium (Risser 4 to 5) averages 2 years. Increasing degrees of ossification result in decreasing likelihood of curvature progression.

To evaluate the various types of scoliosis, certain measurements must be done. Measurement of the severity of a scoliotic curve has practical application not only in the selection of patients for surgical treatment, but also in monitoring the results of corrective therapy. The most accepted method of measuring the curve is the Cobb method (Fig. 3-7), which determines the angle of the curvature only by the ends of the scoliotic curve, depending on the inclination of the end vertebrae. This method, which has been adopted and standardized by the Scoliosis Research Society, classifies the severity of scoliotic curvature into seven groups (Table 3-1). The Cobb method has some drawbacks, such as well-recognized and significant interobserver and intraobserver variability. For this reason, a change of at least 23 degrees has been stated as being necessary to describe any perceived progression as "significant" with complete statistical reliability. This is a fairly marked change that might require too great a progression to be used in day-to-day practice.

It is also necessary to look for rotation of the spine, which is greatest at the level of the apical vertebra but is quite variable in degree from one patient to another.

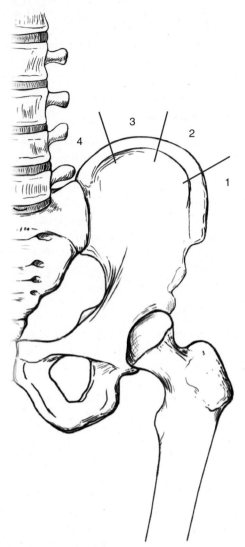

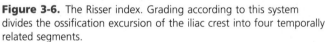

Figure 3-6. The Risser index. Grading according to this system divides the ossification excursion of the iliac crest into four temporally related segments.

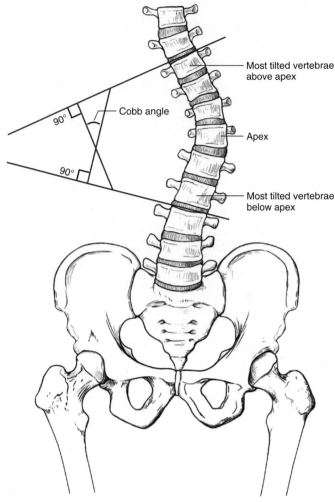

Figure 3-7. The Cobb method.

Scoliotic curves of the same magnitude in two patients may have significant different degrees of vertebral rotation. The degree of rotation can be calculated by various methods (the Cobb and Noe methods).

The Cobb technique for grading rotation uses the position of the spinous process as a point of reference. On the frontal view, the spinous process appears in the center of the body if there is no rotation. The spinous process migrates toward the convexity as the degree of rotation increases.

In the Noe method, vertebral rotation is graded from 0 to 4 on the basis of asymmetry of pedicles as they appear on frontal view. In grade 0, there is no rotation. When the pedicle is toward or two thirds to the midline, it is grade 1 or 2, respectively. In grade 3, the pedicle is in midline, and in grade 4, the pedicle is beyond midline.

A set of lateral bending films are often taken to assess the rigidity or flexibility of the curves, as was discussed

above. Passive lateral bending radiographs in the frontal plane of the thoracic and lumbar spine together are also obtained with the patient supine and recumbent, bending maximally to the left and then to the right. This is a preoperative radiograph and enables the surgeon to measure

Table 3-1. The Scoliosis Research Society Classification of Severity of Scoliotic Curvature Using the Cobb Method

Group	Angle of Curvature
I	<20°
II	21°–30°
III	31°–50°
IV	51°–75°
V	76°–100°
VI	101°–125°
VII	>125°

the degree of passive correction that can be achieved and helps to determine the extent of fusion.

Magnetic Resonance Imaging

As was discussed previously, MRI is increasingly being used to investigate children with scoliosis. However, considerable controversy exists regarding the routine use of MRI. A review of the literature suggests that routine MRI is not indicated in patients with adolescent idiopathic scoliosis with a typical right thoracic curve who are neurologically intact. In their study of 140 consecutive adolescent patients with idiopathic scoliosis, Winter and colleagues identified only four patients with an abnormality. However, in the infantile and juvenile age groups, some authors have noted a high incidence of abnormalities. The reported incidence of spinal cord anomalies in this group ranges from 17.6% to 26%. Findings that could indicate a spinal cord abnormality include a left thoracic curve, absent abdominal reflex, lower limb neurologic deficit, foot deformity, and the presence of any cutaneous stigmata of occult dysraphism. The main indications for further diagnostic imaging in scoliosis are listed in Box 3-2.

MRI has had a revolutionary impact on imaging the neural axis. It has the ability to produce detailed images with excellent tissue contrast in any plane without the use of ionizing radiation. Unfortunately, the nature of scoliosis, with different areas of the spine moving into and out of the standard planes of imaging, means that interpretation can be difficult. Young children require sedation and occasionally general anesthesia to have a complete scan. Despite this, MRI is the primary imaging modality in the assessment of scoliosis after plain radiography, particularly in the infantile and juvenile forms, in which the incidence

of spinal cord abnormalities is higher. MRI is useful in identifying hydromyelia, syringomyelia, intramedullary tumors, and dysraphic abnormalities such as a tethered cord, diastematomyelia, or lipoma. In this respect, MRI has replaced CT.

Computed Tomography

Children with underlying congenital skeletal malformations and segmentation abnormalities, such as butterfly vertebra or hemivertebra, or diastematomyelia, require a slightly different imaging approach. MRI will provide excellent detail about the nature of the spinal canal and cord, but details of the osseous anatomy can be evaluated further with localized CT and three-dimensional reconstructed images. With the advent of multislice CT, this can be quickly done even in very young patients without sedation.

Postoperative Imaging

Before discharge from the hospital, it is necessary to be certain that the internal fixation hardware that was used is intact. This is assessed by radiographs in the erect position, with frontal and lateral planes.

In the rare instance of postoperative paraplegia, the spinal instrumentation needs to be assessed to exclude extradural compression on the spinal cord, utilizing CT or MRI.

Optimization of these images because of the severe artifacts generated by the metallic fixation is imperative. On CT, multislice scanners with acquisition of thinner slices minimize the artifacts. On MRI, modification of sequences is important. On MRI, we do not use frequency-selective fat suppression, and we rarely use most gradient echo techniques. We also use mostly turbo or fast spin echo, increase the bandwidth markedly, and use somewhat smaller voxel sizes.

Postoperative spinal infection is a very serious complication. Risk factors include advanced age of the patient, prolonged hospitalization, obesity, diabetes mellitus, malnutrition, immunosuppression, and duration of the operation. The most common organism implicated is *Staphylococcus aureus*, although infection with a variety of other organisms may be encountered. Postoperative infections typically manifest 10 to 15 days after surgery, although longer delays are not unusual.

Early conventional radiographic findings of disc space loss, osteopenia, and vertebral end plate erosion may be difficult to distinguish from some postoperative changes. With progressive infection, vertebral destruction, osseous fragmentation, and reactive sclerosis may occur. Loss of fixation and loosening of spinal hardware are also seen in advanced infection.

In the early stages of infection, CT is not reliable, and scintigraphy is nonspecific, particularly in the early postoperative period. The normally increased activity that is seen on scintigraphic studies limits their usefulness in detecting postoperative spinal infection.

BOX 3-2 Main Indications for Further Imaging in Scoliosis

Congenital causes
Dysraphic states
Developmental causes (neurofibromatosis)
Painful deformity
Idiopathic scoliosis*
   Clinical
      Age (<10 years)
      Headache
      Neurologic signs or symptoms
      Neck symptoms
      Foot deformity
   Radiographic
      Atypical curves (left)
      Wide spinal canal
      Thin pedicle(s)
      Increased kyphosis
Rapid progression (>15 degrees a year)
Abnormal somatosensory evoked potential study
Preoperative
Postoperative

*Indications for MRI in idiopathic scoliosis.

In a study evaluating MRI, plain films, and radionuclide studies in the evaluation of vertebral osteomyelitis, MRI was shown to be as accurate and as sensitive as combined bone and gallium scanning and more sensitive than plain films. The MRI appearance of pyogenic infection is characteristic, making MRI a rapid, noninvasive method for the detection of vertebral osteomyelitis. On T1-weighted images, disc space infection shows confluent decreased signal intensity from the intervertebral disc space and contiguous vertebral bodies relative to the normal vertebral body marrow signal. On T2-weighted images, there is increased signal intensity of these tissues. The intervertebral disc shows abnormal increased signal intensity in a nonanatomic morphology.

MRI defines the epidural changes with infection, the most accuracy occurring after contrast administration. Epidural abscess is seen as a central nonenhancing region surrounded by enhancing inflammatory tissue. Phlegmon is seen as diffusely enhancing soft tissue.

Additionally, MRI provides a means of differentiating neoplasm and degenerative disease from osteomyelitis. In neoplastic disease, the disc space is almost always spared. Degenerative disease usually shows decreased signal from the disc space on T2-weighted images to desiccation of the nucleus. A couple of pitfalls can occur in the diagnosis of disc space infection with MRI and are related to the changes that may occur in the vertebral bodies and end plates in association with disc degeneration. The first problem that can occur is the potential masking of the usual low-signal-intensity changes of disc space infection on T1-weighted magnetic resonance images by superimposed high-signal-intensity Modic type II degenerative end plate changes on both T1 and T2-weighted images. Correlation with the T2-weighted images would help to make the diagnosis in this scenario, showing abnormal increased signal intensity within the disc space with disc space infection. Second, Modic type I end plate changes associated with degeneration have signal changes involving the vertebral bodies similar to those of disc space infection with decreased T1 and increased T2 signal in the adjacent end plates.

Acute hemorrhage is typically characterized by isointensity to increased signal in the epidural space on T1-weighted images and diminished signal on gradient echo or T2-weighted images. Very acute blood collections, however, may have different signal intensity characteristics. Most musculoskeletal hemorrhage appears in MRI imaging like fairly simple fluid.

LUMBAR INSTABILITY AND SPONDYLOLISTHESIS

Definition

Segmental lumbar instability generally is due to a degenerative or listhesic process of the lumbar spine, and radiologic imaging is essential to its diagnosis.

The radiographic criterion for instability of the middle and lower cervical spine is the presence of sagittal translation greater than 3.5 mm or sagittal plane angulation greater than 20 degrees on flexion-extension radiographs. In the lumbar spine, instability may be present when there are sagittal angulations of greater than 15 degrees at L1-2, L2-3, and L3-4, greater than 20 degrees at L4-5, and greater than 25 degrees at L5-S1 or when translation movement exceeds 4.5 mm from flexion to extension. Studying 1090 outpatients with low back and/or leg pain, Iguchi and colleagues concluded that translation of the lumbar segment has a greater influence than does angulation on lumbar symptoms.

Lumbar spine segmental mobility has commonly been studied by dynamic radiographic methods. Dynamic radiographs, with maximal extension and flexion of the lumbar tract, represent the most widely used technique and a valid method to estimate sagittal segmental lumbar motion.

Spondylolisthesis is related to spinal instability and is due to abnormal movement of one vertebral body relative to the vertebral body below, often causing clinical symptoms such as low back pain. This movement can be anterior (anterior spondylolisthesis), posterior (retrolisthesis), or lateral (lateral listhesis). With scoliosis, lateral listhesis is not uncommon adjacent to the epicenter of the curve.

Classification

Spondylolisthesis can be divided into five types: dysplastic (related to congenital abnormalities of the upper portion of the sacrum), isthmic (caused by fatigue or acute fractures or elongation of the pars interarticularis) (Figs. 3-8 and 3-9), degenerative (Fig. 3-10), traumatic (fractures of structures other than the isthmus) and pathologic (resulting from generalized or localized bone disease).

It is important to distinguish between spondylolisthesis that is associated with spondylolysis and spondylolisthesis that occurs without an associated defect in the pars interarticularis. As a rule, the latter form is associated with degenerative disc disease and degenerative changes and subluxation of the facet joints and is referred to as degenerative spondylolisthesis.

Degenerative Anterior Spondylolisthesis

A degenerative listhesis is seen in approximately 4% of elderly patients and predominates at the interspace between the fourth and fifth lumbar vertebrae, usually in older women. The facets at the L4-5 level are oriented more sagittally than are those at the L5-S1 level and are therefore more capable of allowing anterior movement. In the presence of degenerative joint changes, this sagittal orientation may become even more striking. The inferior facets of the fourth lumbar vertebra gradually erode between the superior facets of the fifth lumbar vertebra and produce forward displacement of L4. It is frequently associated with either

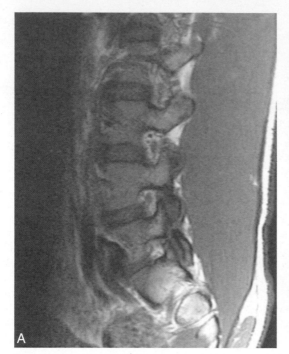 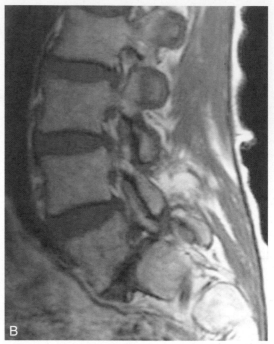

Figure 3-8. Spondylolysis. Two different sagittal T1-weighted MR images (**A** and **B**) show bilateral L5 pars defects with a spondylolisthesis.

partial or complete sacralization of the fifth lumbar vertebra. The predisposing factor is thought to be a very stable lumbosacral facet joint with unusually heavy stress on the L4-5 facet joint. Radiographic findings include osteoarthritis of the apophyseal joints (articular space narrowing, sclerosis, and osteophyte formation), forward slipping of the superior vertebra on the inferior one, and, in some instances, intervertebral osteochondrosis (vacuum phenomenon, disc space narrowing, and end plate sclerosis).

Degenerative Retrolisthesis

Another pattern of spondylolisthesis without spondylolysis is a degenerative type associated with intervertebral osteochondrosis. This type is characterized by posterior displacement of the superior vertebra. This is most commonly seen at L5-S1 and, although seen at many levels, is somewhat uncommon at L4-5. The cause of the retrolisthesis appears to be degeneration of the intervertebral disc, which results in decreased height of the involved disc space, closer approximation of adjacent vertebral bodies, and gliding of corresponding articular processes. Frequent associated radiographic findings include changes of osteochondrosis (vacuum phenomenon, disc space loss, vertebral body marginal sclerosis, and osteophyte formation).

Spondylolysis

Spondylolysis represents a defect in the pars interarticularis of the vertebra that may be unilateral or bilateral. It is classically considered a stress fracture and is thought to

begin in adolescence. Spondylolysis might or might not be associated with spondylolisthesis and is most frequent in the lumbar region of the spine, the fifth lumbar vertebra being most commonly affected. The frequency of spondylolysis appears to be greater in athletes, especially those who are involved in gymnastics, diving, weightlifting, and American football.

Unilateral spondylolysis commonly occurs in 15% to 30% of spondylolysis cases. It has been considered to be clinically benign and is not likely to be associated with forward slippage. Sairyo and colleagues studied 20 athletes with unilateral spondylosis and concluded that it could lead to stress fracture or sclerosis with enlargement of the contralateral lamina and pedicle due to an increase in stresses in this region also known as Wilkinson syndrome (see Fig. 3-10).

The cause of lumbar spondylolysis has long been discussed. The current consensus supports an acquired traumatic lesion originating sometime between infancy and early adulthood.

Isthmic spondylolysis is present in 5% to 6% of the population. The incidence is zero at birth but rises sharply to 5% at age 4 to 5 years. The origin of the lesion is unknown; however, the current theory states that isthmic spondylolysis results from a fatigue fracture through a congenitally weak pars interarticularis.

Postoperative Spondylolisthesis

Postsurgical spondylolisthesis includes iatrogenic lumbar instabilities that can lead to postoperative spondylolisthe-

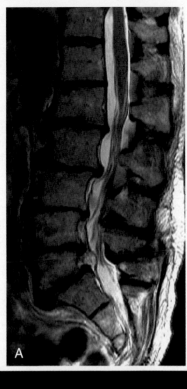

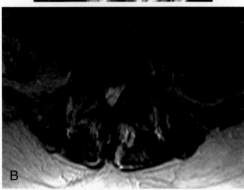

Figure 3-9. Degenerative spondylolisthesis. Sagittal (**A**) and axial (**B**) T2-weighted images of the lumbar spine show spondylolisthesis at L5-S1 secondary to degenerative facet changes. There are multilevel disc and facet joint degenerative changes.

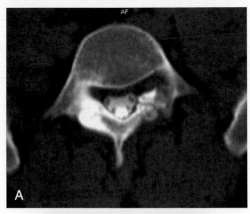

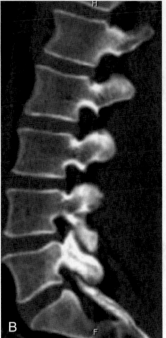

Figure 3-10. Wilkinson syndrome. Axial (**A**) and sagittal (**B**) CT images of the lumbar spine. There is a defect in the left pars interarticularis, and there are sclerosis and enlargement of the contralateral right lamina (stress reaction) of L5.

sis. This usually occurs above the level of the fusion. The incidence is between 3% and 5%. The instability may be secondary to a fatigue fracture of the pars at the upper end of a lumbar spinal fusion or secondary to an acute injury during surgery (posterior structures). More commonly, it is secondary to extensive removal of the supporting structures (lamina, articular processes, spinous processes) in an effort to decompress adequately in the case of neoplasm, stenosis, or multiple disc herniations. This pathology is of great importance, but it is often underestimated and has scarcely been studied. Moreover, postoperative spondylolisthesis has been shown to be responsible for serious clinical findings with a high potential for evolution, and the correction of such findings is a difficult challenge to surgeons.

Epidemiology

Spondylolysis with or without spondylolisthesis occurs in 5% to 8% of adults. It is commonly believed that spondylolysis does not exist at birth. The incidence is 4.4% to 5% at the age of 6 years, increasing to 6% at the age of 18 years, which is quite similar to that observed in adulthood. There are rare adult acquired cases. These usually occur in three situations: postoperatively, in high-performance athletes, and occasionally related to malignancy.

Spondylolysis is rare in patients under 5 years of age, frequent in those between 7 and 10 years of age, and very rare after the age of 20 years. While spondylolysis has a male-to-female ratio of 2:1 (the highest, 6.4%, in white men and the lowest, 1.1%, in black women), spondylolisthesis is more common in females.

Progression of spondylolisthesis increases with age, beginning at about 8 years in girls and 12 years in boys. At first, spondylolysis is asymptomatic, and by the time pain is experienced, 90% of the patients show slippage by less than 30%.

Imaging

Lumbar spine segmental mobility has commonly been studied by dynamic radiographic methods. Dynamic radiographs, with maximal extension and flexion of the lumbar tract, represent the most widely used technique and a valid method to estimate sagittal segmental lumbar motion.

Spondylolisthesis has been graded as follows, according to the degree of forward slippage of a vertebra on the one below it: grade I, 0% to 25%; grade II, 25% to 50%; grade III, 50% to 75%; and grade IV, 75% to 100%.

Spondylolysis is usually evident on lateral radiographic projection (see Fig. 3-8A); however, oblique views are particularly helpful. The vertebral body has a "Scottie dog" appearance on oblique projections. A unilateral or bilateral radiolucent area through the neck of the "Scottie dog" can be identified, corresponding to a pars interarticularis defect (see Fig. 3-8B). Reactive sclerosis about the radiolucent band may be seen, although true callus is unusual. However, although chronic nonunion may be demonstrated, radiography is unreliable for detection of early and acute lesions.

Isotope imaging with single photon emission tomography (SPECT) is considered to be an extremely sensitive technique for early diagnosis of acute lysis and may be predictive of the ability for lysis to heal. Unfortunately SPECT is nonspecific, detects only 17% of chronic lesions, and cannot distinguish between stress reaction and overt fractures. Developmental lesions that are acquired in the first decade are often asymptomatic and usually inactive on isotope studies.

CT is probably the best method for demonstrating spondylolytic defects and may also be used for assessment of healing. Reverse-angle axial oblique CT has been utilized successfully for identifying defects by demonstrating discontinuity in the bony ring of the posterior elements of the vertebra (Fig. 3-11). However, CT is limited in detection of other pathologic processes. Healing pars defects show sclerosis at the fracture margins and, when remote, contralateral pedicle sclerosis.

MRI is a useful method to demonstrate spondylolysis (see Fig. 3-8), but in some cases, the pars defect can be difficult to detect, particularly if nonangulated axial images are not obtained through the area of interest. On axial CT and MRI, the continuous facet sign is used where one can follow the L4-5 facets straight through to the L5-S1 facets on these nonangulated axial images. Sagittal images are somewhat easier to read for this disorder than axial images. Activity can be assessed on MRI by the presence of marrow edema.

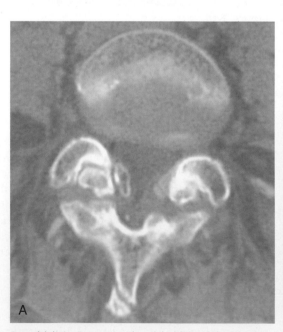
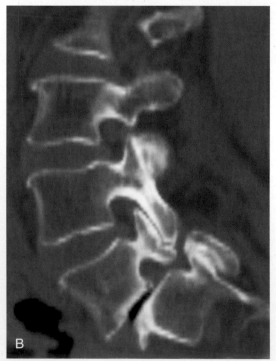

Figure 3-11. Spondylolysis. Reverse-angle axial oblique (**A**) and sagittal reconstruction (**B**) CT images of the lumbar spine demonstrate spondylolisthesis of L5-S1 secondary to bilateral defects in the pars interarticularis of L5.

In children, bone scan with SPECT is probably the best test to perform because it shows uptake in an active spondylolysis.

KYPHOSIS

The term *kyphosis* is used to refer to excessive curvature in the thoracic spine. Kyphosis can be the result of many causes (e.g., trauma, developmental problems, degenerative disc disease, infection). When viewed from one side, a kyphosis deformity can be gradual and smooth, as in postural roundback, or it can be a sharp and angular (gibbus) deformity, as in congenital kyphosis, Potts disease, or, to a lesser extent, Scheuermann's kyphosis. Other causes of spinal kyphosis include those that occur with disorders of the nervous system and muscle disorders (cerebral palsy, muscular dystrophy, spinal muscular atrophy, and myelomeningocele), neurofibromatosis, connective tissue disorders, Paget's disease, tumors, and after surgery. Kyphosis can also be seen in association with scoliosis. In these cases, kyphosis is usually related to an underlying cause of the scoliosis, such as neurofibromatosis. In idiopathic scoliosis, there is more often straightening rather than accentuation of the kyphosis.

In the postoperative correction of kyphosis, it is important to assess the spine curvature on the frontal views and the sagittal balance on the lateral views of the patient's spine. Flat-back syndrome results from an iatrogenic loss of lumbar lordosis with forward inclination of the trunk and is frequently recognized as a complication following placement of thoracolumbar instrumentation.

Scheuermann's Disease

Scheuermann's disease is a structural deformity of the spine that develops prior to puberty and becomes most prominent during the adolescent growth spurt. The cause is unknown.

Initial descriptions focused on thoracic kyphosis; however, it was noted that thoracolumbar and lumbar variants also occur. A minimal scoliosis may be associated in about one third of cases. Classic radiographic descriptions (Fig. 3-12) include irregular vertebral end plates, narrowing of the intervertebral disc spaces, three or more vertebrae wedged 5 degrees or more, and an increase in normal thoracic kyphosis to greater than 45 degrees.

The prevalence of Scheuermann's disease varies depending on inclusion criteria and has been reported to be between 0.4% and 8%.

Imaging

Radiography. A standard radiographic evaluation of a patient with Scheuermann's disease or other causes of kyphosis includes anteroposterior and lateral standing radiographs on long films, which would incorporate the entire thoracolumbar spine on one film. The patient should be standing in a neutral position with hips and knees fully extended to allow for a true evaluation of the sagittal balance. The lateral view should be taken with the arms elevated at 90 degrees in front of the subject to prevent the bony outlines of the upper extremities from obscuring the vertebral body images.

The diagnosis of Scheuermann's kyphosis is confirmed on the lateral radiographs (Fig. 3-12). The angle between the end plates of each respective vertebral body should be measured by using the Cobb technique. The presence of three adjacent vertebral bodies with 5 or more degrees of anterior wedging confirms the diagnosis of Scheuermann's kyphosis.

The Cobb technique should be used to measure the overall degree of kyphosis of the thoracic spine. The end vertebral bodies, which are defined as the last vertebral body tilting into the kyphotic deformity, should be selected both proximally and distally. The levels of these particular vertebral bodies should be noted, as they are the same vertebral bodies that should be selected on subsequent films to ensure that the examiner is consistent with follow-up evaluations.

Secondary changes of Scheuermann's kyphosis should be noted, such as the necessary presence of Schmorl's nodes, irregular vertebral end plates, and disc space narrow-

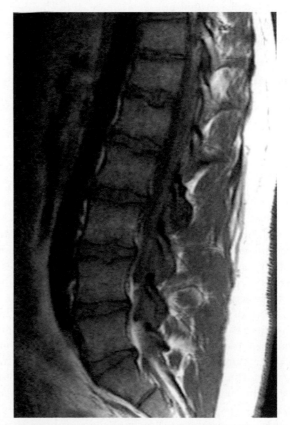

Figure 3-12. Lumbar Scheuermann's disease. Sagittal T1-weighted MR image demonstrates multiple Schmorl's nodes throughout the lumbar spine.

ing. Scoliosis and spondylolisthesis have been associated with Scheuermann's kyphosis. These should be documented on plain radiographs and treated as separate entities.

Other entities that share the differential diagnosis of Scheuermann's kyphosis can be excluded radiographically as well. Congenital kyphosis, ankylosing spondylitis, multiple compression fractures, tumor, infection, tuberculosis, and postlaminectomy kyphosis can be distinguished by clinical history and confirmed by radiographic evaluation.

The dynamic quality of the kyphosis should be assessed to distinguish Scheuermann's kyphosis from postural kyphosis. A lateral radiograph can be obtained in hyperextension. Should the deformity correct entirely, postural kyphosis is the most likely diagnosis, rather than Scheuermann's kyphosis.

It is necessary to account for the rigidity of the curve in treatment decisions, as the ability for correction with bracing and surgical intervention will be affected.

Magnetic Resonance Imaging, Computed Tomography, and CT Myelography. MRI, CT scan, and CT myelography can be helpful adjunctive studies in planning the care of a patient with Scheuermann's disease or other types of kyphosis. MRI, in particular, helps the surgeon to further define the local anatomy. In particular, attention should be given to the coexistence of thoracic spinal stenosis, syrinx, or any other intrathecal abnormalities that would affect surgical care.

Additionally, an anatomic assessment of the lumbar discs can be made, and it may affect surgical decision making in terms of which levels to incorporate in the fusion.

Postlaminectomy Kyphosis

In the cervical spine, the most frequently encountered deformity is that of kyphosis, and the most frequent cause of cervical kyphosis is iatrogenic or postlaminectomy kyphosis. The causes of postlaminectomy kyphosis range from neglect of preoperative kyphosis to removal of the tethering posterior restraints in the cervical spine or inadequacy of posterior restraints caused by radiation for tumors.

Instability following spinal surgery is an important determinant leading to an unsuccessful outcome. Spinal instability is well recognized following decompressive spinal procedures that excise bone. The amount of bone that is resected is a significant factor in determining the likelihood of developing postoperative instability. Surgeons agree that resection should be limited to the minimal amount of bone necessary for adequate visualization or decompression. At present, simple disc resection is typically performed through a small unilateral laminotomy defect. The major advantage of laminotomy versus laminectomy is less bone removal and a lower likelihood of postoperative instability. Resectional procedures that are limited to the region of the lamina are rarely complicated by instability.

Extensive cervical laminectomy can also lead to progressive spinal instability. Postoperative cervical instability is rarely seen after single-level laminectomy or multiple unilateral hemilaminectomies. However, surgical excision of multiple laminae leads to loss of normal posterior ligamentous integrity, resulting in progressive anterior subluxation and exaggerated kyphosis, producing the "swan-neck" deformity. The kyphosis is probably aggravated by concomitant muscle weakness.

Imaging

Plain radiographs, including flexion-extension views, are necessary to measure the kyphosis from the most tilted cranial vertebra sagittally to the most caudally tilted vertebra. This implies identification of the end and neutral vertebrae. Ankylosis must be ruled out, because its presence would necessitate preemptive posterior release. Although facet ankylosis often can be ruled out with oblique plain radiographic films, CT might be necessary. MRI is useful to evaluate cord changes, including myelomalacia, syrinx formation, or cord atrophy. These findings can significantly increase the risk of neurologic deficit with surgery or correction. MRI can also help to assess the degenerative status of the discs at the end levels of the fusion. Although myelography and postmyelography CT scanning add specificity in the diagnosis of cord and root impingement, the postmyelogram CT is informative in the exact detailing of the vertebral artery anatomy, the status of the facet joints, and the pedicle anatomy at C7 to determine whether there is a vertebral artery entering at that level and whether the pedicle will accept a screw.

Traumatic Kyphosis

Traumatic kyphosis is a traumatic compression of one or more vertebrae and may occur in the cervical, thoracic, thoracolumbar, or lumbar spine. The most commonly affected location is the thoracolumbar junction. It may lead to either cosmetic or symptomatic kyphosis. This may be prevented by early stabilization of high-grade unstable traumatic spinal injuries. Although the majority of posttraumatic deformities usually occur after spinal column trauma, which is initially treated nonoperatively, several miscellaneous causes of posttraumatic deformity may occur after surgery. These include nonunion, implant failure, Charcot spine, and technical error.

In the thoracic spine, an injury to the anterior column resulting from a flexion-compression injury will produce a decrease in the height of the anterior portion of the vertebral body, resulting in a focal kyphosis at this level. This deformity will cause hyperextension of adjacent spinal regions, resulting in altered facet joint motion, instability, and worsening of the degenerative process.

Each year in the United States, there are more than 1 million acute injuries to the spine, approximately 50,000 of these resulting in fractures to the bony spinal column. The improvements in emergency medical services and the increased safety standards have been increasing the trend for improved patient survival with incomplete and complete spinal cord injuries. Ironically, this has been associated with a greater number of patients presenting with symptoms related to loss of normal spinal alignment or worsening of spinal deformity.

Imaging

Plain radiographs, including anteroposterior and lateral views, are essential. Flexion and extension lateral and anteroposterior bending views are important in assessing the flexibility of any spinal deformity.

CT offers detailed evaluation of spinal bony architecture, and multislice CT has added advantages for spinal trauma imaging, including volume imaging, the ability to acquire multiplanar reconstructions, three-dimensional images, and thick-slice (wedge) multiplanar reconstructions that mimic conventional radiographs. This allows the visualization of subtle structural abnormalities, especially involving the posterior element bony structures that are often difficult to visualize on plain radiography.

Imaging postoperative patients with metallic implants often presents a challenge. Metal causes artifacts such as beam hardening. The metal artifacts depend on the composition of the hardware (titanium produces the least amount of artifact, and cobalt chrome alloys produce the most). Artifacts also depend on the geometry of the implant (its thickness and orientation) and are most severe in the direction of the thickest portion of the implant. Metal artifacts also depend on peak kilovoltage and current, the reconstruction algorithm, and the slice thickness and orientation of the multiplanar reconstruction. Optimization of these parameters can help to reduce metal artifacts.

MRI is useful in visualizing spinal soft tissue structures in detail and to evaluate the canal and neural structures but can be limited by susceptibility to artifacts related to hardware.

Infectious Kyphosis

The term *infectious kyphosis* refers to septic destruction of vertebral bodies, which can lead to severe kyphosis. In particular, tuberculous vertebral osteomyelitis can produce soft-tissue abscess, high-grade kyphosis, and a sharp gibbus deformity with an exaggerated kyphosis epicentered in the lower thoracic spine.

LORDOSIS

A somewhat lordotic curve is normal in the cervical and lumbar spine. Causes of increased lumbar lordosis include postural, congenital, postoperative, achondroplasia, fixed flexion deformity of the hip, and neuromuscular scoliosis.

Postural lumbar lordosis refers to accentuated lumbar lordosis with no fixed deformity and full correction on forward flexion. This condition is typically seen in 8- to 10-year-old girls and may be associated with ligamentous laxity. Management is with reassurance that the posture will resolve with time.

Plain radiographs, including anteroposterior and lateral views, are the most important imaging method. Flexion and extension lateral radiographic views are important in assessing the flexibility of the spinal deformity.

REFERENCES

Aaro S, Dahlborn M: Estimation of vertebral rotation and the spinal and rib cage deformity in scoliosis by computer tomography. Spine 1981;6:460–467.

Ali RM, Green DW, Patel TC: Scheuermann's kyphosis. Curr Opin Pediatr 1999;11:70–75.

Boachie-Adjei O, Lonner B: Spinal deformity. Pediatr Clin North Am 1996;43:883–897.

Connelly PA, Abitbol JJ, Martin RJ: Spine: Trauma. Rosemont, IL: American Academy of Orthopaedic Surgeons, 1997.

D'Andrea G, Ferrante L, Dinia L, et al: "Supine-prone" dynamic X-ray examination: New method to evaluate low-grade lumbar spondylolisthesis. J Spinal Disord Tech 2005;18:80–83.

DeSmet AA, Goin JE, Asher MA, Scheuch HG: A clinical study of the differences between the scoliotic angles measured on posteroanterior and anteroposterior radiographs. J Bone Joint Surg Am 1982;64:489–493.

Dupuis PR, Yong-Hing K, Cassidy JD, Kirkaldy-Willis WH: Radiologic diagnosis of degenerative lumbar spinal instability. Spine 1985;10:262–276.

Fernbach SK: Urethral abnormalities in male neonates with VATER association. AJR Am J Roentgenol 1991;156:137–140.

Fredrickson BE, Baker D, McHolick WJ, et al: The natural history of spondylolysis and spondylolisthesis. J Bone Joint Surg Am 1984;66:699–707.

Goldstein LA, Waugh TR: Classification and terminology of scoliosis. Clin Orthop Relat Res 1973;93:10–22.

Gupta R, Sharma R, Vashisht S, et al: Magnetic resonance evaluation of idiopathic scoliosis: A prospective study. Australas Radiol 1999;43:461–465.

Hensinger RN: Spondylolysis and spondylolisthesis in children. Instr Course Lect 1983;32:132–151.

Katz JN, Lipson SJ, Larson MG, et al: The outcome of decompressive laminectomy for degenerative lumbar stenosis. J Bone Joint Surg Am 1991;73:809–816.

Kirkaldy-Willis WH, Farfan HF: Instability of the lumbar spine. Clin Orthop Relat Res 1982;165:110–123.

Kim CW, Perry A, Garfin SR: Spinal instability: The orthopedic approach. Semin Musculoskelet Radiol 2005;9:77–87.

Kose N, Campbell RM: Congenital scoliosis. Med Sci Monit 2004;10:RA104–RA110.

Lee SW, Wong KW, Chan MK, et al: Development and validation of a new technique for assessing lumbar spine motion. Spine 2002;27:E215–E220.

Lewonowski K, King JD, Nelson MD: Routine use of magnetic resonance imaging in idiopathic scoliosis patients less than eleven years of age. Spine 1992;17(6 suppl):S109–S116.

Loder RT, Urquhart A, Steen H, et al: Variability in Cobb angle measurements in children with congenital scoliosis. J Bone Joint Surg Br 1995;77:768–770.

Lonstein JE: Natural history and school screening for scoliosis. Orthop Clin North Am 1988;19:227–237.

McMaster MJ: Infantile idiopathic scoliosis: Can it be prevented? J Bone Joint Surg Br 1983;65:612–617.

Nissinen M: Spinal posture during pubertal growth. Acta Paediatr 1995;84:308–312.

Nokes SR, Murtagh FR, Jones JD 3rd, et al: Childhood scoliosis: MR imaging. Radiology 1987;164:791–797.

Noordeen MH, Taylor BA, Edgar MA: Syringomyelia: A potential risk factor in scoliosis surgery. Spine 1994;19:1406–1409.

Papanicolaou N, Wilkinson RH, Emans JB, et al: Bone scintigraphy and radiography in young athletes with low back pain. AJR Am J Roentgenol 1985;145:1039–1044.

Pennell RG, Maurer AH, Bonakdarpour A: Stress injuries of the pars interarticularis: Radiologic classification and indications for scintigraphy. AJR Am J Roentgenol 1985;145:763–766.

Putto E, Tallroth K: Extension-flexion radiographs for motion studies of the lumbar spine: A comparison of two methods. Spine 1990;15:107–110.

Ramirez N, Johnston CE, Browne RH: The prevalence of back pain in children who have idiopathic scoliosis. J Bone Joint Surg Am 1997;79:364–368.

Redla S, Sikdar T, Saifuddin A: Magnetic resonance imaging of scoliosis. Clin Radiol 2001;56:360–371.

Resnick D, Kransdorf M: Bone and Joint Imaging, 3rd ed. Philadelphia: Elsevier Saunders, 2005.

Risser JC: The iliac apophysis: An invaluable sign in the management of scoliosis. Clin Orthop 1958;11:111–119.

Ross JS: Magnetic resonance imaging of the postoperative spine. Semin Musculoskelet Radiol 2000;4:281–291.

Sagi HC, Jarvis JG, Uhthoff HK: Histomorphic analysis of the development of the pars interarticularis and its association with isthmic spondylolysis. Spine 1998;23:1635–1639; discussion 1640.

Sairyo K, Katoh S, Sasa T, et al: Athletes with unilateral spondylolysis are at risk of stress fracture at the contralateral pedicle and pars interarticularis: A clinical and biomechanical study. Am J Sports Med 2005;33:583–590.

Schwend RM, Hennrikus W, Hall JE, Emans JB: Childhood scoliosis: Clinical indications for magnetic resonance imaging. J Bone Joint Surg Am 1995;77:46–53.

Stokes IA, Frymoyer JW: Segmental motion and instability. Spine 1987;12:688–691.

Urbaniak JR, Schaefer WW, Stelling FH 3rd: Iliac apophyses: Prognostic value in idiopathic scoliosis. Clin Orthop Relat Res 1976;116: 80–85.

Vaccaro AR, Silber JS: Post-traumatic spinal deformity. Spine 2001;26(24 suppl):S111–S118.

Wiltse L: Spondylolisthesis Classification and Etiology. St Louis: Mosby, 1969.

Wiltse LL, Rothman SLG, Milanowska K, et al: Lumbar and lumbosacral spondylolisthesis. Philadelphia: Saunders, 1990.

Wynne-Davies R: Congenital vertebral anomalies: Aetiology and relationship to spina bifida cystica. J Med Genet 1975;12:280–288.

Young LW, Oestreich AE, Goldstein LA: Roentgenology in scoliosis: Contribution to evaluation and management. Am J Roentgenol Radium Ther Nucl Med 1970;108:778–795.

SUGGESTED READINGS

Albert TJ, Vacarro A: Postlaminectomy kyphosis. Spine 1998;23: 2738–2745.

This is a review of the risk factors, biomechanics, workup, and surgical treatment of postlaminectomy kyphosis.

Armstrong GW, Livermore NB 3rd, Suzuki N, Armstrong JG: Nonstandard vertebral rotation in scoliosis screening patients: Its prevalence and relation to the clinical deformity. Spine 1982;7:50–54.

A total of 6321 schoolchildren were screened in this study using Moire topography in Ottawa in 1979. Analyses of 400 roentgenograms showed that 39% had rotation of a nonstandard variety. This study also describes the different types of curves and their prevalence.

Beutler WJ, Fredrickson BE, Murtland A, et al: The natural history of spondylolysis and spondylolisthesis: 45-year follow-up evaluation. Spine 2003;28:1027–1035; discussion 1035.

This is a prospective study of spondylolysis and spondylolisthesis that was initiated in 1955 with a radiographic and clinical study of 500 first-grade children. This report is the only prospective study to document the natural history of spondylolysis and spondylolisthesis from onset through more than 45 years of life in a population that was unselected for pain.

Borenstein D: Epidemiology, etiology, diagnostic evaluation, and therapy of low back pain. Curr Opin Rheumatol 1994;6:217–222.

This is a complete review of data concerning the epidemiology, etiology, diagnostic evaluation, and treatment of low back pain that have been reported over the one year. Patients who have a longer period of pain during the initial episode of pain are at greatest risk of recurrence of pain.

Cassar-Pullicino VN, Eisenstein SM: Imaging in scoliosis: What, why and how? Clin Radiol 2002;57:543–562.

Scoliosis may be a spinal manifestation of underlying disease, and although most cases of scoliosis are idiopathic, imaging plays a very important role in determining the underlying etiology and in monitoring the changes of the deformity that take place with growth. This review focuses on descriptions of different imaging techniques and how and why the techniques should be applied.

Davis PC, Hoffman JC Jr, Ball TI, et al: Spinal abnormalities in pediatric patients: MR imaging findings compared with clinical, myelographic, and surgical findings. Radiology 1988;166:679–685.

Eighty-one pediatric patients with a variety of spinal disorders, including suspected dysraphism, scoliosis, neoplasia, and neurofibromatosis, underwent magnetic resonance imaging. The results were retrospectively compared in this study with those of myelography followed by computed tomography and surgery.

Evans SC, Edgar MA, Hall-Craggs MA, et al: MRI of "idiopathic" juvenile scoliosis: A prospective study. J Bone Joint Surg Br 1996;78: 314–317.

In this prospective trial, the authors performed an MRI of the spine and hindbrain in 31 patients with scoliosis of onset between the ages of 4 and 12 years. On the basis of their findings, the authors conclude that an MRI of all patients with scoliosis of juvenile onset should be obligatory.

Gundry CR, Fritts HM Jr: MR imaging of the spine in sports injuries. Magn Reson Imaging Clin N Am 1999;7:85–103.

This review describes the advantages and utilities of MRI in sports medicine. It remains the mainstay in the noninvasive diagnosis of most soft-tissue abnormalities occurring within and about the spine. The role of MRI in the evaluation of central spinal stenosis, the central spinal canal, and the spinal cord is unsurpassed by other noninvasive imaging modalities.

Iguchi T, Kanemura A, Kasahara K, et al: Lumbar instability and clinical symptoms: Which is the more critical factor for symptoms: Sagittal translation or segment angulation? J Spinal Disord Tech 2004;17: 284–290.

In this report, sagittal translation and angulation at the L4-5 segment were measured in flexion-extension films in 1090 outpatients with low back and/or leg pain using a three-landmark measuring method. The authors conclude that translation of the lumbar segment has a greater influence than does angulation on lumbar symptoms and that the presence of both radiologic factors could be an indicator for persistence of the symptoms.

Katsumi Y, Honma T, Nakamura T: Analysis of cervical instability resulting from laminectomies for removal of spinal cord tumor. Spine 1989;14:1171–1176.

In this prospective study, 34 patients with cervical cord tumor were followed to investigate the incidence of postoperative deformity or instability after laminectomies.

Modic MT, Feiglin DH, Piraino DW, et al: Vertebral osteomyelitis: Assessment using MR. Radiology 1985;157:157–166.

Thirty-seven patients who were clinically suspected of having vertebral osteomyelitis were prospectively evaluated with magnetic resonance imaging, radiography, and radionuclide studies in this prospective study.

Prahinski JR, Polly DW Jr, McHale KA, Ellenbogen RG: Occult intraspinal anomalies in congenital scoliosis. J Pediatr Orthop 2000; 20:59–63.

Thirty consecutive patients with congenital spinal deformity underwent magnetic resonance imaging to determine the incidence of occult intraspinal anomaly in this prospective study.

Teplick JG, Laffey PA, Berman A, Haskin ME: Diagnosis and evaluation of spondylolisthesis and/or spondylolysis on axial CT. AJNR Am J Neuroradiol 1986;7:479–491.

This study reviews the CT findings in 300 patients who underwent axial CT of the lumbar spine in which spondylolysis and/or spondylolisthesis had been diagnosed. It concludes that axial CT is a highly accurate method for diagnosing and evaluating spondylolysis and all types of spondylolisthesis.

Watura R, Cobby M, Taylor J: Multislice CT in imaging of trauma of the spine, pelvis and complex foot injuries. Br J Radiol 2004;77(spec no 1):S46–S63.

This review discusses the principles of when, where, and why multislice CT imaging of the spine, pelvis, and complex foot injuries should be performed.

Winter RB, Lonstein JE, Heithoff KB, Kirkham JA: Magnetic resonance imaging evaluation of the adolescent patient with idiopathic scoliosis before spinal instrumentation and fusion: A prospective, double-blinded study of 140 patients. Spine 1997;22:855–858.

This is a prospective, double-blinded study of the magnetic resonance imaging findings in the neural axis of 140 neurologically normal typical adolescents with idiopathic scoliosis who were scheduled for scoliosis surgery.

CHAPTER 4

Spinal Deformity in the Clinical Setting

BARON S. LONNER

The clinical evaluation of the patient with a spinal deformity consists of a thorough history and physical examination supplemented by imaging studies. The evaluation allows the practitioner to make or confirm a diagnosis and to determine prognosis and natural history of the deformity, and it guides the treatment plan.

HISTORY

The history is tailored to the patient on the basis of age and presenting information. As part of the initial history, it is important for the surgeon to determine the patient's chief complaint and personal needs when recommending a treatment plan. The patient initially is questioned about the onset of the spinal deformity. A majority of disorders have an indolent onset; however, a minor trauma or significant injury resulting in acute-onset deformity may indicate fracture, either pathologic through a neoplasm or osteoporotic bone or traumatic as a result of a significant injury to the spine (Fig. 4-1). By way of example, the patient with ankylosing spondylitis who has had a mild trauma and acute worsening of a kyphotic deformity should raise suspicion for occult fracture requiring immediate treatment.

Deformity associated with constitutional symptoms such as fevers, chills, or night sweats may indicate an infectious etiology. Travel to an endemic area in which tuberculosis is present may point to this entity, for example (Fig. 4-2).

The most common pathology seen in the pediatric patient is idiopathic scoliosis. In adults, idiopathic scoliosis of long standing or adult-onset degenerative scoliosis are the most commonly encountered disorders. The clinical presentation of a pediatric patient differs in several respects from that of the adult. Adolescents are most likely to present with idiopathic scoliosis. This is often discovered on a school screening examination or an examination by the patient's pediatrician or by family members who note a deformity. Although children and adolescents do not typically have severe pain, a relatively mild to moderate backache is not uncommon, particularly in patients who have thoracolumbar curvature. Their pain may be exacerbated by activities and by the use of a heavy book bag for school. The adult patient, on the other hand, most commonly has pain as the primary complaint to a varying degree.

The patterns and location of pain and its severity are instructive to the examining physician. The pain may be localized to the convexity of the curvature as a result of strain of convex paraspinal musculature or may be on the concavity, possibly related to asymmetric facet loading and arthrosis. Intercostal neuralgia may occur, most commonly on the concavity as a result of foraminal narrowing and intercostal nerve impingement. In severe deformity, the caudal ribs may impinge on the iliac crest, resulting in localized pain (Fig. 4-3). In addition, degenerative changes in the lumbar spine may result in radiculopathy and pain along a dermatomal pattern as well as axial back pain from disc and/or facet pathology (Fig. 4-4). Patients with adult-onset degenerative scoliosis or with childhood-onset idiopathic scoliosis may develop secondary lumbar spinal stenosis and present with neurogenic claudication.

Any treatment the patient has received is also an essential part of the history. If the patient presents for the first time without any treatment, a nonoperative approach might be more appropriate, and if the patient has exhausted modalities such as nonsteroidal anti-inflammatory medication, physical therapy, and bracing, consideration is given to operative management. The patient should be queried about bowel and bladder function; gait disturbance and limitations in the distance the patient can ambulate should also be discussed with the patient. Bowel or bladder dysfunction and gait abnormalities may occur as a result of severe spinal stenosis in the cervical, thoracic, or lumbar spine. Myelopathy is characterized by an unsteady gait and spasticity, whereas cauda equina compression is associated with loss of endurance and often burning or pain in the buttocks and thighs. An antalgic gait or a Trendelenburg gait could be related to hip pathology. The adult patient should be questioned about changes in height or waistline

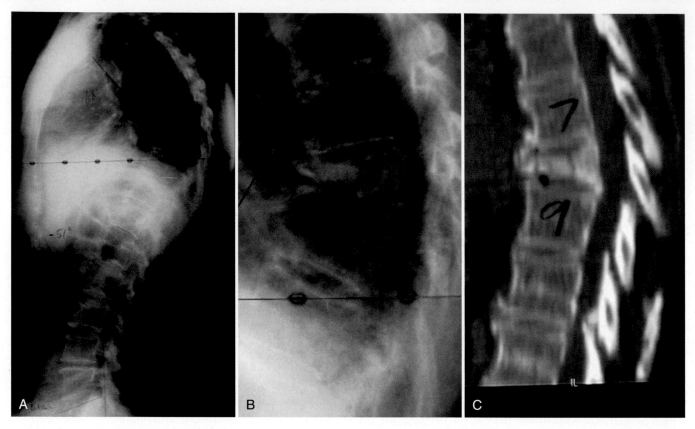

Figure 4-1. A compression fracture of the eighth thoracic vertebra through osteoporotic bone seen in a 60-year-old woman. Lateral radiograph (**A**), coned-down view (**B**), and sagittal reformat CT scan (**C**) illustrate the fracture.

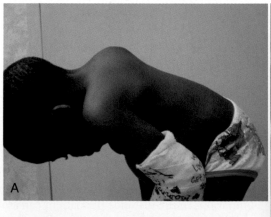

Figure 4-2. A 6-year-old Liberian boy with pulmonary tuberculosis that also involved the proximal thoracic spine and resulted in gibbus formation and subtle neurologic findings. The boy is seen from the side (**A**), and the severe collapse and deformity with the spinal cord draped over the involved vertebrae are visualized on the sagittal MR image (**B**).

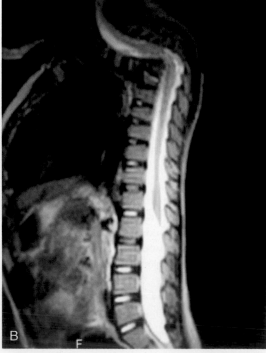

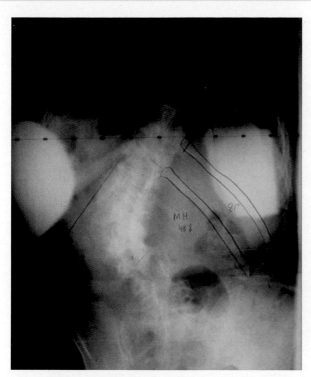

Figure 4-3. Rib impingement on the iliac crest can be a source of pain, as occurred in this adult woman with long-standing idiopathic scoliosis.

and posture over time, findings that are indicative of progression of deformity. If the patient has prior radiographs, the patient should be encouraged to bring those to the attention of the examining physician so that progression of deformity or change in spinal alignment over time can be ascertained. A history of shortness of breath and loss of endurance could indicate restrictive lung disease due to severe deformity in the thoracic spine (Fig. 4-5). Pulmonary problems, of course, might also be related to medical comorbidities such as asthma or congestive heart disease or other intrinsic disease.

A detailed medical history should be taken. A history of osteopenia or osteoporosis may affect treatment decisions, and medical conditions may determine whether or not a patient is an operative candidate or whether additional medical evaluation and treatment are required. A family history should be elicited. Familial disorders include idiopathic scoliosis, kyphosis, Marfan syndrome, and neurofibromatosis. A review of systems should be conducted. The following examples indicate the importance of targeted questioning. Weight loss, fevers, or chills may be indicative of neoplasm or infectious disease. Patients with congenital scoliosis should be asked about any knowledge of cardiac, genitourinary, neurologic, or auditory system abnormalities, as associated anomalies are common in con-

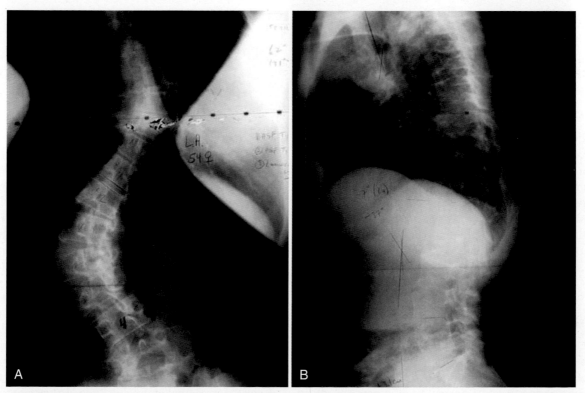

Figure 4-4. Marked diffuse degenerative disc disease associated with adult idiopathic scoliosis. **A,** Lateral listhesis of L3-4, concave end plate sclerosis, and osteophyte formation are common findings, as seen in this patient. **B,** Flattening of lumbar lordosis is common in degenerative collapse and contributes to sagittal plane imbalance in some individuals.

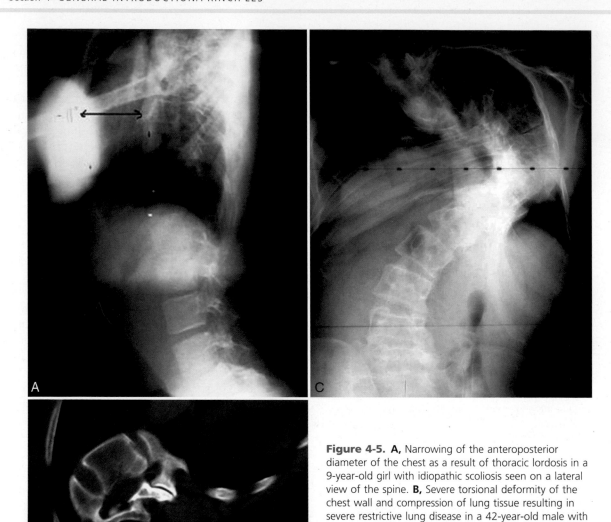

Figure 4-5. A, Narrowing of the anteroposterior diameter of the chest as a result of thoracic lordosis in a 9-year-old girl with idiopathic scoliosis seen on a lateral view of the spine. **B,** Severe torsional deformity of the chest wall and compression of lung tissue resulting in severe restrictive lung disease in a 42-year-old male with untreated scoliosis as seen on a CT scan. **C,** The corresponding posteroanterior radiograph.

genital deformity. Patients with neuromuscular scoliosis might have a history of aspiration pneumonia, and the extent and nature of this should be discussed, as should the patient's feeding habits. Nutritional depletion is common in this patient group. Often, patients have been treated with gastrostomy for feeding in the setting of gastroesophageal reflux and aspiration pneumonia. A thorough history begins to guide the surgeon to diagnosis and treatment options based on the specific needs of the individual patient.

PHYSICAL EXAMINATION

Physical examination begins with standard evaluation of height, weight, and the patient's arm span. Arm span measurements are useful in evaluating pulmonary function for determining percentages of normal to eliminate the effect of loss of trunk height due to curvature. Arm span measurements are increased in the patient with Marfan syndrome. The patient should undress and wear a gown placed with the opening in the back to allow for full evaluation. The gown may later be removed in a discreet fashion to assess the patient's skin and anterior chest. Alternatively, a bikini-style bathing suit or sport bra may be worn by the female patient and shorts by the male. Gait should then be evaluated. Subtle abnormalities may indicate leg-length inequality, neurologic deficits, or hip pathology. The patient should be asked to walk on the heels and toes to assess the strength and endurance of the dorsiflexors and plantar flexors of the ankle joint. An antalgic or shortened stance phase on one side might point to painful hip pathology or leg pain due to radiculopathy. The skin should be thoroughly evaluated for abnormalities such as café au lait spots or inguinal and axillary freckling or neurofibromas that are seen in neurofibromatosis, midline abnormalities such as skin dimpling, nevi, hair tufts, or sinuses that could indicate intraspinal anomalies such as diastematomyelia or lipoma.

A neurologic evaluation should include motor, sensory, and reflex testing of the lower extremities; in cases of cervi-

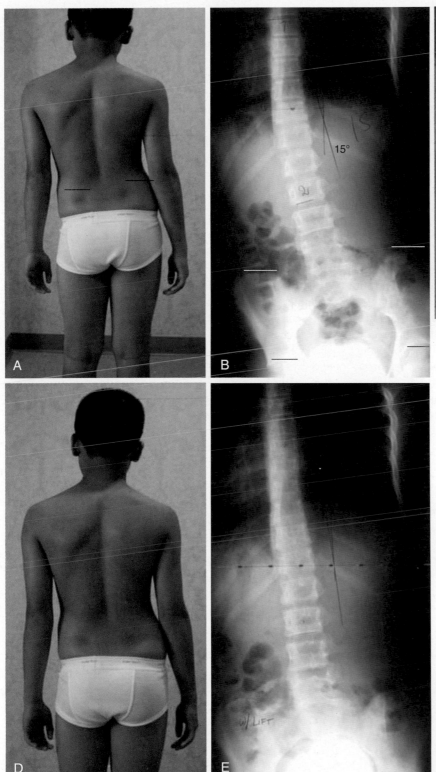

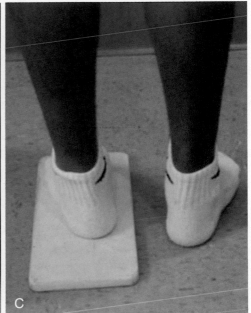

Figure 4-6. Leg-length inequality results in pelvic obliquity and secondary scoliosis when significant. Pelvic obliquity (**A**) and secondary scoliosis (**B**) are noted in this boy with unequal leg lengths. Correction of the clinical deformity is noted with placement of a lift beneath the foot of the short leg (**C** and **D**) with near complete correction of the scoliosis on radiograph (**E**).

cal or cervicothoracic deformity or upper extremity symptoms, the upper extremities should be thoroughly evaluated as well. Ankle clonus and Babinski (plantar-flexor response) as well as abdominal reflexes should be assessed and might, when abnormal, indicate neural element compression or tethering. Neurologic findings can be subtle and can be manifested by differences in calf or thigh circumference or cavus foot or curling of the toes.

Leg lengths should be evaluated, and the hip should be examined for range of motion and the presence of pain. Spinal deformity related to leg length inequality will be at least partially corrected when the patient is reexamined in the seated position or when a lift is placed under the short extremity (Fig. 4-6).

A spinal deformity evaluation should then be undertaken. The patient is examined from the back in the standing position. Asymmetry of the shoulders and waistline, scapular prominence, and pelvic obliquity might be noted. The presence of kyphosis or scoliosis, particularly when severe, can be readily noted, and the flexibility of these deformities can be assessed clinically with lateral bending as well as hyperextension. A forward bend test is performed to bring out chest wall or lumbar deformity associated with the torsional component of scoliosis and can be quantified with the use of a scoliometer (Fig. 4-7). The difference in posterior chest wall height can also be assessed by a linear measurement with the patient in the forward bend position. Sagittal plane deformities such as lordosis and kyphosis are best assessed with the patient standing with the side to the examiner.

Angular kyphosis may be better appreciated with the patient in the forward bend position assessed from the side (Fig. 4-8). Coronal balance can be assessed with a plumbline dropped from the base of the neck and measuring from the gluteal cleft.

As a specific diagnosis comes into view, additional targeted examination can be performed, as will be outlined in future chapters. For example, in patients with ankylosing spondylitis, spinal flexibility (Schober's test), chin-brow angle, and chest expansion evaluation are useful. In patients with Marfan syndrome, the following findings are characteristic: high-arched palate, hallux valgus, chest wall deformities (pectus excavatum or carinatum), genu valgum, and arachnodactyly.

Chest wall inspection should be done from an anterior perspective as well, since patients may have significant pectus carinatum or excavatum, which might or might not be symptomatic or require treatment but can be of significant concern to the patient and family (Fig. 4-9).

Thorough history taking and physical examination of the patient lay the foundation for a comprehensive understanding of the patient's spinal deformity, which is then further delineated by imaging studies.

IMAGING

Radiographic analysis of the patient's spinal deformity should begin with standing full-length (14 × 36 inch) radiographs of the spine. For patients who are unable to stand owing to neuromuscular disease or paralysis, the study should be done in a seated upright position whenever possible. The radiographs should include the cervical, thoracic, lumbar, and sacral spines as well as the iliac crest and hips (Fig. 4-10). This allows the practitioner to determine skeletal maturity based on the ossification of the iliac apophysis (Risser sign) and the triradiate cartilage. In addition, pathology of the hip can be evaluated. Coned-down views of regions of the spine can then be obtained on the basis of anomalies encountered on the long radiograph. For example, if a hemivertebra is noted, this may be more clearly delineated on a localized view.

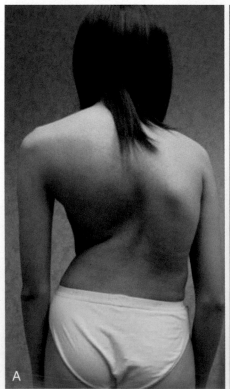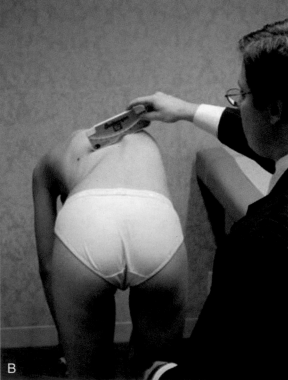

Figure 4-7. A, Shoulder, waistline, and scapular asymmetry are all noted in this patient with idiopathic scoliosis evaluated in the standing position. **B,** On forward bending, the rotational rib prominence is more pronounced, and the angle of trunk rotation can be measured.

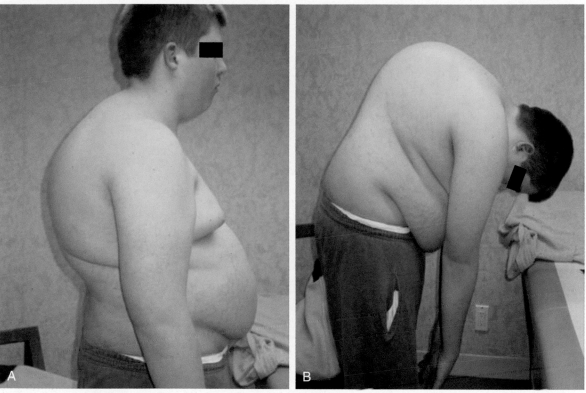

Figure 4-8. This adolescent boy has Scheuermann's kyphosis as noted on a side view in the standing (**A**) and forward bend (**B**) positions.

Radiographs are then analyzed for location and magnitude of curvature in addition to the nature of the pathology and underlying diagnosis. Careful counting of the number

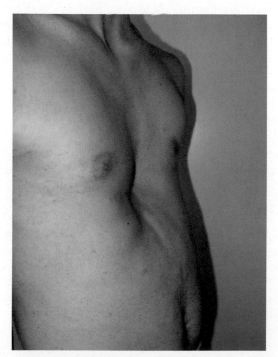

Figure 4-9. Pectus excavatum often is asymptomatic but can be of significant personal concern to the patient and family.

of vertebrae in each region of the spine is important, particularly if surgical intervention is considered so as to avoid wrong-level surgery. Supine bending radiographs, AP traction views, fulcrum bending, and push-prone views in addition to hyperextension radiographs over a bolster to assess flexibility of kyphosis all have a place in determining the flexibility of the curvature and deciding on operative levels when appropriate.

Magnetic resonance imaging (MRI) is indicated in the following circumstances. Patients with infantile or juvenile idiopathic scoliosis have an increased incidence of intraspinal anomalies, such as tethered cord or syrinx, and should have a screening MRI to include the occiput down to the sacrum, particularly if surgery is contemplated even in the absence of neurologic abnormalities (Fig. 4-11). The same applies to a patient with congenital scoliosis who is scheduled for surgery, as there is an elevated prevalence of intraspinal anomalies that could increase operative risk in these patients. The patient with a neurologic deficit or back pain should have evaluation with MRI of the appropriate regions of the spine. For most adults undergoing surgery, MRI of the lumbar spine is indicated to assess the caudal lumbar discs for integrity in terms of presence of disc degeneration or desiccation or compressive neural element lesions. Determination of distal fusion level is often affected by this information.

Computed tomography (CT) evaluation is beneficial to delineate bony architecture in the patient with congenital

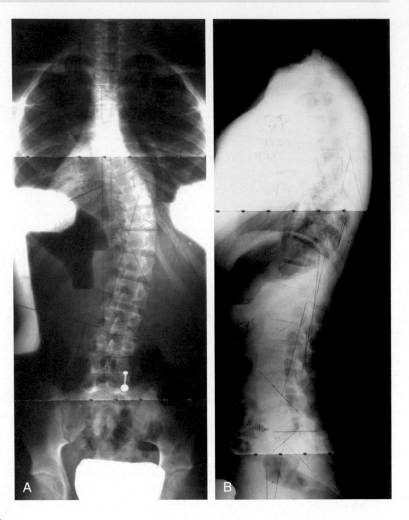

Figure 4-10. Full-length standing posteroanterior (**A**) and lateral (**B**) radiographs of the spine should include the cervical, thoracic, lumbar, and sacral spines and the pelvis and hips.

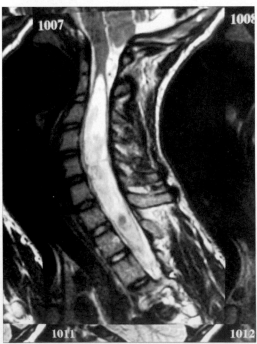

Figure 4-11. This adolescent girl presented with rapidly progressive scoliosis with a typical idiopathic curvature pattern. Subsequent evaluation with MRI performed owing to rapid progression revealed a sizable cervical spinal cord syrinx.

deformity, for example, and may also be used to template the pedicle diameter and length in patients who are expected to undergo spinal instrumentation with pedicle screws (Fig. 4-12). Myelography coupled with CT scan is beneficial for the patient with neural compressive symptomatology with lesions that might not be readily diagnosed by MRI, particularly in the face of severe deformity or revision surgery.

These imaging studies in addition to the history and physical examination allow the surgeon to plan treatment and, in the case of surgery, map out an operative plan.

FURTHER EVALUATION

Each patient must be considered individually for the possibility of further diagnostic evaluation. In the adult patient, a thorough general medical evaluation is required. Cardiac stress testing and echocardiography could be indicated even in the absence of cardiac symptoms, owing to the extensive nature of the planned surgery.

Nutritional evaluation should be considered in elderly patients and in pediatric patients in whom nutritional intake is questionable. This should include evaluation of albumen, total lymphocyte count, and transferrin levels.

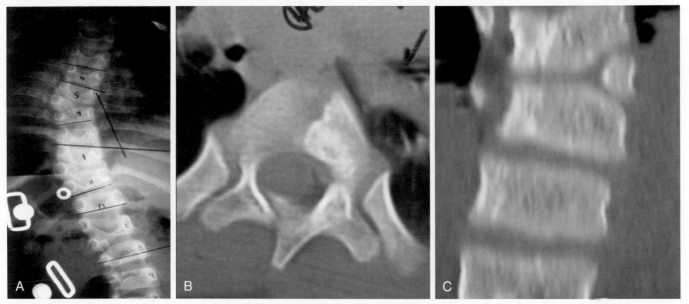

Figure 4-12. This 3-year-old girl had two thoracic hemivertebrae noted on posteroanterior radiograph (**A**) and axial and coronal CT views (**B** and **C**).

Nutritional supplementation perioperatively might be indicated and could help to lower the infection rate in a nutritionally depleted individual.

Pulmonary function evaluation should be considered in all patients, particularly those with significant thoracic deformity. In the idiopathic scoliosis patient, choice of an anterior or posterior operative approach may be directed by the results of pulmonary function testing. This will be addressed further in the section on idiopathic scoliosis.

The patient with congenital scoliosis should have echocardiography and renal sonography to rule out associated cardiac and genitourinary anomalies. The patient with neuromuscular scoliosis as a result of cerebral palsy, for example, might require evaluation with either a barium swallow or a pH probe to rule out gastroesophageal reflux, which might require gastrostomy tube placement. The patient with Marfan syndrome is sent for slit lamp examination of the eyes to rule out superior lens dislocation as well as routine echocardiography to evaluate for aortic root dilation and cardiac valvular abnormalities that can occur. Genetic testing may also be indicated. Many children present with a constellation of findings that might suggest a genetic syndrome; they should be referred to a geneticist for further evaluation.

SUMMARY

The clinical evaluation of the patient with a spinal deformity from history to physical examination and finally to imaging and further diagnostic studies is utilized to ascertain the diagnosis, determine prognosis, and guide treatment decisions.

REFERENCES

Beals RK, Robbins JR, Rolfe B: Anomalies associated with vertebral malformations. Spine 1993;18:1329–1332.

Birch JG, Herring JA: Spinal deformity in Marfan syndrome. J Pediatr Orthop 1987;7:546–552.

Bleck E: Orthopedic Management in Cerebral Palsy. Philadelphia: JB Lippincott, 1987.

Bradford DS, Tay BK, Hu SS: Adult scoliosis: Surgical indications, operative management, complications, and outcomes. Spine 1999;24: 2617–2629.

Bunnell WP: The natural history of idiopathic scoliosis before skeletal maturity. Spine 1986;11:773–776.

Burwell RG, James JN, Johnson F, et al: The rib hump score: A guide to referral and prognosis? J Bone Joint Surg Br 1982;64:248.

Cheung KM, Luk KD: Prediction of correction of scoliosis with use of the fulcrum bending radiograph. J Bone Joint Surg Am 1997;79: 1144–1150.

Dvarik D, Roberts J, Burke S: Gastroesophageal evaluation in totally involved cerebral palsy patients. Paper presented at AAOS meeting, New Orleans, LA, 1986.

Joseph KN, Kane HA, Milner RS, et al: Orthopedic aspects of the Marfan phenotype. Clin Orthop 1992;277:251–261.

MacEwen GD, Winter RB, Hardy JH: Evaluation of kidney anomalies in congenital scoliosis. J Bone Joint Surg Am 1972;54:1341–1454.

Pruijs JE, van Tol MJ, van Kesteren RG, van Nieuwenhuizen O: Neuromuscular scoliosis: Clinical evaluation pre-and postoperative. J Pediatr Orthop 2000;9B:217–220.

SUGGESTED READINGS

Goldberg MJ: Marfan and the marfanoid habitus. In Goldberg MJ (ed): The Dysmorphic Child: An Orthopaedic Perspective. New York: Raven Press, 1987, pp 83–108.

A synopsis of clinical manifestations of Marfan syndrome is provided in this chapter.

Lonstein JE: Patient evaluation. In Lonstein JE, Bradford DS, Winter RB, Ogilvie JW (eds): Moe's Textbook of Scoliosis and Other Spinal Deformities, 3rd ed. Philadelphia: WB Saunders, 1995, pp 45–86.

An overview of patient evaluation for individuals with spinal deformity is provided in this classic textbook.

Newton PO, Faro FD, Gollogly S, et al: Results of preoperative pulmonary function testing of adolescents with idiopathic scoliosis. J Bone Joint Surg Am 2005;87:1937–1946.

The impact of adolescent idiopathic scoliosis is evaluated in a large patient cohort.

Weinstein SL: Natural history. Spine 1999;24:2592–2600.

This article represents a synopsis of natural history studies of probability of progression and clinical impact of adolescent idiopathic scoliosis.

Winter S: Preoperative assessment of the child with neuromuscular scoliosis. Orthop Clin North Am 1994;25:239–245.

Clinical evaluation and preoperative workup of the child with neuromuscular scoliosis is discussed in this article.

CHAPTER 5

Biomechanics of Spinal Instrumentation

THOMAS R. HAHER *and* ANTONIO VALDEVIT

Although spinal instrumentation design is a dynamically evolving process, the mechanical behavior of devices with the spine remains unaltered. It is imperative that the contemporary spine surgeon not only be aware of recent developments in surgical techniques and instrumentation but also be familiar with the underlying mechanical principles associated with the instrumentation and deformity correction. The surgeon will then be able to establish the efficacy of the instrumentation under the intended use and avoid the potential pitfalls that occur in applying the instrumentation under less than ideal specifications. Understanding the mechanical behavior of present-day devices will help clinicians to differentiate between the emergence of technical fads and an innovative device with novel concepts. The spine is a complex and interconnected assembly of joints. It is not an independent series of functional spinal units. Surgical intervention on one element of the spine will generate mechanical and biologic perturbations in adjacent anatomic members. Thus, a cascade of biomechanical ramifications throughout the spine is initiated. The clinician can minimize the biomechanical cascade in the spine when a mechanical basis with respect to the implanted instrumentation exists.

The aim of this chapter is not to provide clinicians with cumbersome analytic arguments favoring one or more systems for implantation. Rather, this chapter is focused on exposure to basic mechanics and its relationship to techniques and devices that have been reported in the literature. In this manner, a clinician can make personal judgments in his or her practice with regard to achieving a surgical goal based on the instrumentation or procedure to be undertaken. The mechanical behavior, however, is only a single component in the surgical decision-making process. Other factors, such as patient selection, bone quality, patient compliance, patient lifestyle, and comorbidity, must also be addressed. The components that make up spinal instrumentation include screws/hooks (defined as anchors), rods/plates (defined as longitudinal members), cross-links (defined as horizontal members), and intervertebral devices (defined as a structure that is placed between two adjacent vertebral bodies). The proper combination of one or more of these components (subassembly) in a particular spinal implant assembly can lead to a successful outcome, while these same components can yield clinical failures if they are arranged in mechanical opposition to the applied forces.

IMPLANT MECHANICS

Concepts

Rheology

Rheology deals with deformation and flow of materials under load with respect to elasticity, plasticity, viscosity, and strength. These terms apply not only to elements of the applied instrumentation but also to the spinal column. Proper interaction of these fundamental material properties between the instrumentation and spinal column are important in establishing the mechanical stability that is required for healing.

Elasticity

An elastic element has full recovery from deformation. An applied force (F) will deform the structure, but when the force is removed, the structure will regain its original dimensions. The linear portion of the load-deformation curve represents elasticity of a structure. The slope of this portion of the curve defines the unique stiffness of the structure (k) (Fig. 5-1).

Plasticity (Coulomb Element)

Plastic deformation represents permanent deformation. There is no recovery and no return to the original dimension. The plastic region of the load-deformation curve follows the elastic region. The transformation point from elastic to plastic is referred to as the *yield point* (see Fig. 5-1). Deformation beyond the yield point is permanent by definition. The amount of deformation may be calculated

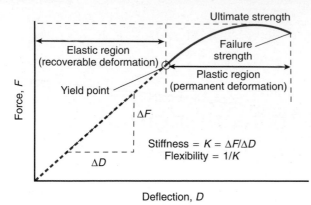

Figure 5-1. Characteristic load versus deflection plot for a material.

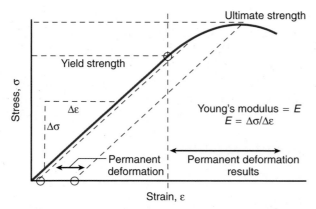

Figure 5-2. Characteristic stress versus strain plot for a material. In this case, the geometry of the material does not affect the output.

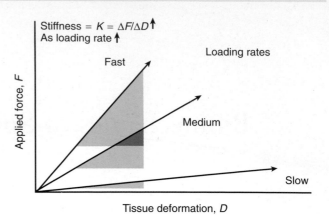

Figure 5-3. Effects of loading on viscoelastic materials.

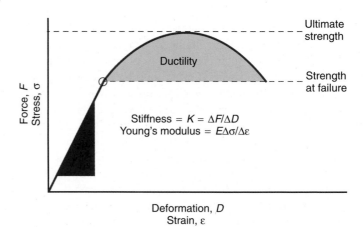

Figure 5-4. An implant can be stiff, strong, and ductile simultaneously.

along the stress-strain or load-deformation curve. When the load is released in the elastic portion of the curve, the curve will return to zero deformation. When the load is released in the plastic portion of the curve, a line drawn from the point of load release parallel to the slope of the elastic portion of the curve will intersect the x-axis (deformation). This value is the permanent deformation resulting for the applied load (Fig. 5-2).

Viscosity

Viscosity is a time-dependent property that resists shear and flow. Deformation depends not only on the applied force but also on the rate of force application (Fig. 5-3). The rate of deformation varies directly with the magnitude of the force. There is no elastic return when the force is removed. All human tissues exhibit viscous properties.

Strength

Strength defines the point at which the material will fail. It is a function of the amount of force or stress needed to break the material. The term *ultimate tensile strength* is often used to describe the strength of a material. The ultimate tensile strength is the maximum tensile

force per unit area that a material can develop prior to failure.

The implant should be stiff, strong, and ductile. Each mechanical property of the implant is unique and not a function of the other properties. In the load-deflection curve or a stress-strain curve, the stiffness (or modulus in the stress-strain curve) is defined as the slope of the elastic portion of the curve (Fig. 5-4). The strength is defined as the load needed to reach failure of the implant, and the ductility is the amount of plastic deformation the implant is able to achieve prior to failure. Therefore, an implant may be stiff to control the curve, strong to prevent failure of the implant under physiologic loads, and ductile so that the surgeon may bend the implant in situ if desired or needed.

The Effect of Implant Geometry on Spinal Stability

The moment of inertia is a geometric property regarding the cross-sectional area of the structure. It describes the spatial distribution of the material in a structural section in relation to its neutral axis. It is not related to the mate-

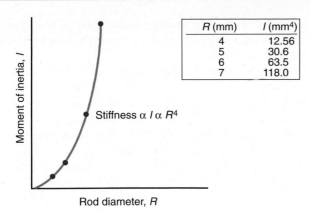

R (mm)	I (mm⁴)
4	12.56
5	30.6
6	63.5
7	118.0

Stiffness $\alpha\ I \alpha\ R^4$

Figure 5-5. The moment of inertia for a rod and hence its strength is proportional to the fourth power of the radius.

rial of the structure but reflects the ability of the structure to resist bending. A small change in the rod diameter has a large effect on the resistance to bending (Fig. 5-5).

The moment of inertia is defined by I and is proportional to the fourth power of the rod radius (r):

$$I : 1/4\pi r^4$$

A very small increase in radius has a large effect of the resistance to bending. The moment of inertia for a 4-mm solid rod is 12.56 mm⁴, while the moment of inertia for a 7-mm rod is 118.0 mm⁴. The moment of inertia for a 7-mm rod is approximately 10 times that of a 4-mm rod.

Mechanics of the Instrumented Spine

Effect of the Moment of Inertia on Spinal Mechanics

When rod diameter is increased in a composite construct such as an instrumented spine, a much lower difference in bending stiffness is realized than would be expected for a cylinder only. The use of rods with larger diameters to achieve stability can be overcompensatory. The resulting stiffness is a combination of the inherent stiffness of the native spinal column and the reduced stiffness of a contoured rod. In such cases, the reduced-diameter rod may display a decreased number of stress cracks during contouring, since it is more ductile. However, this must be balanced by the need for sufficient stability. Appropriate stability can be achieved through the use of cross-links, bracing, and an increased rod diameter.

The Effects of the Yield Point on Implant Mechanics

The yield point is defined as the stress needed to achieve permanent deformation in an implant. It is the point where elastic deformation ends and plastic deformation begins. Implants with an elevated yield point are difficult to bend

in situ. When the yield point is lowered, the implant is much easier to bend in situ. Lowering the yield point has no effect on implant stiffness. Overall stiffness might even be increased with the addition of multiple anchors. The effect of rod size and hook numbers on construct stiffness has been addressed. In simple three-point bending tests, the stiffness values of 4.8-mm, 5.5-mm, and 6.35-mm stainless steel and titanium rods were proportional to those expected from the area moment of inertia formulation. However, increasing the rod diameter of the instrumentation/spinal model construct produced a much smaller increase in bending stiffness. Commercially pure titanium (CPTi) is an example of a metal that has a low yield point and adequate strength.

Forces in the Creation of a Deformity

The function of the spine is to support applied physiologic loads and allow controlled ranges of motion. The forces allowing these functions must be in equilibrium. The failure or flow of a long column (such as the spine) when loaded axially is through buckling.

Buckling of a Column. The spine is a long, slender column and thereby tends to fail by buckling. The critical buckling load is defined by Euler's formula:

$$F_{cr} = EI\pi^2/L^2$$

where L is the length of the column and E and I are material and property constants. Therefore, the critical force to cause buckling is inversely proportional to the length of the column (Fig. 5-6). The longer the column, the less

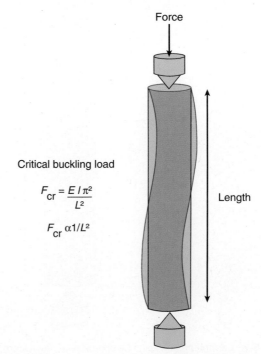

Force

Critical buckling load

$$F_{cr} = \frac{E\,I\,\pi^2}{L^2}$$

$$F_{cr}\ \alpha\,1/L^2$$

Length

Figure 5-6. The buckling theory of a long, slender column.

force is needed for buckling. These conditions are present in a rapidly growing adolescent.

The above formula can predict the behavior of a true homogeneous column. The spine, however, cannot be considered a true column. The spine is a nonhomogeneous structure. It is composed of discs and bone with interposed soft tissue. Buckling is already present in the normal spine, as evidenced by the sagittal contour. Normal cervical lordosis, thoracic kyphosis, and lumbar lordosis represent physiologic buckling. When buckling does occur as predicted by Euler's formula it is usually catastrophic in nature. Scoliosis (buckling) occurs slowly over time. The critical force for buckling can be important, however, when the curve is initiated by other factors and then progresses as the critical buckling force is reached by weight of the trunk, upper extremities, and head (Fig. 5-7).

Uncoupling of Anterior and Posterior Spinal Growth. The spine grows or elongates by anterior and posterior vertebral growth. A balance between these growths will result in the normal coronal and sagittal planes. Uncoupled growth as seen with anterior overgrowth, however, will result in a deformity.

Force Application in the Creation of a Deformity. A three-dimensional spinal deformity may be simulated by force application. The application of forces to the spine can result in scoliosis; however, these forces must be applied in a distinct order. The most severe scoliosis occurs with loading performed in the order of rotation followed by lordosis and finally lateral flexion. Relative anterior overgrowth initiating a lordosing effect is thought to be a mechanism of idiopathic scoliosis creation, particularly in thoracic curvature.

Coupled Motion

Motion about one axis that is consistently associated with motion about a second axis is defined as coupled motion. Coupled motion exists between coronal and sagittal motion in the spine. When the lumbar spine undergoes rotation, lateral bending also occurs. The reverse is also true: Lateral bending of the spine results in rotation. This principle helps to explain the three-dimensional properties of spinal deformities. For example, derotation of the spine will decrease scoliosis. Removing the structures that resist correction or produce the deformity will allow the spine to rotate about its normal axis of rotation. The coupled motion that follows will decrease the curvature. The force coupling of the vertebrae with respect to bending and subsequent rotation produces the rib cage deformity in scoliosis. It is also the basis for the Adam's forward-bending test.

The Two-Stage Hypothesis

Initiation of the Curve by Neuromuscular Deficits. An underlying neuromuscular condition or a defect in the neuromuscular control system as evidenced by postural disequilibrium of a vestibular or visual basis may initiate curve progression. Curve initiation from a neuromuscular condition may be caused by asymmetry of the transversospinalis muscle, resulting in axial rotation and lateral deviation. Curve propagation follows as the curve increases secondary to biomechanical factors such as achieving the force needed for column buckling.

Forces in the Correction of a Deformity. There is an intimate relationship between coronal and sagittal motion. Rotation produces lateral bending, and lateral bending produces rotation. Therefore, spinal rotation is also a precipitating factor in the development of scoliosis. The structures that control spinal rotation are important in determining the etiology as well as the treatment of scoliosis (Fig. 5-8). Loss of rotation stability of the spine is associated with destruction of the anterior column of the spine. Ninety percent of rotational stability is lost with the destruction of the anterior column, while only 30% of

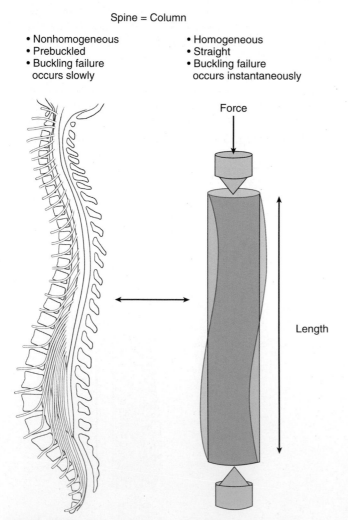

Spine = Column

- Nonhomogeneous
- Prebuckled
- Buckling failure occurs slowly

- Homogeneous
- Straight
- Buckling failure occurs instantaneously

Force

Length

Figure 5-7. Can the human spine be approximated by a long, slender column?

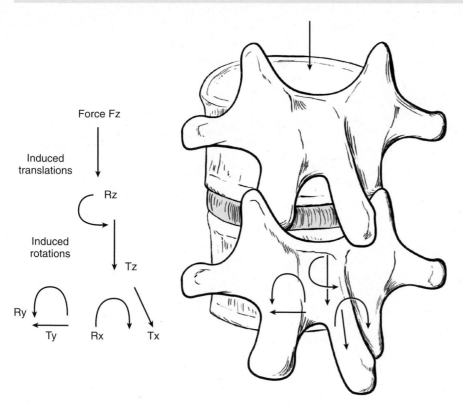

Force Fz

Induced
translations

Rz

Induced
rotations

Tz

Ry

Ty   Rx   Tx

Figure 5-8. In coupled motion, the application of a force in a single direction can also generate translations and/or rotations in other directions.

rotational stability is lost with the destruction of the posterior column. Destruction of the anterior column has a significant effect on reducing the rotational stiffness of the spine. The relationship of anterior column to rotational stability can be explained by understanding its relation to the axis of rotation.

The Axis of Rotation

The axis of rotation is a point about which all other all other parts rotate (Fig. 5-9). Structures at a distance from the axis will have an advantage in controlling motion. The axis of rotation of the spine in rotation is located in the vicinity of the spinal canal. Therefore, the anterior aspect of the spine, being the farthest from the axis, will have a mechanical advantage in resisting rotation. Control of the anterior column will facilitate the correction of the deformity by eliminating the resistance to derotation. This can be achieved by anterior release with or without instrumentation or segmental posterior instrumentation in a supple curve. Laminar hooks may have a mechanical disadvantage in controlling rotation owing to their proximity to the axis of rotation.

Control of the Sagittal Plane

The axis of rotation for flexion and extension is located posterior to the disc space. When the magnitude of the force, the point and line of application of the force, and the location of the axis of rotation are known, the response of the spine to the force can be predicted. The implant's ability to resist the applied force can also be determined. If a distraction force is applied posterior to the axis of rotation in the sagittal plane, lumbar lordosis will be decreased or kyphosis will be created. A compressive force anterior to the axis will have the same effect. Compression applied posterior to the axis will result in lumbar lordosis. The response of the spine to an applied force will also be a function of the distance of the force to the axis of rotation. The greater the distance, the larger is the effect of the force. This is the mechanical basis for anterior spinal surgery.

Instrumentation systems have tendencies to produce predictable effects on the sagittal profile of the spine. Anterior instrumentation in compression produces kyphosis in the thoracic and lumbar spines. This is due to the location of the compression in relation to the axis of rotation. Anterior instrumentation is indicated for thoracic curves with hypokyphosis or thoracic lordosis. It is contraindicated with thoracic kyphosis greater than 40 degrees unless the sagittal profile is recreated with structural interbody grafts. When used in the lumbar spine, anchors must be placed posteriorly in the vertebral body as close to the axis of rotation as possible, and rods must be contoured into lordosis to avoid creating kyphosis. Interbody structural support with cages or structural bone graft can also help to minimize this problem. Posterior instrumentation is usually lordotic in nature and should not be used for the

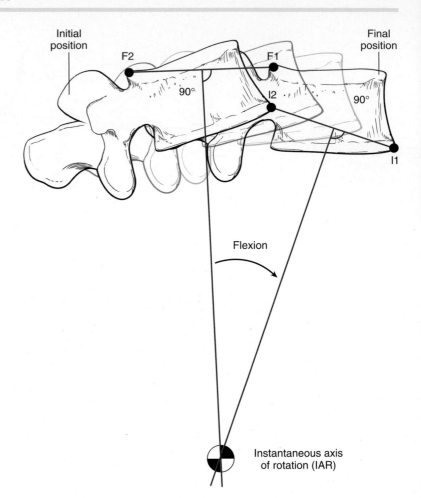

Figure 5-9. The instantaneous axis of rotation can be computed by knowing the initial and final positions of any two unique points on a vertebral body.

treatment of lordotic curves unless the rods are prebent to achieve a normal sagittal profile.

Posterior Column Shortening in the Treatment of Thoracic Kyphosis

Posterior column shortening over each level will effectively reduce kyphosis while sparing the middle and anterior columns. The axis of rotation migrates anteriorly to the anterior aspect of the disc with destruction (facet and lamina resection) of the posterior column. The correction is harmonious over the entire length of the curve. Stress concentrations at the distal anchor sites are reduced, thereby eliminating distal junctional kyphosis.

With some knowledge of rudimentary mechanics, the basic elements of spinal constructs can be discussed.

THE AMERICAN SOCIETY FOR TESTING AND MATERIALS MODEL

In vitro tests are limited by bone quality, specimen geometry, and specimen alignment. In addition, there is rarely a universal consensus with regard to loading conditions. Although individual testing facilities employ different testing methodologies and philosophies, spinal instrumen-

tation can be accurately compared to established devices using the American Society for Testing and Materials (ASTM) model. ASTM has been established and is charged with determining and establishing standardized testing and procedural practices in order to compare not only new and established instrumentation systems but also different instrumentation systems. Standards are proposed, revised, debated, and voted on for acceptance by members of the society, which include representatives from academia, industry, and government agencies. Prior to discussing some of the in vitro literature associated with spinal instrumentation, it is important to present a brief overview of some of the terms that are associated with spinal instrumentation and mechanical testing.

Screws

As defined by ASTM, there are unique definitions of the screws that make up spinal instrumentation:
1. Expansion head screw: a threaded anchor that is designed so that the head can be elastically deformed to establish a connection with another element
2. Locking head screw: a threaded anchor that is rigidly connected to a longitudinal element (such as a rod)

3. Self-locking screw: a threaded anchor design that deforms at the end of the insertion process and results in locking the screw to the mating spinal element
4. Shaft screw: a threaded anchor that has an unthreaded shank equal to the threaded diameter

Metallic bone screws in general are defined by several characteristics and include the following:

1. Buttress thread: an asymmetrical thread profile characterized by a pressure flank that is nearly perpendicular to the screw axis
2. Cancellous screw: a screw that is designed primarily to gain purchase into cancellous bone, typically HB (see #8 below) in thread design and might or might not be fully threaded
3. Cortical screw: a screw that is designed primarily to gain bicortical purchase into cortical bone, typically HA (see #7 below) in thread design and fully threaded
4. Pitch: the length between thread crests
5. Nontapping screw: a screw whose tip does not contain a flute; usually requires that a tap be inserted into a pilot hole prior to screw insertion in moderate or hard bone
6. Self-tapping screw: a screw that has any number of flutes at the thread tip and is intended to cut the screw thread in the bone during insertion
7. Type HA: a screw that has a spherical undersurface of the head, shallow asymmetrical buttress thread, and deep screw head
8. Type HB: a screw that has a spherical undersurface of the head, shallow asymmetrical buttress thread, and shallow screw head
9. Type HC: a screw that has a conical undersurface of the head and symmetrical thread
10. Type HD: a screw that has a conical undersurface of the head and asymmetrical thread

Screws make up the base from which all forces are transferred to and from the rods in an assembly. By ASTM definition, a spinal assembly is considered a complete spinal configuration as intended for surgical use. For posterior forces to be transferred, the screws must remain fixed and secure within bone. Loosening of the screws will redistribute the loads to other members within the posterior construct that are not designed to bear the additional loading. Through repeated loading cycles, the entire construct will loosen and thus lead to a clinical failure. To avoid this scenario, contemporary screws have evolved with variations in thread, head, and shaft design. The most obvious of these innovations is that of the conical shaft. The concept behind such a design is that an increased diameter is engaged within the strong cortical bone outer shell of the vertebral body in an attempt to increase fixation of the screw. The moment of inertia changes through the length of the screw. Resistance to bending is greatest at the anchor/rod boundary or the cortical bone/screw boundary. In contrast, a cylindrical screw will possess uniform moment of inertia (and hence strength) except near the screw head. In such a design, the rod may induce significant bending in the screw head region and thereby initiate a toggling phenomenon that can be a predicate to screw loosening. With the use of high- and low-density polyurethane as a test medium, the pullout strength between conical and cylindrical pedicle screws has been examined. Significantly increased pullout strengths and insertion torques were reported for conical screws with respect to cylindrical screws in both test media. Although the increased pullout strength and insertion torque for conical screws lends credence to the cortical bone being engaged with a larger-diameter thread, the latter finding might be somewhat troublesome clinically. The increased insertion torque may induce bending moments on the spine segment during surgery. Clinically, predrilling or reducing the screw size, both of which can compromise the integrity of fixation, could resolve this issue. Further, the likelihood of fracture during insertion might be increased. At this point, clinical experience and technique are invoked to achieve optimal fixation using this particular screw design.

One must be aware of two aspects regarding these conical screws. The first is the possibility of strength loss during insertion or positioning should the screw have to be backed out to mate with the connecting rod; the second is that during loading, the connecting rods will induce bending at the screw head and that a toggle mechanism could be induced with the cortical bone contact region as the fulcrum. A comparison of conical screws that were fully seated to those that were fully seated but then backed out one half turn and one full turn has been performed by using a porcine model. At full insertion, pullout load and stiffness were increased by 17% ($P < 0.1$) and 50% ($P < 0.05$), respectively, using conical screws as compared to cylindrical screws. No loss in pullout load, stiffness, or energy to failure was noted between conical screws that were backed out up to one full turn following full insertion and conical screws that were fully inserted. The change in diameter between successive threads is minimal; therefore, a single turn back out should not provide a significant loss of bony contact. According to this study, under clinical conditions, one can back out a conical screw up to one complete turn without a significant loss in fixation that would occur under fully seated conditions. Screws with a narrowing flute could lead to the compaction of trabecular bone and thus to a favorable effect on pullout.

The susceptibility to loosening via toggle was determined by applying continuous cyclic loads to calf specimens with conical screws backed out 180 degrees and comparing these to standard cylindrical screws. Conical screws resulted in significantly increased deflections: approximately 47% above those displaced by cylindrical screws. This finding illustrates the potential for toggle associated with these screws. While they engage the strong cortical bone with a large diameter, the internal region of the vertebral body containing the trabecular bone is anchored with a continuously reducing diameter thread

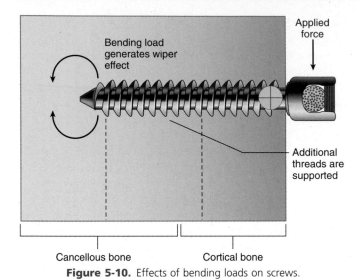

Figure 5-10. Effects of bending loads on screws.

and shaft. Loading at the head of the screw will pivot the small thread through the soft trabecular bone and induce toggling of the screw. It remains to be determined whether this condition occurs clinically, especially in the case of a polyaxial conical screws. In a polyaxial screw, the locking mechanism might provide a sufficient amount of induced micromotion to provide stress relief at the screw tip and hence possibly avoid this toggle condition. Although pullout tests are a standard by which screws are evaluated and compared, clinically, direct axial pullout does not occur. While an axial force is directed along the screw axis, owing to the presence of a stiff rod and significant kyphosis, the dominant loading due to the interconnecting rod is a bending moment. Continued bending of the screw head due to flexion and extension motions of the spine can generate micromotion of the threads in the cortical and trabecular bone. Although trabecular bone is weaker, the volume of trabecular bone that is in contact with the screw is substantially greater than the amount of cortical bone. Per unit volume, the cortical bone/screw thread interface is stronger, but the increased number of threads within the trabecular bone leads to a substantial contribution in overall toggle resistance. In axial pullout, strength is primarily due to cortical bone purchase. In bending, both bone components contribute to overall screw stability (Fig. 5-10).

Screw Placement

In addition to screw design, screw placement plays an important role in resulting construct stiffness. Screws were placed at 10-mm (protruding by 10 mm), 5-mm, 0-mm, and –5-mm (countersunk by 5 mm) depths relative to the dorsal surface of a polyethylene corpectomy model. In flexion and extension, stiffness increases of approximately 230% were observed at –5-mm levels as compared to 10-mm levels. Mechanically, this is not an unexpected result. Loading takes place at the model/screw interface. The

screw head containing the interconnecting rod is located at a greater distance from this loading axis. The increased distance contributes to an increase in the moment arm and hence an increased moment. In the case of polyaxial screws, this places increased demands to load resistance on the locking mechanism of the screw. In monoaxial screws, the rod retention mechanism is placed under increased stress as well as the rod itself. In polyaxial screws, micromotion in the screw head can act to reduce the resultant load that is placed on the rod and rod retention mechanism. Regardless of whether monoaxial or polyaxial screws are employed, the incorporation of the rod retention and head-locking mechanism must be maintained in close proximity to the bone surface. It follows that the clinician should attempt to maintain the resulting posterior construct as close to the spine as possible. Posterior systems that remain distant from the spine must be mechanically enhanced through structural support or load sharing to ensure a stable construct.

Cross-Links

Cross-links pose another mechanical member that has seen development. Although cross-links employed in a construct increase rigidity by shortening the length of the construct, the effects are not overly significant until a torsional load is applied through the spine. Under torsional loads, inclusion of cross-links within the screw/rod construct significantly enhances stability. In flexion, extension, and lateral bending modes, both rods in the construct move in the same plane at the same time; therefore, at any point in the motion, the relative distance between the rods is essentially unchanged. However, in rotation, the rotation axis is not at a point between the rods; it rests within or near the spinal canal. Therefore, the separation distance between the rods will change owing to a twisting of the construct in conjunction with the rotation and bending of the spine due to the coupled motion between functional spinal units (Fig. 5-11). Clinically speaking, in all hook constructs or those with a majority of hooks, cross-links can be useful or necessary; however, in configurations in which segmental screw fixation is utilized, this might not be required.

Rods

Screws may provide the anchor for spinal constructs, but it is the rods that provide the stability. Rods transmit loads to the spine via the anchors. While screws and cross-links can be variable in design, rods are limited to material properties, diameter, and geometry. With respect to the latter, currently utilized rods are cylindrical, although a square rod has been previously utilized. Material properties are generally limited to two options: titanium and stainless steel. Recently, CPTi has emerged as a material that is suitable for use as rods in spinal constructs. In a

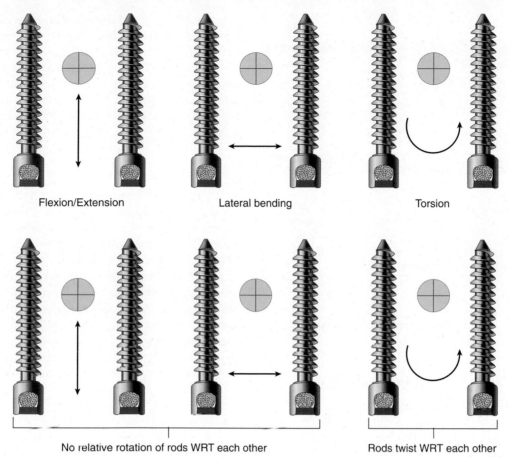

Figure 5-11. Cross-links minimize the effects of torsional loads but display minimal effects in other loading modes.

comparison of 4-mm and 5-mm stainless steel rods to 4.5-mm CPTi rods using intervertebral spacers in a human cadaveric model, no significant differences in compression, flexion, extension, lateral bending, and torsion between rod constructs were found. This leads one to conclude that CPTi rods display a reduced yield point yet can provide sufficient rigidity with respect to stainless steel rods of comparable diameter. However, a rod that is employed in a long construct without anterior column support is subject to greater loads than is one that is utilized in a single-level fusion with anterior structural support. The reduced-yield point of CPTi rods permits permanent deformation with low force and results in a consequent reduction in the direct load transferred to the screw anchors. In the condition in which high-yield load materials are employed as rods, increased load is transferred to the screws and can result in screw backout or toggle initiation, since the rod will not deform from the preset contouring within the construct. In addition, a reduced-diameter rod will permit increased load sharing between the construct and the spine. Mechanically, the strength of a rod is related to the moment of inertia, a measure of how much material is located about a central axis (or point of motion). Specifically, the moment of inertia for a rod is related to the strength by the fourth

power of the radius of the rod, as was previously noted. An increase of 1 mm in diameter from a 4-mm to a 5-mm diameter rod changes the moment of inertia (and the stiffness) by almost 250%.

A large-diameter rod posteriorly can stabilize the posterior column via load transfer. However, if anterior column support is not addressed, bending moments in flexion and axially compressive loads will subject the construct to increased stresses. The effects of increasing rod diameter in a seven-level construct did not significantly alter the construct stiffness with the addition of interbody cages in one study. This then raises the issue of employing large-diameter rods in cases in which anterior instrumentation will be used to supplement the construct. Anterior instrumentation generates two-column support and results in a reduction of posterior moments under flexion, compression, and lateral bending in isolation. Consider a long horizontal beam that is securely constrained at one end (Fig. 5-12). Application of even a small load at the free end will generate a bending moment at the fixed end and will result in increased stresses within the beam to resist bending. If the same condition were applied with a support located under the beam at the free end, a large load would be required to induce bending in the beam. The inclusion

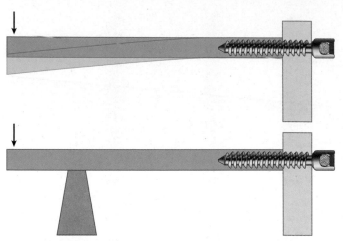

Figure 5-12. Bending within a rod can be minimized if supplemental support is placed near the point of load application.

of the support effectively shortens the moment arm through which the moment will act.

Single-Rod Versus Dual-Rod Construct

With the use of smaller rods, one could make the argument that a single large-diameter rod may suffice to establish construct rigidity rather than using two small rods. While this concept is intriguing, one must also consider symmetry with respect to load distribution. The use of a single-rod construct versus a dual-rod construct with and without intervertebral spacers has been investigated, and as was expected, the addition of the second rod does significantly increase construct stiffness. More specifically, the effects of increased rod diameter from 4.75 mm to 6.35 mm under single- and dual-rod configuration used in conjunction with intervertebral cages has been studied. It was determined that the dual 4.75-mm construct resulted in increased construct stiffness in comparison to either single-rod construct. No significant differences in stiffness were noted between the rod diameters when the single-rod configuration was employed with the spacers. The dual-rod configurations displayed reduced screw/rod strain compared to the single-rod constructs.

Statically, dual-rod systems provided increased stability in comparison to single-rod systems in flexion-extension and torsion. Single- and dual-rod systems were comparable in lateral bending. Following cyclic loading, a significant decrease in flexion-extension construct stability was seen for the single-rod systems as compared to dual-rod systems. A dual-rod system reduces screw/rod strain and hence minimizes the effect of toggle. In addition the large-diameter single-rod systems have a large moment of inertia with respect to most of the rods employed in the dual-rod systems. With the large rod stiffness, screws become the point at which load is concentrated. With less stiff rods, the load sharing between rod and screw can

occur and thus reduce the concentration of moment at the screw/bone interface. It is important to recognize that in a laboratory setting, only initial stability and performance are measurable. Clinical functionality and long-term performance are the subject of outcome studies and require many years of clinical follow-up to accurately complete, and of course, they rely in part on a biologic component of fusion.

Cages

In any construct, bending is minimized or reduced when more than one support is included. In the case of isolated posterior rod/screw constructs, flexion induces bending, since a deformable intervertebral disc does not rigidly support the anterior region of the spine. While in the case of a healthy disc, sufficient anterior column support is generated, in the case of a degenerated disc, increased bending will be induced, owing to the loss of mechanical integrity of the disc (Fig. 5-13). Interbody support initially emerged as stand-alone devices. Placement of a solid body between the intervertebral end plates would suffice to initiate fusion, provided that the material/bone interface was conducive to bone ingrowth. Such a device could also be fabricated with a prespecified lordotic angle. These devices, while restoring lordosis, disc height, and increased resistance to bending, displayed instability within the disc space in extension and torsion. This inherent instability not only reduced fusion rates but also led to migration of the interbody devices. In cases in which the device footprint was small and located near the central region of the vertebral end plate, subsidence would become evident because the device would bear the entire flexural bending load, thereby advancing the device into the weakest region of the end plate. Combining the interbody spacer with posterior screw/rod constructs provided clinicians the benefits of anterior support while also pro-

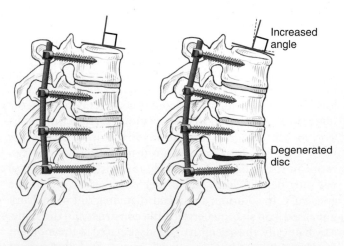

Figure 5-13. Increased degeneration can increase spinal deflection (or angulation) and result in instability, thereby perpetuating additional degeneration.

viding increased resistance to motion in extension, thereby stabilizing the device.

Cage stability can be related directly to fusion rate and quality. The limitations of migration and micromotion are important factors in cage design. The resistance to pullout is then the ability of this mechanism to resist axial tensile loading. Cage dynamics are a function of end plate contact area, contact geometry (such as spikes and threads), penetration depth, cage stiffness, and the quality of the adjacent bone and soft tissues.

The use of intervertebral spacers is common in the treatment of lumbar fusion. Although considerable work has been done in evaluating the properties of these devices with respect to mechanical performance, the parameterization of these results with respect to the geometry of the device is generally uninvestigated. In a study by Gödde involving 42 patients (18 months mean follow-up), undergoing primary posterior lumbar fusion with rectangular and wedge-shaped spacers, segmental lordosis decreased 8 degrees at L3-4, 5 degrees at L4-5, and 3 degrees at L5-S1. In the wedge-shaped cage group, segmental lordosis increased 3 degrees at L3-4, 6 degrees at L4-5, and 8 degrees at L5-S1. The authors concluded that, with rectangular cages, the segmental lordosis of the fused segments decreases, with sagittal balance compensating by changes in sacral tilt, which uses up the patient's hip extension reserve. Conversely, wedge-shaped cages significantly increased segmental lordosis and therefore are preferred in restoration of sagittal alignment in instrumented posterior lumbar interbody fusion procedures. It must be noted that several factors come into play with cage geometry and individual in vivo clinical results. Bone density is an element to be considered. A wedge-shaped spacer might be susceptible to stress concentrations on the end plate. In restoring lordosis, the anterior aspect of the vertebral body will be placed in a condition of increased stress at the contact point when the patent induces flexion. The rectangular spacer might reduce the compensatory motions of the adjacent segments as the segmental lordotic angles may be less. Another concern is that of facet distraction. In the case of a rectangular implant, posterior distraction opens up the facets, which must be counteracted by compression of the posterior instrumentation. This is less necessary with lordotic implants. The Gödde study was not able to statistically differentiate changes in overall lumbar lordosis and sacral tilt between the two designs. This indicates that while local differences might be apparent, the overall functionality of the spine might not be varied between the two device designs. To establish better parameterization, a longer follow-up with segmental and overall geometric measurements at periodic time points could be warranted. The surgical approach is another aspect that must be considered. A single posterior approach using wedged implants might be less effective than an anterior spacer insertion for height restoration followed by posterior stabilization. Critical thinking is necessary to develop a rationale for any surgical procedure, especially in the context of local and global deformity.

American Society for Testing and Materials Testing of Spinal Instrumentation

All of the material that has been discussed thus far has dealt with clinical or basic science studies of spinal instrumentation. These studies involve an in vitro model that may consist of one or more spinal segments from either cadaveric or animal specimens. Although the testing and loading methodology within a specific study might be reproducible, the specimens, although similar, are less so. In the case of human specimens, the bone mineral density can vary widely, as can the geometric dimensions. These variables are less dramatic with respect to animal models but are nonetheless present. As well, one can see that it is often difficult to directly compare the results of one study with those of another, owing to differences in testing methodology. To alleviate comparison problems as well as to establish standards that governing agencies could reference, the American Society for Testing and Materials (ASTM) was established. The society is not intended for the evaluation of device superiority or clinical efficacy. Rather, it is concerned with development of testing methodologies, practices, and standards for characterization of devices and materials. These standards provide researchers, governing agencies, and manufacturers with methods by which new devices can be compared to other, similar predicate devices or to historical data for quality control. With respect to spinal instrumentation, there are four basic standards in effect. They are listed in Table 5-1.

Each standard will be described here in brief to expose the clinician to the mechanical limits to which these devices are subjected during development. Specifics with respect to specimen labeling, alignment, fixture material, and reporting are beyond the scope of this chapter.

F2193-02: Standard Specifications and Test Methods for Components Used in the Surgical Fixation of the Spinal Skeletal System. This document specifically addresses specifications and test methods to the evaluation of spinal screws, plates, and rods as individual components rather

TABLE 5-1. ASTM Spinal Instrumentation Standards

Number	Title
F2193-02	Standard Specifications and Test Methods for Components Used in the Surgical Fixation of the Spinal Skeletal System
F1717-04	Standard Test Methods for Spinal Implant Constructs in a Vertebrectomy Model
F2077-03	Standard Test Methods for Intervertebral Body Fusion Devices
F2346-05	Standard Test Methods for Static and Dynamic Characterization of Spinal Artificial Discs

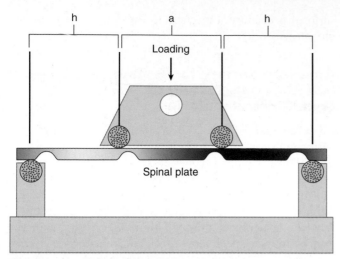

Figure 5-14. Four-point bending and compression testing of a spinal plate according to ASTM 2193.

than as a construct. For all of these components, both static and dynamic (fatigue) tests are specified under one or more loading modes. In the case of spinal plates, two tests are stipulated: one each in static and dynamic modes. The static test is shown in Figure 5-14 and is loaded to failure in displacement control (10 mm/min) until failure. The separation distances are prespecified depending on the intended anatomic location of the plate (cervical or lumbar). The dynamic or fatigue test is similar but requires that the plate be subjected to different R ratio values. The R value is the ratio between the maximum load and the minimum load. In the case of lumbar or thoracic plates, the R value is 0.1. For cervical plates, the R value is −1; that is, the plate must be subjected to compressive and tensile loading on the anatomic contact surface. Figure 5-15 illustrates a test setup that can achieve an R value of −1. Unlike static testing, fatigue or dynamic tests are conducted in load

control. The initial load values for dynamic tests are predetermined from the static test results. Plates are tested dynamically starting at 75% of the ultimate failure load (or moment) recorded during the static test. The test is conducted until fatigue failure of the plate or achievement of 2.5 million cycles. When plate specimens fail, subsequent fatigue tests are initiated at 50% and 25% of the static ultimate failure load. The fatigue test is designed to establish a load (moment) versus number of cycles to failure. (Often, this is termed the *S/N* curve, with *S* designating stress or strain, depending on application.) Generally, two specimens are required to pass this fatigue test. The load at which specimens pass the test is termed the *runout load*. Fatigue testing should be continued until the difference between the maximum load resulting in failure and the runout load is less than 10% of the ultimate failure load. In this particular standard, the maximum frequency for testing has been set at 30 Hz. With respect to spinal rods, the testing is quite similar. The major difference is that the static testing rollers that are used in the evaluation of spinal plates possess a notch to stabilize yet not unduly constrain the rod during load application. The fatigue testing procedure is conducted in a fashion similar to that described for spinal plates. The setup to evaluate spinal screws is shown in Figure 5-16. As with rods and plates, both static and fatigue tests are stipulated. The screw is inserted to a depth of 10 mm within the test block and loaded at the midpoint of the block while the screw head is maintained fixed. Static tests are applied at a maximum rate of 25 mm/min; fatigue tests are conducted as previously described.

F1717-04: Standard Test Methods for Spinal Implant Constructs in a Vertebrectomy Model. The previous standard was specific to construct components. This particular standard is designated to examine the use of spinal instrumentation as a construct. The test configuration is depicted in Figure 5-17. The test blocks are altered depending on

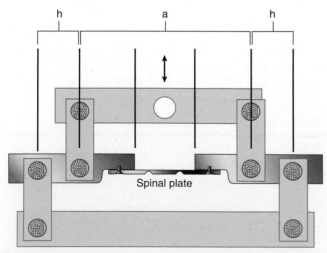

Figure 5-15. Four-point bending, compression, and tension testing of a spinal plate according to ASTM 2193. This fixture will permit loading in both directions (tension and compression).

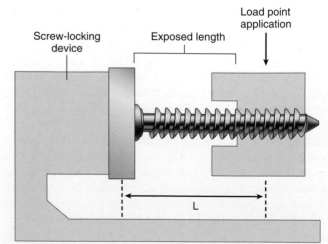

Figure 5-16. Bending test setup for spinal screws as described in ASTM 2193.

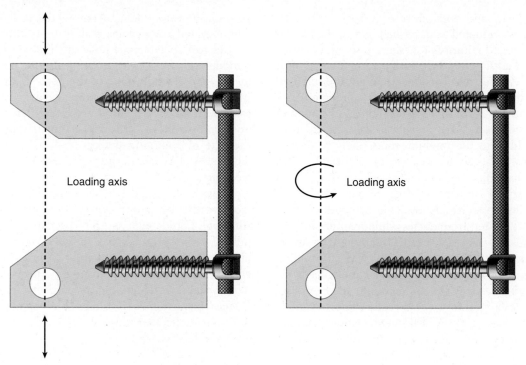

Figure 5-17. Standard test setup for compression-tension, bending, and torsion in a vertebrectomy model as described in ASTM 1717. The blocks and screw separation dimensions are dictated by the intended use of the spinal construct (cervical, thoracic, or lumbar).

the anatomic application site (lumbar or cervical) and whether the user is evaluating constructs involving screws or hooks in conjunction with rods, hooks, or cables. In this standard, several static tests are cited. They include compression, tension, and torsion. The tension and compression tests are conducted at a rate of 25 mm/min. In the case of compression, the construct is loaded in flexion, while tension is represented in the case of extension. The rate for torsion tests is 60 degrees/min. It must be noted that at times, the construct will not fail catastrophically. That is, rods and screws or hooks might not break but might instead deform under loading. In this case, one must determine the yield point as a starting point for the conduction of the fatigue tests. The yield point is the load at which permanent deformation is imparted to the construct. Mechanically, the construct is weakened and will display a decrease in load resistance (stiffness). The fatigue test is conducted as previously described, but in this case, the spinal construct must endure 5 million cycles to achieve runout condition. In addition, the fatigue test is to be conducted at only 5 Hz, resulting in a test duration in excess of 11 days.

F2077-03: Standard Test Methods for Intervertebral Body Fusion Devices; F2346-05: Standard Test Methods for Static and Dynamic Characterization of Spinal Artificial Discs. These standards are the most recent. F2346 for intervertebral disc devices has emerged owing to the development of total disc arthroplasty and is based on F2077. F2077 is a standard regarding the testing of interbody devices such as cages and spacers, whether they are used

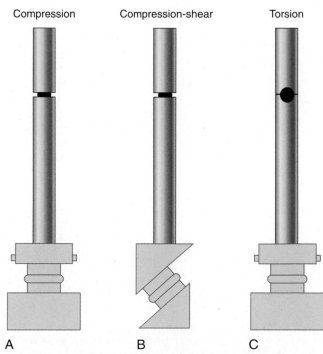

Figure 5-18. The experimental setup for mechanical evaluation of an interbody spinal device. The ball joint permits axial application of loads. **A,** Compression. **B,** Compression-shear. **C,** Torsion.

in anterior or posterior procedures. In these standards, three tests are proposed: compression (Fig. 5-18A), compression-shear (Fig. 5-18B), and torsion (Fig. 5-18C) in both static and fatigue modes. The static loading rates are 25 mm/min and 60 degrees/min for the compression,

compression-shear, and torsion tests, respectively. The fatigue tests are conducted as described, but in the case of the compression and compression-shear tests, the R value must be at least a value of 10. In torsion, the R value must be −1, that is, left and right torsion. Although the standard recommends that these fatigue tests be conducted in a 37°C saline bath at 2 Hz or less, it is left to the user to select a test frequency. With respect to the test environment, air would pose the medium most likely to display wear problems. The wear component associated with testing of artificial discs is best addressed through design and development of simulators. With respect to test frequency, a testing apparatus is available to conduct these fatigue tests at elevated frequencies while maintaining the prescribed loads. In the case of F2077, fatigue tests are to achieve a runout load at 5 million cycles, while 10 million cycles of fatigue are required to achieve runout loads for intervertebral disc devices. At the recommended test rate of 2 Hz, a single fatigue test would require approximately 29 and 58 days, respectively. As was stated, testing machines are available that can reproducibly and accurately apply the prescribed load yet run at elevated frequency. Figure 5-19 illustrates a load and deformation versus time graph with the sinusoidal loading frequency at 60 Hz. At this rate,

10 million cycles could be completed in less than 2 days. The elevated frequencies may impart additional burdens on the test specimen. These can include excess thermal buildup and stress concentration due to the possibility of increased deflection. One of the goals associated with any ASTM standard is that historical data can be compared to current devices. Testing at elevated frequencies might not lend itself to historical comparison. However, in the case of emerging devices such as intervertebral disc devices, ASTM has permitted the user to select the test frequency.

As with all medical fields, emerging technologies are faced with regulatory issues to acquire marketability. Although bodies such as ASTM strive to establish testing practices and protocols, it is the governing bodies that ultimately dictate the load levels, durability, and fatigue endurance to gain some insight with respect to in vivo performance. Independent researchers evaluate medical devices through in vitro studies based on personal mechanical and intellectual ideology. If regulating bodies are to evaluate devices, standardized testing is also a component that must be satisfied. The standardized tests might not reflect a clinical condition. Standardized test are used only to compare devices rather than to determine effectiveness.

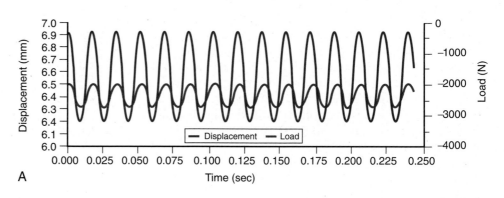

A

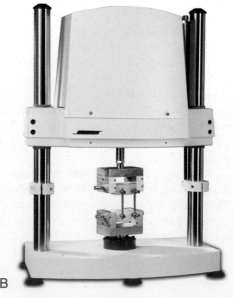

Figure 5-19. A, Load and displacement plotted versus time. **B,** Electromagnetic machines can achieve high load control combined with high frequency. (**B,** *Courtesy of ElectroForce Systems Group [Bose Corporation], Eden Prairie, MN.*)

B

The design of any new device, whether intended for the spine or other anatomic site, requires mechanical input from engineering personnel as well as an equal contribution from clinical staff. In this manner, the mechanical requirements to conduct and pass the standardized tests can be merged with the clinical demands of the device required to effectively treat patients.

SUGGESTED READINGS

Abshire BB, McLain RF, Valdevit A, Kambic HE: Characteristics of pullout failure in conical and cylindrical pedicle screws after full insertion and back-out. Spine J 2001;1:408–414.

Conical screws may be backed out up to a full turn without loss of pullout strength.

Button G, Gupta M, Barrett C, et al: Three- to six-year follow-up of stand-alone BAK cages implanted by a single surgeon. Spine J 2005;5:155–160.

The stability of intervertebral cages is increased with posterior instrumentation and results in decreased morbidity.

Dick JC, Zdeblick TA, Bartel BD, Kunz DN: Mechanical evaluation of cross-link designs in rigid pedicle screw systems. Spine 1997;22:370–375.

The use of rod cross-links can increase construct stability. The effect is most significant in torsion.

Dietl RH, Krammer M, Kettler A, et al: Pullout test with three lumbar interbody fusion cages. Spine 2002;27:1029–1036.

The design of lumbar intervertebral cages affects the in vitro mechanical properties of the device.

Haher T, O'Brien M, Orchowski J, et al: The role of the lumbar facet joints in spinal stability: Identification of alternate paths of loading. Spine 1994;19:2667–2671.

Although the effect or rod diameter resulted in bending stiffness values according to the inertia formula, increases in spinal construct bending stiffness were not as dramatic.

Haher T, Ottaviano D, Lapman P, et al: A comparison of stainless steel and CP titanium rods for the anterior instrumentation of scoliosis. Biomed Mater Eng 2004;14:71–77.

Selection of a reduced-diameter rod can provide sufficient construct stiffness if the correct material is also chosen.

Hsu CC, Chao CK, Wang JL, et al: Increase of pullout strength of spinal pedicle screws with conical core: Biomechanical tests and finite element analyses. J Orthop Res 2005;23:788–794.

In test models of varying density, conical screws displayed increased pullout strengths and insertion torques compared to cylindrical pedicle screws.

Lill CA, Schlegel U, Wahl D, Schneider E: Comparison of the in vitro holding strengths of conical and cylindrical pedicle screws in a fully inserted setting and backed out 180 degrees. J Spinal Disord 2000;13:259–266.

The decreasing diameter of the screw within the bone can make conical screws susceptible to loosening through cyclic toggling.

Mikles MR, Asghar FA, Frankenburg EP, et al: Biomechanical study of lumbar pedicle screws in a corpectomy model assessing significance of screw height. J Spinal Disord Tech 2004;17:272–276.

The depth of screw insertion relative to the dorsal surface can dramatically affect the strength of a construct.

Oda I, Abumi K, Yu BS, Sudo H, Minami A: Types of spinal instability that require interbody support in posterior lumbar reconstruction: An in vitro biomechanical investigation. Spine 2003;28:1573–1580.

Posterior pedicle systems might not be sufficient to restore stability to the anterior column of the spine.

Oda I, Cunningham BW, Lee GA, et al: Biomechanical properties of anterior thoracolumbar multisegmental fixation: An analysis of construct stiffness and screw-rod strain. Spine 2000;25:2303–2311.

A dual-rod configuration results in a more stable construct as compared to a single-rod construct, regardless of rod diameter.

Pitzen T, Geisler FH, Matthis D, et al: Motion of threaded cages in posterior lumbar interbody fusion. Eur Spine J 2000;9:571–576.

Posterior column support through pedicle systems is required to stabilize intervertebral cages.

Polly DW Jr, Cunningham BW, Kuklo TR, et al: Anterior thoracic scoliosis constructs: Effect of rod diameter and intervertebral cages on multi-segmental construct stability. Spine J 2003;3:213–219.

Increasing the rod diameter posteriorly can provide anterior column support mechanically. One must consider the bending moment generation at the rod/screw interface.

Shimamoto N, Kotani Y, Shono Y, et al: Static and dynamic analysis of five anterior instrumentation systems for thoracolumbar scoliosis. Spine 2003;28:1678–1685.

Under cyclic loading, dual-rod systems generate less overall toggle and hence reduced moments at the rod/screw interface. This results in a more stable construct.

Takemura Y, Yamamoto H, Tani T: Biomechanical study of the development of scoliosis, using a thoracolumbar spine model. J Orthop Sci 1999;4:439–445.

Scoliosis can be reproduced in vitro. The most clinically representative model is achieved through rotation followed by flexion and lateral bending.

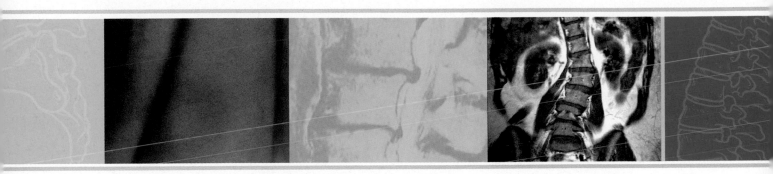

Pediatric Deformity

CHAPTER 6

Infantile and Juvenile Idiopathic Scoliosis

Amer F. Samdani *and* Randal R. Betz

Idiopathic scoliosis is classified according to the age of onset: infantile (0 to 3 years), juvenile (4 to 9 years), and adolescent (10 years to maturity). This categorization was formulated to coincide with periods of increased growth velocity. However, growth velocity is relatively steady during the juvenile period. Therefore, the term *early-onset scoliosis* has been used for children younger than 5 years old. Children who manifest scoliosis prior to the age of 5 years appear to be at highest risk for developing cardiopulmonary problems such as restrictive pulmonary disease, hypertension, or cor pulmonale. In this chapter, we discuss the epidemiology, clinical features, and management of infantile and juvenile scoliosis. Treatment of progressive scoliosis in the developing child poses unique challenges. We discuss the latest surgical options, such as stapling and vertical expandable prosthetic titanium rib (VEPTR), for these challenging curves.

INFANTILE IDIOPATHIC SCOLIOSIS

Epidemiology

Infantile idiopathic scoliosis is a structural spinal deformity with apical rotation and wedging that presents in the first 3 years of life. It represents fewer than 1% of all cases of idiopathic scoliosis in the United States and is less common in the United States than in Europe. Males are more commonly affected than females; some authors report a ratio of 3.5 boys to 1 girl. Most curves develop within the first year of life and usually are left sided.

Harenstein first described infantile scoliosis in 1930. In 1954, James and colleagues reported on a series of 212 patients with infantile scoliosis. They noted the preponderance of left-sided thoracic curves. Thirty-three percent of the curves resolved spontaneously. The patients with resolving curves all had onset prior to 1 year of age, and none developed compensatory curves. Higher rates of resolution were reported in the 1960s: Lloyd-Roberts and Picher reported 92 out of 100 patients resolving spontaneously.

Two theories have been proposed to explain the pathogenesis of infantile scoliosis: intrauterine molding and postnatal pressure on the spine from supine positioning. Browne first postulated that intrauterine pressures might mold the spine and result in not only scoliosis but also, ipsilateral to the convexity, plagiocephaly, limited hip abduction, and rib molding. An objection to this theory is that the abnormalities are not present at birth but rather develop over time. Because the incidence of infantile scoliosis is higher in Europe, Mau postulated that postnatal pressure and molding caused by supine positioning might be responsible. This is supported by the association of ipsilateral plagiocephaly, hip flattening, and contractures of the neck and feet in these children. The prone position is associated with sudden infant death syndrome, and more American children are positioned supine, which might increase the incidence of infantile scoliosis.

Clinical Features

The differential diagnosis of an infant who presents with scoliosis includes congenital, neuromuscular (myelomeningocele, muscular dystrophies, intraspinal anomaly), syndromic (neurofibromatosis), and idiopathic scoliosis. The latter is a diagnosis of exclusion. Therefore, a detailed history and physical examination make up a first and essential step to rule out these alternative etiologies. The history should include detailed questions of birth record, achievement of developmental milestones, and relatives with similar conditions.

The physical examination begins with a general assessment of infant health, including height and weight on every visit. Undressing the infant facilitates a thorough examination of the skin for markers such as café au lait spots, sacral dimples, or hairy patches. The former is concerning for neurofibromatosis, and the latter is concerning for an intraspinal anomaly. The infant's shoulders, chest, and pelvis are evaluated for asymmetry. In addition, the presence of plagiocephaly should be noted. This most often occurs ipsilateral to the concavity of the curve. Laying the infant convex side down over the examiner's knee assesses rigidity of the curve.

In addition, the evaluation of extraocular muscle movement is essential; the presence of nystagmus has alerted us to the presence of a Chiari malformation in two patients.

Imaging

The infant who presents with scoliosis should undergo an anteroposterior and lateral full spine radiograph. These images may detect vertebral anomalies and diagnose a congenital basis for the scoliosis. Radiographs that provide suspicion for congenital anomalies require computed tomography with two- and three-dimensional reconstructions to delineate the anatomy. Plain radiographs are adequate for serial documentation of curve progression. These should be performed in the same position during every visit. Infant position during the radiograph should be duly marked (supine, sitting, standing) as this will affect spine curvature. When the child is able to stand, the authors obtain two radiographs: one supine to compare with earlier supine films and one erect to serve as a new baseline. These radiographs should be examined to measure the rib-vertebral angle difference (RVAD) as described by Mehta. She identified the apical vertebrae and measured the angle formed by the rib with a perpendicular line drawn through the inferior end plate (Fig. 6-1). This measurement is taken for both the concave and convex sides. If the difference between the concave and convex sides exceeds 20 degrees, there is a high probability of curve progression.

For double major curves, the RVAD is measured at T12. Furthermore, Mehta classified the rib heads as either phase I or II. In phase I, there is separation of the rib head from the vertebral body, whereas as the curvature progresses, there is overlap of the rib head with the vertebral body on the convex side. Apical vertebrae in phase II implies certain progression. Mehta reported 46 of 86 curves in phase I resolved. In a study by Ferreira and colleagues in 1972, 37 of the 40 curves that progressed had an RVAD greater than 20 degrees.

Every child who presents at or progresses past 20 degrees undergoes a full spine MRI from the posterior fossa (to assess for a Chiari malformation) to the sacrum (to evaluate for a tethered cord). The presence of neural axis abnormalities in scoliotic infants ranges from 20% to 50%. Gupta and colleagues in 1998 reported three of six patients harboring an intraspinal anomaly. Dobbs and colleagues reviewed the records of 46 infants who presented with normal neurologic findings and a curve magnitude greater than 20 degrees. They reported that 10 of these patients (21.7%) harbored an intraspinal anomaly. These included five patients with Arnold-Chiari malformation, three with syringomyelia, one with a low-lying conus, and one with a brain stem tumor. Interestingly, eight of these patients required neurosurgical intervention. Therefore, Dobbs and colleagues advocate a total spine MRI in any infant who presents with a curve greater than 20 degrees. Computed tomography scans with two- and three-dimensional reformats are useful for children under consideration for the VEPTR device. These images are studied

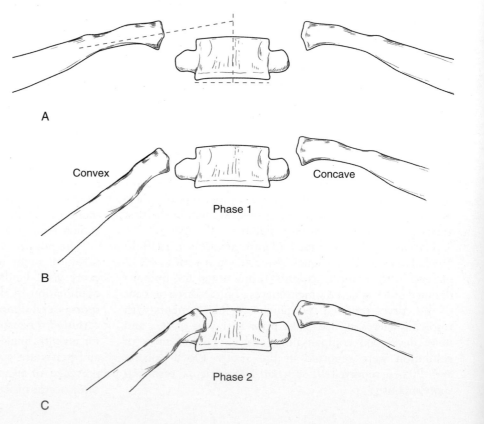

Figure 6-1. The rib-vertebral angle (**A**) is constructed by the intersection of a line perpendicular to the apical vertebral end plate with a line drawn from the midneck to the midhead of the corresponding rib. The rib-vertebral angle difference (RVAD) is the difference between the rib-vertebral angles of the concave and convex ribs of the apical vertebra. In a straight spine, the RVAD is 0. In a scoliotic spine, the convex ribs form a more acute angle with the vertebral body than do the concave ribs, thereby producing an RVAD that is greater than 0. In addition to the RVAD, Mehta described two phases that helped to distinguish between progressive and resolving infantile curves. Phase 1 (**B**) is the early stage of infantile scoliosis in which the convex rib head does not overlap the vertebral body on the posteroanterior radiograph. Phase 2 (**C**) is the next stage of progressive deformity, in which the rib head overlaps the vertebral body on the posteroanterior radiograph.

to evaluate lung volumes and the presence of appropriate attachment sites for the device. The authors believe that most children with infantile scoliosis harbor an underlying syndrome that geneticists have not yet classified.

JUVENILE SCOLIOSIS

Epidemiology

The prevalence of juvenile scoliosis is estimated to be between 8% and 16% of all patients with idiopathic scoliosis. Juvenile idiopathic scoliosis by definition occurs in patients between 4 and 10 years of age. The cause remains elusive; theories include posterior column dysfunction, deficiency of neurotransmitters suggesting a pineal gland abnormality, and genetic, with several authors documenting an increased familial occurrence.

Juvenile idiopathic scoliosis shares similarities with both infantile and adolescent idiopathic scoliosis. Infantile scoliosis is most commonly seen in males and is most often a left spontaneous curve that might resolve. Adolescent scoliosis shows a female predominance with a right thoracic curve that progresses during the adolescent growth spurt. Overall, the juvenile form is more common among girls with a girl:boy ratio ranging from 2:1 to 4:1. However, when one breaks down the juvenile group into ages 3 to 6 years and 6 to 10 years, the results change, the girl:boy ratio in the former being 1:1 and in the latter being 8:1. This might reflect infantile curves that were detected later; thus the male predominance. Furthermore, the younger age group (3 to 6 years) tends to have left thoracic curves, and resolving curves are diagnosed at a younger age.

The curve patterns of juvenile scoliosis resemble those of adolescent patients. The ratio of right thoracic to left thoracic curves is 3:1. Robinson and colleagues described curve patterns in 109 patients with juvenile scoliosis. They reported a right thoracic to left thoracic ratio of 1:1 for patients between 3 and 6 years of age. The ratio of girls to boys was 1:1.6, the boys having a mean age of 5 years and 8 months and the girls having a mean age of 7 years and 2 months. Curve progression was noted in 104 of the 109 patients (95%). They reported follow-up until skeletal maturity in 89 patients, and 77 of these required a spinal arthrodesis. Others have reported a high rate of progression in juvenile scoliosis, although not as high as in the Robinson and colleagues series. Tolo and Gillespie in 1978 found curve progression in 42 of 59 curves (16 required surgery). Mannherz and colleagues found that 26 of 43 progressed, with 13 requiring surgery. Furthermore, Mannherz found left-sided curves to have the highest potential for resolving without treatment (6 of 12). They also reported that if the RVAD improved to 10 degrees or less, there was high probability for curve resolution.

Clinical Features

Juvenile idiopathic scoliosis is a diagnosis of exclusion. A thorough history and physical examination should be per-formed to exclude any underlying reason for the curvature. Questions addressing pain, motor, sensory, urine, and bowel symptoms should be included.

Not only should the physical examination include a thorough examination of the back for deformity, but also note should be made of any cutinized abnormalities, such as a dimple or hairy patch, which could signal an underlying etiology. A complete neurologic examination, including motor nerves, sensory nerves, and reflexes, should be performed. The presence of a spinal syrinx might be suggested by subtle neurologic findings such as asymmetric abdominal reflexes or absent gag reflex.

Imaging

Initial radiographic evaluation includes standing postero-anterior and lateral views of the whole spine. Serial Cobb angle measurements are taken to document curve progression. The Risser sign is usually zero, and bone age radiographs are recommended if there is discrepancy between chronologic age and physical features. Bending radiographs aid in determining effectiveness of brace therapy, and are useful prior to surgical intervention. Mehta's RVAD measurements do not prognosticate progression in juvenile patients as well as in infantile patients. However, the RVAD is useful in predicting response to brace treatment. Risk factors for progression include thoracic hypokyphosis (less than 20 degrees) and curves greater than 45 degrees at presentation. Similar to infantile scoliosis, the high incidence of neural axis abnormalities in this age group warrants an MRI of the entire neural axis. Gupta and colleagues reported on 34 patients between 0 and 10 years of age with curves greater than 20 degrees and without neurologic findings and reported an incidence of 17.6%.

TREATMENT OPTIONS

Progressive scoliosis in the developing spine poses unique management challenges. The importance of maintaining, if not correcting, the scoliosis is vital to prevent cardiopulmonary compromise. Furthermore, traditional treatments such as casting, bracing, and spinal fusion may have negative effects on the growing spine and chest cavity. The crankshaft phenomenon is well described in skeletally immature patients who undergo posterior spinal fusion. The latest treatment strategies, such as vertebral body stapling and the VEPTR, attempt fusionless curve control.

Nonsurgical Treatment

According to the criteria set forth by Mehta, curves with Cobb angles less than 25 degrees and an RVAD less than 20 degrees are at low risk for progression. These patients can be followed closely with serial radiographs every 4 to 6 months. Long-term follow-up of patients with resolving scoliosis demonstrates that there was no advantage of plaster casting over physiotherapy with regard to functional outcome. Even after curve resolution, the patient should be followed every 1 to 2 years until skeletal maturity. Patients with progressive scoliosis or curves greater than 25 degrees on initial presentation warrant immediate treatment. Progression is indicated by an increase in the Cobb angle or RVAD of 5 to 10 degrees.

The main nonsurgical treatment options include casting and bracing. Casting is performed under general anesthesia and in successive stages. With the child on a Cotrel frame, the spine is gently corrected, and the plaster of Paris jacket is applied over two layers of stockinet. The plaster is then contoured over the rib hump to help flatten it. The jackets are changed at intervals of 6 to 12 weeks. Once the spine has attained adequate correction, the child is transitioned to a removable brace. The brace is removed once the spine remains straight for 6 months. Patients should be followed until skeletal maturity. Mehta reported on 136 patients with progressive infantile scoliosis who were treated with casting. Patients who were referred early (mean age of 1 year and 7 months) with smaller curves (mean Cobb angle of 32 degrees) had the best prognosis for resolving their scoliosis.

Bracing remains a mainstay of conservative treatment of scoliosis, although its efficacy has not been demonstrated definitively in a prospective or randomized study. In a meta-analysis of 1910 patients with idiopathic scoliosis, Rowe and colleagues found a success rate of 60% for bracing in the juvenile population. Others report lower success rates. Brace wear is often necessary for 16 to 23 hours per day over a span of 5 years. Studies show decreased quality of life and self-esteem in braced patients, and brace compliance is poor.

Surgical Treatment

Fusion

Many surgical procedures have been developed to control curve progression in the skeletally immature spine. The general principle of earlier procedures was that a short, straight spine is better than a long, curved one. The crankshaft phenomenon occurs when a developing spine undergoes a posterior-only fusion. The anterior spinal column continues to grow in spite of the posterior tether, resulting in marked vertebral rotation. A combined anterior/posterior procedure is necessary to prevent the crankshaft phenomenon. However, this approach entails negative effects on the developing thorax and lungs. Open triradiate cartilages appear to be a good indictor of which patients will develop the crankshaft phenomenon and therefore should undergo anterior growth arrest.

Convex epiphysiodesis is based on the principle that spinal deformity results from overgrowth on the convex side of the spine. In 1963, Roaf reported on convex spinal epiphysiodesis. Although 23% of his patients demonstrated significant improvement, 40% remained essentially unchanged. Marks and colleagues recently published a report substantiating the limited effectiveness of both anterior and posterior convex epiphysiodesis.

Owing to the inherent problems of fusing the immature spine, including creating a short trunk, several techniques to accomplish nonfusion stabilization have been developed. The main goals of these techniques include obtaining control of curve progression with some initial correction while preserving spinal growth.

Growing Rods

Harrington first described the single-rod instrumentation technique in 1962. Harrington used a subperiosteal approach and placed a single distraction rod connected to hooks at the distal ends. Moe modified Harrington's technique in several ways. The subperiosteal exposure was limited to the areas of hook placement, and these sites were not fused. Patients wore a Milwaukee brace postoperatively, and patients underwent expansion when greater than 10 degrees of loss of correction occurred. Reported complications, including hook dislodgement and rod breakage, occurred in 50% of patients. In 1997, Klemme and colleagues reported on their 20-year experience using the Moe technique. Sixty-seven patients underwent an average of 6.1 procedures. The average curve reduction was 30%, and in 44 of the 67 patients, the curve stabilized. Blakemore and colleagues modified the technique by placing the rod submuscularly to allow for better contour and alignment without causing unintended fusion. In addition, they performed an apical fusion in patients with stiff curves and those with curves over 70 degrees. Curves improved from a mean Cobb angle of 66 degrees to 38 degrees. Complications occurred in 24% of the patients.

Akbarnia and Marks developed the dual-rod technique to improve on hardware-related complications. In this technique, subperiosteal dissection is limited to the upper and lower anchor sites. Hooks and screws are used in a clawlike configuration and may be fused with bone graft. The rod is placed subcutaneously and joined on each side with tandem connectors. Patients are braced until final fusion occurs. Lengthenings are done at approximately 6-month intervals. Thompson and colleagues compared the dual-rod technique with the single-rod technique in a retrospective comparison and found that the dual-rod systems produced better initial correction and allowed more growth. However, the overall complication rate appeared similar (48%).

Stapling

Long bone stapling across the physis is used to treat limb discrepancy in young children. In 1951, Nachlas and Borden tested vertebral body stapling in a canine model of scoliosis. They demonstrated either stabilization or improvement in many of the animals. Some staples failed because they spanned three vertebrae. In 1954, Smith and colleagues reported on the use of stapling for congenital scoliosis. The early results were disappointing, as many of the children had little growth remaining and the curves were severe with severe rotation. Some staples loosened and broke, decreasing the enthusiasm for this procedure.

Braun and colleagues tested a newly developed Nitinol staple in a goat scoliosis model. This staple has been developed by Medtronic Sofamor Danek (Memphis, TN). These staples conform to a "C" shape when at body temperature, providing stronger fixation. Nitinol is a shape memory metal alloy of 50% nickel and 50% titanium. Injury to surrounding tissues has not been observed in human experience in cervical spine fusions. Implant studies in animals have shown only minimal elevation in tissue that is in contact with the metal, and titanium is considered a safe implant material. Nickel allergy occurs in a very small percentage of the population and is not expected to occur through the use of this staple. The U.S. Food and Drug Administration has approved this staple for use in the anterior spine as a vertebral body staple, along with the more traditional usage in hand and foot osteotomies.

The surgical procedure can be performed by a spine surgeon who is familiar with thoracoscopy or in collaboration with a general surgeon. This would be a clinician-directed application, or so-called off-label use, of an FDA-approved device. The patient is positioned with the side of the convex curve facing up. A double-lumen endotracheal tube is inserted so that the convex lung can be collapsed. Fluoroscopic imaging is used to confirm levels. All the vertebrae in the Cobb undergo stapling. If thoracoscopy is being utilized, small portal incisions are made; otherwise, two mini-thoracotomy incisions (less than 5 cm) are used. A trial inserter is used to measure the dimensions of the staple. The smallest staple that spans the disc space is used. Maximum correction occurs in the operating room through proper positioning and by pushing with the staple trial instrument. The patients do not wear a brace postoperatively and have no activity restrictions. Betz and colleagues recently reported on 39 patients who underwent vertebral body stapling of 52 curves. Progression was defined as loss of correction greater than 10 degrees. For the group of patients under age 8 years with less than 50-degree curves and at least 1 year follow-up, curve stability was attained in 87%. One patient (2.6%) experienced a major complication of developing a diaphragmatic hernia, and minor complications occurred in five patients (13%). In this report, four patients had curves greater than 50 degrees, and three failed. Therefore, our current recommendations are vertebral stapling for immature patients (Risser 2 or less) with curves between 20 and 45 degrees. Curves less than 25 degrees are considered if they have shown 5 degrees of progression. These results are encouraging, but a randomized, prospective study is needed to establish the efficacy and indications of vertebral body stapling in juvenile idiopathic scoliosis.

Vertical Expandable Prosthetic Titanium Rib

The spine, lungs, and chest grow interdependently. In progressive early-onset scoliosis, the rib and chest wall deformities can be severe. Decreased pulmonary function in the patients who require early fusion is well documented. Campbell and colleagues developed the vertical expandable prosthetic titanium rib (VEPTR) to address both spine and chest wall deformity with the need for a fusion. The original indication for this device was for the treatment of thoracic insufficiency syndrome, which is defined as the inability of the thorax to support normal respiration and growth. This is diagnosed by a history of respiratory difficulties, on physical examination by lack of motion as demonstrated by the thumb excursion test, and radiographically by a restricted hemithorax. The major categories of this syndrome include flail chest, rib fusion and scoliosis, and hypoplastic thorax syndrome as seen in Jeune's and Jarcho-Levin syndromes. The VEPTR device does not involve spinal arthrodesis but rather an opening wedge thoracostomy and implantation. The device can be attached rib to rib, rib to spine, or rib to pelvis, depending on the individual patient. After initial implantation and correction, the patient undergoes serial lengthenings every 4 to 6 months. Once the original device has been maximized (after approximately 6 to 8 lengthenings), the device is exchanged out. In patients with congenital scoliosis and fused ribs, the longitudinal growth of the thoracic spine after VEPTR was 7.1 mm per year, compared with a normal of 6 mm per year. Both the concave and convex sides of the spine showed growth, as did the unilateral unsegmented bar.

In 2006, the FDA expanded the uses of the VEPTR device to include children with infantile and juvenile scoliosis with constrictive chest walls. We have attained good success in treating over 30 such infants with the VEPTR device. The majority of the correction is attained at the time of the initial surgery. Patients return every 4 to 6 months for routine lengthening procedures. The most common complications are seen in children with low body mass in whom the hardware is prominent. This can result in skin breakdown. This issue is avoided by performing a meticulous, multilayer closure.

PEARLS & PITFALLS

- A detailed neurologic examination is mandatory, as subtle findings such as loss of abdominal reflexes might be the only indication of an underlying anomaly.
- When obtaining the history, the clinician should ask about previous operations on the chest, as these patients are at higher risk for progression and less responsive to brace treatment.

Illustrative Case Presentations

CASE 1. A 10-Year-Old Boy with Right Thoracic Curve

A 10-year-old boy presented to our institution with a 35-degree right thoracic curve (Fig. 6-2). Radiographically, his triradiates were open, and he was a Risser 0. Neurologic examination was nonfocal. MRI scan revealed no abnormalities. Initially, the patient was placed in a thoracolumbosacral orthosis and was followed with serial radiographs. His radiographs at 1 year showed progression to 42 degrees. Therefore, after a lengthy discussion with the family concerning the various options, including continued observation in the brace, the patient underwent a vertebral body stapling of T6 through L1. He tolerated the procedure well and was placed in a brace for 1 month postoperatively, after which we imposed no limitations on his physical activity. Currently, he is 2 years post–vertebral body stapling and is actively participating in sports. His curve has stabilized at 28 degrees.

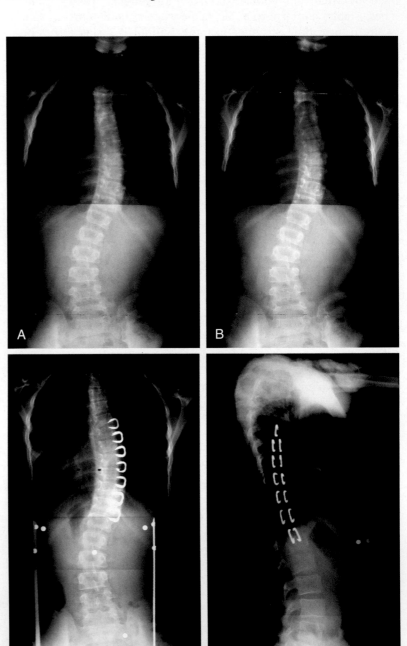

Figure 6-2. A, Anteroposterior spine radiograph at 10 years of age demonstrating a 35-degree right thoracic curve. The patient was prescribed a brace and was followed with serial radiographs. **B,** Anteroposterior spine film at 11 years of age demonstrating progression to 42 degrees. At this point, the patient's family elected vertebral body stapling. **C** and **D,** Anteroposterior and lateral films taken 2 years after the stapling procedure demonstrating the maintenance of 28 degrees of curvature.

CASE 2. A 2-Year-Old Boy with Generalized Hypotonia and Progressive Scoliosis

N.R. is a 2-year-old boy with the diagnosis of generalized hypotonia and a progressive scoliosis (Fig. 6-3). He presented to us with a 93-degree thoracic curve, which had progressed from 64 degrees. The patient underwent placement of bilateral T2 to T3 to the pelvis VEPTR devices. His postoperative radiographs demonstrated a correction to 50 degrees. He will undergo repeated expansions of his VEPTR devices every 4 to 6 months to allow continued spinal growth. These procedures are done through small incisions and usually require a one-night stay in the hospital. Once maximal lengthening has been obtained on the VEPTR devices, they will be exchanged, allowing another series of lengthenings.

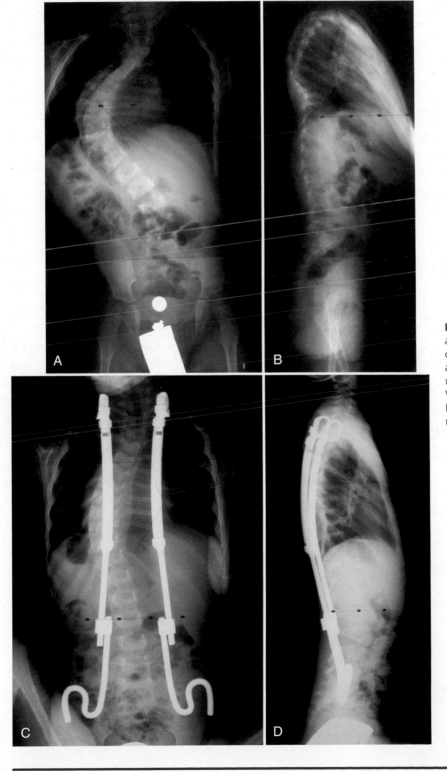

Figure 6-3. A and **B,** Preoperative anteroposterior and lateral radiographs demonstrating a 93-degree curvature in a 2-year-old boy. **C** and **D,** Postoperative anteroposterior and lateral films. The patient underwent placement of bilateral T2 to T3 to pelvis VEPTR devices. His curve now measures 50 degrees. He will undergo expansion procedures every 4 to 6 months to allow continued spinal growth.

REFERENCES

Browne D: Infantile scoliosis. Clin Proc Child Hosp Dist Columbia 1969;25:157–177.

Climent JM, Sanchez J: Impact of the type of brace on the quality of life of adolescents with spine deformities. Spine 1999;24:1903–1908.

Ferreira JH, de Janeiro R, James JI: Progressive and resolving infantile idiopathic scoliosis: The differential diagnosis. J Bone Joint Surg Br 1972;54:648–655.

Harrenstein R: Die Skoliose bei Sauglingen und ihre Behandlung. Z Orthop Chir 1930;52:1–40.

Harrington PR: Treatment of scoliosis: Correction and internal fixation by spine instrumentation. J Bone Joint Surg Am 1962;44-A: 591–610.

Lloyd-Roberts GC, Pilcher MF: Structural idiopathic scoliosis in infancy: A study of the natural history of 100 patients. J Bone Joint Surg Br 1965;47:520–523.

Mau H: Etiology of idiopathic infantile scoliosis. Reconstr Surg Traumatol 1972;13:184–190.

Nachlas IW, Borden JN: The cure of experimental scoliosis by directed growth control. J Bone Joint Surg Am 1951;33:24–34.

Roaf R: The treatment of progressive scoliosis by unilateral growth-arrest. J Bone Joint Surg Br 1963;45:637–651.

Smith AD, Von Lackum WH, Wylie R: An operation for stapling vertebral bodies in congenital scoliosis. J Bone Joint Surg Am 1954; 36:342–348.

Tolo VT, Gillespie R: The characteristics of juvenile idiopathic scoliosis and results of its treatment. J Bone Joint Surg Br 1978;60-B: 181–188.

SUGGESTED READINGS

Akbarnia BA, Marks DS, Boachie-Adjei O, et al: Dual growing rod technique for the treatment of progressive early-onset scoliosis: A multicenter study. Spine 2005;30:S46–S57.

A retrospective review of 23 children who underwent the dual-rod technique to control progressive scoliosis. The authors document the safety and efficacy of this technique.

Betz RR, D'Andrea LP, Mulcahey MJ, Chafetz RS: Vertebral body stapling procedure for the treatment of scoliosis in the growing child. Clin Orthop Relat Res 2005;434:55–60.

The authors describe their experience in 39 patients with scoliosis who were treated with vertebral body stapling. Eighty-seven percent of the curves were well controlled.

Blakemore LC, Scoles PV, Poe-Kochert C, Thompson GH: Submuscular Isola rod with or without limited apical fusion in the management of severe spinal deformities in young children: Preliminary report. Spine 2001;26:2044–2048.

A retrospective review of 29 young children treated with a submuscular growing rod with or without apical fusion. The authors conclude that this is a worthwhile technique in children who do not tolerate orthotic treatment.

Braun JT, Ogilvie JW, Akyuz E, et al: Fusionless scoliosis correction using a shape memory alloy staple in the anterior thoracic spine of the immature goat. Spine 2004;29:1980–1989.

The authors report excellent results using a shape memory alloy staple in treatment of experimental scoliosis in a goat model.

Campbell RM Jr, Hell-Vocke AK: Growth of the thoracic spine in congenital scoliosis after expansion thoracoplasty. J Bone Joint Surg Am 2003;85-A:409–420.

The authors report on 21 patients with congenital scoliosis treated with expansion thoracoplasty and VEPTR. They report the continued growth of the spine in these patients.

Dobbs MB, Lenke LG, Szymanski DA, et al: Prevalence of neural axis abnormalities in patients with infantile idiopathic scoliosis. J Bone Joint Surg Am 2002;84-A:2230–2234.

The authors describe the largest series of patients with infantile scoliosis who were evaluated with a spine MRI. Ten of 46 patients harbored an intraspinal anomaly.

Gupta P, Lenke LG, Bridwell KH: Incidence of neural axis abnormalities in infantile and juvenile patients with spinal deformity: Is a magnetic resonance image screening necessary? Spine 1998;23:206–210.

The authors report a combined prospective and retrospective review of patients with infantile and juvenile scoliosis. They conclude that a total spine MRI is indicated in these patients because of the high incidence of neural axis abnormalities.

James JI: Idiopathic scoliosis: The prognosis, diagnosis, and operative indications related to curve patterns and the age at onset. J Bone Joint Surg Br 1954;36-B:36–49.

An early review of curve patterns and natural history of 212 patients with scoliosis.

Klemme WR, Denis F, Winter RB, et al: Spinal instrumentation without fusion for progressive scoliosis in young children. J Pediatr Orthop 1997;17:734–742.

The authors describe a mixed group of 67 patients with progressive scoliosis who were managed with spinal instrumentation without fusion.

Mannherz RE, Betz RR, Clancy M, Steel HH: Juvenile idiopathic scoliosis followed to skeletal maturity. Spine 1988;13:1087–1090.

The authors reviewed 43 patients with juvenile scoliosis who were followed to skeletal maturity. The authors describe the natural history, effects of bracing, and risk factors for progression.

Marks DS, Iqbal MJ, Thompson AG, Piggott H: Convex spinal epiphysiodesis in the management of progressive infantile idiopathic scoliosis. Spine 1996;21:1884–1888.

A retrospective review of 22 patients with infantile scoliosis who underwent anterior and posterior convex spinal epiphysiodesis. The authors conclude that this procedure does not prevent progression in patients with infantile idiopathic scoliosis.

Mehta MH: Growth as a corrective force in the early treatment of progressive infantile scoliosis. J Bone Joint Surg Br 2005;87: 1237–1247.

The author reviews the results of serial plastic jacket applications in 136 patients with infantile scoliosis.

Mehta MH: The rib-vertebra angle in the early diagnosis between resolving and progressive infantile scoliosis. J Bone Joint Surg Br 1972;54:230–243.

Mehta's original description of the RVAD and its prognostic value in determining resolving and progressive infantile scoliosis.

Robinson CM, McMaster MJ: Juvenile idiopathic scoliosis: Curve patterns and prognosis in one hundred and nine patients. J Bone Joint Surg Am 1996;78:1140–1148.

The authors describe the major curve patterns observed in 109 patients with juvenile scoliosis.

Rowe DE, Bernstein SM, Riddick MF, et al: A meta-analysis of the efficacy of non-operative treatments for idiopathic scoliosis. J Bone Joint Surg Am 1997;79:664–674.

A meta analysis of 1910 patients with idiopathic scoliosis who were managed with either bracing, electrical stimulation, or observation. In this study, the 23 hours a day bracing regimen was most successful.

Thompson GH, Akbarnia BA, Kostial P, et al: Comparison of single and dual growing rod techniques followed through definitive surgery: A preliminary study. Spine 2005;30:2039–2044.

The authors conducted a retrospective study of 28 patients who underwent placement of growing rods. The authors concluded that dual rods provided better initial correction and maintenance of the correction than did single rods.

CHAPTER 7

Adolescent Idiopathic Scoliosis

Fernando E. Silva *and* Lawrence G. Lenke

OVERVIEW

Idiopathic scoliosis exists in three forms: infantile, juvenile, and adolescent. Our focus is on idiopathic scoliosis in adolescence, which includes the ages between 10 and 18 years. Adolescent idiopathic scoliosis (AIS) is a diagnosis of exclusion, and its radiographic diagnosis necessitates measuring a coronal plane angle, using the Cobb method, of 10 degrees or more.

The prevalence of 10-degree curves in adolescent patients is 2% to 3%. This prevalence decreases as a function of curve magnitude to about 0.3% to 0.5% and 0.1% in curves measuring 20 degrees and 40 degrees, respectively. Furthermore, although the overall prevalence is equal between genders, the prevalence is higher among females when curves greater than 10 degrees are considered, with a 4:1 ratio of females to males.

Several studies have looked at different factors as possible etiologies of AIS. Neurologic anomalies ranging from dysfunction in proprioception to maldevelopment in central pattern generators in spinal cord have been implicated. Disorders of connective tissue, hormonal factors including melatonin, and muscle structural changes have been investigated as possible causes. From a biomechanical standpoint, AIS could theoretically occur as a critical buckling load (F) is reached during a patient's growth spurt. Such a critical buckling load can occur as the spine lengthens during a growth spurt and is defined by Euler's formula: $F = EI\,\pi^2/L^2$, where E and I are material and property constants, respectively, and L is the column's length, in this case the patient's precipitous increase in height. However, the etiology of AIS remains elusive.

In contrast, it appears clear that AIS has a hereditary basis. The incidence is 11% in first-degree relatives, 2.4% in second-degree relatives, and 1.4% in third-degree relatives. Additionally, concordance among monozygotic and dizygotic twins is 73% and 36%, respectively. However, heredity is not a factor as a prognosticator for curve progression, although genetic modifiers that play a role in curve progression might be identified in the future; if they are, they will be useful in determining optimal timing for brace treatment or surgery.

EVALUATION

Assessment of AIS begins with history taking, including any associated symptoms such as pain and weakness. The patient is also asked about how she or he perceives her or his appearance as related to the deformity. Following a general medical history, inquiry into how the curve was detected and any treatment to date is undertaken. It is imperative to obtain a family history of scoliosis. The patient should also be asked about age of menarche, voice changes in males, and any growth spurts that have been noted in both genders. Neurologic complaints such as weakness and clumsiness demand further workup, as do left-sided curves. The ultimate diagnosis of AIS, again, is that of exclusion. Hence, other possible causes of scoliosis must be discounted, such as congenital, neuromuscular, and syndromic types.

The oral cavity is examined for any palatal anomalies, a high-arched palate being associated with Marfan syndrome. The integument is evaluated for café au lait spots, and any dimples and/or hair patches over the lumbodorsal spine are noted. Limb laxity is evaluated, and if it is present, further genetic counseling or testing is requested. With the patient standing and her or his hips and knees fully extended, the relationship of the patient's head to the pelvis from a coronal and sagittal profile is evaluated, and any trunk shift is noted. Shoulder, breast, and pelvic asymmetry are noted. An Adams forward-bending test is performed to get a clinical sense of curve rotation, and this is further quantified with the aid of a scoliometer. A neurologic examination, including all cranial nerves, with emphasis on motor strength, reflexes, including abdominal reflexes, sensory modalities, and gait, is carried out. With the patient supine, limbs are measured if a leg-length discrepancy is suspected, especially if pelvic obliquity is suspected or present. If the leg-length discrepancy is the possible culprit, the patient is reevaluated with an appropriate-height shoe lift.

Radiographic evaluation entails erect posterior anterior and lateral 36- × 14-inch long-cassette views, including bending films for further curve classification and planning surgical intervention. Unusual curves and salient neurologic findings also demand total-spine magnetic resonance imaging. Neurosurgical consultation is requested if any anomalies of the neural elements are evident clinically and/or from magnetic resonance imaging.

CLASSIFICATION

In 1983, King and colleagues analyzed a series of 409 patients with AIS. Their work led to the first treatment-based AIS classification (Fig. 7-1). It also further developed the important concept of selectively fusing only the thoracic curve in King II curves (double thoracic and lumbar curvature with larger or stiffer thoracic curve). The deficiency in this classification system is that it included only thoracic curves, analyzing them only in the coronal plane. Although its interobserver and intraobserver reliability is fair at best, it has remained the gold standard for 20 years.

In 2001, Lenke and colleagues published a new, more comprehensive AIS classification system. This treatment-based classification not only encompasses thoracic curves but also includes thoracolumbar/lumbar curves. Additionally, it is biplanar, as it assesses curves in both the coronal and sagittal planes. This practical and easy-to-use system is reliable in terms of interobserver and intraobserver reliability. Its definition of the structural characteristics of a proximal thoracic (PT) curve has been deemed reliable, leading to shorter proximal fusions when the curve is not considered structural. Furthermore, it allows a stricter curve evaluation, permitting a more objective analysis of when a given curve pattern will tolerate a selective fusion that will lead to a balanced outcome to avoid postoperative decompensation.

The three-tiered classification of Lenke and coworkers combines a curve type (1 through 6) and lumbar and sagittal modifiers to produce a complete curve classification (e.g., 1A−) (Table 7-1). First, a curve type, 1 through 6, is determined following assessment of the upright coronal, lateral, and side-bending radiographs (Figs. 7-2 and 7-3). The main thoracic (MT) or thoracolumbar/lumbar (T/TL) regions are designated either as the major curve (largest Cobb measurement) or as a minor structural or

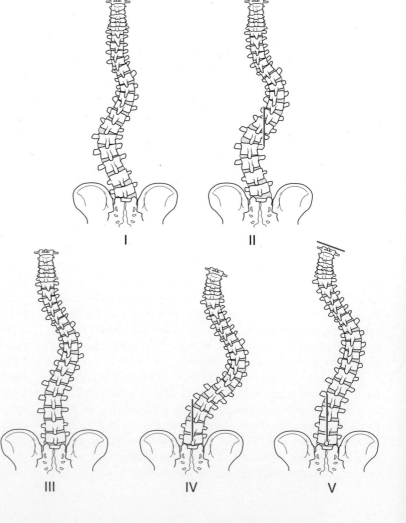

Figure 7-1. The King-Moe classification scheme. **I,** Lumbar > thoracic (both cross midline). **II,** Thoracic > lumbar (both cross midline). **III,** Thoracic only. **IV,** Thoracic only (L4 tilted into curve). **V,** Double thoracic (+ T1 tilt).

TABLE 7-1. Lenke Classification Scheme

THE LENKE CLASSIFICATION SYSTEM FOR AIS

Curve Type	Proximal Thoracic	Main Thoracic	Thoracolumbar/Lumbar	Description
1	Nonstructural	Structural*	Nonstructural	Main Thoracic (MT)
2	Structural	Structural*	Nonstructural	Double Thoracic (DT)
3	Nonstructural	Structural*	Structural	Double Major (DM)
4	Structural	Structural§	Structural§	Triple Major (TM)
5	Nonstructural	Nonstructural	Structural*	Thoracolumbar/Lumbar (TL/L)
6	Nonstructural	Structural	Structural*	Thoracolumbar/Lumbar-Main Thoracic (TL/L-MT)

*Major = Largest Cobb measure, always structural; Minor = All other curves with structural criteria applied; §Type4 - MT or TL/L can be the major curve

STRUCTURAL CRITERIA
(Minor Curves)

Proximal Thoracic - Side Bending Cobb ≥ 25°
- T2-T5 Kyphosis ≥ +20°

Main Thoracic - Side Bending Cobb ≥ 25°
- T10-L2 Kyphosis ≥ +20°

Thoracolumbar/Lumbar - Side Bending Cobb ≥ 25°
- T10-L2 Kyphosis ≥ +20°

LOCATION OF APEX
(SRS Definition)

CURVE	APEX
Thoracic	T2 -T11-12 Disc
Thoracolumbar	T12 - L1
Lumbar	L1-2 Disc - L4

MODIFIERS

Lumbar Spine Modifier	Center Sacral Vertical Line to Lumbar Apex
A	CSVL between pedicles
B	CSVL touches apical body(ies)
C	CSVL completely medial

Thoracic Sagittal Profile T5 - T12	
Modifier	**Cobb Angle**
− (Hypo)	< 10°
N (Normal)	10° - 40°
+ (Hyper)	> 40°

Curve Type (1-6) + Lumbar Spine Modifier (**A, B, C,**) + Thoracic Sagittal Modifier (−, N, +) = Curve Classification (e.g. **1B+**): _____

From Lenke LG, Betz RR, Harms J, et al: Adolescent idiopathic scoliosis: A new classification to determine extent of spinal arthrodesis. J Bone Joint Surg Am 2001;83:1169–1181. Reprinted with permission from The Journal of Bone and Joint Surgery, Inc.

nonstructural curve. The PT curve is always a minor curve, but whether it is structural or not must be determined. A minor curve is structural if on side bending, it remains 25 degrees or more. Hyperkyphosis in the PT region (T2 to T5 ≥ +20 degrees) or thoracolumbar junction (T10 to L2 ≥ +20 degrees) makes curves in this area structural regardless of the side-bending Cobb measurement. Thus, a schema of six curve types is created on the basis of whether the MT or TL/L regions are the major curves and whether the remaining two regions are minor structural or nonstructural curves (see Fig. 7-2B).

Next, a lumbar spine modifier—A, B, or C—is assigned on the basis of the position of the apex of the lumbar spine relative to the center sacral vertical line (CSVL). The CSVL is the vertical line that is drawn parallel to the radiograph edge and perpendicular to the floor from the geometric center of S1 that depicts the coronal position of the lumbar spine in relation to the pelvis. A shoe lift is used if the pelvis has more than 2 cm of obliquity. If the CSVL falls between the pedicles up to the stable vertebra, then the lumbar modifier A is assigned. The stable vertebra is defined as the most cephalad vertebra below the major curve with a centroid most closely bisected by the CSVL. When the CSVL touches the apical pedicle, the lumbar modifier B is assigned. Finally, if the apex of the lumbar spine is completely off the CSVL, then the lumbar modifier C is assigned. Lastly, a sagittal thoracic modifier, "−," "N," or "+," is assigned on the basis of the T5 to T12 thoracic sagittal alignment. When sagittal kyphosis is less than +10 degrees, the "−" or hypokyphotic sagittal modifier is assigned; for +10 to +40 degrees, the "N" or normal modifier is assigned, and for greater than 40 degrees, the "+" or hyperkyphotic modifier is assigned.

A Lenke 1 curve, the most common curve type, is composed of an MT major curve and nonstructural PT and TL/L regions. In a Lenke 2 curve, the major curve remains the MT region, but the PT region becomes structural, while the TL/L region is nonstructural. Besides the aforementioned structural radiographic criteria, a positive clavicle angle (elevation of the left clavicle in a right main

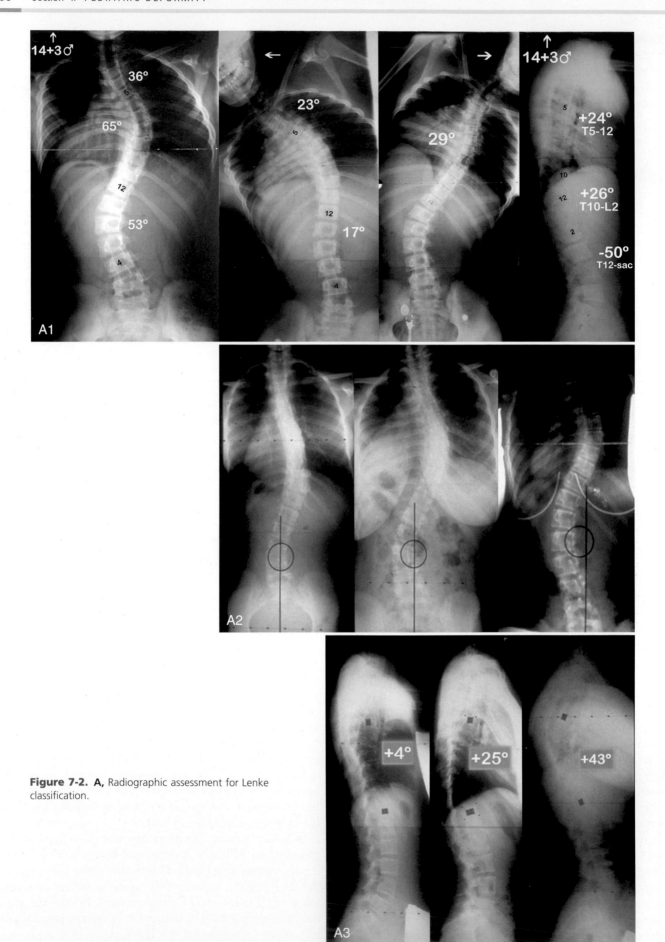

Figure 7-2. A, Radiographic assessment for Lenke classification.

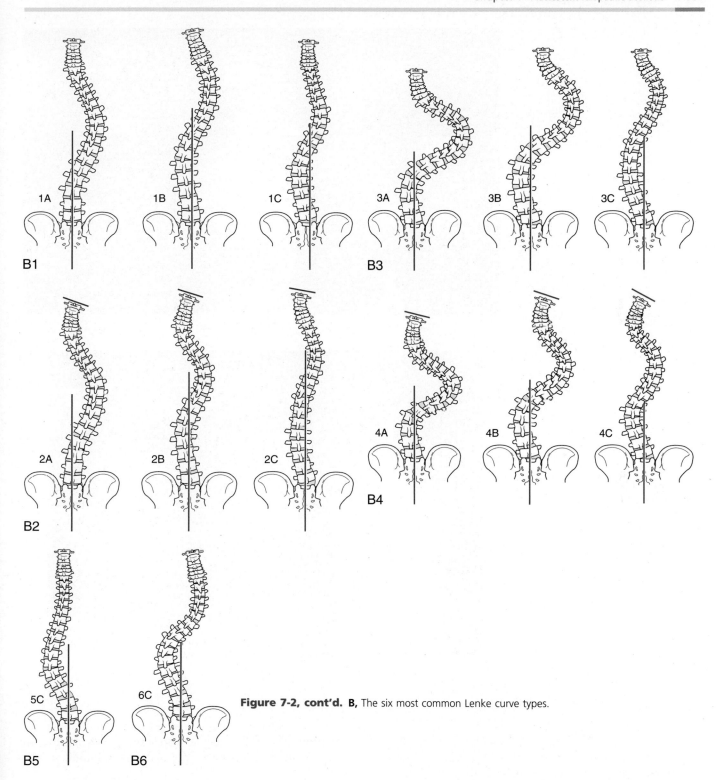

Figure 7-2, cont'd. B, The six most common Lenke curve types.

thoracic, left proximal thoracic curve pattern), and/or left shoulder elevation (for a right MT curve) also potentially renders the PT curve structural. The MT region remains the major curve in Lenke 3 curves, but the TL/L region becomes structural, the PT being nonstructural. The tho-

racic and TL/L curves have similar structural characteristics. But regardless of a TL/L curve's structural criteria on side-bending films, if thoracolumbar junction kyphosis exists (T10 to L2 ≥ 20°), then the curve is considered double major (Fig. 7-4). Although lumbar modifiers A, B,

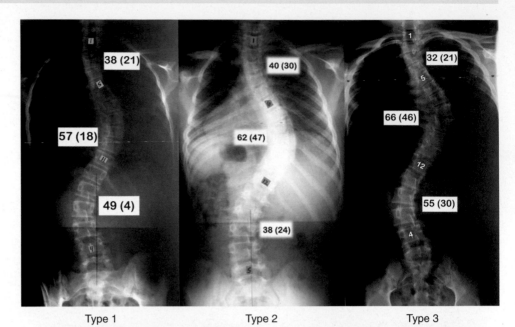

Type 1   Type 2   Type 3

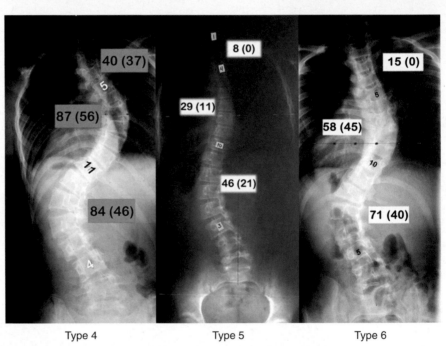

Type 4   Type 5   Type 6

Figure 7-3. Lenke curve types (side-bending Cobb measurements).

or C and sagittal modifiers "–," "N," or "+" can apply to curves 1 to 3, Lenke 3 curves usually have a C lumbar modifier and often a TL/L kyphosis. With Lenke 4 curves, either the MT or the TL/L region is the major curve; however, all three regions are structural in this rare curve type. In accordance with Scoliosis Research Society definitions, a curve is considered thoracolumbar if an apex exists between bodies of T12 and L1 and lumbar if an apex exists between the L1 to L2 disc and the L4 body. In Lenke 5 curves, the major curve is in the TL/L region. Here, the PT and MT regions are nonstructural. In Lenke 6, the major curve is the TL/L region, and the MT region is

structural, the PT being nonstructural. Essentially, all Lenke 5 and 6 curves have a lumbar type C modifier.

TREATMENT OPTIONS

Observation, bracing, and surgery are options in the treatment of AIS. These treatment modalities are based on the natural history of AIS. Curves that are less than 20 degrees at presentation are observed and followed at 4- to 6-month intervals. For 20- to 30-degree curves, bracing is started if there is 5 degrees or more of progression between consecutive visits. In terms of bracing, this is usually instituted

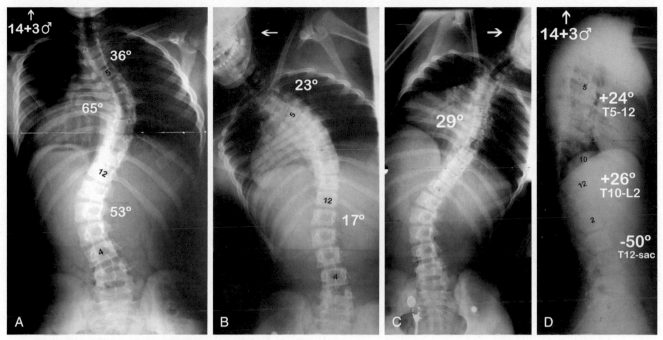

Figure 7-4. A seemingly 1CN curve (**A–C**) that is actually a 3CN curve when the sagittal profile (**D**) is considered.

at the first visit when the patient is skeletally immature (Risser grade 2 or lower) and presents with a 30- to 45-degree curve (Fig. 7-5). Bracing has no role in the skeletally mature patient as an initial mode of treatment. Several brace options exist; deciding which brace to use is a function of the curve's apex. For instance, curves having an apex above T6 would likely require the use of a Milwaukee (cervical thoracolumbosacral orthosis) brace. Conversely, curves with apices below T7 and above L2 do well in a Boston (underarm, thoracolumbosacral orthosis) brace. The latter type is more acceptable to the patient, given the lack of a cervical extension. To be effective, bracing should provide approximately 50% correction at initial fitting and be worn on a full-time basis. Bracing is weaned at skeletal maturity unless the patient's curve progresses while properly braced, at which time the patient likely warrants an operative intervention.

Operative intervention is usually recommended for patients with progressive curves that fail or cannot tolerate bracing as well as those who present with curves that are 45 degrees or more. The classification system of Lenke and coworkers enables the scoliosis surgeon to plan treatment on the basis of the curve types that are generated with this three-tiered system, as previously described.

Lenke Type 1: Main Thoracic Curves

Surgical treatment involves treating only the MT curve posteriorly. All curves can be treated with posterior instrumentation and fusion, regardless of the lumbar and/or sagittal modifier. On the basis of preoperative clinical shoulder balance, fusion levels normally are T3 to T5 proximally, ending distally at one to two levels cephalad to the stable vertebra if the intended lowest instrumented vertebra (LIV) is touched by the CSVL, provided that this is not in the apex of the curve or does not have a significant degree of rotation present (pedicle screws in these situations are required, since maximal apical translation/derotation is essential). With posterior instrumentation, the concave rod is placed first for "–" or "N" sagittal modifiers;

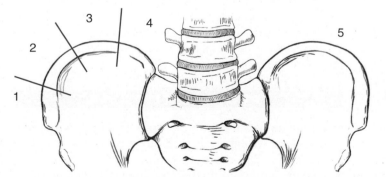

Figure 7-5. The Risser grading system for skeletal maturity.

conversely, the convex rod is placed first for "+" or hyperkyphotic sagittal planes. Corrective maneuvers include a combination of cantilever, rod derotation, in situ contouring, and bilateral apical vertebral derotation—especially in posteriorly fusing proximal to the stable vertebra—and compression/distraction maneuvers. Posterior implants include hooks, wires, or—more commonly utilized at our institution—screws. Anterior surgery may be considered for curves that are associated with normal kyphosis or a hypokyphotic spine. Anterior instrumentation is not recommended in the setting of hyperkyphosis, as this is a kyphogenic construct and will tend to increase kyphosis. This can be performed either thoracoscopically or by open thoracotomy. Anterior release via thoracoscopic or open technique can be utilized as an adjunct to posterior surgery in large, rigid curves.

Lenke Type 2: Double Thoracic Curves

Both the PT and MT curves are addressed posteriorly or circumferentially for double thoracic curves. Correct classification of this curve type is particularly critical so as to render the proper surgical approach without ensuing shoulder malalignment (Fig. 7-6). The instrumentation sequence is a function of each curve's sagittal profile. Proximal instrumentation begins at T2 or T3, according to the size and flexibility of the proximal curve and the preoperative clinical shoulder balance. The LIV is usually one or two levels cephalad to the stable vertebra, but again, with careful analysis, levels proximal to this can be instrumented provided that pedicle screw techniques are used. As with all scoliosis surgery, the goal is coronal and sagittal malalignment correction, leveled shoulders, and a lumbar spine in the best possible position.

Lenke Type 3: Double Major Curves

Although this curve type reveals the least deformity from a clinical standpoint, as both curves tend to offset each other, thoracic and lumbar prominences can be separately noted on the Adams forward-bending test. Both curves require posterior fusion, although a selective thoracic fusion can sometimes be considered on further analysis, as will be discussed later. The thoracic sagittal plane modifier dictates which posterior instrumentation sequence to perform first in the thoracic region.

Lenke Type 4: Triple Major Curves

All three curves require posterior fusion and instrumentation. However, an anterior release and fusion of MT or TL/L may be performed for curves that are greater than 100 degrees, when a curve of more than 80 degrees remains on side bending and with hyperkyphosis in the thoracic and thoracolumbar/lumbar planes. However, with current pedicle screw instrumentation and techniques, this is at times unnecessary. Other authors advocate anterior release

and fusion for curves over 80 degrees when more than 60 degrees remain on side bending.

Lenke Type 5: Thoracolumbar/Lumbar Curves

These curves are usually addressed via an anterior approach to avoid posterior dissection across the TL junction, thus attempting to prevent TL junction kyphosis. Here, the proximal and distal fusion levels are the end vertebrae of the Cobb angle, although bending films can help to determine whether the LIV can be more proximal to the end vertebra of the Cobb if a parallel disc is seen at the lower end of the curve. The latter is accomplished by noting that the vertebra above the parallel disc has less than Nash-Moe grade I rotation. These curve types can also be corrected by using a posterior approach, and the lowest level of instrumentation is usually the lower end vertebra. Posterior correction is usually carried out on the convexity of the curve.

Lenke Type 6: Thoracolumbar/Lumbar– Main Thoracic Curves

Surgical management is similar to that of type 3 curves, with posterior fusion and instrumentation of both the MT and TL/L regions. Anterior release is sometimes necessary for the TL/L component on the basis of the curve magnitude, kyphosis, or curve rigidity. Also, as with type 3 curves, selective fusion of the major TL/L curve can occasionally be considered.

SUMMARY

The etiology of AIS remains unclear, as its diagnosis of exclusion implies. Once it has been diagnosed, follow-up with possible bracing or surgical intervention might be warranted. Proper curve classification is imperative for proper surgical management. Anterior and posterior approaches can be appropriate, and although all curves can be approached posteriorly, we employ an anterior approach in selected Lenke 1A– and Lenke 6CN curves and almost always in Lenke 5CN curves. We also predicate that a selective fusion be carried out whenever possible; hence, curve analysis should be carried out from this perspective. Caring for this group of deformity patients is a very satisfactory undertaking, and when the aforementioned principles are employed, some of the shortcomings of scoliosis surgery, such as decompensation and adding on of a fused curve, can be avoided.

PEARLS & PITFALLS

- Fusion levels are key for preventing decompensation, as fusing the wrong levels is among the culprits of a postoperatively decompensated spine.
- The magnitudes of the rib and lumbar humps are both important during the clinical analysis and decision

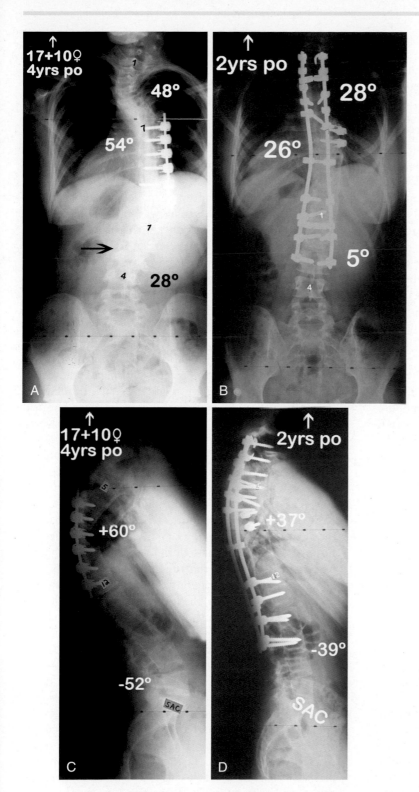

Figure 7-6. A patient with a Lenke 2 curve who initially underwent an anterior approach and required a posterior revision, including vertebral resection. **A,** After a T7-12 ASF, the patient had proximal thoracic and lumbar curve progression. **B,** A postoperative AP radiograph shows improved curves in all three regions of the spine. **C,** A preoperative lateral radiograph demonstrates thoracic hyperkyphosis. **D,** A postoperative lateral radiograph shows normalization of the thoracic kyphosis after the T9 posterior vertebral resection.

making for selective fusion. For example, is the patient willing to accept a moderate lumbar hump when contemplating a selective thoracic fusion and vice versa?

- Do not overlook the thoracolumbar sagittal profile, as this can lead to curve misclassification and incorrect operative management (see Fig. 7-4).
- Paying attention to the shoulders on clinical examination and preoperative radiographs is critical in choosing proximal fusion levels, so as to optimize postoperative shoulder balance and not miss appropriate assessment of a proximal thoracic curve, which might need to be included in the instrumented fusion. The extent of the proximal arthrodesis is based on the clinical assessment of whether or not the shoulders are leveled as well as the size and structural character of the proximal thoracic curve. If the proximal thoracic curve is structural, start

at T2 if the shoulder opposite the major curve is elevated or elevates on push-prone films; start at T3 if the shoulders are balanced; and start at T4 if the contralateral shoulder is depressed. If the proximal thoracic curve is nonstructural, start at a vertebra that is one or two levels above the upper end vertebra of the Cobb angle of the MT; if the shoulders are balanced, start at a vertebra that is one level above the upper end vertebra; if the shoulder opposite the major curve is depressed, start at the upper end vertebra. The upper end vertebra in the MT varies from T4 to T7. Again, if the proximal thoracic curve is hyperkyphotic, it is included in the instrumented fusion regardless of shoulder balance or structural characteristics on posteroanterior bending films.

- Distal fusion levels are essentially based on the relationship between the end, neutral, and stable vertebrae of the distal structural curve to be fused. However, current correction techniques employing pedicular fixation and derotation maneuvers often allow for distal fusion levels to be saved by fusing one or two levels proximal to the stable vertebra.

- In placing thoracic screws, it is essential to follow sequential steps at every screw placement. With small pedicles, take time to expand the pedicle to accommodate a screw. Although we advocate the use of pedicle screws whenever possible, it is imperative, in employing hook/rod segmental instrumentation, to reverse the hook orientation where the discs reverse in orientation, to maintain coronal and sagittal balance. If an all-screw construct is used, the previous principle remains; however, compression forces are used at the endmost part of the construct. In fusing to a vertebra that is proximal to the stable vertebra, this LIV must be touching the CSVL and not have a significant rotation (Nash-Moe grade ≤ 1.5), and the disc below this proximal vertebra must be parallel or closed on the convexity. On the basis of the lumbar modifier, attention must be paid to the degree of tilt left on the LIV in carrying out selective fusions, as will be discussed later.

- As was noted earlier, Lenke 1 curves can be addressed via an anterior approach, but the posterior approach is especially useful with hyperkyphotic curves, in large patients, and when questionable pulmonary function exists. However, curves with Cobb measurements between 40 and 70 degrees, especially those that have a "−" or a hypokyphotic sagittal modifier, and those in the skeletally immature may be treated with endoscopic or open anterior instrumentation and fusion. Rarely, extremely large and/or stiff curves and/or those with severe sagittal plane malalignment may be treated with open or endoscopic releases followed by posterior instrumentation and fusion. However, our trend is to treat these curves via posterior-only techniques.

- In Lenke 2 curves, the sagittal profile of the PT portion of the curve is critical, not only as a criterion for including this curve in the fusion, as was noted above, but also during the correction sequence. In this curve type, the PT tends to by hyperkyphotic, and the MT tends to be hypokyphotic. With use of an all-pedicle-screw construct, a single rod with appropriate coronal and sagittal profiles is bent and placed on the left side. Appropriate coronal in situ bending is carried out to correct the coronal plane. If a rib hump needs to be corrected, an apical derotation maneuver is carried out. Finally, compression of the left PT curve and distraction at the MT curve are carried out to correct and fine-tune the sagittal profile.

- One of the significant advances made by Lenke and colleagues' classification system was that it achieved a deeper understanding of when to carry out selective fusions, especially with curve types 1C to 3C and 6C. Such understanding stems from the development of stricter criteria to define the structural character of individual curves. The latter in turn permits an improved objective ability to analyze and choose which curves can be selectively fused without ensuing clinical imbalance. Several radiographic parameters are important in the preoperative analysis prior to selectively fusing a curve. These parameters help to objectively analyze the structural nature of each curve relative to each other, such that if they match, then both curves require surgical attention. To this effect, relative Cobb angle measurements, apical vertebral rotation, and apical vertebral translation ratios of the thoracic and thoracolumbar/lumbar curves are important in the analysis and decision process. Additionally, skeletal maturity and clinical appearance are important considerations. Again, on the basis of the lumbar modifier, attention must be paid to the degree of tilt left on the LIV in carrying out selective fusions. A rough estimate of the degree of tilt to be left on LIV is equal to the remaining tilt on a supine preoperative film, with intraoperative evaluation always necessary. For type A curves, the lower endplate of the lowest instrumented vertebra should be horizontal, a mild tilt should be left on type B curves, and an appropriate degree of tilt is left on type C curves. Clinical assessment of the deformity cannot be overemphasized, as it plays as important a role as the radiographic findings do in deciding whether or not to carry out a selective fusion.

- Selective anterior fusions of major TL/L curves associated with minor and partially structural thoracic curves and with Lenke curves 5C and especially 6C can occasionally be considered. The latter can be contemplated provided that the thoracic curve is less than 50 degrees, the curve bends out to 20 degrees or less, the TL/L : T Cobb ratio is 1.25 or more, and the triradiate cartilages are closed. Additionally, such selective fusions should not be undertaken when shoulder depression ipsilateral to the TL/L curve exists, in highly skeletal immature patients, and/or when a clinically unacceptable rib hump is present. To prevent decompensation, if the lumbar curve bends out less than the thoracic curve, the lumbar curve should not be overly corrected, as the thoracic curve likely will not compensate.

Illustrative Case Presentations

CASE 1. Type 1AN Curve Left and Right

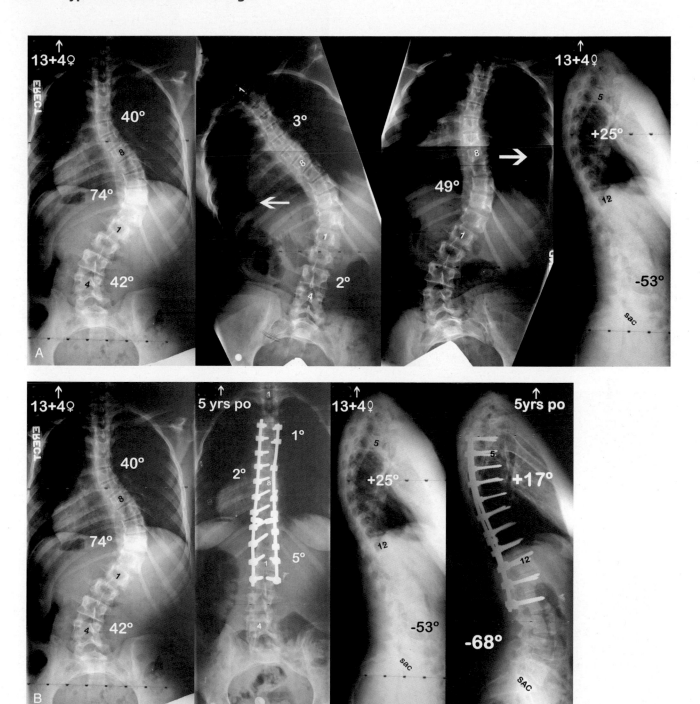

Figure 7-7. **A,** Preoperative posteroanterior, side-bending, and lateral views. **B,** Comparison of postoperative with preoperative radiographs. Note the balanced correction.

Continued

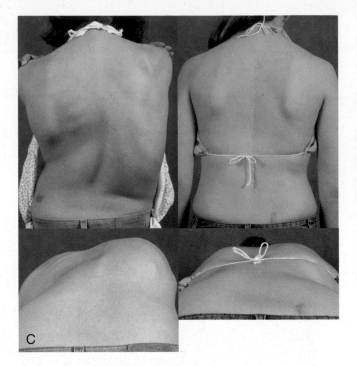

Figure 7-7, cont'd. C, Preoperative clinical trunk shift and significant rib hump, both essentially corrected on the postoperative clinical views.

CASE 2. Type 1BN Curve

Endoscopic instrumentation and fusion were performed from T5 to T11.

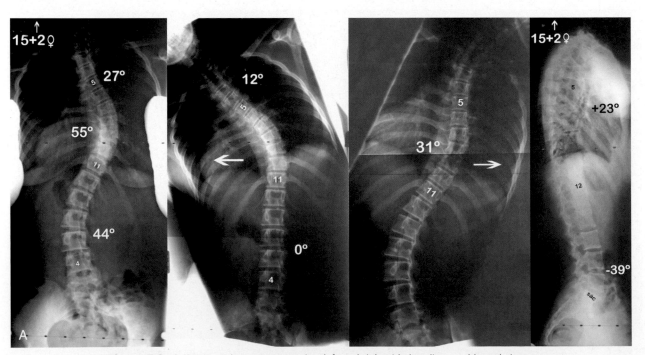

Figure 7-8. A, Preoperative posteroanterior, left and right side-bending, and lateral views.

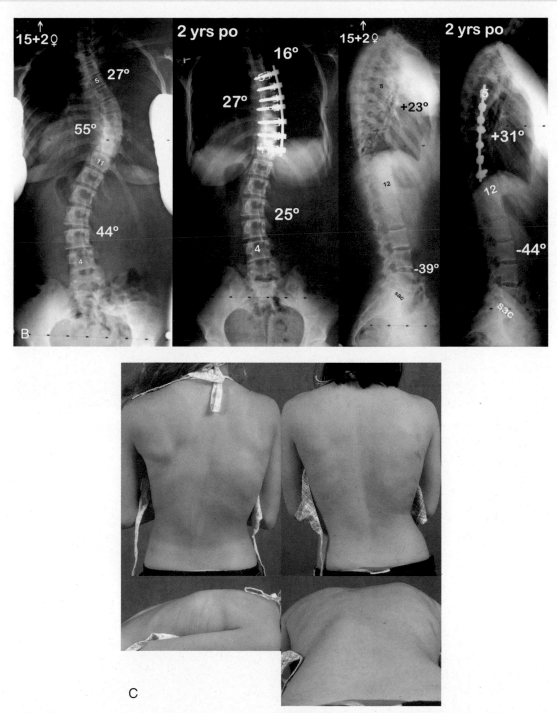

Figure 7-8, cont'd. B, Comparison of preoperative with postoperative radiographs. **C,** Pre- and postoperative clinical photos demonstrate nice correction and overall balance.

CASE 3. Type 2AN Curve

Posterior instrumentation and fusion without thoracoplasty were performed from T2 to L3.

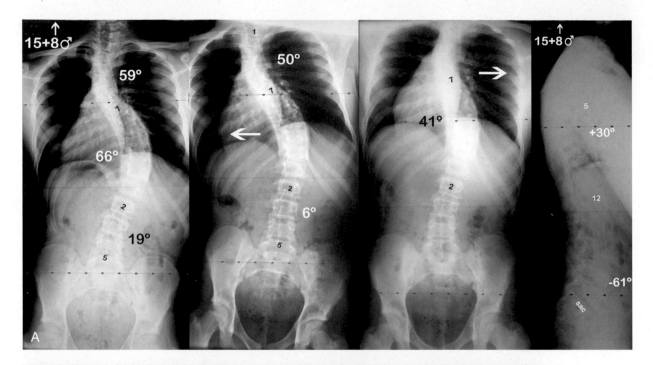

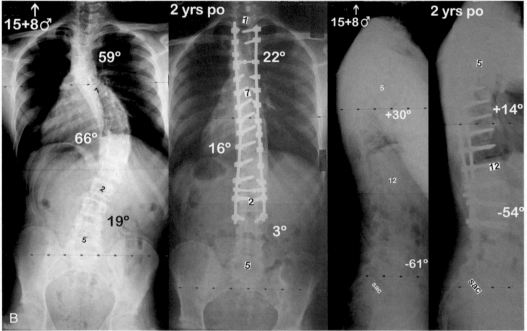

Figure 7-9. A, Preoperative posteroanterior, left and right side-bending, and lateral views. **B,** Comparison of preoperative with postoperative radiographs demonstrates correction and overall coronal and sagittal balance.

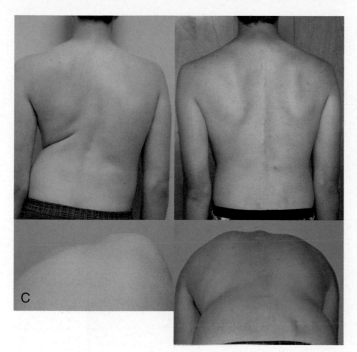

Figure 7-9, cont'd. C, Preoperative and postoperative posteroanterior and forward-bending clinical views demonstrate excellent clinical balance as well as thoracic cage deformity correction.

CASE 4. Type 3CN Curve

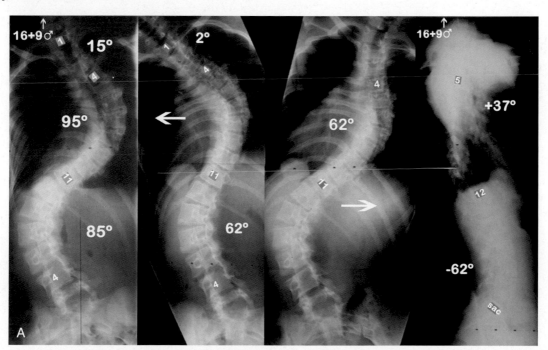

Figure 7-10. A, Preoperative posteroanterior, left and right side-bending, and lateral views.

Continued

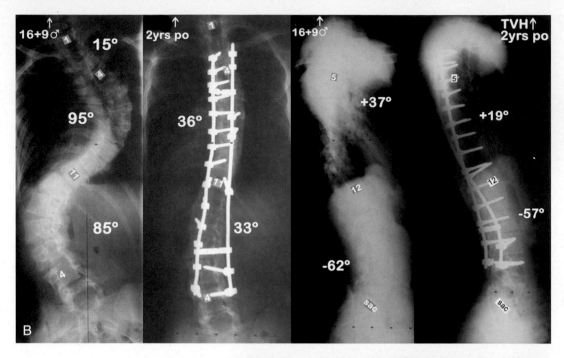

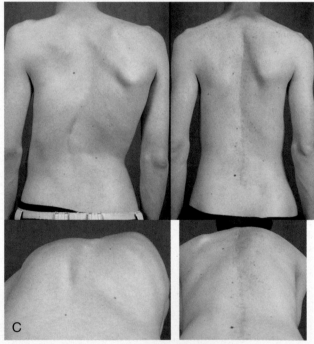

Figure 7-10, cont'd. B, Comparison of preoperative with postoperative radiographs. **C,** Preoperative and postoperative clinical views demonstrate shoulder symmetry, balanced trunk, and significant correction of thoracic cage deformity.

CASE 5. Type 4C+ Curve

Treated posteriorly without anterior releases.

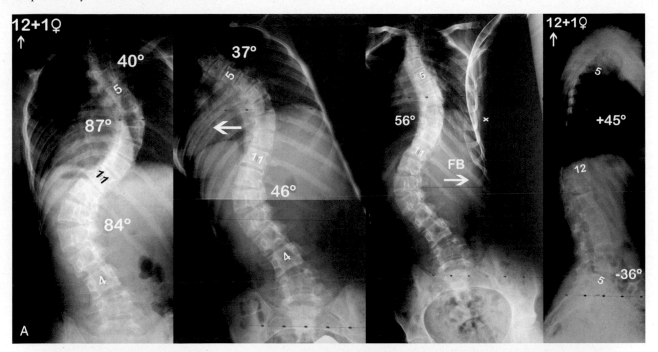

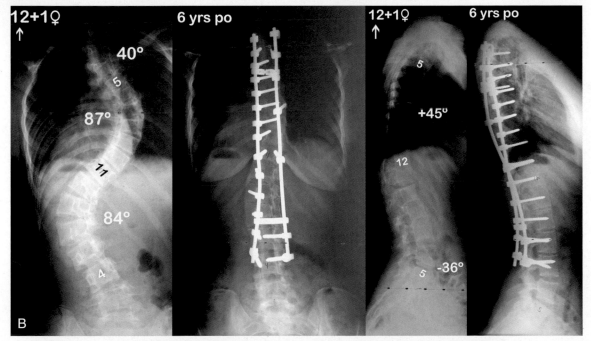

Figure 7-11. A, Preoperative side-bending views demonstrate all three curves to be structural. **B,** Postoperative views reveal excellent radiographic shoulder and overall coronal and sagittal balance when compared with the preoperative views.

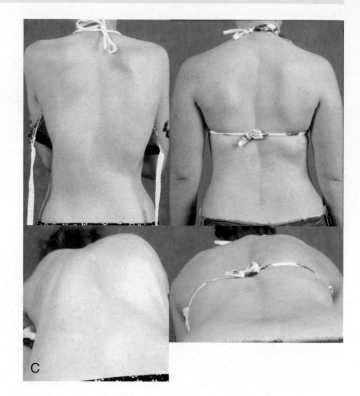

Figure 7-11, cont'd. C, Pre- and postoperative clinical photos demonstrate nice correction and overall balance.

CASE 6. Type 5C– Curve

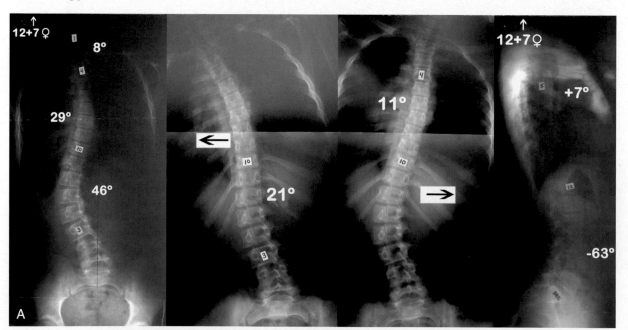

Figure 7-12. A, Preoperative posteroanterior, left and right side-bending, and lateral views.

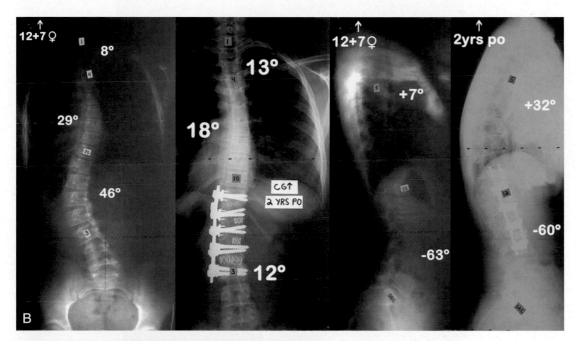

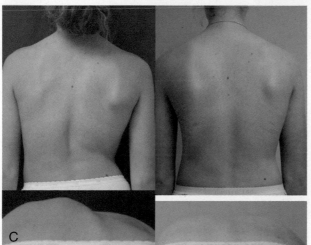

Figure 7-12, cont'd. B, Anterior instrumentation and fusion were performed from T11 to L3 with a dual screw/dual rod system. **C,** Preoperative and postoperative clinical photos. Postoperative forward bend demonstrates significant thoracic cage deformity correction.

CASE 7. Type 5C– Curve

Posterior instrumentation and fusion were performed.

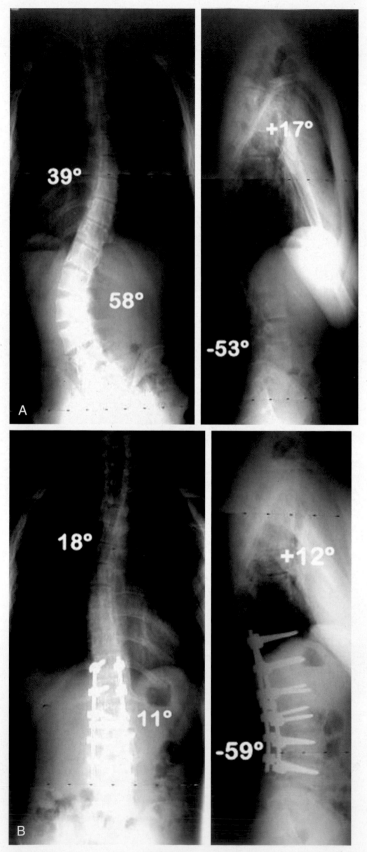

Figure 7-13. A, Preoperative posteroanterior and lateral views. **B,** Postoperative views demonstrate balanced correction with lordosis preservation.

CASE 8. Type 6CN Curve

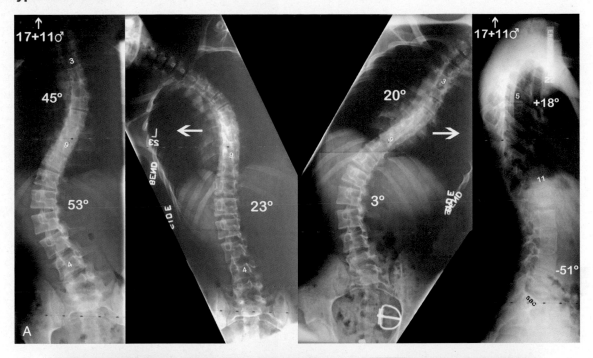

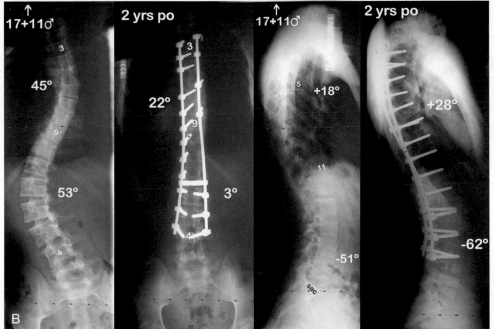

Figure 7-14. A, Preoperative views reveal a lumbar curve of 53 degrees; however, given the lumbar kyphosis, this must be included in the fusion. **B,** Comparison of preoperative to postoperative views demonstrates excellent coronal and sagittal correction, maintenance of thoracic kyphosis, and restoration of lumbar lordosis.

Continued

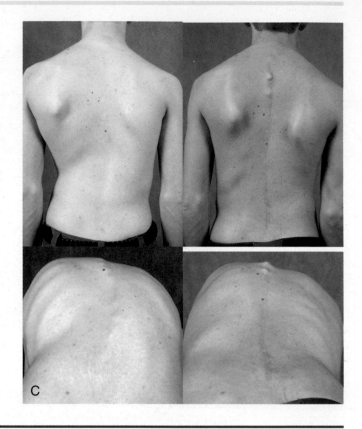

Figure 7-14, cont'd. C, Pre- and postoperative clinical photos demonstrate nice correction and overall balance.

REFERENCES

King HA, Moe JH, Bradford DS, Winter RB: The selection of fusion levels in thoracic idiopathic scoliosis. J Bone Joint Surg Am 1983;65:1302–1313.

Lenke LG, Betz RR, Harms J, et al: Adolescent idiopathic scoliosis: A new classification to determine extent of spinal arthrodesis. J Bone Joint Surg Am 2001;83:1169–1181.

SUGGESTED READINGS

Bridwell KH, McAllister JW, Betz RR, et al: Coronal decompensation produced by Cotrel-Dubousset "derotation" maneuver for idiopathic right thoracic scoliosis. Spine 1991;16:769–777.

This classic article was one of the first to describe the reasons behind coronal decompensation produced by the CD derotation maneuver for thoracic scoliosis.

Edwards CC II, Lenke LG, Peelle MW, et al: Selective thoracic fusion for adolescent idiopathic scoliosis with C modifier lumbar curves: 2- to 16-year radiographic and clinical results. Spine 2004;29:536–546.

This article evaluated 44 patients who underwent a selective thoracic fusion for adolescent idiopathic scoliosis who had a deviated lumbar C modifier. The authors found acceptable coronal and sagittal alignments postoperative without any patients having future surgery with extension into their lumbar spine.

Kesling KL, Reinker KA: Scoliosis in twins: A meta-analysis of the literature and report of six cases. Spine 1997;22:2009–2014.

This article explains the increased occurrence of scoliosis in twins by evaluating six cases and reviewing the literature.

Lenke LG, Betz RR, Bridwell KH, et al: Intraobserver and interobserver reliability of the classification of thoracic adolescent idiopathic scoliosis. J Bone Joint Surg Am 1998;80:97–106.

This article demonstrated poor-to-fair intraobserver as well as interobserver reliability of the King Classification System of thoracic AIS, thus challenging the results of studies utilizing this type of curve classification system.

Lenke LG, Bridwell KH: Achieving coronal balance using Cotrel-Dubousset instrumentation (C-DI). In VIIIth Proceedings of the International Congress on Cotrel-Dubousset Instrumentation. Nimes, France: Sauramps Medical Publishers, 1991, pp 27–32.

This article describes ways of optimizing coronal balance when treating AIS with segmental CDI instrumentation.

O'Brien MF, Kuklo TR, Blanke KM, Lenke LG: Adolescent idiopathic scoliosis. In Radiographic Measurements Manual: Spinal Deformity Study Group. Memphis, TN: Medtronic Sofamor Danek, USA, Inc., 2004, pp 47–70.

This radiographic measurement manual highlights and describes common radiographic measures that are utilized in evaluating scoliosis patients.

O'Brien MF, Kuklo TR, Blanke KM, Lenke LG: Technique for analysis and classification of operative adolescent idiopathic scoliosis. In Radiographic Measurements Manual: Spinal Deformity Study Group. Medtronic Sofamor Danek, USA, Inc., 2004, pp 32–40.

This radiographic measurement manual highlights and describes common radiographic measures that are utilized in evaluating scoliosis patients.

Rinella AS, Cahil P, Ghanayem AM, et al: Thoracic pedicle expansion after pedicle screw placement in a pediatric cadaveric spine: A biomechanical analysis. Paper #35 presented at SRS 39th Annual Meeting, September 6–9, 2004, Buenos Aires, Argentina.

This paper describes the ability of the thoracic pedicles to expand in a pediatric cadaver model, thus accepting a larger screw diameter than would be anticipated on the basis of actual pedicle dimensions.

Sanders AE, Baumann R, Brown H, et al: Selective anterior fusion of thoracolumbar/lumbar curves in adolescents: When can the associated thoracic curve be left unfused? Spine 2003;7:705–714.

This series found that in patients whose thoracic curve preoperatively is less than 50 degrees and patients who are greater than Risser 1, the associated thoracic curve can often be left unfused as the thoracolumbar and lumbar curve is the major deformity.

Sweet FA, Lenke LG: Anterior single-rod CD Horizon instrumentation for scoliosis. In Lenke LG, Betz RR, Harms J (eds): Modern Anterior Scoliosis Surgery. St. Louis: Quality Medical Publishing, 2004, pp 399–409.

Anterior single-rod instrumentation for scoliosis is a viable technique for thoracic, thoracolumbar, and lumbar curves, especially when interbody support is utilized in the thoracolumbar and lumbar junctions.

CHAPTER 8

Scheuermann's Kyphosis

ALOK D. SHARAN, WILLIAM LAVELLE, *and* THOMAS J. ERRICO

OVERVIEW

Scheuermann's disease was first described by Holger Scheuermann in 1920 after he observed a rigid round back deformity in adolescents. He noticed that this deformity was not passively correctable, in contrast to the postural deformities that were more commonly seen in this age group. On radiograph, Scheuermann noticed an anterior wedging of vertebral bodies and end plate irregularities in these patients. Sorenson noted the same irregularities on radiograph and used this observation to define the present-day criteria of Scheuermann's disease of three contiguous thoracic vertebrae with 5 degrees of wedging anteriorly. He believed that the end plate irregularities contributed to the fixed deformity that is now known as *Scheuermann's kyphosis*. No clear etiology of Scheuermann's kyphosis has been elucidated to date. Today, Scheuermann's kyphosis is the most common cause of a rigid thoracic and thoraco-lumbar kyphosis in adolescents.

Epidemiology

Various authors have attempted to report an incidence of Scheuermann's kyphosis. Sorensen reviewed a series of studies and found the prevalence of Scheuermann's kyphosis to be between 0.4% and 8.3%. The largest study to evaluate the incidence of Scheuermann's kyphosis examined 580,000 Danish army recruits. In this study, the authors found the incidence of Scheuermann's kyphosis to be 6%. Scoles and colleagues performed studies on cadavers and found a 7.4% prevalence of Scheuermann's kyphosis.

The gender distribution of Scheuermann's kyphosis has also been debated. It has been suggested that Scheuermann's kyphosis has an equal incidence in both males and females, while others have shown an increased frequency in males. It has generally been accepted now that the ratio of male:female is 2:1 to 7:1. The apparent difference in gender distribution can be explained by the normal growth pattern of the spine. Between the ages of 12 and 14 years, thoracic kyphosis decreases; it then increases until skeletal maturity is reached. The peak growth rate is the period during which the most amount of deformity will occur. In boys, the peak growth rate occurs during the period of increasing kyphosis; in girls, the peak growth rate occurs during a period of increasing lordosis.

Etiology

The true cause of Scheuermann's kyphosis is unknown; however, a number of possible etiologies have been proposed. Scheuermann himself proposed that avascular necrosis of the vertebral ring apophysis results in an arrest of longitudinal growth of the anterior vertebral body. The isolated growth arrest causes a wedging of the anterior portion of the vertebral bodies. This theory was later called into question when the vertebral ring apophysis was found not to contribute to longitudinal vertebral growth.

Schmorl suspected a disturbance in vertebral growth. He theorized that the intervertebral disc material herniated through vertebral end plates, forming the nodes that now bear his name. He felt that these herniations caused a loss of intervertebral disc height as well as inhibited endochondral ossification and therefore caused anterior vertebral wedging. Histologic studies have shown abnormal cartilage at the end plates in patients with Scheuermann's kyphosis, but there have also been reports of Schmorl's nodes found routinely in normal patients.

Growth hormone abnormalities have also been implicated as an etiology. It has been noted in the past that patients with Scheuermann's kyphosis are particularly tall. Ascani and colleagues were able to demonstrate increased growth hormone in these patients, but no direct pathophysiology has ever been described.

Scheuermann was the first to propose a mechanical mechanism for the development of kyphosis. He recognized a high incidence of kyphosis in heavy laborers and theorized that perhaps anterior stress on the vertebral bodies from extrinsic mechanical factors causes an anterior vertebral wedging. This would be supported by the improvement in anterior wedging that is seen in patients who were compliant with brace wear; however, not all patients who are heavy laborers have Scheuermann's kyphosis.

Natural History

The natural history of Scheuermann's kyphosis is believed to be related to its severity. In patients with mild disease (less than 60 degrees), few adverse affects or poor clinical outcomes are expected. The absolute degree of deformity has been found to progress in the majority of untreated patients. Murray and colleagues followed 67 patients with an average kyphotic deformity of 71 degrees for 32 years. These patients were evaluated by physical examination, pulmonary function testing, and a questionnaire. There were no differences between the patients with kyphotic deformity and age-matched controls with respect to days missed from work due to back pain, self-esteem, social function, activities of daily living, level of education, or pulmonary function. Despite these optimistic findings, the patients with kyphotic deformity had more spine tenderness on physical examination and limited thoracic extension. These patients also sought employment that was deemed "less physically strenuous" and reported a passive level of activity on the job.

The association of back pain in patients with untreated kyphotic deformity has been confirmed in multiple other studies and was found to have an incidence as high as 50% of patients. A comparatively high rate of spondylosis has also been reported in patients with Scheuermann's kyphosis. Back pain in patients with Scheuermann's kyphosis is often recalcitrant to conservative treatment. The degree of deformity is likely related to the extent of back pain; few patients experienced disabling pain who had deformities less than 60 degrees.

Neurologic effects are a rare consequence seen with Scheuermann's kyphosis. Paraparesis has been reported either due to the kyphotic deformity itself or as a secondary consequence from disc herniation or a dural cyst. Short segments with particularly severe deformity are considered to be at the highest risk for neurologic compromise.

Cardiopulmonary complications have been reported but are also rare. Extreme kyphotic curves greater than 100 degrees have been shown to develop restrictive pulmonary disease based on pulmonary function testing.

EVALUATION
Clinical Evaluation

Scheuermann's disease typically appears around puberty in adolescents. Growing children may develop a transient back pain; however, pain is more common in the adolescent patient, with an incidence of 20% to 60%. Adult patients with kyphosis typically present with symptoms of pain, while adolescents often present because of referral by their teachers or parents for cosmetic reasons. For the patient who presents with painful Scheuermann's kyphosis or any back pain symptoms, a thorough history of the pain severity, location, chronology, and ameliorating and exacerbating features is necessary. Adolescent patients with Scheuermann's kyphosis and back pain typically have pain distal to the apex of their deformity. The pain is exacerbated by standing, sitting, or strenuous activity and is relieved by rest. If this pain pattern is not seen, then other pathologic conditions must be considered and the diagnosis of Scheuermann's kyphosis should be called into question. In the adult, pain is typically seen in the lumbar region secondary to degenerative changes at levels that have compensated for the thoracic kyphosis.

The cosmetic deformity will likely have a history of gradual progression. In the early stages, parents and teachers might attribute the kyphosis to poor posture. Cosmetic complaints might be the only driving force to patient presentation and might not only entail concerns about spinal deformity. Ill-fitting clothes as well as disproportionately growing limbs can also be the presenting symptoms.

Rare concomitant conditions should also be investigated. Neurologic complaints in patients with Scheuermann's kyphosis show a high degree of variability. Screening for neurologic complaints ranging from unilateral radiculopathy, paresthesias, and paraplegia should occur. Neurologic complaints may be due to a direct compression by the deformity, an epidural cyst, or a thoracic disc herniation. Males between the ages of 14 and 20 years have been reported as having the highest risk of thoracic disc herniation. Symptoms of restrictive pulmonary disease are a possibility but are not common. The study by Murray and colleagues reported restrictive pulmonary disease in patients with curves greater than 100 degrees. Pulmonary function tests are usually not needed for patients with Scheuermann's disease, as most of these patients will have normal pulmonary function or even increased function.

On physical examination, the kyphotic deformity is noted and will demonstrate rigidity in the thoracic and thoracolumbar components in extension. An initial observation of the erect patient from the side will demonstrate a negative sagittal balance as well as rounded shoulders. The patient should also be observed from behind to assess for a rotational component to the deformity, since more than one third of patients with Scheuermann's kyphosis also have some degree of scoliosis. A compensatory lumbar and cervical lordosis will be evident in the patient's normal posture, but this should be correctable with forward bending. The thoracic and thoracolumbar components will remain rigid. A full neurologic evaluation of the upper and lower extremities is critical. The upper extremities should be examined for shoulder girdle tightness, while the patient's lower extremities should be evaluated for hamstring and iliopsoas tightness.

Radiographic Evaluation

Plain films on long cassettes of the entire spine should be obtained in both the anteroposterior and lateral planes. The lateral films should be obtained with the hips and knees fully extended and with the arms flexed forward to 90 degrees. Hyperextension films of the thoracic deformity should be obtained with a bump placed under the apex of the deformity to determine the flexibility of the curve. Utilizing the Cobb technique, the overall degree of kyphosis of the thoracic spine should be measured. The superior and inferior vertebral bodies are selected on the basis of their tilt into the kyphotic deformity. A dot should be placed on the anterior and posterior corners of the end plate of the superior vertebral body. A line connecting these two points is drawn. The same should be completed for the inferior vertebral body. The angle subtended by the perpendicular of these two lines determines the kyphotic deformity. It is important to select the same vertebral bodies in examining serial radiographs. Classically, the presence of three adjacent vertebral bodies with 5 degrees of anterior wedging confirms the diagnosis of Scheuermann's kyphosis. Recently, Bradford has proposed that the presence of only one wedged vertebral body is all that is needed for the diagnosis of Scheuermann's kyphosis. The findings of Schmorl's nodes, disc space narrowing, and end plate changes may also be seen. Two curve patterns are typically seen in Scheuermann's kyphosis. The most common type typically extends from T1-2 to T12-L1. The second type is thoracolumbar and typically extends from T4-5 to L2-3. The second pattern typically progresses into adulthood, owing to the lack of support from the thoracic cage.

Any patient with neurologic symptoms should be considered for MRI evaluation to examine the spinal cord and exiting nerve roots. In addition, an MRI should be obtained to evaluate for the presence of a thoracic disc herniation or cyst in a patient who presents with pain. Computed tomography and myelography may also be ordered as deemed necessary to complete the radiologic evaluation. The presence of other pathologic findings on a radiographic analysis of the patient effectively rules out a diagnosis of Scheuermann's kyphosis.

TREATMENT OPTIONS
Nonoperative Treatment

The natural history of Scheuermann's kyphosis is not as clear as that of scoliosis. Once the diagnosis has been made, it is important to maintain close observation until skeletal maturity. Bracing is indicated for passively correctable curves that are greater than 45 degrees.

The most common type of bracing used in Scheuermann's kyphosis is the Milwaukee brace. With the use of three-point bending, the brace applies an extension force to the thoracic spine via posterior pads placed on the apex of the curve. It is typically used for curves that have an apex at T6 to T9. Braces should be worn full time for at least 12 months and sometimes for 18 months. The goal of brace treatment is reconstitution of the anterior height of the vertebral body. Once this has been achieved, the brace can be worn on a part-time basis. Bradford and colleagues reported on the use of the Milwaukee brace in Scheuermann's disease in 75 patients. After an average of 34 months of brace wear, the authors documented a 40% decrease in the thoracic kyphosis and a 35% decrease in the lumbar lordosis. In one of the larger series looking at long-term results of the Milwaukee brace for Scheuermann's disease, Sachs and colleagues reported on 120 patients who wore the brace for an average of 14 months full time and 18 months part time. After a minimum 5-year follow-up, they observed an initial correction of 50% followed by a loss of correction of an average of 20 degrees. Unfortunately, 31% of compliant patients failed treatment and required surgery.

For curves that are not flexible, some authors have advocated the use of a corrective cast. Ponte and colleagues treated 1043 individuals who presented with irregular vertebral bodies that were consistent with a diagnosis of Scheuermann's disease. They applied either an antigravity type of cast or a localizer type of cast for a mean period of 8 months (83%), 12 months (16%), and 16 months (1%). They were able to obtain a 4% angular improvement with the antigravity cast and 42% with the localizer cast. They followed cast placement with a nighttime Milwaukee brace and intense physical therapy. They reported a mean loss of correction of 4 degrees at the 3-year follow-up. Although cast treatment did not achieve as much correction as a brace did, the cast was able to maintain the correction. Brace treatment has been shown to be successful in individuals who have not attained skeletal maturity. The goal is to prevent a progression of the curve and reconstitute the height of the anterior vertebral body. Failure of treatment is defined as progression of deformity with brace treatment or rigid curves greater than 75 degrees. After this point, surgery could be indicated.

Surgery

Surgery for Scheuermann's kyphosis has evolved with the advent of newer instrumentation and a better understanding of spine biomechanics. In planning for surgical correction of Scheuermann's disease, three main issues should be evaluated: (1) the approach that should be used for correction (anterior only, posterior only, combined anterior/posterior), (2) the levels to be included in the fusion, and (3) the type of correction maneuver to be used.

Biomechanics of Kyphosis

To understand the principles of surgical correction, it is important to understand the mechanics of the deforming forces that are involved. The structural deformity in Scheuermann's disease is a concave curve anteriorly and a convex curve posteriorly. This places tremendous tensile forces on the posterior elements and compressive forces on the anterior vertebral bodies. These forces contribute to further progression of the deformity. Correction of the kyphosis requires a lengthening of the anterior column and a shortening of the posterior column to prevent further progression.

It is also important to note that the neutral axis of the deformity lies in the spinal canal; therefore, the vertebral bodies at the ends of the curve have large lever forces. Failure to fuse to the appropriate levels can result in tremendous forces at the end of the instrumentation and can result in fatigue failure. This can result in the instrumentation breaking or pulling out of the spine. In addition, it is important to remember that the formation of a pseudarthrosis posterior is more likely, since bone graft will be placed in a region of tensile forces. Meticulous decortication of the posterior elements should be performed, along with the placement of abundant bone graft. The formation of a solid fusion will ensure maintenance of the correction. In addition, the instrumentation that is used should be able to convert the tensile forces into compressive forces to provide an appropriate mechanical environment for fusion.

Goals and Approach

The goal of surgery for Scheuermann's disease is to prevent further progression of the kyphosis via a solid fusion. In addition, some form of deformity correction is preferable while always protecting the neural elements. It is important to note that the Scoliosis Research Society defines normal kyphosis from T2 to T12 to vary from 20 to 45 degrees as measured by the Cobb method. Although it might seem preferable to try to correct the deformity to the normal range, there is a risk to overcorrection. This might be evident in the cervicothoracic region, where a junctional kyphosis may occur. Current recommendations include limiting the correction to 50% of the original deformity. It is also important to note that the only absolute indication for surgery is a neurologic deficit. This would require a formal decompressive procedure along with deformity correction. The relative indications for surgery include curves greater than 75 degrees that are resistant to nonoperative treatment, progressive pain that has failed conservative treatment, and/or respiratory problems due to curves greater than 100 degrees.

It is commonly believed that rigid curves should be managed with an anterior release and posterior spinal fusion. More flexible curves could be managed with only posterior spinal fusion. Lowe and Kasten suggest obtaining a supine hyperextension film with a wedge at the apex of the curve. It has been a traditional belief that curves that can be corrected to less than 50 degrees could be managed with posterior spinal fusion; otherwise, an anterior release has to be combined with posterior spinal fusion. With the advent of newer, more rigid instrumentation, many surgeons have begun to use only posterior instrumentation for correction of the deformity.

It is also important to remember that kyphotic deformities tend to displace the spinal cord anteriorly. In performing correction posteriorly, the vessels can be stretched, attenuating the blood supply to the spine. Whenever possible, it is important to try to preserve the segmental vessels anteriorly to allow adequate perfusion of the spinal cord.

Posterior Spinal Fusion

Posterior spinal fusion with instrumentation is the most common procedure typically performed for Scheuermann's kyphosis. A fusion posteriorly relies on continued growth of the anterior column to stabilize and possibly correct the kyphotic deformity. The upper and lower Cobb levels should be involved in the fusion to avoid a junctional kyphosis (Fig. 8-1). It is recommended that the fusion extend to the vertebra above the first lordotic disc.

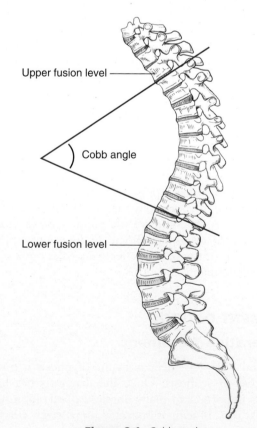

Upper fusion level

Cobb angle

Lower fusion level

Figure 8-1. Cobb angle.

Lowe and Kasten recommend a minimum of eight anchors above and below the apex of the kyphosis. This can be accomplished by using pedicle-transverse process claws with hooks or by using pedicle screws. After placement of the anchors, two 5.5-mm or 6.0-mm smooth rods are contoured to an anticipated kyphosis as seen on the hyperextension lateral radiograph. The rods are inserted into the hooks and/or pedicle screws above the apex and are then cantilevered into the distal implants (Fig. 8-2). The set screws are placed to hold the rod in position temporarily. Compression is then applied toward the apex to reduce the kyphosis. Sometimes the use of in situ benders can help in positioning the rod into the anchors. It is important during the procedure to perform a thorough decortication, facetectomy, and placement of abundant bone graft.

Some surgeons use the double-rod technique in reducing the kyphosis. In this technique, a total of four smooth rods are used. One rod is contoured to match the curve above the apex of the deformity, while another rod is contoured to match the lower part of the curve. The overlapping parts of the rods are then brought together and connected with a double domino connector (Fig. 8-3). Typically, two or three domino connectors are used. These connectors are typically near the apex of the curve, and it is important to ensure that they are not too prominent.

For some rigid curves, an osteotomy might help to realign the spine into a more neutral position. The two types of osteotomies that are typically used are the Smith-Peterson osteotomy and the pedicle subtraction osteotomy. The Smith-Peterson osteotomy is an osteotomy that hinges on the middle column and closes the posterior column. It is useful for thoracic and thoracolumbar curves to obtain a modest amount of correction over multiple segments. The pedicle subtraction osteotomy is a more extensive osteotomy. It can achieve 30 to 40 degrees of kyphosis correction by resecting bone only at one level. It is typically performed in the lumbar spine, below the spinal cord, to minimize injury to the cord. In cases of Scheuermann's disease, a pedicle subtraction osteotomy might be required at the thoracic level, making it a riskier option.

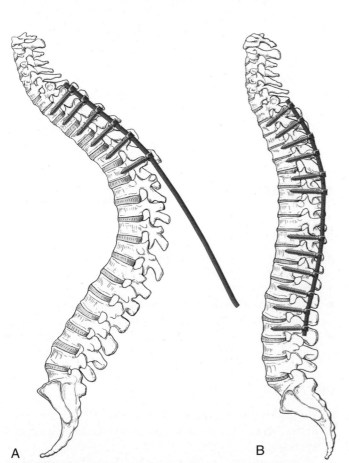

Figure 8-2. Posterior spinal fusion. After the placement of anchors, two 5.5-mm or 6.0-mm smooth rods contoured to an anticipated kyphosis are inserted into the hooks and/or pedicle screws above the apex (**A**) and then cantilevered into the distal implants (**B**).

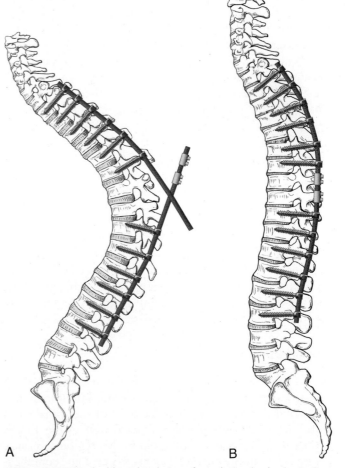

Figure 8-3. The double-rod technique for reducing kyphosis. **A,** One rod is contoured to match the curve above the apex of the deformity, while another rod is contoured to match the lower part of the curve. **B,** The overlapping parts of the rods are then brought together and connected with double domino connectors.

Combined Anterior/Posterior Spinal Fusion

A combined anterior release and instrumented posterior fusion is indicated for patients who have a rigid curve that will not correct to less than 50 degrees on the hyperextension lateral radiograph. These procedures are typically performed on the same day to avoid the morbidity of two separate anesthetic procedures. The anterior release is typically performed first. This should be performed at the apex of the curve, and the adjacent six to eight segments should also be released when possible. A complete discectomy should be performed, including resection of the anterior longitudinal ligament. This will allow the bony elements of the spine to have more flexibility and will make it easier to perform the correction for the posterior part of the procedure. Ideally, all levels that will be involved in the fusion should be released.

Exposure can be performed through a formal open thoracotomy or a retroperitoneal approach, depending on the levels that need to be exposed. Unless instrumentation is being performed, it is important to try to preserve the segmental vessels to allow for adequate perfusion of the spinal cord. Single-lung ventilation is preferred to allow for adequate exposure of the disc spaces. Once a thorough discectomy has been performed, morselized rib autograft can be placed into the disc spaces. Cages may sometimes be used if a significant lengthening of the anterior column is needed. A chest tube is inserted into the thoracic cavity, and the wound is then closed. The patient is then positioned for a formal posterior fusion as described above.

Anterior Instrumented Fusion

In patients with very flexible curves, an anterior instrumented fusion can be performed to correct the deformity. This technique is useful to save fusion levels both posteriorly and anteriorly. A complete anterior release of soft tissues should be performed. Vertebral body screws are then placed, achieving bicortical purchase. A single 6.5- to 7-mm precontoured rod is then placed to achieve correction of the deformity. Structural allografts or cages are recommended to correct the deformity.

Complications

Surgery for Scheuermann's kyphosis is not benign and has a significant risk of complications. It is important to understand that the cross-sectional diameter of the spinal canal at the apex of the deformity is narrowed owing to the kyphosis. The placement of hooks in this region can cause compression of the neural elements. Neurologic complications have been reported in surgery for Scheuermann's kyphosis, but the exact rate is unknown. Complications can arise during the placement of instrumentation or during the correction procedure itself. Continuous electrophysiologic monitoring is critical to evaluate for this. If there are any questions about the validity of the monitoring, a wake-up test should be performed.

Junctional kyphosis has been reported to be 20% to 30% in the series of Lowe and Kasten. It was initially believed to be a result of cutting the superior or inferior supraspinous ligament. Unfortunately, this problem persisted with better surgical technique and the use of newer instrumentation. It is now believed to be a result of not ending at the level above the first lordotic disc or the proper proximal vertebrae. In addition it has been noted that screw pullout at the lowest instrumented vertebrae can result in subsequent junctional kyphosis. This can occur if the screw is too short or if a hook is used at the lowest vertebral level.

CONCLUSION

The treatment of Scheuermann's kyphosis requires a comprehensive understanding of the natural history of the disease and the various methods for treatment. Nonoperative treatment can be successful in the properly chosen patient. If this fails, surgery has been shown to provide satisfying results. Many studies have shown an improvement in back pain with surgery. One study has even been able to show a marked improvement in Oswestry Disability Scores. This surgery involves significant risks, but with proper patient selection and proper surgical technique, the outcomes for the treatment of Scheuermann's kyphosis can lead to a tremendous impact and satisfaction for the affected individual.

PEARLS & PITFALLS

PEARLS

- A Milwaukee brace is recommended for adolescents who have curves greater than 45 degrees and still have growth potential.
- The advent of pedicle screw instrumentation has helped to decrease the need for anterior release.
- In deciding on the distal level, the instrumentation should end at the level above the first lordotic disc.

PITFALLS

- Failure to include the whole curve in the instrumented levels can result in instrument failure and/or junctional kyphosis.
- Maintaining the anterior segmental vessels is critical, as the spinal cord is stretched during kyphosis correction and can result in an attenuated blood supply.

Illustrative Case Presentations

CASE 1. A 16-Year-Old Male with a Progressive and Painful Kyphosis of 120 Degrees

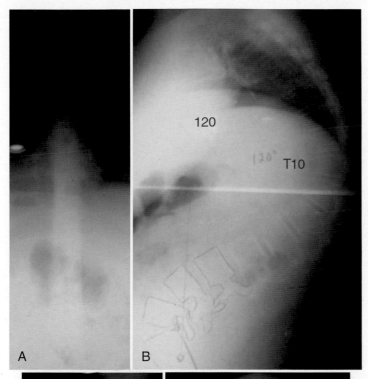

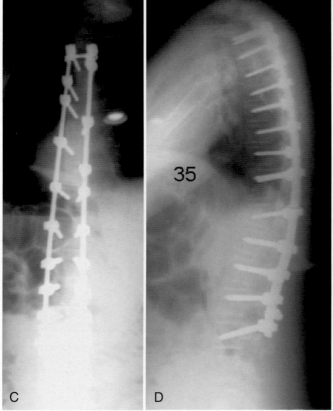

Figure 8-4. A and **B,** Preoperative posteroanterior and lateral radiographs of the spine. **C** and **D,** Postoperative posteroanterior and lateral radiographs of the spine following corrective posterior surgery utilizing Ponte osteotomies and T10 corpectomy. *(Courtesy of Baron S. Lonner, MD.)*

CASE 2. A 16-Year-Old Female with Kyphosis of 94 Degrees Treated with Anterior Thoracoscopic Release and Fusion and Posterior Instrumented Fusion

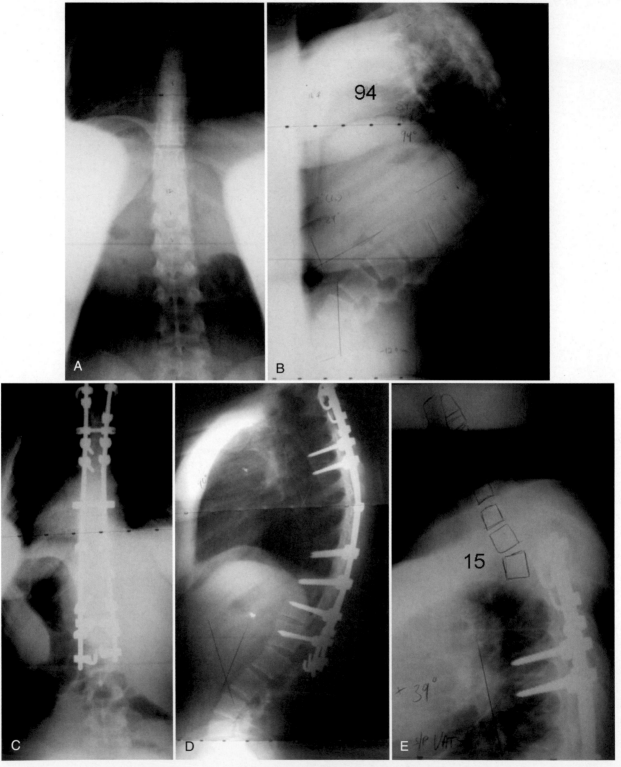

Figure 8-5. Preoperative (**A** and **B**) and postoperative (**C–E**) posteroanterior, lateral radiographs. Proximal and distal junctional kyphosis was noted radiographically at follow-up but did not require treatment. *(Courtesy of Baron S. Lonner, MD.)*

CASE 3. A 16-Year-Old Male with a Progressive and Painful Kyphosis of 74 Degrees

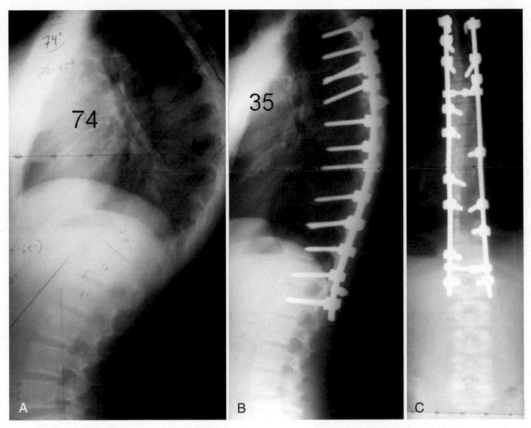

Figure 8-6. Preoperative lateral (**A**) and postoperative lateral (**B**) and posteroanterior (**C**) radiographs. *(Courtesy of Baron S. Lonner, MD.)*

REFERENCES

Ascani E, Borelli P, La Rosa G, et al: Malattia de Sheuermann I: Studio ormonale progressi in patologia vertebrale. In Gaggi A (ed): Le Cifosi. Bologna, Italy, 1982, p 97.

Bradford DS: Scheuermann's kyphosis and roundback deformity: Results of Milwaukee brace treatment. J Bone Joint Surg Am 1974;56: 740–758.

Lowe TG: Kyphosis of the thoracic and thoracolumbar spine in the pediatric patient: Surgical treatment. Instr Course Lect 2004;53: 493–500.

Lowe TG: Mortality Morbidity Committee Report. Read at the 22nd Annual Meeting of the Scoliosis Research Society, Vancouver, British Columbia, Canada, September 1987.

Ponte A, Gebbia F, Elisea F: Nonoperative treatment of adolescent hyperkyphosis. Presentation at the 19th Scoliosis Research Society, Orlando, Florida, September 1984.

Scheuermann H: Kyfosis dorsalis juveniles. Ugeskr Lager 1920;82:385.

Scoles PV, Latimer BM, DiGiovanni BF, et al: Vertebral alterations in Scheuermann's kyphosis. Spine 1991;16:509–515.

Sorensen KH: Scheuermann's Juvenile Kyphosis: Clinical Appearances, Radiography, Etiology, Pathology. Copenhagen: Munksgaard, 1964.

Wassmann K: Kyphosis juvenilis Scheuermann: An occupational disorder. Acta Orthop Scan 1951;21:65.

SUGGESTED READINGS

Arlet V, Schlenzka D: Scheuermann's kyphosis: Surgical management. Eur Spine J 2005;14:817–827.

This review article discusses the use of newer segmental instrumentation used to correct kyphosis. The four-rod technique and various compression techniques are also presented.

Boachie-Adjei O, Sarwahi V: Scheuermann's kyphosis. In Dewald R (ed): Spinal Deformities: A Comprehensive Text. New York: Thieme Medical Publishers, 2003, pp 777–786.

This chapter describes some of the surgical concepts and techniques that are used in correcting kyphosis in Scheuermann's disease.

Hosman AJ, Langebo DD, deKleuver M: Analysis of the sagittal plane after surgical management for Scheuermann's disease: A view on overcorrection and the use of an anterior release. Spine 2002;27: 167–175.

This paper analyses the difference in curve morphometry after an anterior-posterior procedure vs. posterior only. In this cohort of 33 patients, there were no differences in Cobb angle, correction, or sagittal balance.

Lenke LG: Kyphosis of the thoracic and thoracolumbar spine in the pediatric patient: Prevention and treatment of surgical complications. Instr Course Lect 2004;53:501–510.

This article discusses successful strategies for operative intervention for kyphosis surgery. Included in the article is a discussion on proper preoperative planning, including choosing the appropriate levels. This article reviews causes of unsuccessful outcomes including choosing inappropriate levels, failure to provide adequate anterior support when necessary, and inadequate spinal fixation.

Lowe TG, Kasten MD: An analysis of sagittal curves and balance after Cotrel-Dubousset instrumentation for kyphosis secondary to Scheuermann's disease: A review of 32 patients. Spine 1994;19: 168–1685.

This paper analyzed curve correction in 32 patients with curves greater than 75 degrees. The authors found that there was an appropriate correction of the unfused lumbar curve. Junctional kyphosis was avoided if the correction did not exceed 50% or if the fusion did not reach the first lordotic level.

Murray PM, Weinstein SL, Spratt KF: The natural history and long-term follow-up of Scheuermann kyphosis. J Bone Joint Surg Am 1993;75:236–248.

This classic article describes the long-term follow-up of 67 patients with Scheuermann's kyphosis who were followed for an average of 32 years compared to a control group. The patients with Scheuermann's kyphosis had more intense back pain, jobs that require less activity, and less range of motion of extension of their trunk.

Poolman RW, Been HD, Ubags LH: Clinical outcome and radiographic results after operative treatment of Scheuermann's disease. Eur Spine J 2002;11:561–569.

This article describes the operative results of patients with Scheuermann's kyphosis, correlating it with improved SRS scores. In this series, patients whose hardware was removed experienced a loss of the correction even after radiologic examination of the fusion was completed.

Sachs B, Bradford D, Winter R, et al: Scheuermann's kyphosis: Follow-up of Milwaukee-brace treatment. J Bone Joint Surg Am 1987;69: 50–57.

This classic article is one of the most comprehensive articles that have evaluated the use of the Milwaukee brace for the treatment of kyphosis.

Tribus CB: Scheuermann's kyphosis in adolescents and adults: Diagnosis and management. J Am Acad Orthop Surg 1998;6:36–43.

This article gives an overview of the natural history, etiology, nonoperative, and operative procedures for the surgical correction of Scheuermann's kyphosis.

CHAPTER 9

Congenital Scoliosis

David S. Feldman, Aaron K. Schachter, Daniel Alfonso, Baron S. Lonner, *and* Afshin E. Razi

Congenital scoliosis is defined as a lateral curvature of the spine resulting from abnormal vertebral development. Congenital scoliosis is often not clinically detectable at birth and may become evident later in life if and when there is progression of the curve. Eighty percent of infants who present with scoliosis will have a congenital scoliosis, that is, an abnormal architecture of the spine. The scoliosis may be due to failure of formation of elements of the spine, failure of segmentation of the vertebrae, or a combination of the two. In the other 20% of infants with scoliosis, there is normal vertebral formation.

ETIOLOGY

The etiology of most vertebral anomalies is multifactorial. Intrauterine environmental factors, such as hypoxia in the first 2 months of gestation, play a critical role in the development of congenital scoliosis. Animal studies have demonstrated that hypoxic insult at the developmental stage equivalent to a 6-week human embryo causes spinal anomalies similar to those seen in congenital scoliosis. Additionally, fetal exposure to thalidomide, lovastatin, and certain progesterone/estrogen compounds might increase the incidence of these anomalies. Environmental abnormalities and, less commonly, genetic factors lead to anomalous somite segmentation, causing congenital vertebral abnormalities and eventually a scoliotic curve. In rare cases, such as Jarcho-Levin syndrome, spondylocostal dysostosis, and Klippel-Feil syndrome, genetic factors are the sole cause. Studies have shown that a spinal anomaly that is present in one monozygotic twin is usually not present in the other.

CLASSIFICATION OF CONGENITAL SCOLIOSIS

The classification of congenital scoliosis is largely descriptive. The scoliosis is described in terms of location in the spine and whether or not it represents a failure of formation or segmentation, or both.

Failure of Vertebral Formation

Failure of formation of the spinal elements can be represented by absence of any portion of the vertebra. The most common form of this is the presence of a hemivertebra. This involves a complete failure of formation at a specific site on one side of the spine. The side with the hemivertebra will become the convexity of the curvature, as growth will be disproportionate.

Classification of the hemivertebra aids in the prediction of progression of the curve. Complete failure of formation will have variable growth potential that often depends on the segmentation of the intact hemivertebra. Segmentation is determined by the presence or absence of a disc space and concomitant ring epiphysis growth plate above or below the hemivertebra. The hemivertebra may be classified as segmented (a disc space above and below), semisegmented (a disc space above or below), or nonsegmented hemivertebra (no disc spaces).

The hemivertebra may also be classified by whether or not the lateral portion of the hemivertebra is contained within the arc of the curve drawn on the convexity of the curve. This is described as incarcerated (within the curve) or nonincarcerated (outside of the curve). An incarcerated hemivertebra is one in which the adjacent vertebral bodies conform in their shape, that is ovoid, and that appears trapped between the normal vertebrae. The pedicle of an incarcerated hemivertebra is in line with adjacent pedicles. This tends to compensate for the maldeveloped hemivertebra, which is "tucked into" the spinal column. A nonincarcerated hemivertebra has a pedicle that is outside the pedicle line of adjacent levels and tends to be fully segmented.

The presence of more than one hemivertebra may represent a hemimetameric shift (HMMS). This term refers to two offsetting deformities. In HMMS, two or more hemivertebrae are present on contralateral sides of the spine, and there is at least one normal vertebra between them. This is found in up to 11% to 15% of cases of congenital scoliosis. HMMS is more common in the thoracic region. The distance between the levels on each side is important in determining the type of curve that is created. The farther apart the opposite hemivertebrae are from each other, the worse is the prognosis.

Finally, a partial failure of formation produces a wedge-shaped vertebra, which produces disproportionate growth on the convexity. The presence or absence of normal disc spaces above and below the wedge vertebra plays an important role in determining progression and treatment.

Defects of Vertebral Segmentation

Failure of segmentation occurs when adjacent somites and associated mesenchyme fail to fully separate. This results in the partial or complete loss of a growth plate in the affected area. Fusion of the facet joints and/or disc spaces occurs on the affected side of the vertebral column. Curve progression is dependent on the location and the number of vertebrae affected. Defects of vertebral segmentation can occur unilaterally or bilaterally.

Unilateral Failure of Segmentation

Unilateral failure of segmentation results in the formation of a unilateral bar. A unilateral bar leads to scoliosis because while the bar prevents longitudinal growth ipsilaterally, the unaffected side continues to grow.

Bilateral Failure of Segmentation

Bilateral failure of vertebral segmentation leads to the formation of a block vertebra. The symmetrical bilateral restriction of longitudinal growth leads to the development of a shortened segment without significant scoliosis. Bilateral failure of segmentation anomaly may occur in the cervical spine. If multiple cervical vertebrae are involved, it is termed *Klippel-Feil syndrome*. A clinical triad of short neck, low posterior hairline, and decreased range of motion is seen in some patients with Klippel-Feil syndrome.

Defects of Vertebral Formation and Segmentation

A small percentage of patients may possess a combination of defects of both formation and segmentation, creating a complex structural abnormality. A unilateral nonsegmented bar and a contralateral hemivertebra located in the convexity of the curve occur in approximately 11%

of cases of congenital scoliosis; this defect carries the worst prognosis.

RATE OF PROGRESSION

The prognosis for curve progression in patients with congenital scoliosis is based on three factors: age of the patient, the location of the curve, and the type of anomaly.

Age

Curve progression is most likely to occur during two periods of accelerated growth. The first of these periods is within the first 2 years of life, during which most curves become evident. The second period occurs during the adolescent growth spurt, between ages 10 to 13 years in females and approximately 2 years later in males. Progression may also be seen after maturity in the presence of a severe deformity.

Location of the Curve

Thoracolumbar curves have the greatest tendency to progress, followed by lower thoracic and upper thoracic curves. An important consideration in the management of a hemivertebra is the location of the defect in the spine. Spinal decompensation becomes more problematic the more caudad the location of the hemivertebra. This will become particularly important during the discussion of treatment of the congenital scoliotic curve.

Type of Anomaly

The fully segmented hemivertebra acts as a wedge as it grows, producing a curve that commonly progresses at a rate of 1 to 2 degrees per year. Lower thoracic and thoracolumbar region anomalies may progress faster. If two hemivertebrae are located on one side within a curve, progression is likely to be greater than it would be if only one defect is present.

A semisegmented hemivertebra has only one functional disc, its accompanying growth centers being either cephalad or caudad. These curves progress less rapidly and are often less than 40 degrees at skeletal maturity.

A nonsegmented hemivertebra is fused to the neighboring vertebrae at both the cephalad and caudad poles. Therefore, no disc spaces and growth plates are associated with this type of anomaly. There is little growth potential, and it is associated with minimal progression.

The degree of deterioration from failure of segmentation is based on the rate of growth of the unaffected side and the extent of involvement of the nonsegmented bar. Associated curves tend to progress rapidly at a rate of 2 to 6 degrees per year. By 10 years of age, most curves exceed 50 degrees. This anomaly might not be evident on radiographs until the bar ossifies around the age of 3 to 4 years.

Although incarcerated hemivertebrae may be associated with cephalad and caudad disc spaces, these spaces are usually narrow and have poor growth potential. Curvature associated with this anomaly may slowly progress but rarely exceeds 20 degrees in magnitude. Incarcerated hemivertebrae have less potential for causing scoliosis than do fully segmented hemivertebrae that are not incarcerated.

In the case of a hemivertebra located at the lumbosacral junction or the two hemivertebrae that make up an HMMS located far from each other, there tends to be a more rapid progression of the deformity, often requiring surgical intervention.

A unilateral nonsegmented bar with contralateral hemivertebra carries the worst prognosis for curve progression, while block vertebra has the most benign course. The most aggressive curves progress at an average of 6 degrees per year, and those in the thoracolumbar spine progress at a rate of up to 14 degrees per year. Unilateral nonsegmented bar with contralateral hemivertebra often exceeds 60 degrees by age 4 years.

NATURAL HISTORY

Congenital scoliosis is not a benign condition. Up to 10% to 25% of cases are not progressive, 15% to 25% progress slowly, and 50% to 75% progress rapidly. Up to 40% of patients who are treated nonoperatively will have curvature between 40 and 60 degrees, and up to 30% will have a curve greater than 60 degrees at skeletal maturity. Congenital deformity tends to be more rigid and structural than in other types of pediatric scoliosis.

ASSOCIATED ANOMALIES

Various intraspinal and extraspinal abnormalities are associated with congenital scoliosis. The incidence of any associated anomaly has been estimated to be from 30% to 60%. The frequency of intraspinal abnormalities noted in patients with congenital scoliosis varies from 18% to 58%.

Intraspinal abnormalities may include tethering of the spinal cord, diastematomyelia, lipoma, dermoid cyst, syringomyelia, diplomyelia, and a low-lying conus medullaris. The incidence of intraspinal abnormality may be higher among patients with deformities that are classified as failure of formation.

A tethered cord can be caused by fibrous bands, a tight filum terminale, ectopic nerve roots, or arachnoid adhesions. It can also be associated with diastematomyelia, a sagittal split in either the spinal cord or the cauda equina. An osseous or fibrocartilaginous spur arising from the posterior aspect of adjacent vertebral bodies causes this split. Diastematomyelia is often associated with a unilateral bar with a contralateral hemivertebra. Interestingly, HMMS has a low association (6%) with intraspinal anomalies.

Although spina bifida occulta and more significant vertebral anomalies have similar etiologies, studies have shown no significant relationship between them.

The most common extraspinal anomalies involve the ribs and the genitourinary and cardiac systems.

Rib anomalies may be acquired or congenital. Congenital rib abnormalities include absent ribs, extra ribs, and rib synostoses. Severe deformation of the rib cage can occur as a result of a large thoracic curvature. If this occurs before age 8 years, it can interfere with pulmonary development and result in restrictive lung disease. All are commonly found associated with congenital scoliosis. In spondylothoracic dysplasia (Jarcho-Levin syndrome), there are multiple associated posterior rib fusions, which constrict the thorax and eventually result in respiratory failure and death. In spondylocostal dysostosis, the ribs are not severely involved, but there is marked shortening of the trunk, which could impair lung development.

Defects of other organ systems are found in up to 30% to 60% of patients with congenital scoliosis. Genitourinary system anomalies are present in 20% to 40% of patients. Horseshoe kidney, unilateral renal agenesis, ectopic kidney, duplication, urethral anomalies, and reflux are also found. Recognition of genitourinary system anomalies is important because up to 25% of patients require interventional therapy, such as surgery or hemodialysis.

Congenital heart defects occur in up to 26% of patients who have congenital scoliosis. In addition, severe curvature may exacerbate existing cardiopulmonary dysfunction. These anomalies may be fatal, and early recognition is essential.

Other rare anomalies that are associated with congenital scoliosis include absent uterus and vagina, cleft palate, cleft lip, preauricular ear tags, and mandibular hypoplasia. Some of these abnormalities occur with significant consistency to be classified as syndromes.

The VACTERL syndrome is one of the most commonly associated syndromes. It includes vertebral anomalies, imperforate anus, cardiac abnormalities, tracheoesophageal fistula, renal dysplasia, and limb malformations. Klippel-Feil syndrome, congenital fusion of multiple cervical vertebrae, may be noted. Its triad of a low posterior hairline with a short and stiff neck has classically identified this syndrome. Sprengel deformity, an elevation of the scapula, is caused by failure of proper descent of the scapula in utero. This is believed to be due to a process of failure of segmentation similar to that seen in congenital spinal anomalies. Goldenhar syndrome, or oculoauricular vertebral dysplasia, is uncommonly found. It consists of unilateral malformation of the ear and facial hypoplasia with congenital scoliosis.

PATIENT EVALUATION

The evaluation of the patient with congenital scoliosis must include an assessment for associated anomalies. A thorough history should be taken to identify prenatal drug exposure, prenatal and postnatal development, past medical history, ambulatory status and balance, and neurologic development. Complete systemic reviews, including those of the genitourinary and cardiopulmonary systems, should be performed.

Physical examination should include an assessment of general appearance to observe for facial and trunk abnormalities or limb deficiency. The skin should be assessed. Midline skin abnormalities such as a dimple, nevus, hairy patch, sinus tract, or lipoma might indicate the presence of an intraspinal anomaly. Gait is evaluated to rule out neurologic or lower-extremity abnormalities. A thorough neurologic evaluation, including motor, sensory, and reflex examination, should be done. Pathologic reflexes such as ankle clonus and Babinski signs are assessed. Subtle neurologic abnormality may be noted by the presence of asymmetric calf and/or thigh circumference, asymmetric abdominal reflex, cavus foot, curled toes, and/or a mild limp.

The spine is evaluated with the patient in a standing position. Shoulder, scapula, and waist asymmetry and torso decompensation are often noted. The shoulder is elevated on the side of the curve convexity, and the head is often tilted toward the concavity. A forward-bending test is done to evaluate for associated rib deformity. In some cases, the rib deformity will be minimal despite significant scoliosis, owing to a lack of rotational deformity. Pelvic obliquity may be seen with rigid lumbar or lumbosacral curves.

Spinal radiographs should be performed in all patients with suspected congenital scoliosis. These radiographs are necessary to identify the type, location, and magnitude of curvature. High-quality standing or sitting upright (for nonambulators) posteroanterior and lateral radiographs on a 14 × 36 inch film should be obtained. The lateral radiograph should be examined carefully for the presence of concomitant kyphosis or lordosis. A posterolateral quadrant or corner hemivertebra, resulting in kyphoscoliosis, can be difficult to detect prior to the occurrence of significant deformity. A coned-down radiograph is helpful in defining spinal anomalies. After the type of anomaly on the anteroposterior radiograph has been identified, the number of viable growth plates adjacent to the anomalous vertebrae should be determined to assess the potential for growth imbalance and progressive curvature. A high-quality magnetic resonance image (MRI) or computed tomography scan with coronal and sagittal reformats can assist in this regard.

Curve description is based on the direction in which the apex points, the region of the spine in which the primary curve or curves occur, the location of compensatory curves, and sagittal deformity and sagittal balance. The degree of curvature is established by using the standard Cobb method.

Follow-up radiographic assessment should be performed with serial standing radiographs at 3- to 6-month intervals, depending on the age of the child and the degree of curvature. At each visit, the current radiograph should be compared with both the previous radiograph and the original radiograph so that an accurate assessment of curve progression can be determined. If there is more than 5 degrees of progression, this should be considered significant.

All patients with congenital scoliosis are indicated to undergo an MRI evaluation of the complete spine. This is particularly important in the patient who exhibits positive neurologic findings or if surgery is planned. The MRI is utilized to identify the presence of intraspinal anomalies as well as the presence of a Chiari malformation. This is crucial, since congenital scoliosis or kyphosis is associated with the highest rate of neurologic injury following operative correction compared with other forms of scoliosis. The study should include the brain to rule out Chiari malformation or hydrocephalus and the cervical, thoracic, and lumbosacral spines.

The need for MRI of the spine in the absence of neurologic finding has been considered. Several recent studies have documented poor correlation between physical examination and MRI findings. The incidence of occult intraspinal anomalies on MRI is noted to be 30% to 41%, with neurologic findings detected in only 36% to 65% of those patients.

Echocardiography should be employed to evaluate the heart. B-mode ultrasonography has been shown to be a reliable replacement for intravenous pyelogram as a screening tool for genitourinary anomalies.

TREATMENT

The goals of treatment of congenital scoliosis are to (1) prevent or arrest curve progression, (2) preserve spinal function and mobility, (3) treat or prevent cardiopulmonary disease, and (4) correct spinal deformity. Three key factors in gaining optimal results in these patients are early recognition, anticipation of prognosis, and prevention of deterioration. This may be achieved by nonoperative or operative methods.

Nonoperative Treatment

Bracing is not nearly as successful in the treatment of congenital scoliosis as it is in the treatment of idiopathic scoliosis. It can be helpful in controlling long, flexible congenital or compensatory curves in the preadolescent stage. Bracing may be utilized in the postoperative period to control compensatory curves. Bracing should not be employed in situations of severe imbalance, in congenital lordosis or kyphosis, in skeletally mature patients, or in the presence of a rigid curve, such as those associated with unilateral failure of segmentation. Some clinicians have recommended the use of the Milwaukee brace, when appropriate, which has a less adverse effect on pulmonary function. A head extension can also be used to treat upper thoracic curvature and to control abnormal head tilt.

Operative Treatment

Surgical intervention is indicated for proven progressive curves in the skeletally immature patient. The curve does not need to approach the threshold of 40 degrees, as is often mentioned with regard to adolescent idiopathic scoliosis. Operative management can be classified into four categories, which often can be combined to treat a single patient with a congenital scoliosis. These are fusion in situ, fusion with correction, osteotomies, and growing instrumentation systems.

Hemiepiphyseodesis/Hemiarthrodesis

The anterior hemiepiphyseodesis and posterior hemiarthrodesis are performed together to arrest growth on the convexity of the curve. This combination is the ideal surgical procedure to manage curves that are caused by unilateral failure of vertebral formation. The goal of this procedure is to stop curve progression and to allow slow correction of deformity by taking advantage of continued growth on the concavity of the curve.

It is best suited for patients younger than 5 years of age with a fully segmented hemivertebra with curvature of less than 70 degrees that corrects to less than 40 degrees on side-bending films. Contraindications to this procedure include local kyphosis and unilateral failure of segmentation. Disadvantages are the slow process of correction and the unpredictability due to the uncertainty of growth potential on the concavity.

The procedure is performed as a combined anterior and posterior growth arrest. The anterior spine is approached by utilizing a method that allows for optimal exposure of the defect, whether by thoracotomy, thoracoscopy, or a thoracoabdominal or retroperitoneal abdominal approach. Discectomy and bone grafting are performed at the level and the side of the hemivertebra as well as at a level above and a level below. A posterior approach and convex fusion are then performed. This is accomplished by stripping the posterior musculature over the convexity of the curve. Care is taken to strip the musculature and decorticate only the convex-sided facet joints and posterior elements, as done anteriorly. Patients are immobilized for 3 to 6 months postoperatively with either a cast or a brace.

Transpedicular hemiepiphyseodesis and posterior arthrodesis have been advocated as a single approach that avoids the morbidity associated with the anterior approach. Although the outcome of this technique is promising,

there has been no report on long-term follow-up to maturity at this time.

Arthrodesis in Situ

The goals of early fusion in situ are to stabilize mild to moderate curvature to prevent severe deformity and its associated problems. This is optimally applied to cases of unilateral bar, which is recognized to have a poor prognosis if left untreated. The best outcomes are obtained if the surgical intervention is undertaken as soon as the anomaly is recognized. The upper and lower end vertebrae of the Cobb angle of the curvature should be included in the fusion. In situ arthrodesis may be performed by a posterior or combined anterior-posterior approach.

Posterior spinal arthrodesis alone includes posterior stripping of the muscles and fusion of the posterior elements in situ without correction, leaving the anterior structures intact. Postoperative cast immobilization or instrumentation is performed if there are adequate bony elements. Posterior fusion alone is rarely indicated in this population due to the high incidence of the crankshaft phenomenon with persistent anterior growth in the young child. The exception is the case of kyphoscoliosis with anterior or anterolateral failure of segmentation.

Combined anterior and posterior arthrodesis in situ is a better alternative than posterior arthrodesis alone in most cases. This approach limits the possibility of the crankshaft phenomenon. The indications are age less than 10 years, marked growth imbalance, and unilateral unsegmented bar with contralateral hemivertebra.

Apical fusion alone has not demonstrated good long-term outcome and is not recommended in the treatment of congenital scoliosis.

Deformity Correction and Arthrodesis

Large, flexible congenital curvatures over 40 degrees can be treated with instrumented or uninstrumented corrective surgery. A posterior approach is indicated for curvatures less than 70 degrees in patients over 10 years of age, while more rigid curves over 70 degrees or curvature in young patients with open triradiate cartilage and Risser 0 or 1 skeletal maturity may be treated by anterior release and fusion followed by posterior fusion. The goal of surgery is to restore coronal and sagittal balance, similar to the goal in adolescent idiopathic scoliosis. Instrumentation is often complicated by anatomic variation of the congenital spine. Computed tomography can be helpful to determine the presence and size of pedicles if screw instrumentation is desired.

Owing to concern about neurologic complications, compressive maneuvers are favored over direct distraction when instrumentation is employed, so as not to lengthen the spine in congenital scoliosis. In addition to preoperative MRI screening of the spine, multimodality intraoperative spinal cord monitoring and the Stagnara wake-up test or ankle clonus test should be routinely utilized to monitor spinal cord integrity during surgery.

Uninstrumented fusion with corrective casting has a very low neurologic complication rate; however, curve correction is lower than with instrumented procedures and pseudarthrosis rates are higher.

Excision of Hemivertebra

The goal of the procedure is to remove the anomaly prophylactically and to achieve deformity correction by using the excision as a wedge osteotomy. The accepted indications for this procedure are for the treatment of lumbosacral hemivertebra with fixed imbalance, apparent leg-length discrepancy as a result of pelvic obliquity secondary to lumbosacral deformity, and truncal imbalance in patients at an early stage of growth before the compensatory curves have become rigid. It has become more aggressively applied recently to optimize spinal correction and minimize levels that are fused. Hemivertebra excision is performed by removing the hemivertebra and its adjacent discs. The vertebra is removed anteriorly to the dura and anterior half of the pedicle, and morselized graft is placed in the defect. This is followed by removal of the remaining pedicle and hemilamina by a posterior approach. Instrumentation is performed if the local anatomy allows. Otherwise, cast immobilization is performed. The procedure may be performed in one or two stages. Correction ranging from 40% to 67% without significant neurologic complication using the one- or two-stage technique has been reported. Hemivertebra excision may also be performed from a posterior approach alone, removing the pedicle and body of the hemivertebra through this approach.

Osteotomy and Arthrodesis

Severe, rigid scoliosis as a result of untreated congenital scoliosis is characterized by marked truncal decompensation and, at times, fixed pelvic obliquity. The most severe deformities are often associated with mixed vertebral anomalies and rib anomalies, such as synostosis. These are optimally treated with osteotomy and arthrodesis. Options include multiple posterior osteotomies such as Smith-Peterson osteotomies with posterior instrumentation, pedicle subtraction osteotomies, vertebral column resection performed from an anterior-posterior approach, posterior-based decancellation procedures, or posterior-based vertebral column resections.

The goals of surgery are to restore spinal balance and to preserve or restore pulmonary function. These patients will have significant restrictive lung disease and are at risk for pulmonary failure. In some cases, pulmonary function can be stabilized or improved by these procedures. Complication rates are elevated in comparison to those in non-

resection procedures and include neurologic injury, severe blood loss, and pseudarthrosis.

Growing Instrumentation Systems

Intermittent Rod Distraction. Because many congenital scoliotic curves can be quite severe in very young patients, nonfusion systems allow for growth of the spine to allow chest wall and spine development. A number of procedures employ posteriorly placed subcutaneous/subfascial rods to correct curves by intermittent distraction. These systems include hooks or pedicle screws placed at the extremes of the curve and neither stripping nor fusing the middle segment and allowing, through rod connectors, for distraction every 6 months. Arthrodesis is performed at the end of the process of repeated distractions. Curve correction ranged from 48% to 62% in their series. Neurologic complications are rare in this group, but infection, hardware failure, and junctional kyphosis are problems. A similar procedure is a Luque trolley, which consists of segmental sublaminar wires without fusion. This has been associated with premature fusion and a high complication rate. Newer systems that are under experimentation include pedicle screw systems that allow for growth of the rod and spine. Clinical outcome with these systems is lacking.

Expansion Thoracoplasty. Thoracic insufficiency syndrome can be found in the setting of congenital scoliosis. Thoracic insufficiency syndrome can be caused by primary deformities, such as rib absence or synostoses, or secondary deformities resulting from degree of curvature, rotation, or foreshortening of the affected side. The effects of these deformities are aberrant lung function and development. The end result is extensive extrinsic restrictive lung disease that leads to poor exercise tolerance, recurrent respiratory infections, and eventually profound respiratory compromise that could require ventilatory support.

Thorax expansion is meant to mechanically stabilize and distract the thorax, thereby correcting three-dimensional thoracic deformity and improving volume available for respiration and lung growth.

One such device that was designed for this purpose is the vertical expandable prosthetic titanium rib (Synthes Spine Co., West Chester, PA). This was developed to expand the thorax and indirectly corrects spinal deformity, thus allowing spinal, thoracic, and probably lung growth to occur. It was also developed to prevent the respiratory compromise caused by thoracic insufficiency syndrome. It has been used in the United States since the late 1980s. The limited reported results demonstrate positive effects on both lung function and development.

Instrumentation is currently available as a rib-to-rib implant, a hybrid implant (rib-to-lumbar hook), and a rib-to-pelvis implant. Thorax expansion is applied to the affected ribs on the concavity of the curve, and distraction results in expansion of the thoracic cavity on the ipsilateral side as well as an indirect correction of the spinal deformity without instrumentation of the spine itself, thereby preserving longitudinal growth of the spine. This also can be utilized bilaterally for primary thoracic insufficiency syndromes such as spondylothoracic dysplasia and Jeune syndrome.

Campbell and colleagues reported on 27 patients with thoracic insufficiency syndrome secondary to congenital scoliosis with a mean age of 3.2 years at the time of initial surgery (range: 0.6 to 12.5 years). They found that the patients had a mean of 10.4 procedures over the 5.7-year follow-up period. The mean height of the thoracic spine increased by a mean of 0.71 cm per year. No significant change was noted in regard to primary or secondary respiration or oxygen saturation; however, they found a significant decrease in mean respiratory rate, and one patient on preoperative continuous positive airway pressure was successfully weaned postoperatively. There were 52 complications reported in 22 patients. The complications included component migration (seven), skin complications (four), wound infection, pulmonary infection, and two cases of brachial plexopathy.

Smith and colleagues reported a multicenter review of 257 patients who were operated on from 1990 to 2003. They identified 455 adverse events in 154 patients (60%). Seventy-five percent were classified as minor to moderate and included wound infection (17%), pulmonary infection (15%), and device migration (15%). Twenty-one percent were classified as severe and included gastrointestinal or urologic problems (9%), cardiac problems (8%), device failure (5%), and neurologic problems (5%). Five percent were classified as life-threatening or fatal.

Expansion thoracostomy with serial lengthening could be the preferred treatment for young children with chest wall deformity and scoliosis associated with fused ribs. The potential serious complications that are associated with this procedure require multidisciplinary care and attention to details of soft-tissue management.

Adjunctive Treatment

Halofemoral Traction. Arlet and colleagues reported the use of halofemoral traction to progressively correct a 145-degree curve in a patient with preoperative restrictive lung disease and cor pulmonale. After adequate correction over a period of 3 weeks, instrumented fusion was performed, obtaining satisfactory curve correction and improving lung vital capacity. The authors suggest the usefulness of this procedure in patients with high-risk, very severe congenital scoliosis.

Thoracoscopy. Multiple authors have reported on the efficacy of thoracoscopic surgery employed in the correction of idiopathic scoliosis. Thoracoscopy is associated with a lower level of morbidity in comparison to traditional thoracotomy when anterior release is necessary for curve correction. Although some studies have included patients with congenital scoliosis, no exclusive series of congenital scoliosis has been reported to date. Thoracoscopic hemivertebra resection has also been reported.

SUMMARY

Congenital scoliosis is a potentially serious condition. Early diagnosis is essential to anticipate prognosis based on the type and site of anomaly, the amount of spinal growth remaining, and the degree of growth imbalance anticipated. Congenital scoliosis is associated with other systemic defects, including genitourinary, cardiac, and intraspinal anomalies. Appropriate screening for these abnormalities should be performed. Deterioration of the deformity must be prevented. Deformity that is at risk for progression, such as segmentation failure, requires immediate surgical treatment. It is much better to do a simple operation to balance spinal growth early on than to wait and perform a more complex salvage procedure when the deformity is severe and the patient's cardiopulmonary status might be compromised. New developments such as thoracoscopic techniques and expansion thoracoplasty could play an increasingly important role in the treatment of severe curves.

PEARLS & PITFALLS

PEARLS

- The prognosis for curve progression in congenital scoliosis is based on three factors: the age of the patient, the location of the curve, and the type of anomaly.
- A coned-down radiograph is helpful in defining spinal anomalies.
- All patients with congenital scoliosis are indicated to undergo an MRI evaluation of the complete spine.
- Three key factors in gaining optimal results in these patients are early recognition, anticipation of prognosis, and prevention of deterioration.
- It is much better to do a simple operation to balance spinal growth early on than to wait and perform a more complex salvage procedure when the deformity is severe and the patient's cardiopulmonary status might be compromised.

PITFALLS

- Beware of intraspinal and extraspinal abnormalities that can be associated with congenital scoliosis.
- Congenital scoliosis/kyphosis is associated with the highest rate of neurologic injury following operative correction compared with other forms of scoliosis.
- Bracing should not be employed in situations of severe imbalance, in congenital lordosis or kyphosis, in skeletally mature patients, or in the presence of a rigid curve such as those associated with unilateral failure of segmentation.
- Beware of the crankshaft phenomenon in performing posterior fusion alone.
- Thoracic insufficiency syndrome with impaired lung function can affect surgical outcome.

Illustrative Case Presentations

CASE 1. A 3½-Year-Old Boy with Fused Ribs and Thoracic Insufficiency

The child was managed with thoracostomy and vertical expandable prosthetic titanium rib placement.

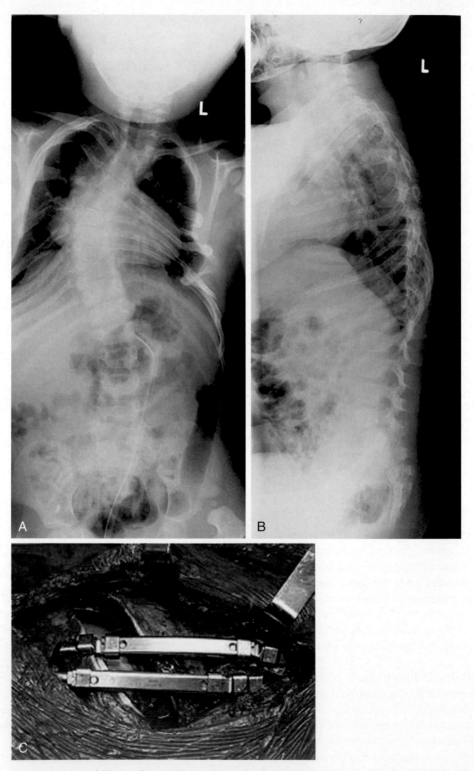

Figure 9-1. Posteroanterior (**A**) and lateral (**B**) standing scoliosis radiographs. **C,** Thoracostomy and vertical expandable prosthetic titanium rib placement.

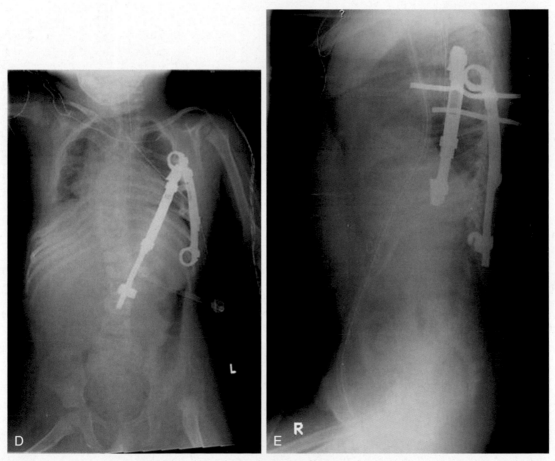

Figure 9-1, cont'd. Posteroanterior (**D**) and lateral (**E**) radiographs after vertical expandable prosthetic titanium rib placement.

CASE 2. An Adolescent, Skeletally Mature Boy with Progressive Scoliosis and Kyphosis
The patient was treated by combined thoracoscopic release and posterior instrumented fusion.

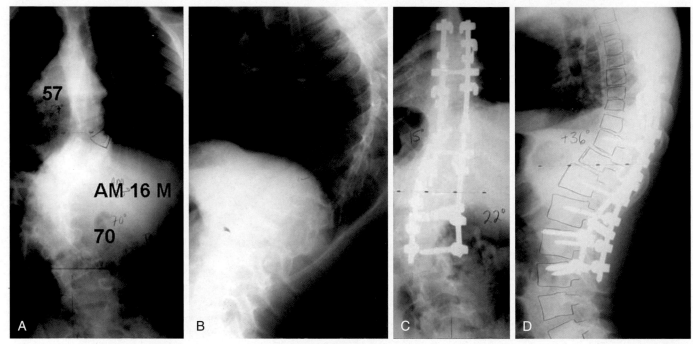

Figure 9-2. Preoperative posteroanterior (**A**) radiograph demonstrating scoliosis and lateral radiograph (**B**) demonstrating kyphosis. Postoperative posteroanterior (**C**) and lateral (**D**) radiographs following thoracoscopic release and posterior instrumented fusion.

CASE 3. A 5-Year-Old Boy Demonstrated Progression of a Congenital Curvature Due to Fully Segmented Midlumbar Hemivertebrae
Posterior-based hemivertebrae excision was performed, resulting in near 100% correction that was maintained 3 years postoperatively. The procedure allows for maximal correction with minimal impact on growth and function.

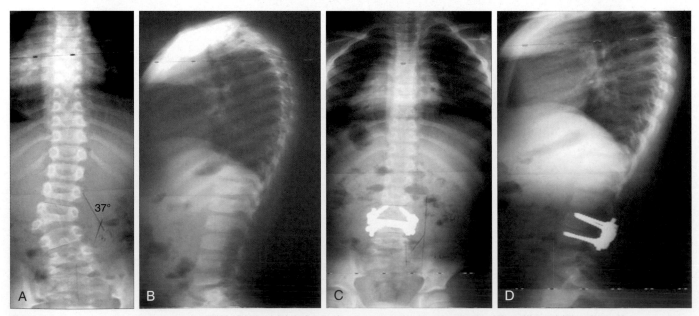

Figure 9-3. Preoperative posteroanterior (**A**) and lateral (**B**) radiographs. Postoperative posteroanterior (**C**) and lateral (**D**) radiographs demonstrating a near 100% correction.

CASE 4. A 7-Year-Old with Failure of Segmentation of Multiple Thoracic Segments and Progressive Curvature of the Thoracic Spine

Treatment consisted of a vertebral column resection procedure through the apex of the congenital fusion and instrumentation of the anomalous spine only to maintain growth and function through normal spinal segments, resulting in 70% correction of the deformity at the index procedure. As is not uncommon in a young child who is treated surgically, adding-on to the proximal and distal ends of the curvature was noted 2 years postoperatively. The plan of treatment is for bracing to control the relatively flexible ends of the curvature, but the possibility of further curve progression and surgery remains high.

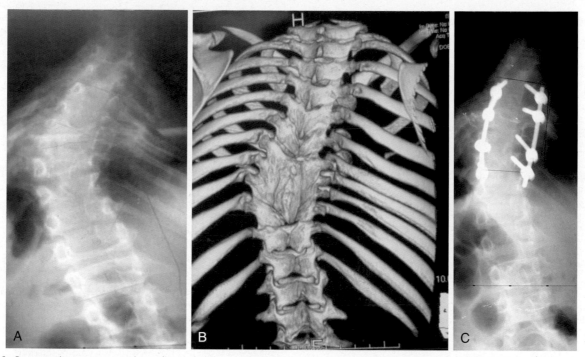

Figure 9-4. Preoperative posteroanterior radiograph (**A**) and coronal reformatted computed tomography scan (**B**). **C,** Postoperative posteroanterior radiograph.

CASE 5. A 7-Year-Old Boy with Multiple Mixed Congenital Spinal Anomalies and Progressive Scoliosis

The patient was treated with a growing rod procedure. A vertical expandable prosthetic titanium rib would have been another option for treatment of this child.

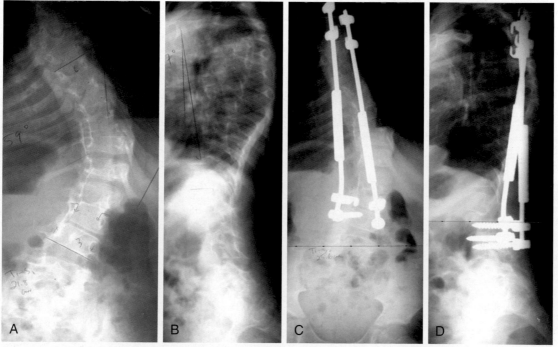

Figure 9-5. Preoperative (**A**) and lateral (**B**) radiographs. Postoperative posteroanterior (**C**) and lateral (**D**) radiographs after treatment.

REFERENCE

Smith JT, Skaggs DL, Smart M: Adverse events associated with the Vertical Expandable Prosthetic Titanium Rib (VEPTR): A multicenter review of 257 patients. Paper presented at the Scoliosis Research Society 39th Annual Meeting, Buenos Aires, Argentina, September 6–9, 2004.

SUGGESTED READINGS

Artlet V, Papin P, Marchesi D: Halofemoral traction and sliding rods in the treatment of neurologically compromised congenital scoliosis: Technique. Eur Spine J 1999;8:329–331.

This study focuses on severe congenital scoliosis, in which traction (whether with a halo or instrumental) is known to expose patients to neurologic complications. However, patients with restrictive lung disease might benefit from halo traction during the course of the surgical treatment. The authors conclude that the technique that they describe using sliding rods in combination with halofemoral traction can be useful in high-risk, very severe congenital scoliosis.

Basu PS, Elsebaie H, Noordeen MNH: Congenital spinal deformity: A comprehensive assessment at presentation. Spine 2002;27: 2255–2259.

A series of 126 consecutive patients with congenital spinal deformity is presented. The main objective is to assess the incidence of intraspinal anomaly and other organic defects associated with different types of spine deformity at presentation. MRI and echocardiography should be an essential part of the evaluation of patients with congenital spinal deformity, and special attention should be paid to patients with segmentation abnormalities, mixed defects, and kyphosis.

Boachie-Adjei O, Bradford DS: Vertebral column resection and arthrodesis for complex spinal deformities. J Spinal Disord 1991;4: 193–202.

Sixteen patients aged 13 to 55 with severe rigid spine deformities were treated by two-stage anterior and posterior vertebral column resection, fusion, and segmental spinal instrumentation. They conclude that decancellation, which includes radical vertebral column resection, spinal shortening, and segmental instrumentation posteriorly, can achieve a balanced correction and significant pain relief for the select patient who presents with severe rigid spine deformity that is not adequately treatable by more established techniques.

Campbell RM Jr, Smith MD, Mayes TC, et al: The effect of opening wedge thoracostomy on thoracic insufficiency syndrome associated with fused ribs and congenital scoliosis. J Bone Joint Surg Am 2004;86-A:1659–1674.

Opening wedge thoracostomy with use of a chest wall distractor directly treats segmental hypoplasia of the hemithorax, which results from fused ribs associated with congenital scoliosis. The operation addresses thoracic insufficiency syndrome by lengthening and expanding the constricted hemithorax and allowing growth of the thoracic spine and the rib cage. The procedure corrects most components of chest wall deformity and indirectly corrects congenital scoliosis, without the need for spine fusion. The technique requires special training and should be performed by a multispecialty team.

Hedequist D, Emans J: Congenital scoliosis. J Am Acad Orthop Surg 2004;12:266–274.

This review concludes that congenital scoliosis is caused by early embryologic errors in vertebral column formation. Defining the deformity, predicting the natural history, and applying the correct treatment can help to ensure successful management. Most congenital spine anomalies can be classified, and many have a predictable natural history. Because the deformities are associated with other organ system anomalies in more than half of patients, the surgeon should look for cardiac, auditory, genitourinary, and renal anomalies. Intraspinal abnormalities are present in approximately one third of patients with congenital spine deformities. Curve progression is best documented by measuring identical landmarks on sequential radiographs. MRI is warranted when curve progression is established or when surgical intervention is planned. Management of progressive deformity is generally by early in situ fusion because orthotic treatment is rarely appropriate. Other surgical techniques include combined anterior and posterior epiphysiodesis, hemivertebra resection, and reconstructive osteotomies.

Hoppenfeld S, Gross A, Andrews C, Lonner B: The ankle clonus test for assessment of the integrity of the spinal cord during operations for scoliosis. J Bone Joint Surg Am 1997;79:208–212.

The ankle clonus test, a method for evaluating the integrity of the spinal cord during operations for scoliosis, is predicated on the finding that patients who are recovering from general anesthesia normally have temporary ankle clonus bilaterally. An absence of transient ankle clonus has been shown to indicate neurologic compromise. The test was performed on 1006 patients whose conditions were managed with spinal arthrodesis and instrumentation and 115 control patients who had an operation under general anesthesia because of a condition that was unrelated to the spine. It concludes that the ankle clonus test was found to be more accurate than the wake-up test and monitoring of somatosensory evoked potentials for predicting neurologic compromise.

Kesling KL, Lonstein JE, Denis F, et al: The crankshaft phenomenon after posterior spinal arthrodesis for congenital scoliosis. Spine 2003;38:267–271.

This study identifies the incidence of any possible risk factors for the crankshaft phenomenon after posterior spinal arthrodesis for congenital scoliosis. It concludes that crankshafting was observed in 15% of the patients, more often with larger curves and earlier fusions.

Leatherman KD, Dickson R: Two-stage corrective surgery for congenital deformities of the spine. J Bone Joint Surg Br 1979;61:324–328.

This study describes 60 patients who had a two-stage procedure to correct congenital deformities of the spine. In the 50 patients with scoliosis, half of the deformities were due to hemivertebrae and half to unilateral bars. The average correction of the deformity was 47%. Early neurologic signs that were observed in two patients with a diastematomyelia resolved. Posterior spinal fusion alone in the rapidly progressing congenital deformity might not prevent further progression, particularly in cases with unilateral bars. The study concludes that anterior resection of the vertebral body with later posterior fusion with Harrington instrumentation is safe and effective.

Lopez-Sosa F, Guille JT, Bowen JR: Rotation of the spine in congenital scoliosis. J Pediatr Orthop 1995;15:528–534.

This study reviewed the progression of spinal rotation in 100 consecutive patients with 119 curves. Eighty-four patients with a single curve were included in this study. Thirty-nine cases were due to failure of segmentation, 38 cases were due to failure of formation, and 7 cases were unclassifiable. The study concludes that because of the uncertainty of remaining growth potential in congenitally dysplastic vertebrae, possible future growth in the spine should be considered before undertaking operative procedures.

McMaster MJ: Congenital scoliosis. In Weinstein SL (ed): The Pediatric Spine: Principles and Practice, 2nd ed. Philadelphia: Lippincott Williams & Wilkins, 2001, pp 161–177.

This textbook is organized around 12 sections, each consisting of one or more chapters. The major sections are devoted to disease groups: Congenital Anomalies, Developmental Abnormalities, Traumatic Conditions, Inflammatory and Infectious Conditions, Neoplasms and Malformations, Metabolic Disease, and Neuromuscular Disease. Each of these sections gives the reader a comprehensive framework for surgical decision making when managing children with these disorders. While several chapters are devoted to idiopathic scoliosis, for which neurosurgeons are rarely consulted, the coverage of congenital anomalies, trauma, infections, and neoplasms is broad and well done.

Niemeyer T, Freeman BJC, Grevitt MP, Webb JK: Anterior throacoscopic surgery followed by posterior instrumentation and fusion in spinal deformity. Eur Spine J 2000;9:299–304.

This study evaluated the clinical results, radiologic correction, and morbidity following anterior thoracoscopic surgery followed by posterior instrumentation and fusion, to determine whether there is evidence to support the efficacy of this technique. Twenty-nine patients undergoing thoracoscopic anterior release or growth arrest followed by posterior fusion and instrumentation were evaluated from clinical and radiologic viewpoints.

Rittler M, Paz JE, Castilla EE: VACTERL association: Epidemiologic definition and delineation. Am J Med Genet 1996;63:529–536.

This study departed from a preconceived definition of VACTERL by including more than one of these six anomalies in the same infant: V (vertebral anomalies), A (anal atresia), C (congenital heart disease), TE (tracheo-esophageal fistula or esophageal atresia), R (renourinary anomalies), and L (radial limb defect). Under this definition, 524 infants were identified by ECLAMC out of almost 3,000,000 births between 1967 and 1990. Observed association rates among VACTERL components, as well as between VACTERL and other defects, were compared to randomly expected values obtained from 10,084 multiply malformed infants (casuistic method) from the same birth sample.

Ruf M, Harms J: Hemivertebra resection by a posterior approach: Innovative operative technique and first results. Spine 2002;27: 1116–1123.

This is a retrospective study of hemivertebra resection using transpedicular instrumentation by a posterior approach in young children. The objective was to assess a new method of early intervention in congenital scoliosis by a posterior approach. It concludes that posterior resection of hemivertebrae with transpedicular instrumentation is a safe and promising procedure that offers significant advantages for controlling congenital deformity: excellent correction in both the frontal and sagittal planes, short segment of fusion, high stability, no need for an anterior approach, and low neurologic risk.

Winter RB, Lonstein J, Denis F, Santa-Ana de la Rosa H: Convex growth arrest for progressive congenital scoliosis due to hemivertebrae. J Pediatr Orthop 1988;8:633–638.

This study looks at 13 patients with progressive congenital scoliosis due to hemivertebrae or hemivertebrae associated with other spinal anomalies who were treated by convex anterior and posterior hemiarthrodesis and hemiepiphysiodesis. It concludes that this procedure is a valuable treatment modality for selected patients with congenital scoliosis.

Winter RB, Moe JH, Lonstein JE: Posterior spinal arthrodesis for congenital scoliosis. An analysis of two hundred and ninety patients, five to nineteen years old. J Bone Joint Surg Am 1984;66:1188–1197.

This study analyzed the results of posterior arthrodesis of the spine for congenital scoliosis, with or without Harrington instrumentation, in 290 of 323 surgical patients between the ages of 5 and 19 years. The length of follow-up averaged 6 years and ranged from 2 to 28 years. The average curve before surgery was 55 degrees (range: 13 to 155 degrees), the average curve at correction was 38 degrees (range: 5 to 102 degrees), and the average curve at final follow-up was 44 degrees (range: 5 to 103 degrees). It describes the different surgical procedures that were performed and their complications.

Cerebral Palsy and Other Neuromuscular Disorders in Children

Roy M. Nuzzo *and* Thomas J. Errico

Unfortunately, some children have neurologic pathology that physically disables them more and more as the neuropathology progresses. Typically, each variant has a complex name or even a group of names with historical, eponymic, and etiologic underpinnings. In a way, these many names draw attention to the scope of our ignorance of complex biochemical interactions.

In contrast, some children have a nonprogressive neuropathology that impairs physical development and movement as the most obvious specific findings in a cluster of many. One term, *cerebral palsy*, collectively denotes this neurologically nonprogressive category. Also different is the practice of distinguishing members of the group by the scope of impairment rather than by the esoteric chemical or genetic features. For this reason, whereas the progressive disorders are many, by count of their categories and names, each disorder being tiny in individual membership, cerebral palsy is a lone fuzzy designation with huge membership.

SAVVY AND WIT

Cerebral palsy thus becomes the 800-pound gorilla that gets attention. Do you doubt this? Go into any hospital and ask where the CP clinic is. Somebody, very practiced, without looking up, gestures at the posted sign with the arrow. Then see what happens when you ask where the clinic for metachromatic leukodystrophy is. If you persist in your descriptions, you eventually get asked whether that is anything like cerebral palsy. With a sigh you say, "Well yessss, sort of." That same sign with the same arrow directs you. You can hear, from behind you, in a perturbed whisper, "Why didn't you just say that in the first place?"

It should not be surprising, then, that in clinical practice, there is a coming together of those who share similar needs of resources and, to a lesser degree, a history of early onset. Scattered through the defined disorders of perinatal onset that are referred to as *cerebral palsy* are found victims of near drowning, unsuccessful hanging, bubble gum

aspiration, electrocution, burst cerebral aneurysms, post-neurosurgical tumor resection, head trauma from automobile accidents, and so forth. Even excluding these, almost 40% of the core group will be found to have an inborn metabolic or genetic anomaly. Genetic interference with developing neurons may be directly causal, or genes may act merely by inciting prematurity, the claimed cause of about 30% of cases of "true" cerebral palsy.

For the obsessive categorist, it is a problem. Patients with progressive disorders intermingle in cerebral palsy facilities. Distinctions, clear in print, are simply not found in the treatment facility structure.

With cerebral palsy, the greatest dangers are intellectual momentum and diagnostic overgeneralization. Broad rules of thumb fail. Pitfalls are plentiful but not obvious or intuitive. Generalities send us on resource-sapping unproductive forays, while subtlety beckons our recognition. No single treatment method or device can be effectively and safely uniformly applied. Our art of medicine is nowhere as artful or as intuitive as it must be in managing this population.

Scoliosis treatment does not demand highly convoluted formulations of elaborate goals. To the initiated, they are simply too obvious. We know what we want and where it is that we want to go. What requires our attention is constant awareness of what we don't want to happen in the process. We enter each surgical venture with a clearly thought-out concept of avoidance of complications. Mental shopping lists have value, but when everybody on the block has a dog, the wise shopper carefully scrutinizes the sidewalk while walking to the store!

DEFINITIONS

Cerebral palsy is a historical term that arose specifically to dispel the stigma that children who moved in an awkward way were not doing that because of idiocy. The public, at that time, did know what a palsy was. Anybody with an industrial mishap or a touch of polio could come by one.

The palsy designation played up the motor weakness or inability to control movement. As a term, *cerebral palsy* has been so integrated into our language that some have sought to dodge its own stigma by further wordplay. *Static encephalopathy* is a synonym. Although in actuality more inclusive of nonmotor features, this term is used exclusively by some neurologists and occasionally by parents who deny that their child has cerebral palsy.

SAVVY AND WIT

No, it is that other "whatchamacallit," as they dig for their slip of paper on which this obfuscating term has been carefully written down with pronunciation helpers. We can repeat our test! Where is the static encephalopathy clinic? Where do you land? Oh—the CP clinic.

So, grading them like olives or eggs, we segregate children with cerebral palsy.

The olives: How large is the palsy? One limb? Two? Three? Four? This classification does not make sense but is thoroughly ingrained in bureaucracy. One affected limb is *monoplegia*. Two can be *hemiplegia* or *diplegia*. Three is *triplegia*. Four affected limbs used to be referred to as *quadriplegia*; however, this term has been preempted by patients with cervical spinal, not cerebral, injury. Those with four limbs involved are currently referred to as having *total-body cerebral palsy*, because in no one with four limbs affected are the head and neck spared. *Paraplegia*, in this context, is also no longer used, as it has come to refer to lower spinal injury. Die-hards who cling to quadriplegia reassert that term by using *spastic quadriplegia* interchangeably with *total-body cerebral palsy*.

The eggs: What is the grade or quality of the palsy itself? *Spastic*: reacts to stretch with spasm. *Athetoid*: continuous writhing, snakelike movements of the limbs. *Chorea*: fidgety excessive movement that is tremulous under resistive tension. *Dystonia*: rigidity with postures generating other postures in other places. A clearer and more useful way of looking at cerebral palsy will be addressed later in the chapter.

Designating cerebral palsy in this way is akin to describing stars by their magnitude—how bright they look from here. It helps you point, but it tells you little about the thing itself. As with comprehensive star catalogs, guides to the constellations of infantile neurologic syndromes are weighty and ever subjected to update.

GENERALITIES OF NEUROMUSCULAR CONDITIONS

Static Conditions

By definition, the brain pathology of cerebral palsy does not worsen. Outward manifestations, however, do worsen and can confuse the issue. Uneven muscle tone and growth over time cause twisting and odd bending of limbs and postures and flattening and dislocation of joints, as well as progressive loss of equality with normal children. One must beware, however, because medical comorbidities such as aspiration, status epilepticus, lurking cardiac defects, brain ventricle obstruction, and cyst expansion can indeed further worsen the underlying static cause. An anoxic event that damaged the brain might also have damaged the heart. Structural heart defects commonly damage the brain. If the initial cause was a major inborn error, that gun is still loaded; it could fire again.

Progressive Disorders

Progressive disorders are set apart, not just out of academic compulsion, but because there is even more certainty of what else will eventually fail and when. Possible association of deficits in other systems, if lurking, can affect surgery or recovery and healing. Although progressive disorders tend to be listed like entries in a telephone book, there is a white pages/yellow pages subdivision. Generally, the quest for diagnosis looks along lines of primarily neurologic versus muscle degeneration. Even when so divided, distinctions may be artificial, as genetic anomalies can be multifaceted. Certain variants of muscular dystrophy show substantial neurologic involvement.

Faced with a scoliosis that is worsening, where do these categorizations leave us? Progressive cause or not, case by case, we need to think about the actual problems at hand, and those problems are not diagnostic labels. Is this particular scoliosis going to harm or, given other considerations, not change the patient's ultimate quality of life? What is the speed of this process? Is this patient going to be able to appreciate an improvement if it is attained? If treatment goes well, will the patient perceive it or will the family reap any benefits? If it goes badly, can the patient's condition become even worse? The important maxim "No situation is so bad that it can't be made worse" must be remembered! With all these lists of findings, which one is most at work here? We need to know, or at least guess at, the mechanics of deformation when figuring how to counter the effects of progression and time the surgery that may result.

Active Deformation

Active deformation is caused by generally asymmetric muscle balance or the unrelenting motor action of a specific group. A lumbar hip-hiking reflex has an extraordinary association with structural scoliosis. When the index finger is run up the lower right paraspinal area, does a prominent reflex elevation of the right pelvis follow? That lumbar arcing or hip hike is called *incurvatum* or the *Gallant sign*. If this response is one-sided, scoliosis is almost assured. It is just a question of how much and when. Chances are, given even a loud noise, that the incurvatum that was elicited by your finger stroke will again be seen.

It isn't just a "sign"; it is what happens! This built-in predisposition will be prominent during any chronic noxious stimulus, so chronic bladder or urethral inflammation or infection or colon distention can cause scoliosis to worsen. A finger stroke is low on the list of potential stimuli.

Anything that is noxious in cerebral palsy brings out predisposed posturing. Treat it, and you treat the scoliosis. In the very young, we prescribe hard-to-tolerate braces and then give up, blaming noncompliance. Or we lessen the active deforming pull—directly—with medication and try again. Treatment tries to stay below the threshold of reactive posturing. You can guarantee that if a child turns blue and holds his or her breath when a brace is applied, the caretaker will remove it. Period. You can get all bent out of shape over noncompliance or rethink the problem. What underpins the reluctance to follow prescription?

Bracing

With our most difficult patients, we commonly use two different braces for scoliosis, which we swap back and forth. Typically, one is based on horizontal derotation, whereas the other is a side-bending type. In no case do we allow pressure on the abdomen. Between gastroesophageal reflux and aspiration, braces that cause significant abdominal pressure are losers from the beginning. The brace cannot decrease overall body volume. Any "push" in one place needs to allow a "response to push" somewhere else. We displace body parts in the direction we want them to go, creating space with the brace to accept the displacement.

How can we make the push less nasty? Knowing the source of the forces helps. Visualize this: A child with suddenly prominent lumbar scoliosis is placed supine. One thigh is held flat to the table. The other leg is then passively flexed at the hip and knee by the examiner, bringing the knee toward the chest before it is then returned to being extended. With repetition of this passive, single-sided hip flexion-extension motion, the child might bend at the waist laterally rightward then leftward, looking like a windshield wiper in the process. As the psoas pulls and then relaxes with the alternating hip position, a reaction of intermittent lumbar curvature occurs. Treat the psoas spasm, and you treat the scoliosis. That is the scoliosis. Then brace the scoliosis to try to prevent it from recurring. Botulinum toxin type A (Botox) can be injected into the psoas (posterior approach at tip of transverse process of L4). Although the botulinum toxin effect fades over time, this does not mean that there is necessarily a need for drug injections at 3-month intervals. It is the intention to get the brace tolerated and back into the game. A brief respite from difficult forces by medication, physical therapy, or whatever allows resumption of conservative measures. Your knowledge and clinical intuition supply the "whatever."

We don't know exactly why, but fibrosis is common in muscles that are under faulty neurologic control. Such fibrosis acts as a passive constraint around which growth deforms. Such fibrosis will not respond to relaxing drugs or to neurochemical blockers. Such fibrosis hides within neurologically driven overcontracted muscles and confounds the understanding of what is doing what. Block the neurologic signal driving the spasticity, yet the "spasm" doesn't go away! What's up with that? Now we know!

Approaching puberty, we expect rapid growth. Sure, idiopathic scoliosis worsens with rapid growth, but so might a seizure disorder in a child with a neurologic syndrome, which then worsens the deformity. In fact, the seizure disorder might be subclinical for a long time before it becomes recognized as "seizures." In the meantime, asymmetric neural activity is curving the spine. We need to pester our neurologists when we suspect this association. Be suspicious. Botulinum toxin might well provide a reprieve, but the underlying seething neural focus needs attention.

We have even witnessed cases in which scoliosis was made to go away by drugs given to arrest precocious puberty. How? By turning off the low-grade seizure activity, which was in turn brought on by the premature hormonal change. Pubertal hormonal change, clearly, is contributory to seizure activity, and seizure activity can rapidly worsen paralytic scoliosis.

When a child has asymmetric background tone generation, any stimulus becomes deforming. A child with sinusitis presents with one arm waving overhead while leaning strongly. A child with a toothache does the same. Ear problems produce striking sudden odd postures. We have also diagnosed and treated many cases of scoliosis caused by belly ache. On the list of causes of neuromuscular scoliosis, one needs to include colon distention, bladder infection, kidney stones, ureteritis, appendicitis, and splinter, among others. Although these problems appear to be within the domain of general pediatrics, an odd posture in a child severely involved with cerebral palsy who can't verbalize the cause tends to get seen first by an orthopedist. We have determined Lyme disease and juvenile rheumatism to be causes of cerebral palsy "worsening."

PEARL

Cobb is also a salad. Never merely apply the Cobb angle measurement in treating paralytic scoliosis without a consideration of the ingredients that might be in it. Are you measuring an angle or in reality a complex reaction to other medical conditions?

Passive Growth Restraint

Muscles or ligaments that fibrose do not grow sufficiently and thus act as tethers around which growth will deform. Bone growth tethers, such as bar formation in congenital scoliosis, are clear enough. But how do we find, so as to divide, paraspinal soft-tissue growth constraints? A very nasty example of this is seen with severe paralytic lordosis. In some patients, the spine has such a forward arc that the patient appears to have an abdominal tumor or aneurysm protruding through the anterior abdominal wall. Neurosurgical procedures performed on posterior elements can be followed by this forward arcing as a result of either fibrotic changes or spontaneous bony fusions, but so can unremitting tension in low-back extensors. We have used percutaneous transverse fasciotomy in some of these cases as a temporizing measure. Injection of botulinum toxin can test the concept if the fibrosis is partial and hyperactive muscle tone is predominant.

Collapse

Failure to support or weakness of control against gravity can produce scoliosis. Whether it goes to the right or to the left, the key factor is that within the longer floppy curve may lurk a shorter stiff segment that changes little when the longer curve is reversed by bending, bracing, or instrumentation. Is that short segment the real culprit? Is it just an aggravating issue? Either way, it must be addressed. When treating long C-curves, we employ worst-case measurements to identify problem segments. That is, we measure the worst portion found in any given radiographic image regardless of what levels were measured earlier. Also, we measure the original span. Occasionally, a brace might be found to reduce the overall curve while a central portion does not change or even worsens. This tells you that that limited area is out to get you. Occasionally, in a very young child, we fuse a short segment within a larger curve to allow the continuation of conservative management of the rest of the spine rather than getting into long instrumentations with or without fusion. It is a choice made on savvy. When confronted with a very thin, sickly, young-looking child

with such a curve, thin musculature, and nearly zero body fat, would one really want to put long, thick, high-profile metal in that skinny place?

PATIENT APPEARANCE

Age is a designation that entraps. In the cerebral palsy population, chronologic age confuses. It might be better not to know the patient's age. In seeking advice, you quote chronologic age, and advice from cookbooks follows. Such advice is doomed. More important is the age that your patient seems to be. Maturation is key, but maturation is all over the board in neuromuscular patients. There are 19-year-olds weighing 25 pounds with the physiology of a 6-year-old. Such a patient cannot be treated as a 19-year-old.

Imagine a 14-year-old girl with 25 degrees of lumbar scoliosis. Is your mental picture good or bad? You might think, "Fourteen years old with only a 25-degree curve—not so bad." However, consider the following description of the same patient: a 14-year-old girl but looking only 5 years old with 25 degrees of lumbar scoliosis. Have a different mental picture? Now is it good or bad? Physiologically, this is a very immature patient with a 25-degree curve—worse than you thought! Some will refer to certain growth plates to make easy communication sound more elevated, though also susceptible to misinterpretation. A simple description of the general chronologic appearance in the conjunction with actual chronology communicates important critical information to the clinicians.

While you are looking, look at other general features. Consider the following description: This 8-year-old-looking cachectic male has sunken cheeks with retraction of the flesh beneath the mandible. DANGER!! There are many signs of catabolic state (Fig. 10-1). But the most

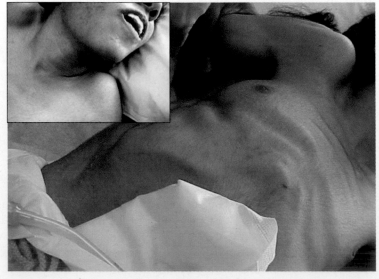

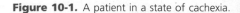
Figure 10-1. A patient in a state of cachexia.

dangerous sign, in a child, is the visibility of the inner surface sunken contour under the jaw, especially at the angle of the jaw. This is an emergency admission. These children can and do code before you get them admitted.

Look very closely. Waxy skin that lacks fine surface texture, like that of a mannequin, is seen in states of chronic nutritional depletion. Beware of the "Tinkertoy" child—one with a succession of prominent joints interconnected by skinny shafts. Generalized loss of muscle (protein) such that unupholstered limbs look to be all joints is a danger sign of both catabolic state and poor reserves. How can we expect the huge anabolic response that is necessary to render our surgery successful in a child who is so drained of substance? Even giving drugs becomes dangerous when they are prescribed by patient weight. Assumptions about distribution volume for that drug might be well off the mark. What water volume is represented in an all-bones-looking person? In this group, we do not push the upper limits of drug dosage without careful reconsideration. Don't ignore difficult medication dosing problems in the history, as it can be an important clue.

PEARL

Force yourself to give the history based on the patient's appearance, as in "a 7-year-old-looking male with features of chronic starvation." Observe the texture of the skin and the degree of muscle tone. The mantra is "Looking, Looking, Looking!"

Morbidity will vary with referral logistics, so specific numbers have little meaning. But as a generalization, children who fit the descriptions of depletion have just about the same mortality and morbidity as do children with untreated leukemia. What we need to know about them is hard or even impossible to measure in a practical way. Our sensitivity in observation is our best clinical tool.

PEARL

Ask this question: Would this child survive a 30% body burn? Minus the infection and damage issues, based on estimates of fluids and weight loss seen postoperatively, posterior spinal fusion is about the metabolic equivalent of a 25% body burn, and anterior-posterior surgery is the equivalent of perhaps 30% or more. The patient's metabolic reserve is critical to the ability to heal the surgical insults we create by our spinal surgical interventions.

TIMING OF SURGICAL INTERVENTION

Besides absolute Cobb angle measurements, a worsening of physiologic vitality despite a static neurologic condition can be a signal to entertain surgical stabilization. Pulmonary function may slip away progressively even with a stable neurologic underpinning. The progressive thoracic curve might be the cause.

The only way to treat a parade of ever-worsening pneumonias and to stop malnutrition might well be to correct spinal deformity. It is common to hear perplexed parents relate that after spinal surgery, their child can now have regular bowel movements and eat regular meals. Why? Because the youngster is no longer chronically obstructed by a tortuous lumbar spine or compressive brace.

We worry about the typical 10-pound weight loss that follows spinal deformity correction and the caloric demands of healing. This loss, however, is then followed by substantial sustained weight gain without any sign of obesity. Body mass is restored with useful proteins restoring strength to an otherwise debilitated patient. Interestingly, spasticity lessens substantially as body mass is restored. We do not know just how malnutrition makes for more spasticity. It does. Restoration of body mass acts like a wonder drug against spasticity. It isn't subtle. Hypoxia and hypercarbia from chronic pulmonary loss and malnutrition are just two elements of the vicious cycle.

Muscular dystrophy presents a special situation. In muscular dystrophy, a progressive disorder, we know that scoliosis, once initiated, simply progresses relentlessly to death or surgery, whichever comes first. To cling to a specific degree of curvature required to advise surgery is simply silly. When a jumper hurls himself from the top of a tall building, his prognosis does not alter floor by floor. Curve prognosis? There is no difference between a 20-degree curve and a 40-degree curve in this disease. Once again, the floor you are passing at that moment is not relevant—it is the sidewalk that should be the concern!

We do know, with muscular dystrophy, that the more prolonged the required surgery and the more pulmonary compromise (intercostal and diaphragm muscle fibrosis and rib cage bellows loss to deformation), the greater is the risk of operative morbidity. In this group, simple operations early on make far more sense than do complicated demanding operations done late. Respiratory compromise in this group is lethal. Spinal deformation is respiratory compromise. Spinal deterioration quickly heralds the end by bringing it on.

In addition, as muscular dystrophy progresses, the use of corticosteroids becomes more aggressive. Spinal surgeons know that corticosteroids tremendously impair bone formation and quality. Spontaneous long bone fractures do occur as steroids are pressed to defend cardiac and vital muscle in this ever-losing battle. The more osteopenic bone gets, the more metal-to-bone fixation points are required in order to not cut out. Time is not your friend.

CHRONIC NUTRITIONAL AND VOLUME RESERVE DEFICIENCY

Healthy scoliosis patients without neurologic issues are quite likely to lose weight after scoliosis surgery despite good appetite. A 10-pound weight loss is common even in patients with smaller frames. As described above, we can infer that the metabolic cost of scoliosis surgery is very high. Nutritional deficits worsen everything in the neurologic patient population, who often have the coexisting problems of low body mass for length. Metabolic reserve, as with circulatory reserve, might be nil.

Scoliosis in neuromuscular patients contributes to all manner of gastrointestinal propulsion difficulties, including constipation, reflux, and quirky eating behaviors. Although few need to have pulmonary insufficiency pointed out, many families are not aware of the scope of ongoing difficulty with feeding. This becomes apparent only in retrospect, well after surgery, when it typically resolves. Months later, families will confide just how transformed bowel function has become and how so many only-now-appreciated feeding issues have gone away.

But that's later. Now, in the preoperative holding area, a patient with poor tissue and metabolic reserves is waiting to be exposed to the most enormous metabolic demand that any surgery can dish out. We are faced with a well-perceived progression of loss of pulmonary function that will worsen with delay. There is a strong desire to proceed.

Yet outcomes may be compromised by problems relating to circulatory and nutritional poverty that have not been addressed. These complications will not be called *chronic volume depletion* or *metabolic insufficiency*; rather, they will be called *wound infection, dehiscence, pseudarthrosis, fixation failure, metal failure,* or *unexplained systemic failure and vascular collapse from anesthesia.*

People with chronic neurologic impairments who depend on the reckoning of others often fail to reconcile their hydration needs. So they adapt. Venous volume, where fluid reserve resides and which is nominally six times arterial volume, diminishes gradually, invisibly, until it is nearly equal to arterial volume. On examination, fluid deficit is not appreciated. Blood components measure as normal in concentration. Yet each component of blood is substantially reduced in total quantity.

Sudden vascular collapse might follow minimal blood loss or anesthetic-induced vasodilatation. Acute shock is often prevented by the anesthesiologist, who intervenes with fluids.

In large-scope surgery, such as spinal fusion, total circulating platelet quantity might be insufficient. Likewise, fibrin and clotting factors in general are decreased. In the course of uneventful surgery, late-onset bleeding can develop from many surfaces that were once dry. "Rebleeding" might be interpreted as intravascular coagulopathy rather than paucity of factors.

Loading with fluids that lack osmotic substance, that is, protein staying power, may transiently distend the vascular space. That further dilutes clotting factors. Poorly held fluid escapes into the lungs, intestines, abdomen, eyes, and dependent areas.

Patients who make it through the operation can wind up boggy with fluid. Over the next few days, as extravasated fluid gets pulled back into the vascular system, we witness a falling blood count. It might not get noticed that other parameters, such as sodium, potassium, and chloride levels, are falling in proportion as well. The urine, which had earlier been deep in color, is now looking like tap water. That might not get noticed as a herald of third-space fluid mobilization. If it is not noticed, blood transfusion in response to a dropping hematocrit might get layered on top of this fluid mobilization, producing pulmonary edema.

PITFALL

It does us no good to know exactly, precisely what to do if we don't know when to do it. Don't just look at angulation and X-ray films. Look at the patient! Evaluate the patient's metabolic reserve with regard to nutrition and circulating volumes with the same critical eye that is given to the latest spinal equipment trays on the operating room nurse's surgical back table!

FALSE CURVATURE

Do X-rays lie? Yes! *False curvature* refers to a spinal curvature that is not as bad as the radiographic image would have you believe. Not infrequently, insurer prearrangements have made it hopeless to get thoughtfully planned radiographs. Approved providers seem to vie for finding ever-new ways to confound the clinician's ability to provide high-quality care.

PEARLS

The sound of the X-ray unit revving up might startle a normal child, but it will launch the spastic child. Many X-ray films of spinal curves are merely images of a child in flight from yet another noxious stimulus. It's like shooting clay pigeons: Pull, then shoot, catching the target at the height of a motion trajectory. By simply asking the technician to hold the warm-up button at half press until the startled birdie lands and settles in, the number of oddball radiograph postures can be cut in half.

Radiologists, fearful of the legal ramifications of missing anything, often give equal verbiage to insignificant details and, given 3 degrees of tilt, invariably mention scoliosis being present. This incendiary report arrives about 2 weeks after you have sent the patient home without that label. The phone starts ringing, and more needless radiographs get taken—all "approved"—to better assess what you missed. This scenario can be headed off by stating in a written note that artifactual curvature was seen in the X-ray film but does not correlate with the clinical examination. Tell the parents, who have been through this endlessly and appreciate your consideration. A week later, you might not remember and will concede to the unnecessary X-ray exposure.

Children with crooked legs will stand in a crooked way. Obtain images of them that way, and you will get misinformation that is nearly useless unless you are out to show the relationship of stance anomaly to the posture.

If you want to know the "upright" spinal specific mechanics that are eliminating the affect of the lower extremities, then have the image obtained with the patient sitting. Sitting how? The patient should be sitting in whatever way sitting normally occurs in daily life. If the daily grind is sitting in a wheelchair, the film can be shot through the back of the wheelchair with a cassette behind the seat back. Some patients require narrow cassettes dropped between the back rest and the back. Whatever recline is normal is what you use. Capture and evaluate the patient's own particular reality. Side-bending films, of course, are taken with the patient supine on the table.

When ordering magnetic resonance imaging (MRI) studies, remember that many of these patients have pumps that need to be turned off. Also, nerve stimulators and the like might need special attention. An experienced person needs to check the function of the unit immediately afterward for possible reprogramming. Arrange for the MR image to be scheduled when a provider who has experience with the particular units involved is available. This simple consideration wins friends and assures against malfunction of electronic devices.

False curves are also produced by pushing a passive supine patient onto the radiograph table from a stretcher in an awkward position. Be willing to repeat the radiograph if it seems out of keeping with what you see. Real curves can be lost by these same mechanisms. A healthy dose of skepticism ought to accompany radiograph interpretation. This does not mean disbelief in the reality of the curve but disbelief in the default assumption that the curve is a curve inherent to the spine rather than imposed on the spine.

Just how did a spinal curve that was imaged at 4-month intervals, stable at 30 degrees, suddenly jolt, in one visit, to 60 degrees? Possibly by an increase in horizontal rotation. That curve was worsening in the sagittal plane as, say, lumbar lordosis, and now has twisted so as to be visible in the anteroposterior plane. What you were calling *lordosis* you are now calling *scoliosis*.

A right hip abduction contracture will show up as a right lumbar curve. A left hip adduction contracture will also appear as a right lumbar spinal curvature. When legs are centered in the chair or aligned by the technician on a radiograph table, hip contracture tilts the pelvis. Surgical spinal correction of pelvic obliquity without regard to hip contracture will result in a pelvis attached to very long crowbars (femurs) that are just waiting to lever that spinal construct away from the spine through the skin.

PITFALL

Beware of the sitting patient with one knee (let's say the right one) protruding more forward than the other. That longer-looking right thigh is most likely an abducted right hip, and the short left thigh results from an adducted hip. The pelvis is rotated forward away from the back rest on the right and is set flush against the back rest on the left. It is, in all probability, also hiked on the adducted side. An "anteroposterior" radiograph of the spine, in reality not anteroposterior to anything, images an oblique pelvis (nicely obscured by lead shields). Surgical derotation of the lumbar spine squares the pelvis in the chair, which would, were it possible, now direct the legs through the chair armrests and through the side wheel spokes. Side thigh guides instead direct the thighs forward, torquing the pelvis back to what it was doing preoperatively. If the postoperative patient isn't facing fully sideways, then the spinal instrumentation has probably failed. Would you ever need a crowbar longer than a femur to wreck anything? Beware of constrained hips. They severely stress spinal instrumentation.

PEARL

How about that left hip subluxation? The left hip is 30% "out." So? So maybe it is all adduction, and the pelvic obliquity is the real basis of the uncovering. An innominate osteotomy couldn't attain coverage of that hip nearly as well as simple adductor lengthening at the time of spinal pelvis leveling if indeed the motion or bending studies found that the pelvis obliquity is secondary to real structural lumbar scoliosis. Leveling the pelvis is a hip coverage operation.

The most important thing to derive from the pelvic radiograph is the depth (volume) of the socket and its verticality. Take the X-ray film and rotate it until a line between the two acetabular centers is horizontal (à la Hilgenreiner's line). Then visualize the femoral head that is supported in this less adducted posture. Make a tracing if you need to (chances are, as a spinal surgeon, you do this mentally). Does its volume look adequate? But if the socket still seems too shallow, too much like a saucer and not enough like a cup, and perhaps too vertical even with the pelvis leveled, then know that deepening the socket might later be needed. But bracing the at-risk hip in abduction after adductor lengthening can be very helpful to your spinal surgery as well as to the hip. As a spinal surgeon, to the degree that pelvic obliquity affects hip coverage and stability, you are a hip surgeon, like it or not.

Abduction? A wedge between the thighs is not abduction. It is leg separation. Both legs can be substantially adducted despite a wide wedge between them as they stack vertically, one above the other. In a windswept patient—

one leg abducted, the other adducted—the abducted leg will merely pull the adducted leg further. Don't do that. Hip abduction is always relative to the pelvis—or at least to the trunk. Abduction bracing considers one leg at a time relative to an effective purchase on the trunk. Forget what braces are called. Most brace names are misleading. Think! One thigh at a time.

FORCES

Gravity does not produce only curvature in weakness; it also produces acceleration. Watch many patients with cerebral palsy and most with spina bifida as they sit. They back up to the chair and then just let go—at 32 ft/sec^2—to impact with the seat. Beanbag floor seats, very popular with children, allow a longer and more exhilarating drop. Don't let the softness fool you.

Skeletal deformity may be primary, but in neuromuscular disorders, skeletal deformity may represent dissipation of abnormal soft tissue forces that were vented through skeletal deformity. We tend to better notice the visibly abnormal: the bone. That's natural. It is also a pitfall.

If the muscles or ligaments adjacent to the spine are so tight that the bone alignment fails, then the tension is reduced. But to straighten the bones to where they had been might reestablish the forces that deformed the spine in the first place. A mental exercise: If you loop a ring of elastic around your neck and run it to your wristwatch, your elbow might bend—deformity. In that deformity, the elastic forces are resolved when your hand is resting on your face. An elbow extension brace corrects the elbow flexion deformity—and securely so. A weird new head posture follows, with gurgling throat sounds as those reset forces find another way, a different way, to exert themselves.

Forces are created or recreated when a deformation is undone with corrective devices. If the deformation, scoliosis, is an effect rather than a cause (crooked growth of bone), straightening the spine might be synonymous with reloading. Abnormal forces, such as spanning muscular tendon tension asymmetry, that have been dissipated by deformation could be recharged by correction. If such muscular forces are active over a long span but were dissipated through a short span, yielding deformation, then correction with a short construct will be followed by very rapid adding on of curvature beyond the fusion.

A curvature may be followed for years, as it was in the following case (Fig. 10-2). An isolated angulation between T6 and L1 slowly drifted beyond brace control. A short, well-targeted correction of T4-L1 was executed perfectly, according to the surgeon's notes, which you are given to review. The notes state that the patient was in perfect alignment in the operating room. The youngster standing before you, not even a year after his surgery, looks just awful—worse than he did before correction of the original deformity. Not one but two different spinal curves, one

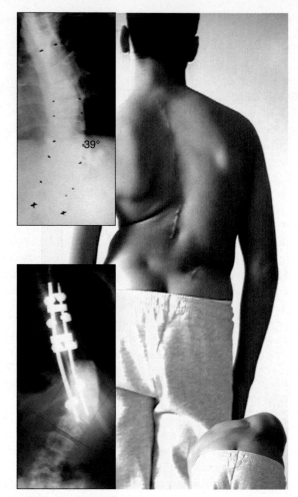

Figure 10-2. A patient who developed isolated angulation between T6 and L1 that slowly drifted beyond brace control. A short, well-targeted correction of T4-L1 had been executed. One year following surgical correction, he is worse than he was before correction of the original deformity. Not one but two different spinal curves, one above T4 and the other below L1, can be seen. The T2 to L1 segment is now unyielding, so the new curves cannot balance through neighboring anatomy.

above T4 and the other below L1, have sprung into existence. Because that original T2 to L1 segment is now unyielding, these new curves cannot balance through neighboring anatomy. His equally crooked brother is in the other room with the exact same story and postsurgical outcome. What was sudden was not the process but the realization of what the process was. A boy with scoliosis is suspicious. Two brothers with scoliosis: an alarm goes off. Mild discoordination and speech oddities: very alarming. This Cobb was a salad.

Even failed conservative treatments, thoughtfully applied, help to sort out the "how" of failure, which reveals the lurking scope of the deforming force. Know your enemy. Have a sense of what the deformation actually is. In cerebral palsy spinal surgery, it is amazing to see how much spinal curvature relaxes when soft-tissue releases are performed in the paraspinal ligaments and intertransverse regions before skeletal instrumentation is even addressed. Why not address the obvious?

KINDS: CODES, WORDS, AND TONES

Codes

In treating pediatric neuromuscular disorders, you will be requested to supply ICD9 codes, which requires forming fog into firm cubes. Naming neurologic disorders, you might think, would reflect what we know about neurology. Half a brain: hemiplegia. Consider, then, a child whose only problem seems to be a bit of awkwardness at certain tasks when pushed to the limit. The MRI scan shows that one side of the brain does not even exist. Plot that on your homunculus. This anomaly occurred before function was assigned. Genetics of neurologic repair and of localization of function are important. Babies with obvious neurologic defects at birth might well show nothing amiss by age 7 years. Yet many seemingly mild deficits in other babies go on unchanged. A static deficit, initially unworrisome, might manifest as worsening in relation to the advancing function of peers. The bottom line is: The scope of apparent neurologic abnormality might not correlate one to one with functional progression. Repair counts, and some babies can do that. Which ones? Mmmmm.

Words

Hemiplegia is used, practically speaking, as a synonym for adult-like stroke. There is a difference between occlusion of the middle cerebral artery and unilateral hemispheric hemorrhage in both scope and quality of loss. The fetus has extensive skull to brain surface arterial and venous bridging vascularity. This disappears in preparation for birth. There is no brain surface watershed early preterm for that reason. You would not expect adult-type "watershed" stroke in prematurity by way of flow loss. The preemie does have a perfusion watershed, but it is adjacent to the ventricles. For this reason, spotty periventricular necrosis (periventricular leukomalacia, PVL) would be expected when blood is diverted (cardiac defects, shunts, pump failure, etc.). The more baby there is to supply, the bigger is the pump job. So the larger preemie twin often gets the PVL.

That aside, adult-like stroke pattern, when seen in children, is what gets called *hemiplegia*. These are typically full-term youngsters, not preemies. Hemiplegia is characterized by greater loss of upper limb function than lower, with legs tending to extension. Loss typically includes sensibility. The hand might become ignored. A loss of global space on one side causes the patient to center in what is left. The patient feels straight when centered in the intact wedge of sensibility. In other words, the patient seeks a tilt and feels tilted when straight.

Diplegia abnormality, better called PVL, might involve only the feet. It extends upward with increasing scope of injury around the periventricular area, spreading until hand and arm representation begins to be seen. The upper limb representation embraces associative areas. So when diplegia has hand involvement, it is common that associative areas are trapped within the neurologic scope of injury. Learning issues, rare in pure hemiplegias and in pure lower-limb diplegia, are common in extended diplegia. Even so, spatial unawareness is still unusual. The exact process that causes diplegia (PVL) can spare one side or the other, in which case, sorry to say, a designation of hemiplegia, so utterly different in quality and treatment, gets misapplied. Fine, wink, wink. As a spinal surgeon, you will not get a vote in this terminology. Just know better. Diplegia pattern is made obvious by hamstring knee flexion in combination with medial leg rotation: medial rotation crouch, for short.

In spastic diplegia, mild medial leg rotation posture implicates mild overactivity of medial hamstrings and certain adductors. However, severe medial rotation does not necessarily mean just a more severe level of the same thing. Severe medial rotation reflects, in addition, an absence: absence of active outward rotation. This magnifying absence reflects an inability to recruit gluteus maximus function, the nearly lone outward rotator of magnitude. It is an important antigravity muscle. Severe medial leg rotation ought to shout low hip extension power.

The reverse—severe hip external rotation—may follow gluteus maximus contracture. These are rare in diplegia and tend to occur in anoxic cases (total-body cerebral palsy, discussed later in the chapter). They can complicate rigidity or dystonia. Such outward contractures are really difficult to eradicate. Any severe hip contracture is of interest to you. That includes hip flexion contractures. Severe lumbar scoliosis can be totally from this cause. The forces on what you do are very high.

Severe anoxic states with asphyxiation (low O_2 and high CO_2) damage the brain broadly and especially in areas of high metabolic rate (cell bodies and ganglia, etc.). The base of the brain, rich in this type of neural structure, gets badly involved, as does the cerebellum. These structures are highly eleptogenic, that is, more prone to seizure activity as an aftermath of injury. But the specifics of reality are quite complex.

Many patients with this form of damage have seizure disorder with widespread foci and with difficult medical management. Hypothalamic functions can be quite disturbed, along with functions that coordinate swallowing, breathing, and basic functions. Once called *spastic quadriplegia*, this condition is now called *total-body cerebral palsy*. Many patients objected to ignoring very vexing head-neck control issues. So quadriplegia is now relegated to spinal cord neck injury.

Because the total-body type of cerebral palsy includes significant basal ganglia damage, rigidity is the common feel to limb resistance. Rigidity tends to stiffen into primitive postures such that limbs both point either left or right in a combined hip and knee flexion, known as *windswept limbs*. When deformity comes from higher centers, an element of will seeps in. Very typical of windswept limbs is that the patients are actively seeking that posture. They complain when out of it. Cut the muscles that enable the posture, and these children will use passive means (e.g., a bed rail) to remaneuver the limbs back to where they feel the limbs belong. Their spinal asymmetries are severe and unrelenting. As with the other kinds of neurologic loss, one side of the brain might recover or somehow be less damaged. Hemiplegia again gets wrongly applied as a label. It does not look anything like a stroke.

A very special form of muscle overactivity occurs in the term infant who has a nearly pure anoxic event (also seen in adults after carbon monoxide poisoning). Status marmoratus is a pathology term for a kind of damage to the basal ganglia. It manifests late, even after 2 years, as it is tied to neuronal loss secondary to the more immediate loss of neuronal supportive cells. Alternating continuous movement such as athetosis results. But the worst version, for us, is dystonia. As a group, these oddly changing muscle tone syndromes are beastly to control and very driven by sensory events. Even good postural intervention can trigger aggravation. These patients become like the subject of the exorcist when they are rigidly constrained. A child who wails for days into weeks without a minute of sleep and who must be in horrible unremitting pain abruptly smiles and stays smiling when a perfectly good brace is removed. This is dystonia. It tips itself off by zigzagging alternating direction postures of sequential joints. Fingers look like "Ws" at times and then later go another way. The ones who do this with tension are real trouble. You can reasonably argue the pros and cons of fusing the scoliotic spine to the pelvis in hemiplegics or the rare diplegic who comes to spinal fusion. The differences will be minute. But dystonics who are left room to distort will distort, so fusions to the sacrum are often necessary.

Tone

Contracture does not imply resistive movement, that is, a quality or feel of range. It implies a stop, an end of possible range. That's clear enough. Contracture is passive stoppage—a joint or fibrosis endpoint. Drugs won't help. Stretching, blindly applied without regard to the level of force of resistance, could crush a joint instead or even hurry a dislocation. Fibrosis occurs within muscles or within myofascia as longitudinal unyielding cords. Following selective dorsal rhizotomy, it is common, probably universal, to see fibrosis occur within muscles that used to be spastic but are now supple. Yet range, though supple, seems to diminish (stop point) with time. This is commonly misinterpreted to be recurrence of the spasticity or some other unfortunate development. What range there is

feels OK. It just stops sooner. True contracture. Fibrosis. Simple and small contracture release fixes it. The key feature is that the finding behaves like any inanimate inelastic constraint: supple up to a stop point, then sudden cessation of motion. Contracture really is not tone. This is confused all the time and is wrong far more often than it is right.

Tone is a term that is used often, but almost never in the same way and nearly always as a wild card for a better, more descriptive but unmentioned term. After more than 30 years of practice, I have no idea what I will see when told that a child has high tone. It implies resistance through the range of motion. Everything and anything gets called tone; therefore, the word has no prognostic value. Forget the words—more often than not they are wrong. Let the forces be with you.

Grab a limb, and put it through a slow joint movement. Note where it stops. Do it again, but quickly. A big difference in range is spasticity: range loss caused by speed. Spasticity is quite stereotypic, that is, easily reproduced with specific evocative examination measures. What you see it do when you fiddle with it is what it is. Spasticity is gamma efferent mediated and thus responds to everything in the loop of high-speed performance and reaction.

Other muscles that are not high-speed muscles also act to restrict motion. They kick in under the reflex outpouring of neural activity of the spinal internuncial pool in response to velocity detection in the high-speed muscles. An attack on high-velocity muscles narrowly will diminish spasticity broadly, as the broad resistance is a reflex second stage response. First is afferent signal (elicited by rapid motion); then comes the efferent response to signal, the kickback that stops the motion. Spasticity responds to reduction in gamma efferent input pathways (SDR), to gamma internuncial communication (GABA inhibitors such as baclofen), or to attack on high-speed muscle components. For botulinum toxin to work most effectively against spasticity, it makes sense to concentrate it in the high-speed muscles at the motor end plate areas where the spindle units concentrate. The botulinum toxin effect on spindles will produce a far better effect than will botulinum toxin that is sprayed about randomly.

Perhaps when you do that examination, it resists right from the start but then suddenly lets go as you persist at attempting to bend the joint. Resists but lets go—that's rigidity. Rigidity tends to be stereotypic as well. It is not speed related, and the origin is not spinal reflex mediated but brain stem. Some will respond to drugs such as L-dopa (Sinemet, etc.). The pharmacology for rigidity is just now beginning to have offerings. Intrathecal baclofen does have effectiveness in rigidity, suggesting that at least some of what is felt has GABA contribution via the internuncials.

If there is significant tone and you are not getting a real handle on it, reposition a nearby joint and repeat the examination. For example, try range of the knee with the hip held still and flexed 60 degrees. Do it again with the hip instead at 30 degrees. If the hip resistance alters by having an adjacent joint in another posture, then you most likely have dystonic response. If the patient has been looking to the right most of the time, turn the head to face the left. Does everything change? Flex the neck while testing that limb; then extend the neck and try again. There are asymmetric tonic neck reflexes (fencing posture to one side as the head turns). There are symmetric tonic neck reflexes (the flexed neck rolls the body like a rug). Neck extension thrusts the patient into extension that has them as the hypotenuse to the wheelchair.

Don't be fooled by mixtures. Fibrotic cords of contracture are common. There are often shades of rigidity along with dystonia. But when dystonia predominates, watch it! Dystonia is not merely tested by changing tension brought on by nearby joints. That is the disease. If you alter the hip joint shape, dystonics will suddenly do bizarre stuff with the opposite hip or hike the pelvis into extreme lumbar scoliosis.

PEARLS & PITFALLS

PEARLS

- Exclude medical conditions that could be causing the scoliosis.
- Observe the patient's physical condition and general health.
- Radiographs can give a false curvature unless the correct posture is assumed.
- MRI scans can affect electronic devices, which must be checked before and after the scans.
- Scoliosis causing pelvic obliquity can give an appearance of hip subluxation.

PITFALLS

- Do not perform surgery in patients whose metabolic reserve cannot withstand the surgery.
- Beware of constrained hips that can severely stress spinal instrumentation.

Illustrative Case Presentation

CASE 1. A 15-Year-Old Male with a History of Cerebral Palsy

A 15-year-old male with a history of cerebral palsy was a part-time ambulator but was mostly dependent on his wheelchair. He was noted to have a rapidly progressive scoliosis which was resistant to bracing (Fig. 10-3). He was found to have a significant lumbar scoliosis with severe pelvic obliquity on physical examination; findings on neurologic examination were consistent with his spastic disorder. Correction of deformity was achieved with a T10 to L3 anterior release and fusion followed by a T5 to sacrum instrumentation and fusion (Fig. 10-4).

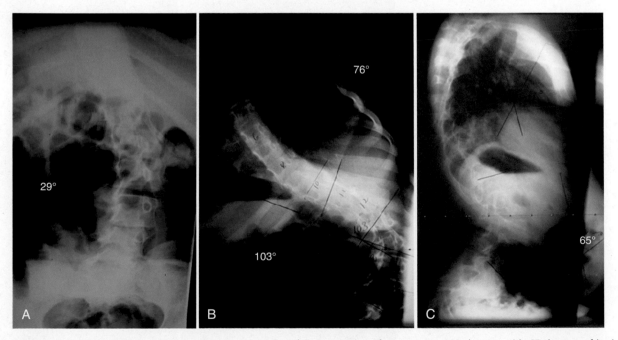

Figure 10-3. A, A 29-degree curve 2 years prior to surgery. **B** and **C,** Progression of curvature to 103 degrees with 65 degrees of lordosis.

Continued

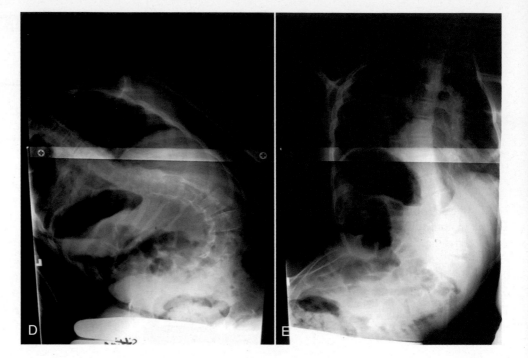

Figure 10-3, cont'd. D and **E,** Left- and right-bending radiographs.

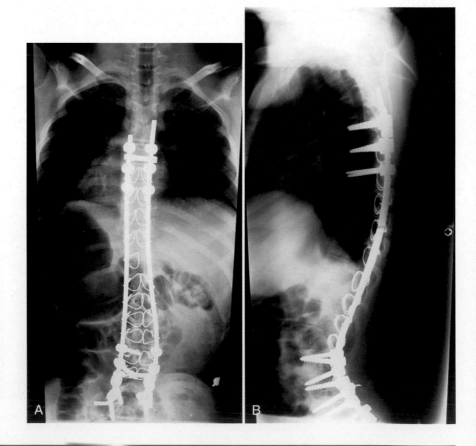

Figure 10-4. A and **B,** Correction of deformity after a T10 to L3 anterior release and fusion followed by a T5 to sacrum instrumentation and fusion.

CONCLUSION

Spinal surgeons, both pediatric and adult, will fall in time, as human nature predicts, into comfortable methodologies and patterns of intervention. Given specified curves with specified flexibility, appropriate surgical intervention can be recommended. The neuromuscular patient represents significant challenges to standard treatment protocols. Difficult questions need to be asked. What is driving the scoliosis at this moment in time is the curvature "inherent" to the spine or "imposed" on the spine by outside factors, some not even musculoskeletal or neurologic! What is the overall health of the patient who is about to undergo a major surgical procedure? What is the best timing of the procedure? Is the diagnosis that was given to the patient accurate? Is there a missed diagnosis or a catchall diagnosis that is missing important nuances?

The treatment of the neuromuscular patient requires much more than technical surgical know-how. It requires savvy, judgment, and a mind that is open to the wide variety of medical factors involved in these patients.

REFERENCES

Freud S: Die infantile cerebrallahmung. In Nothnagel H (ed): Specielle Pathologie und Therapie, vol 9, no 3. Vienna: Alfred Holder, 1897.

Karasawa J, Kikuchi H, Furuse S: Subependymal hematoma in moyamoya disease. Surg Neurol 1980;13:118–120.

Little WJ: On the influence of abnormal parturition, difficult labors, premature birth and asphyxia neonatorum on the mental and physical condition of the child, especially in relation to deformities. Lancet 1861;2:378. Also in Trans Obstet Soc Lond 1862; 3:293–345.

Takeuchi K, Shimizu K: Hypoplasia of the bilateral internal carotid arteries. Brain Nerve 1957;9:37–43.

Volpe JJ: Neonatal seizures. In Neurology of the Newborn, 3rd ed. Philadelphia: WB Saunders, 1981, pp. 172–202.

Volpe JJ: Neurology of the Newborn, 3rd ed. Philadelphia: WB Saunders, 1981.

SUGGESTED READINGS

Berven S, Bradford DS: Neuromuscular scoliosis: Causes of deformity and principles for evaluation and management. Semin Neurol 2002;22:167–178.

Contained herein is a discussion of the spectrum of neuromuscular disorders that have been associated with scoliosis and related spinal deformities and its management.

Birch JG: Orthopedic management of neuromuscular disorders in children. Semin Pediatr Neurol 1998;5:78–91.

This article reviews the clinical manifestation and orthopedic management of Duchenne's muscular dystrophy, spinal muscular atrophy, facioscapulohumeral dystrophy, and Charcot-Marie-Tooth disease.

Hart DA, McDonald CM: Spinal deformity in progressive neuromuscular disease: Natural history and management. Phys Med Rehabil Clin N Am 1998;9:213–232, viii.

This article reviews the prevalence, natural history, and management of scoliosis in neuromuscular diseases that offer the greatest risk for progressive spinal deformity.

McCarthy RE: Management of neuromuscular scoliosis. Orthop Clin North Am 1999;30:435–449, viii.

This article shows that careful preoperative planning and surgery can achieve a well-balanced spine over a level pelvis with a good functional result.

Nuzzo RM, Walsh S, Boucherit T, Massood S: Counterparalysis for treatment of paralytic scoliosis with botulinum toxin type A. Am J Orthop 1997;26:201–207.

This article proves that regarding short-term results using botulinum toxin type A, all of the patients had some reduction in curve measurement (up to >50 degrees). This remains a viable technique to help control difficult-to-manage curves.

Ramcharitar SI, Koslow P, Simpson DM: Lower extremity manifestations of neuromuscular diseases. Clin Podiatr Med Surg 1998;15: 705–737, vi-vii.

This article gives key observations that aid in the recognition of neuromuscular dysfunction, along with an approach to diagnostic evaluation and management for these patients.

Sawin PD, Menezes AH: Neuromuscular scoliosis: Diagnostic and therapeutic considerations. Semin Pediatr Neurol 1997;4:224–242.

This article concludes that neuromuscular scoliosis is a symptom and that the diseases leading to the deformity must be addressed together with the spinal abnormality. The framework of the diagnosis and management is addressed in this article.

Winter S: Preoperative assessment of the child with neuromuscular scoliosis. Orthop Clin North Am 1994;25:239–245.

This article gives an outline of preoperative screening tests and a discussion of common medical issues that should help the surgeon to prepare the child with neuromuscular scoliosis for spinal reconstructive surgery.

CHAPTER 11

Operative Treatment of Neuromuscular Spinal Deformity

SUKEN A. SHAH *and* HARVEY SMITH

Scoliosis is defined as a coronal plane spinal curvature of 10 degrees or more, as assessed by the Cobb method. A scoliotic deformity arising in the clinical setting of muscle imbalance secondary to an underlying neuropathic or myopathic disease can be classified as neuromuscular scoliosis. The associated muscle imbalance in neuromuscular disease causes abnormal biomechanical loading of the spine. According to the Heuter-Volkmann principle, abnormal biomechanical loading secondary to this muscle imbalance and spinal collapse results in asymmetric vertebral body growth in a skeletally immature individual. Progressive deformity is believed to be the result of both progressive muscle imbalance and anatomic deformity.

Of the neuropathic and myopathic disorders associated with scoliosis (Box 11-1), cerebral palsy is the most prevalent. This chapter focuses mainly on the operative treatment of scoliosis due to cerebral palsy. Cerebral palsy has an estimated incidence of 7 per 100,000 live births, with an incidence of scoliosis estimated at between 6.5% and 38%. More severe forms of cerebral palsy, such as spastic quadriplegia, are associated with a higher incidence; Madigan found a 64% incidence in the institutionalized cerebral palsy population. Lonstein and Akbarnia classified scoliotic curves as a result of cerebral palsy into two groups: group I curves, which are double curves with thoracic and lumbar components (S curves), and group II curves, with more lumbar or thoracolumbar curves that extended into the sacrum with associated pelvic obliquity (C curves.)

CLINICAL PRESENTATION AND EVALUATION

Neuromuscular scoliotic curves generally develop at a younger age than idiopathic scoliosis does, and the flexible, postural curve tends to develop into a torsional structural deformity with growth and finally into a stiff curve of considerable magnitude before growth is complete. Cerebral palsy has a broad spectrum of severity; in general, there is a proportional relationship between the severity of involvement of cerebral palsy and curve severity. Dependent sitters with poor head control have a rate of scoliosis approaching 90%. While the rate of curve progression is highly variable, the average progression cited in one report is 0.8 degree a year in curves that are less than 50 degrees and 1.4 degrees a year in curves that are more than 50 degrees; during periods of rapid growth, much more severe progression can occur. Curve progression leads to progressive deformity and trunk imbalance with associated loss of function. Neuromuscular scoliosis may also be associated with significant pain due to sitting difficulties, especially with pelvic obliquity and pressure sores; however, many of these patients are unable to articulate their symptoms.

Initial evaluation should consist of clinical monitoring by physical examination, and when a curve has been identified, standing (when possible) 36-inch posterior-anterior and lateral radiographs of the spine should be obtained. Sitting radiographs may be obtained if the patient is unable to stand; it might be necessary to support the head and trunk in severely affected children with poor truncal control. At our center, we use a standardized sitting frame with lateral support straps to obtain films in the sitting position with minimal external support. Supine bending films can be obtained to assess curve flexibility. Curve magnitude, spinal balance (sagittal and coronal), pelvic obliquity, curve flexibility, and curve progression need to be assessed. A magnetic resonance image should be obtained if there is any suspicion of intraspinal pathology. The patient with established neuromuscular scoliosis requires at least yearly follow-up examination to assess curve progression, but with severe curves or during periods of rapid growth, biannual follow-up is desirable.

In the global planning of disease management, several factors need to be considered. Of paramount importance are the preservation of function, facilitation of daily care, and alleviation of pain. Given the universal progressive nature of neuromuscular scoliosis, early diagnosis of deformity is essential. Curve progression increases the magnitude of deforming forces on the apex of the curve and can

BOX 11-1 Neuromuscular Disorders Associated with Scoliosis and Their Classification

Neuropathic

Upper motor neuron
  Cerebral palsy
  Spinocerebellar degeneration
  Friedreich's ataxia
  Charcot-Marie-Tooth
  Roussy-Levy
  Syringomyelia
  Spinal cord tumor
  Spinal cord trauma
Lower motor neuron
  Poliomyelitis and other viral myelitides
  Traumatic
  Spinal muscle atrophy
  Werdnig-Hoffmann
  Kugelberg-Welander
  Dysautonomia

Myopathic

Arthrogryposis
Muscular dystrophy
  Duchenne
  Limb-girdle
  Facioscapulohumeral
Fiber-type disproportion
Congenital hypotonia
Myotonia dystrophica

lead to progressive muscle imbalance. As the patient's trunk falls forward and there is progressive pelvic obliquity, ambulatory function is compromised. In the wheelchair-bound patient, progressive deformity can compromise sitting.

The role of bracing in neuromuscular scoliosis is questionable. It is generally accepted that bracing is ineffective in significantly altering the ultimate disease progression in the patient with spastic quadriplegia, but some physicians will still recommend a rigid thoracolumbosacral orthosis for a patient with neuromuscular scoliosis. It is important that patient and family understand that the purpose of bracing in this circumstance is not to avoid surgery but to allow further growth before operative intervention. Although it might not alter the final disposition, a soft (polypropylene foam) thoracolumbosacral orthosis can provide seating support and augment function.

Operative intervention in neuromuscular scoliosis is controversial. Given the wide spectrum of disease presentation and progression as well as the concomitant variability in functional status of the patient, the decision to proceed with operative correction and stabilization is based, in large part, on patient-specific factors. For the higher-functioning patient, operative intervention aims to provide a more normal spinal balance and to alter the progression of disease with the goal of preserving function with respect to ambulatory potential. Similarly, in the wheelchair-bound patient, the aim is to maintain

independence in sitting, promote more physiologic respiratory and gastrointestinal functioning, and facilitate overall care.

In the highly functioning child with cerebral palsy, it is intuitively desirable to intervene to halt the progression of deformity and associated loss of function, and the parents or caretakers can make an informed decision, weighing the risks and benefits for their child. Problematically, as Madigan and Wallace observed, the severity of scoliosis is directly proportional to the severity of involvement of cerebral palsy. For the spastic quadriplegic nonambulatory patient, concern has been raised regarding whether the risks of an extensive surgical procedure in a medically compromised patient are warranted. Comstock and colleagues assessed both patient and caregiver satisfaction in a cohort of 100 patients with total-body-involvement spastic cerebral palsy who underwent spinal fusion. The satisfaction of both caregivers and patients was assessed via interview responses to standardized questions, and physical examination was used to assess functional status. Eighty-five percent of the parents who were interviewed indicated that they were satisfied with the results and would repeat the surgery. There was an impression among caregivers that the patients had an improved self-image, and this was confirmed by patients who were able to respond to questions. Both parents and caregivers felt that the surgery had a positive impact on the patient's sitting ability, physical appearance, comfort, and ease of care. Bulman and colleagues and Sussman and colleagues found similar satisfaction rates in their studies.

NONOPERATIVE CARE

Nonoperative management of patients with neuromuscular spinal deformities should be directed at maximizing sitting ability and postural control to facilitate motor and cognitive function. Initial close observation of curves that are less than 20 degrees is reasonable; if progression occurs, initial intervention with a brace might be an option. Bracing is thought to be largely ineffective in stopping curve progression but might slow the rate. Miller and colleagues found no impact on scoliosis curve, shape, or rate of progression in spastic quadriplegic patients who were braced for 23 hours per day over a mean period of 67 months, compared to a similar cohort of patients who were not braced and were followed to spinal fusion. Terejesen and colleagues retrospectively examined a cohort of 86 patients with spastic quadriplegic cerebral palsy and found a mean rate of progression per year of 4.2 degrees with a custom-molded polypropylene thoracolumbosacral orthosis. Interestingly, 25 percent of the patients had no progression or progression of less than 1 degree per year. The degree of curve correction in the orthosis appeared to correlate with nonprogression of the curve. Of note, the patients in Terejesen and colleagues' study had a mean initial Cobb angle of 68.4 degrees.

The bracing studies to date on both neuromuscular and idiopathic scoliosis have had a wide range of inclusion criteria, undefined endpoints, varying methods of assessment, and different follow-up periods. It is generally accepted that in the cerebral palsy patients with scoliosis, bracing likely will not alter the progression of the curve; however, it is reasonable to utilize an orthosis to improve muscle balance and sitting while closely following the curve. Improved sitting could correlate with attentiveness in class, ease of care, improved self-image, and decreased rate of decubitus ulcers.

Another option for patients with flexible curves who need seating support is adjustment of offset lateral chest supports and modular seating systems on the wheelchair. This three-point control of the coronal deformity will prop the child up and address sitting balance; the wheelchair should be the primary seating device. Therapeutic stretching, electrical stimulation, and botulinum toxin lack scientific validity and should have no role in the management of deformity.

OPERATIVE CARE

As was discussed previously, the decision to proceed with operative intervention is complex, and each patient has unique factors to be considered. In general, surgical intervention is considered for patients with a curve magnitude greater than 40 or 50 degrees and significant deterioration in function. There is sufficient evidence that these curves will progress, even if the child has completed his or her growth. The goals of surgery are to correct the spinal deformity, reestablish coronal and sagittal balance, restore pelvic obliquity, and achieve a solid fusion mass.

Managing growth in young children with neuromuscular deformities is challenging, as the scoliosis can be quite progressive during the prepubescent growth spurt. For curves of 60 to 90 degrees, surgery is considered when the deformity becomes stiff by physical examination, and this combination of increasing magnitude and stiffness is an indication for surgery, even if substantial growth remains. If the spine displays continued flexibility on physical examination, surgery can be delayed until the curve reaches 90 degrees and can still be performed with a posterior-only procedure.

For stiff curves or those over 90 degrees, anterior release of the apical levels of the curve is indicated, since it is necessary to gain flexibility to obtain correction. Anterior surgery increases the complication rate and morbidity of spinal surgery in these patients, and it is unclear whether to stage the anterior and posterior procedures separately (1 week apart) or to do both procedures on the same day. Evidence exists to support both strategies, and it is our practice to stage surgeries for patients with severe involvement and multiple medical comorbidities and problems. For relatively healthy patients, we usually perform both stages on the same day, provided that the time under anesthesia or blood loss is not too substantial after the anterior release. Anterior fusion for the so-called crankshaft phenomenon is not necessary, even for young patients, when rigid, segmental instrumentation such as a unit rod is used posteriorly.

Sagittal plane deformities such as pathologic hyperkyphosis or lordosis may develop in patients with neuromuscular disorders, either with or without scoliosis. Flexible, postural deformities can be addressed in younger patients with tight hamstrings by lengthening the posterior thigh musculature and addressing the associated posterior pelvic tilt in these patients or by appropriate modifications to the wheelchair or shoulder harness; but in older children, these adaptations do not work as well. Patients with a previous dorsal rhizotomy can be at particular risk for developing a pathologic hyperlordosis. Fusion and segmental spinal instrumentation are indicated for collapsing deformities and painful sitting when no other alternatives exist.

Historically, fusions with Harrington instrumentation had an unacceptably high rate of pseudarthrosis, occurring in 18% to 27% of cases. The advent of Luque rod segmental instrumentation yielded improved results over the Harrington system. Comstock and colleagues found a mean correction of 51% in a posterior-only instrumentation cohort and 57% in an anterior-posterior cohort. Multiple authors have noted progression of pelvic obliquity if the fusion is not extended to the pelvis. An increased incidence of proximal curve progression, especially proximal junctional kyphosis, has been observed if the proximal level of instrumentation does not extend to at least T2, since most of these children lack sufficient head control.

The Galveston technique to extend the fusion across the pelvis by placing each Luque rod between the pelvic tables has demonstrated acceptable fusion rates across the L5-S1 segment, and appears to provide good control of pelvic obliquity. While the impaction of two Luque rods into the pelvis with associated segmental fusion via sublaminar wires provides a strong construct in the sagittal plane, there exists a moment arm of rotation about the two rods allowing for rod translation with respect to one another and subsequent progression of pelvic obliquity, pseudarthrosis, and implant failure. The use of Luque rods of smaller than a quarter inch in diameter could increase the incidence of implant failure, but the intraoperative bending of quarter-inch-diameter steel rods to the optimal geometry for pelvic implantation presents a technical challenge. Rigid fixation is essential for surgical success. Sanders and colleagues found in their retrospective study of Luque rod instrumentation that a postoperative curve greater than 35 degrees, preoperative curves greater than 60 degrees, crankshaft deformity, and not fusing to the pelvis are factors that are associated with postoperative curve progression.

Historically, there has been debate regarding when to extend the posterior spinal fusion to the pelvis. Pelvic obliquity has been noted to progress in neuromuscular scoliosis if the pelvis is not fused; traditionally, many authors have recommended fusion to the pelvis in nonambulatory patients. In the ambulatory patient with pelvic obliquity, fusion to the pelvis has been traditionally avoided, owing to the belief that it will adversely affect ambulatory function. A recent retrospective study by Tsirikos and colleagues demonstrated preserved ambulatory function in ambulatory patients with cerebral palsy who were fused with unit rod instrumentation. The authors hypothesized that the conventional assumption that ambulatory potential is limited by fusion to the pelvis arose from early attempts at pelvic fixation with Harrington rods that removed lumbar lordosis. This was also possibly caused by the confounding variable of prolonged immobilization and bed rest in earlier segmental systems that did not provide sufficient rigidity for immediate postoperative mobilization and ambulation therapy.

The unit rod that was developed by Bell and colleagues addresses some of the potential limitations of dual Luque rod instrumentation. The implant design of a proximally connected, precontoured rod provides for better rotational control, as the degree of rotational freedom between two independent Luque rods is eliminated. Initial mean curve corrections with the unit rod were reported to be 54.6%, with a mean loss of correction of 6.5% at 2-year follow-up. Westerlund and colleagues more recently found a mean scoliosis correction with the unit rod of 66% and a 75% correction of pelvic obliquity. Twenty-seven of the 28 patients in Westerlund and colleagues' cohort were Risser 2 or less, with preoperative Cobb angles ranging from 45 to 94 degrees. At an average follow-up of 58 months, there was a mean loss of correction of 3 degrees. Dias and colleagues noted similar results in a large group of patients with cerebral palsy scoliosis who were managed with unit rod instrumentation.

Iliac screws perform better in pullout strength than do smooth Galveston rods for pelvic fixation, and the use of segmental pedicle screw constructs has shown substantial correction and fusion rates while accomplishing the goals of leveling pelvic obliquity and addressing seating problems. These newer modular systems can navigate some of the substantial challenges in these patients, such as abnormal pelvic anatomy and hyperlordosis, and can avoid some of the risk in early instrumentation failure but come at a substantial monetary expense. Because of cost issues, the routine use of these modular constructs over the unit rod in the treatment of neuromuscular scoliosis at this time remains an issue of debate.

PREOPERATIVE AND PERIOPERATIVE CONCERNS

The individual with neuromuscular scoliosis is medically complex and can have significant preoperative risk. For a family that is intent on providing maximal medical treatment for a severely involved child with the intent of caring for the child at home and keeping the child involved in school and other outside, community activities, surgical treatment of the spinal deformity will accomplish this goal with the greatest ease and comfort. The risk and complications of a procedure of this magnitude are directly related to the severity of neurologic impairment. Lipton and colleagues have reported that a child who is not fed orally, is severely mentally retarded, cannot speak, has seizures, and cannot sit independently has by far the highest rate of complications. Medical management of seizures, respiratory problems, gastroesophageal reflux and motility issues, and nutrition should be addressed before surgery. Standard preoperative laboratory work, including hematology, metabolic profile, urinalysis, and a coagulation panel, should be obtained, as well as an assessment of nutrition, but we have found the laboratory values are not always a reliable assessment of the preoperative status of the child. Blood loss can be substantial, and a type and cross of 1 to 1.5 times the patient's blood volume should be available prior to the start of surgery. Many parents and caretakers have noted that they were not prepared for the complexity of the patient's postoperative course. Preoperative counseling of the family and caretakers should stress the potential for a prolonged intensive care unit stay as well as the significant possibility of postoperative complications.

Intraoperatively, the surgeon must maintain constant communication with the anesthesia staff. Intraoperative hypotension is frequently secondary to inadequate volume replacement. Correction of a kyphotic deformity can impede venous return to the heart with resultant hypotension. In the event of hypotension during curve correction, an attempt to release pressure on the spine should be made, and an increase in the rate of intravenous fluid and/or blood replacement should be performed; after the blood pressure has been stable for 5 to 10 minutes, it can be safer to proceed with a gradual correction to allow time for the soft tissues to stretch.

Spinal cord monitoring with intraoperative transcranial motor evoked somatosensory evoked potentials should be used. Although it is not uncommon for severely involved children to have weak or absent signals at baseline and therefore for intraoperative neurophysiologic monitoring to be unreliable, children who can stand or ambulate or who have some purposeful lower-extremity movement can and should be monitored intraoperatively to protect function.

SURGICAL TECHNIQUE

After intubation, attachment of appropriate monitoring leads, establishment of large-bore intravenous access, and arterial and central venous catheterization, the patient should be placed prone on a radiolucent table or four-post frame. Care should be taken to ensure that all bony prominences are well padded and that the abdomen hangs free.

The hips can be allowed to gently flex with knee and thigh support to passively correct lumbar hyperlordosis. Intraoperative traction has been described to correct pelvic obliquity, but this is rarely necessary.

A standard posterior exposure of the spine from T1 to the sacrum is performed. Each vertebra must be exposed subperiosteally out to the transverse process. At the inferior margin of the incision, the outer wing of the ilium is subperiosteally exposed down to the sciatic notch. The right and left drill guides for the unit rod are placed in the respective sciatic notch; care should be taken to ensure that the drill guide is as far inferior as possible along the posterior superior iliac spine. The handles of the drill guide are the reference points for alignment; the lateral handle should be parallel with the pelvis, and the axial handle should be parallel with the sacrum. The drill hole is next made by utilizing the guide using a 3/8-inch drill to the predetermined depth; the hole is palpated with a ball-tipped feeler to confirm that there has been no breach of the cortex. Gelfoam should be inserted into the drill holes, and sponges should be packed out over the pelvis to maintain hemostasis.

The spinous process of each level is removed to expose the ligamentum flavum. Care must be taken to preserve the laminae, as they are key to the strength of fixation, especially the supralaminar cortex, which even in osteoporotic bone can be strong. The orientation of the cut will change from lumbar to thoracic vertebrae; this must be recognized to avoid resection of the edge of the lamina. The ligamentum is now opened at each level to expose the sublaminar space and epidural fat.

After removal of all spinous processes and exposure of the sublaminar space, the sublaminar wires are passed at each level. A 16-gauge double Luque wire is passed at each level from T2 to L4, and two wires are placed at T1 and L5. The wire is passed from inferior to superior. After the wire has been passed, it is contoured back over the lamina, and the ends of the wire are contoured to the edges of the incision; this will maintain the intraspinal portion of the wire against the undersurface of the lamina as the remaining levels are instrumented. In passing the wire, care must be taken to avoid levering off the lamina and impinging against the cord; the diameter of the contoured bend should approximate the length of the lamina. In passing the wire, if resistance is felt, remove the wire and alter its curvature.

The length of the rod is measured from T1 to the pelvis. Note that correction of a kyphotic deformity will shorten the spine and correction of a lordotic deformity will lengthen the spine. This can be confirmed by placing the rod upside down with the top of the rod at T1 and confirming that the corner of the rod is at the level of the pelvic drill holes. Intraoperatively, if the rod is noted to be too long (i.e., superior to T1) the limbs at T1 can be secured with cross connectors and the excess rod can be cut. If the rod is noted to be too short, the end can be cut

and a piece of another rod can be joined with rod-to-rod connectors to achieve the necessary length. Both scenarios, however, will weaken the unibody construction of the rod and decrease the ability to generate sufficient cantilever moment.

Facetectomies and decortication are performed, and a preliminary grafting of the area under the rod is performed. After the proper length unit rod has been selected, the pelvic limbs of the rod are crossed and inserted into their respective drill holes. Each limb should be advanced alternatively in 1-cm increments with an impactor. Care must be taken to maintain control of the rod and to ensure that it does not penetrate either table of the pelvis. In the setting of hyperlordosis, the marked anterior inclination of the pelvis increases the risk of the pelvic limb perforating the inner cortex during insertion. The pelvic ends of the rod need to be directed in a more posterior direction to accommodate this angulation; rod placement is facilitated by manual correction of the lordosis prior to rod insertion. In instances of marked lordosis, the pelvic limbs of the rod can be cut and inserted separately and then attached to the rod with rod-to-rod connectors. (Alternatively, iliac screws can be used with modular connectors.)

The spine is manually corrected to the rod, and the wires are tightened sequentially. Pushing the rod to the spine can generate substantial force at the lever arm of the pelvic insertion with subsequent fracture, so a few of the lumbar levels should be wired prior to generating substantial cantilever forces. After the wires have been tightened and retightened, the wires are cut to be 1 cm long and are bent down to the lamina to avoid implant prominence. Copious crushed cancellous allograft is packed, and the wound is meticulously closed. A drain might or might not be used.

Dabney and colleagues noted that when there is marked lordotic deformity, better fixation and correction were achieved with pedicle screws in the lordotic segment. A cadaveric biomechanical study has confirmed that the use of L5 pedicle screws significantly increases the lateral and oblique stiffness of the unit rod construct. McCall and Hayes retrospectively examined a cohort of patients with neuromuscular scoliosis in whom those with a stable lumbosacral articulation were instrumented with a U-rod (unit rod without the pelvic limbs) with L5 pedicle screw fixation. The L5-S1 interspace mobility was assessed on the basis of L5 tilt; patients with more than 15 degrees of L5 tilt were instrumented with a standard unit rod construct. McCall and Hayes found that in follow-up, the patients who were instrumented to L5 with the U-rod had results similar to those of patients who were fused with the standard unit rod construct.

POSTOPERATIVE CARE

Postoperatively, the patient should be maintained, intubated, in an intensive care setting for 24 to 48 hours, and volume status and urine output should be closely monitored. The hemoglobin should be maintained over 9 to ensure adequate perfusion, and the coagulation parameters and platelet count should be corrected as needed, as these patients are frequently coagulopathic. Prophylactic antibiotics are continued for 24 hours. In patients with poor nutritional status, hyperalimentation should be started postoperatively intravenously or via a J-tube. There is no need for immobilization postoperatively, and the patient should be mobilized out of bed and into a wheelchair as soon as medically appropriate. The child's personal wheelchair should be readjusted to accommodate his or her new trunk proportions and pelvic alignment. Children can return to school in 3 to 4 weeks, when sitting tolerance has been attained and no postoperative restrictions or orthoses are employed.

COMPLICATIONS

As was previously discussed, a patient who undergoes spinal fusion for neuromuscular scoliosis frequently has significant associated medical comorbidities, and postoperative complications are prevalent and should be anticipated. The incidence of postoperative complication has been noted to range from 18% to 68%. Curves greater than 70 degrees, severity of neurologic involvement, and severity of recent history of medical problems have been shown to increase the risk of postoperative complications. Respiratory complications are frequent, namely, atelectasis or more severe problems requiring prolonged ventilatory support. Postoperative ileus, pancreatitis, superior mesenteric artery syndrome, pulmonary compromise, and cholelithiasis can occur, and the physician must be vigilant in evaluating any clinical abnormalities. Postoperative wound infections are of particular concern. Infection rates have been reported from 2% to 15%. Most deep infections in the early postoperative period respond well to drainage and irrigation with delayed wound closure over drains or a vacuum-assisted device with intravenous antibiotic therapy and retention of the instrumentation.

OUTCOMES

Correction of neuromuscular scoliosis with the unit rod is typically 75% to 80% with leveling of the pelvis and excellent sagittal alignment. With proper surgical technique and the rigidity of the instrumentation, fusion rates are superior, and pseudarthrosis can be avoided. Parent and caregiver satisfaction is very high for this procedure; over 85% of the caregivers noted benefits beyond sitting and facilitation of care for the child postoperatively. In a group of children that included even the most severely involved,

there was a predicted 70% survival rate at 11 years following surgery.

In summary, scoliosis is common in this group of children with neuromuscular disorders. The majority of these children have progressive spinal deformities that interfere with sitting and other functions and will require surgical stabilization to address these problems and facilitate care. The unit rod is the preferred method of instrumentation; it offers a powerful mechanism of correction in both the coronal and sagittal planes. The risk of complications both perioperatively and postoperatively is substantial but manageable. Caregiver satisfaction is high after this procedure and affords a good long-term outcome.

PEARLS & PITFALLS

PEARLS

- In general, surgical intervention is considered for patients with a curve magnitude greater than 40 or 50 degrees and significant deterioration in function. There is sufficient evidence that these curves will progress, even if the child has completed his or her growth. The goals of surgery are to correct the spinal deformity, reestablish coronal and sagittal balance, restore pelvic obliquity, and achieve a solid fusion mass.
- Correction of neuromuscular scoliosis with the unit rod is typically 75% to 80% with leveling of the pelvis and excellent sagittal alignment. With proper surgical technique and rigidity of the instrumentation, fusion rates are superior, and pseudarthrosis can be avoided.
- Parent and caregiver satisfaction is very high for this procedure; over 85% of the caregivers noted benefits beyond sitting and facilitation of care for the child postoperatively.

PITFALLS

- Significant associated medical comorbidities and postoperative complications are prevalent in the surgical treatment of neuromuscular scoliosis. The incidence of postoperative complications has been noted to range from 18% to 68%.
- Respiratory complications are frequent, namely, atelectasis or more severe problems requiring prolonged ventilatory support. Postoperative ileus, pancreatitis, superior mesenteric artery syndrome, pulmonary compromise, and cholelithiasis can occur, and the physician must be vigilant in evaluating any clinical abnormalities.
- Postoperative wound infections are of particular concern. Infection rates have been reported from 2% to 15%.

Illustrative Case Presentation

CASE 1. A 19-Year-Old Male with Spastic Quadriplegia Cerebral Palsy

A 19-year-old male with spastic quadriplegia cerebral palsy developed a progressive lumbar scoliosis of 90 degrees and pelvic obliquity of 30 degrees. The patient underwent posterior spinal fusion with segmental instrumentation, including iliac fixation. Preoperative seated upright anteroposterior, anteroposterior pelvis, supine traction anteroposterior (Fig. 11-1A–C), and postoperative anteroposterior and lateral radiographs (Fig. 11-1D–F) are illustrated.

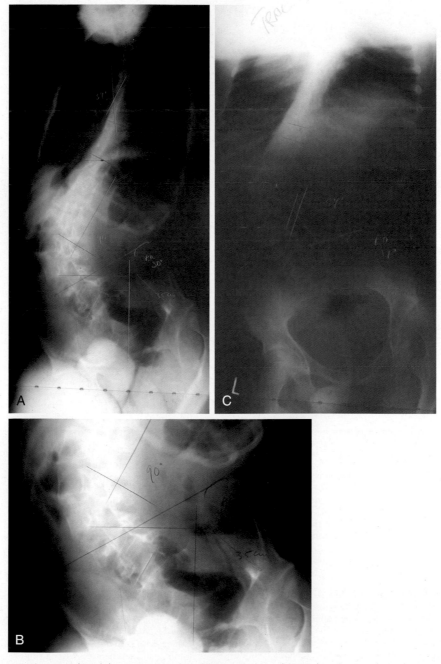

Figure 11-1. Preoperative seated upright anteroposterior, anteroposterior pelvis, and supine traction anteroposterior radiographs.

Continued

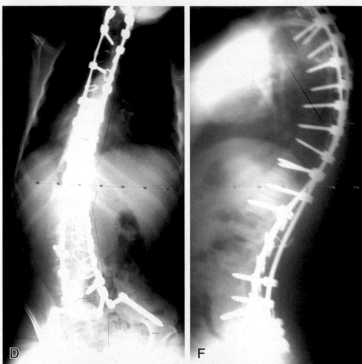

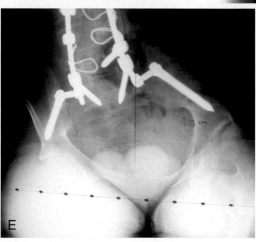

Figure 11-1, cont'd. Postoperative anteroposterior and lateral radiographs.

REFERENCES

Allen BL Jr, Ferguson RL: The Galveston technique for L rod instrumentation of the scoliotic spine. Spine 1982;7:276–284.

Banta JV, Drummond DS, Ferguson RL: The treatment of neuromuscular scoliosis. Instr Course Lect 1999;48:551–562.

Bell DF, Moseley CF, Koreska J: Unit rod segmental spinal instrumentation in the management of patients with progressive neuromuscular spinal deformity. Spine 1989;14:1301–1307.

Bonnett C, Brown JC, Grow T: Thoracolumbar scoliosis in cerebral palsy: Results of surgical treatment. J Bone Joint Surg Am 1976;58: 328–336.

Bradford DS: Neuromuscular spinal deformity. In Bradford DS, Lonstein JE, Ogilvie JW, Winters RB (eds): Moe's Textbook of Scoliosis and Other Spinal Deformities, 2nd ed. Philadelphia: WB Saunders, 1987, pp 271–305.

Broom MJ, Banta JV, Renshaw TS: Spinal fusion augmented by luque-rod segmental instrumentation for neuromuscular scoliosis. J Bone Joint Surg Am 1989;71:32–44.

Dias RC, Miller F, Dabney K, et al: Surgical correction of spinal deformity using a unit rod in children with cerebral palsy. J Pediatr Orthop 1996;16:734–740.

Erickson MA, Oliver T, Baldini T, et al: Biomechanical assessment of conventional unit rod fixation versus a unit rod pedicle screw construct: A human cadaver study. Spine 2004;29:1314–1319.

Herndon WA, Sullivan JA, Yngve DA, et al: Segmental spinal instrumentation with sublaminar wires: A critical appraisal. J Bone Joint Surg Am 1987;69:851–859.

Korovessis PG, Stamatakis M, Baikousis A: Relapsing pancreatitis after combined anterior and posterior instrumentation for neuropathic scoliosis. J Spinal Disord 1996;9:347–350.

Leichtner AM, Banta JV, Etienne N, et al: Pancreatitis following scoliosis surgery in children and young adults. J Pediatr Orthop 1991;11: 594–598.

Lonstein JE: Spine deformities due to cerebral palsy. In Weinstein SL (ed): The Pediatric Spine: Principles and Practice, 2nd ed. Philadelphia: Lippincott Williams & Wilkins, 2001, pp 797–807.

Lonstein JE, Akbarnia A: Operative treatment of spinal deformities in patients with cerebral palsy or mental retardation: An analysis of one hundred and seven cases. J Bone Joint Surg Am 1983;65:43–55.

Madigan RR, Wallace SL: Scoliosis in the institutionalized cerebral palsy population. Spine 1981;6:583–590.

McCall RE, Hayes B: Long-term outcome in neuromuscular scoliosis fused only to lumbar 5. Spine 2005;30:2056–2060.

Miller A, Temple T, Miller F: Impact of orthoses on the rate of scoliosis progression in children with cerebral palsy. J Pediatr Orthop 1996;16:332–335.

Renshaw T: Cerebral palsy. In Morrisy R (ed): Lovell and Winter's Pediatric Orthopaedics. Philadelphia: Lippincott Williams & Wilkins, 2001, pp 563–599.

Robson P: The prevalence of scoliosis in adolescents and young adults with cerebral palsy. Dev Med Child Neurol 1968;10:447–452.

Sanders JO, Evert M, Stanley EA, et al: Mechanisms of curve progression following sublaminar (Luque) spinal instrumentation. Spine 1992;17:781–789.

Shapiro G, Green DW, Fatica NS, et al: Medical complications in scoliosis surgery. Curr Opin Pediatr 2001;13:36–41.

Stanitski CL, Micheli LJ, Hall JE, et al: Surgical correction of spinal deformity in cerebral palsy. Spine 1982;7:563–569.

Sullivan JA, Conner SB: Comparison of Harrington instrumentation and segmental spinal instrumentation in the management of neuromuscular spinal deformity. Spine 1982;7:299–304.

Sussman MD, Little D, Alley RM, et al: Posterior instrumentation and fusion of the thoracolumbar spine for treatment of neuromuscular scoliosis. J Pediatr Orthop 1996;16:304–313.

Szoke G, Lipton G, Miller F, et al: Wound infection after spinal fusion in children with cerebral palsy. J Pediatr Orthop 1998;18:727–733.

Terjesen T, Lange JE, Steen H: Treatment of scoliosis with spinal bracing in quadriplegic cerebral palsy. Dev Med Child Neurol 2000;42:448–454.

Thometz JG, Simon SR: Progression of scoliosis after skeletal maturity in institutionalized adults who have cerebral palsy. J Bone Joint Surg Am 1988;70:1290–1296.

SUGGESTED READINGS

Benson ER, Thomson JD, Smith BG, et al: Results and morbidity in a consecutive series of patients undergoing spinal fusion for neuromuscular scoliosis. Spine 1998;23:2308–2317; discussion 2318.

This study provides the rate of complications of patients who have undergone spinal fusion for neuromuscular scoliosis. It concludes that with surgical techniques and perioperative management in an experienced center, the results for patients undergoing spinal fusion for neuromuscular scoliosis have been improved, and major complications have been minimized.

Bulman WA, Dormans JP, Ecker ML, et al: Posterior spinal fusion for scoliosis in patients with cerebral palsy: A comparison of Luque rod and unit rod instrumentation. J Pediatr Orthop 1996;16:314–323.

In this retrospective study, the results of 15 patients who underwent arthrodesis with dual Luque rod instrumentation are compared with the results of 15 patients in whom unit rod instrumentation was used.

Boachie-Adjei O, Lonstein JE, Winter RB, et al: Management of neuromuscular spinal deformities with Luque segmental instrumentation. J Bone Joint Surg Am 1989;71:548–562.

This study evaluated 46 patients who had neuromuscular spinal deformity and were treated with arthrodesis and Luque segmental spinal instrumentation and followed for an average of 3 years. It provides a descriptive comparison of the results that were obtained for patients with spastic and flaccid deformity. The authors present a rate of complications in 48% of patients treated.

Comstock CP, Leach J, Wenger DR: Scoliosis in total-body-involvement cerebral palsy: Analysis of surgical treatment and patient and caregiver satisfaction. Spine 1998;23:1412–1424; discussion 1424–1425.

This study analyzes the results of spinal fusion in patients with total-body-involvement cerebral palsy to determine early and late outcomes, including caregiver satisfaction. It concludes that avoiding late progression of trunk deformity in skeletally immature patients can be achieved by anterior spinal release and fusion combined with posterior segmental spinal instrumentation and fusion from the upper thoracic spine to the pelvis.

Dabney KW, Miller F, Lipton GE, et al: Correction of sagittal plane spinal deformities with unit rod instrumentation in children with cerebral palsy. J Bone Joint Surg Am 2004;86-A(suppl 1):156–168.

This study looks at patients with cerebral palsy and a severe sagittal plane deformity (70 degrees or more) and concludes that they can be treated successfully with posterior spinal fusion with use of unit rod instrumentation. The authors also conclude that the indications for treatment include loss of sitting ability or balance, back pain, loss of bowel or bladder function, and superior mesenteric artery syndrome that is unresponsive to medical management.

Dias RC, Miller F, Dabney K, et al: Revision spine surgery in children with cerebral palsy. J Spinal Disord 1997;10:132–144.

This study analyzes 10 children with neuromuscular scoliosis and pelvic obliquity who had revision spinal instrumentations and fusions performed at an average age of 14.7 years. According to the authors, the goal of providing symptomatic relief and correction of deformity was accomplished in nine of 10 children; however, two of the nine required two revisions.

Dubousset J, Herring JA, Shufflebarger H: The crankshaft phenomenon. J Pediatr Orthop 1989;9:541–550.

This study was one of the first to evaluate the crankshaft phenomenon. It reviews 40 spinal fusions done prior to Risser stage 1 for idiopathic and paralytic scoliosis to evaluate postoperative curve progression. It concludes that the more immature the patient, the greater is the resultant progression. This progression is an inevitable consequence of continued anterior spinal growth in the presence of a posterior fusion and occurs without pseudarthrosis or hardware failure.

Gersoff WK, Renshaw TS: The treatment of scoliosis in cerebral palsy by posterior spinal fusion with Luque-rod segmental instrumentation. J Bone Joint Surg Am 1988;70:41–44.

This study analyzes the operative procedure and complications in 33 patients who had cerebral palsy and scoliosis and underwent posterior spinal fusion with Luque rod segmental instrumentation.

Lipton GE, Miller F, Dabney KW, et al: Factors predicting postoperative complications following spinal fusions in children with cerebral palsy. J Spinal Disord 1999;12:197–205.

This is a retrospective review of 107 patients with cerebral palsy who had undergone a posterior spinal fusion with unit rod instrumentation by the same two surgeons. This review was done to determine what factors cause complications that lead to delayed recovery time and a longer-than-average hospital stay.

McCarthy RE: Management of neuromuscular scoliosis. Orthop Clin North Am 1999;30:435–449, viii.

This review concludes that neuromuscular scoliosis is classified as a neuropathic or myopathic type. Cerebral palsy is the most common form of neuropathic type, and Duchenne's muscular dystrophy best characterizes the principles and recommended treatment for the myopathic type. Nonoperative measures rarely fully control a progressive scoliosis. Careful preoperative planning and surgery can achieve a well-balanced spine over a level pelvis with a good functional result.

Richards BS, Bernstein RM, D'Amato CR, et al: Standardization of criteria for adolescent idiopathic scoliosis brace studies: SRS Committee on Bracing and Nonoperative Management. Spine 2005;30:2068–2075; discussion 2076–2077.

This review establishes the parameters for future adolescent idiopathic scoliosis bracing studies so that valid and reliable comparisons can be made. It concludes that the optimal inclusion criteria for future adolescent idiopathic scoliosis brace studies consist of age of 10 years or older when the brace is prescribed, Risser 0 to 2, primary curve angles of 25 to 40 degrees, no prior treatment, and, if female, either premenarchal or less than 1 year postmenarchal.

Sponseller PD, LaPorte DM, Hungerford MW, et al: Deep wound infections after neuromuscular scoliosis surgery: A multicenter study of risk factors and treatment outcomes. Spine 2000;25:2461–2466.

This is a retrospective case-control study evaluating risk factors for infection, causative organisms, and results of treatment in patients with cerebral palsy or myelomeningocele who underwent fusion for scoliosis.

Tsirikos AI, Chang WN, Dabney KW, et al: Life expectancy in pediatric patients with cerebral palsy and neuromuscular scoliosis who underwent spinal fusion. Dev Med Child Neurol 2003;45:677–682.

The aim of this study was to document the rate of survival among 288 severely affected pediatric patients (154 females, 134 males) with spasticity and neuromuscular scoliosis who underwent spinal fusion and to identify exposure variables that could significantly predict survival times.

Tsirikos AI, Chang WN, Shah SA, et al: Preserving ambulatory potential in pediatric patients with cerebral palsy who undergo spinal fusion using unit rod instrumentation. Spine 2003;28:480–483.

This is a retrospective study that investigates 24 ambulatory pediatric patients with spastic cerebral palsy and neuromuscular scoliosis. The main objective is to evaluate the effect of spinal fusion from T1 to T2 to the sacrum with pelvic fixation using unit rod instrumentation on the ambulatory potential of these patients.

Westerlund LE, Gill SS, Jarosz TS, et al: Posterior-only unit rod instrumentation and fusion for neuromuscular scoliosis. Spine 2001;26: 1984–1989.

This is a retrospective study that aims to determine the efficacy of posterior-only unit rod instrumentation and fusion in a skeletally immature neuromuscular scoliosis population. It concludes that even in the very young neuromuscular patient, acceptable amounts of curve correction can be achieved and maintained with posterior-only unit rod instrumentation and fusion.

CHAPTER 12

Spinal Surgery in Connective Tissue Disorders

PAUL D. SPONSELLER

Because the spine depends on a balance of forces during growth, many conditions that disrupt the musculoskeletal matrix will cause spinal deformity. In addition, deformities in patients with these conditions have unique natural histories and responses to standard treatments. This chapter will summarize our understanding of these differences. Conditions that are covered include Marfan syndrome, Ehlers-Danlos syndrome, Stickler syndrome, and osteogenesis imperfecta.

MARFAN SYNDROME

The surgeon who is examining the spine must be aware of the manifestations of Marfan syndrome and be able to recognize affected individuals and make the diagnosis. The most apparent clinical findings in Marfan syndrome involve the skeleton (arachnodactyly, scoliosis, dolichostenomelia, sternal deformities, and joint laxity). Taken individually, these findings are not very specific, since they can be seen in the general population. However, Marfan syndrome is a life-threatening disorder, so the presence of multiple findings should prompt a referral to a genetics specialist or the echocardiography lab.

Marfan syndrome is very pleomorphic. One end of the spectrum represents patients who are only mildly affected, and the other end represents patients with a severe neonatal form who usually succumb to cardiovascular complications during the first year of life.

Diagnosis

Although genetic testing is available, it is complex and not highly sensitive. The diagnosis of Marfan syndrome is still clinical. According to the diagnostic (Ghent) criteria, the diagnosis can be made with the presence of two major criteria in addition to involvement of a second system (Box 12-1). The differential diagnosis includes homocystinuria, congenital contractural arachnodactyly, Stickler syn-drome, Ehlers-Danlos syndrome, MASS phenotype, and Schprintzen-Goldberg syndrome. Early diagnosis is of the utmost importance in order to initiate prophylactic β-blockade therapy, which has been shown to be effective in slowing the rate of aortic dilation and reducing the development of aortic complications in patients with Marfan syndrome.

Vertebral Morphology and Dural Ectasia

The classic features of the Marfan spine may include increased vertebral scalloping and lengthened transverse process distance, as well as a reduction in pedicle width and laminar thickness. The pedicles may be reduced to mere slits in some segments. One fourth of Marfan individuals have pedicles of L5 that are too narrow to accept even the smallest pedicle screw (5 mm). Many patients have significant scalloping of the sacrum inside the spinal canal (Fig. 12-1). Therefore, careful preoperative planning of fixation anchors, possibly including computed tomography, is essential.

Dural ectasia is rare in the normal population but has a high prevalence (56% to 92%) in the Marfan population (Fig. 12-2). The consequences of dural ectasia include bony erosion, anterior meningocele, and/or posterior meningocele. The sac is enlarged mainly below the level of L5. There are several definitions of dural ectasia. Fattori used morphologic criteria consisting of bulging of the dural sac to obliterate the epidural fat and contact at least one posterior vertebral body or the presence of nerve root cysts. Villeirs devised a definition of dural ectasia using computed tomography of the spine to define a ratio of the dural sac to the lumbar vertebral bodies. There is also a role for conventional radiographs: They can detect dural ectasia with a very high specificity (91.7%) but a low sensitivity (57.1%).

Scoliosis and Kyphosis

In a large cross-sectional study, there was a 62% prevalence of scoliosis in Marfan syndrome. However, many of the curves were minor, and only 10% to 20% required treatment of any kind. The curve patterns were similar to the pattern that is seen in idiopathic scoliosis. Differences were seen in the sagittal plane, however (see p. 169).

BOX 12-1 The Ghent Diagnostic Criteria for Marfan Syndrome

The index case requires major criteria in two different organ systems and involvement of a third. If the FBN-1 mutation is present, then one major criterion with involvement of a second organ system suffices. A relative of the index case requires one major criterion in family history and one major criterion in an organ system and involvement of a second organ system.

Skeletal System

Major Criteria:

Presence of at least four of the following:

- Pectus carinatum
- Pectus excavatum requiring surgery
- Reduced upper to lower segment ratio or arm span to height ratio > 1.05
- Wrist sign (thumb and fifth digit overlap, circling the wrist) and thumb sign (distal phalanx protrudes beyond border of clenched fist)
- Reduced extension at the elbows (<170 degrees)
- Scoliosis > 20 degrees
- Pes planus
- Protrusio acetabuli of any degree (ascertained on radiographs)

Minor Criteria:

- Pectus excavatum
- Joint hypermobility
- High arched palate
- Facial:
  - Dolichocephaly
  - Malar hypoplasia
  - Enophthalmos
  - Retrognathia
  - Down-slanting palpebral fissures

Ocular System

Major Criterion:

- Ectopia lentis

Minor Criteria:

- Flat cornea
- Increased axial length of the globe (>23.5 mm)

Cardiovascular System

Major Criteria:

- Dilation of the ascending aorta
- Dissection of the ascending aorta

Minor Criteria:

- Mitral valve prolapse with or without mitral valve regurgitation
- Dilation of the main pulmonary artery in the absence of valvular or peripheral pulmonic stenosis (age < 40 years)
- Calcification of the mitral annulus before the age of 40 years
- Dilation or dissection of the descending thoracic or abdominal aorta before the age of 50 years

Pulmonary System

Minor Criteria (Only):

- Spontaneous pneumothorax
- Apical blebs

Skin and Integumentary System

Minor Criteria (Only):

- Striae atrophicae
- Recurrent or incisional hernia

Neurologic System

Major Criterion:

- Lumbosacral dural ectasia by computed tomography or magnetic resonance imaging

Family/Genetic History

Major Criteria:

- First-degree relative who independently meets the diagnostic criteria
- Presence of mutation in FBN1 gene
- Presence of haplotype around FBN1 inherited by descent and unequivocally associated with diagnosed Marfan syndrome in the family

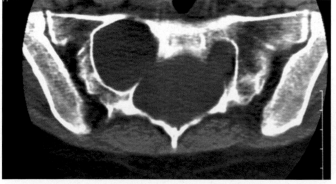

Figure 12-1. Osseous scalloping in Marfan syndrome.

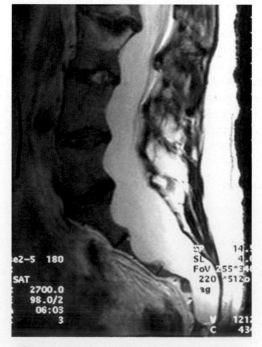

Figure 12-2. Dural ectasia in Marfan syndrome.

Scoliosis progresses at a faster rate in Marfan syndrome than in the general population. Virtually all curves larger than 30 degrees in immature patients will reach at least 40 degrees at maturity. Curves that are larger than 40 degrees increase during adulthood, at a rate slightly higher than that of idiopathic scoliosis. Curves that are greater than 50 degrees progress at a mean rate of 3 degrees per year in adulthood. Marfan patients with scoliosis have been found to have more back pain than do those who do not have scoliosis.

Brace treatment does not seem to have as much success in Marfan syndrome as in idiopathic scoliosis. One study reported a 17% success rate for bracing scoliosis in Marfan syndrome. Thus, bracing is recommended mainly for curves in the range of 15 to 25 degrees. Patients with curves of 25 to 45 degrees may be offered the option of using the brace, but patients and physicians should be aware that there is only a one in five chance of successfully controlling the curve. Bracing is not recommended for curves greater than 40 degrees except as a holding option; the curve will likely increase.

Infantile scoliosis is seen in approximately 2% of people with Marfan syndrome. Bracing has a limited role in this population, especially in smaller curves. It is useful mainly in promoting upright posture in patients with a coexistent kyphosis. In addition, surgery is not usually recommended for patients younger than 4 years of age because of inadequate soft tissue coverage for spinal instrumentation in young Marfan patients. The use of a growing rod employing iliac fixation distally and strong proximal anchorage has been successful in these cases (Fig. 12-3). Fusion will eventually be necessary.

Sagittal plane deformities are also common in Marfan syndrome. The mean kyphosis of the Marfan population is greater than that of the general population. In addition, 40 percent of the Marfan patients have a kyphosis greater than 50 degrees. Different patterns of sagittal alignment can be found: hypokyphosis, hyperkyphosis, and thoracolumbar kyphosis with compensatory thoracic lordosis.

Spine surgery is required in about 10% to 15% of patients. A medical specialist should be involved to comanage cardiac medications and other issues and to assist with anticoagulation management if there is an artificial heart valve. Intraoperative complications specific to these patients include increased bleeding and cerebrospinal fluid leak. We have found aprotinin to be helpful in decreasing blood loss. Cerebrospinal fluid leak occurs because of the dural ectasia. It can be minimized by keeping the patient in slight Trendelenburg position intraoperatively and minimizing dissection inside the canal. If a leak occurs, closure may be possible; if not, a dural patch and postoperative bed rest for 2 to 3 days have been successful. Postoperative complications include failure of fixation, adding on of curvature, and pseudarthrosis. Therefore, in correcting spinal deformity, it is important not to fuse too short a segment of the spine (Fig. 12-4). The surgeon should probably not employ selective thoracic fusion for double major curves unless the lumbar curve is minor. It is also important to take into account any unusual kyphosis that may be present. Failure of fixation is quite common and is due to ligamentous laxity, which allows downgoing hooks to dislodge from lower laminae and upgoing hooks to dislodge from upper laminae. Pedicle screws more often lose fixation owing to thin pedicles; the surgeon should strictly assess the fixation and work to achieve a stable proximal and distal foundation.

Spondylolisthesis

The prevalence of spondylolisthesis in the general population is approximately 3%, and of this population, the mean slip is approximately 15%. In one study, 6% of the Marfan population had spondylolisthesis of the fifth lumbar on the first sacral vertebra with a mean slip of 30%. Although the frequency of spondylolisthesis in Marfan patients might not be markedly higher than that in the general population, if a slip is present, the altered tissue properties allow greater forward slip to occur. It is at this level that the dural ectasia, sacral scalloping, and potential cerebrospinal fluid leaks have the greatest clinical importance.

Cervical Spine Problems

Hobbs and colleagues conducted a radiographic analysis of the cervical spine in patients with Marfan syndrome, which revealed an increased prevalence of focal kyphosis and a slightly increased atlantoaxial movement with flexion and extension. Herzka and colleagues report three cases that suggest that Marfan children could be at risk for atlantoaxial rotatory subluxation when muscle tone is attenuated by general anesthesia or muscle relaxants. Special attention to intubation and positioning, both intraoperatively and postoperatively, could be warranted and rotatory subluxation should be included in the differential diagnosis for Marfan patients with neck pain.

Bone Density

The abnormal fibrillin chromosome 15 in the Marfan population might play a role in the mineralization of bone. Carter and colleagues have demonstrated that there is a reduced axial bone mineral density in men and women with Marfan syndrome. They have postulated that this might be due to mutations of the fibrillin gene or to environmental issues such as reduced exercise, which leads to suboptimal peak bone mass.

Screening and Athletics

It is recommended that Marfan patients avoid physical stress because many aortic dissections occur during these events. Keane and Pyeritz recommend that the physician

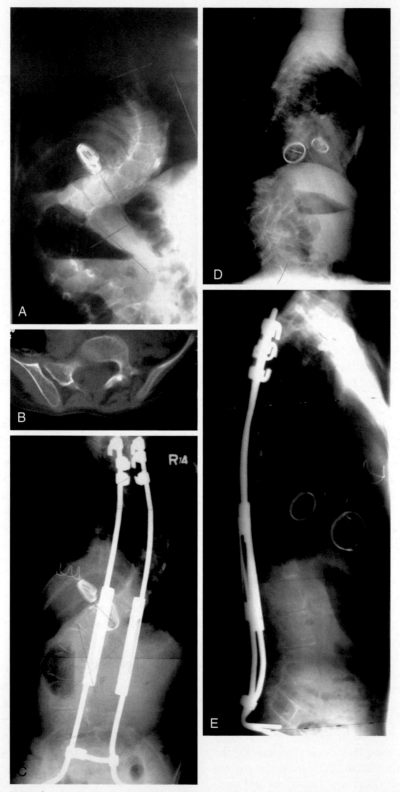

Figure 12-3. Infantile scoliosis in Marfan syndrome. Preoperative anteroposterior radiographic (**A**) and computed tomography (**B**) views. **C,** Anteroposterior radiograph 4 years postoperatively. **D,** Preoperative lateral radiograph. **E,** Lateral radiograph 4 years postoperatively.

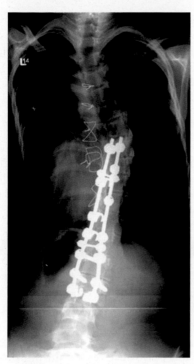

Figure 12-4. Adding-on deformity after correction of scoliosis in a 12-year-old.

counsel on an individual basis. For example, a child with only a slightly dilated aortic root does not need outright restriction but should be counseled away from competitive athletics. On the other hand, an older patient should be advised against any sort of strenuous exertion, especially activities with sudden stops, such as basketball or isometric exercises. Other activities, such as low-intensity isokinetic sports, should be encouraged.

EHLERS-DANLOS SYNDROME

Ehlers-Danlos syndrome (EDS) in most cases is caused by a deficiency in collagen. The most recent classification system is the Berlin nosology, according to which there are nine types of EDS. Scoliosis is most common in types I (classic) and VI (ocular-scoliotic). However, spinal deformity does not appear to be as common as it is in Marfan syndrome. Beighton and colleagues reviewed 100 patients with EDS and found severe scoliosis in only six. Spondylolisthesis is also slightly more common in this condition. Atlantoaxial instability has been reported in type IV EDS but does not often cause impairment or require intervention. Principles of surgical treatment should follow those outlined for Marfan syndrome.

STICKLER SYNDROME

Stickler syndrome (hereditary arthro-ophthalmopathy) is an autosomal dominant disorder of collagen types II or XI. It is characterized by ocular abnormalities (retinal degeneration or myopia), craniofacial abnormalities (cleft palate, retrognathia), hearing loss, and hip and/or spine abnormalities. It is as common as Marfan syndrome but is less frequently recognized. Common spinal abnormalities include vertebral end plate irregularity, disc degeneration, and kyphosis. Severe scoliosis is uncommon. Back pain is very frequent in adults with the syndrome. The occurrence of Scheuermann-like spinal end plate changes along with epiphyseal changes in the hips should make the surgeon suspect Stickler syndrome.

Diagnosis is important because mitral valve prolapse and retinal detachment are also common in this syndrome. Patients should be screened preoperatively for any cardiac or ophthalmologic problems that might require management. The anesthesiologist could experience difficulty in airway management due to a small jaw or midface hypoplasia.

OSTEOGENESIS IMPERFECTA

Osteogenesis imperfecta is due to a defect in type I collagen, the primary collagen of bone matrix. Numerous different mutations have been identified, which in part explain the spectrum of severity and manifestations seen in this disorder. Spinal problems are more common in nonambulatory patients than in ambulatory ones, and bone quality decreases progressively from patients who have straight diaphyses and normal vertebral contours to those with biconcave vertebrae, to thinning of the diaphyses, to absence of a definite diaphyseal cortex. Common spinal problems include basilar invagination, scoliosis, and kyphosis. Bracing is not very effective in controlling curves, except perhaps in ambulatory patients with the most mild osteogenesis imperfecta. In patients with lower bone density, it has been reported to cause rib cage distortion. Spinal surgery may be effective in slowing the decline in pulmonary function due to scoliosis. It also may stabilize or partially reverse neurologic deficits due to basilar invagination.

Preoperative assessment should be extensive to prevent complications. Patients who are undergoing spine surgery at any level should have lateral radiographs of the cervical spine in order to rule out basilar invagination if they have not had these in the past. A detailed history of pulmonary function, such as exercise tolerance and history of pneumonia, should be used to assess the need for postoperative ventilatory support. Pulmonary function tests can be helpful. If there is adequate time (more than 6 months) before surgery dictated by the urgency of the clinical picture, bisphosphonate treatment should be considered to increase bone density in children. Halo-gravity traction can be helpful in providing gradual correction and therefore decreasing the forces on the instrumentation.

Intraoperative Considerations

Anesthetic preparation is often extensive and time-consuming. Exposure of the spine is often difficult, since the ribs usually protrude posteriorly on both sides of the spine and render access to narrow spinal elements difficult. Bleeding tends to be greater than in nonsyndromic cases. In some cases, this can be a factor limiting the performance of same-day anterior and posterior fusion; we recommend the use of trasylol to limit bleeding. However, blood loss is variable, and some patients do not bleed excessively.

Fixation problems are the biggest challenge. Segmental fixation with a hook, wire, or screw at as many levels as possible is recommended. Screws might have an advantage over other anchor types. Intraoperative traction can help to distribute the corrective forces evenly. The rods that are used should be malleable so that they have "give" to match the bone as closely as possible. Large, rigid rods are more likely to cut out of the bone. The surgeon should use discretion in applying corrective force to the spine. A modest amount of correction that is tolerated by the bone is better than a dramatic degree that then causes implement cutout. Care should be especially used in the correction of kyphosis. This correction involves posterior column shortening, which depends significantly on the support of the instrumentation. In osteoporotic bone, this will fail sooner or later. If the surgeon finds himself or herself levering the rod down to meet the spine, that same force will eventually cause a dorsal rod displacement. The use of methylmethacrylate both anteriorly and posteriorly has been advocated when needed to augment fixation. Anteriorly, the surgeon should use it to supplement the vertebral body before a through-and-through hole is prepared. Posteriorly, it is useful for pedicle screws but not as practical for hooks.

Anteriorly, if instrumentation is used, structural anterior column support in the disc spaces can minimize the force on the instrumentation.

Another intraoperative factor for the patient with osteogenesis imperfecta is that the dura is often thin; cerebrospinal leaks may occur. Awareness of this when dissecting around the ligamentum flavum can help to minimize problems.

Occasionally, there are patients with osteogenesis imperfecta whose spines cannot support any instrumentation. The goal of experienced preoperative selection is to counsel these patients against surgery. However, if such a situation occurs, the use of nonresorbable suture tapes to act as sublaminar wires to a thin rod can occasionally salvage some situations. If this is not successful, bone graft with autograft and long allograft struts may permit a fusion to occur after immobilization in a cast.

Postoperative Management

Postoperative bracing for 3 to 6 months might be needed, at the surgeon's discretion. Some loss of correction is common, but it will likely stabilize as long as the fixation is maintained. Dislodgement of fixation at the ends of the construct should be repaired if possible by using alternative means of anchorage (e.g., using pedicle screws or methylmethacrylate or extending the fusion). Prolonged pain is common but usually abates as the fusion matures.

Postoperative Complications

In the consecutive series of McMaster, there were no permanent complications. Postoperative wound hematoma was seen in 40% of patients, and wound dehiscence was common. These responded to secondary closure. Wound infection and pseudarthrosis were not seen.

PEARLS & PITFALLS

- Intraoperative complications primarily involve bleeding. McMaster described five patients with spinal deformity in EDS who were treated by posterior spinal fusion. There is an increased incidence of vascular fragility in this condition, leading to bleeding from small muscular and periosteal vessels during posterior spine fusion. This is usually possible to control by using standard methods. Adequate blood replacement, as well as an intraoperative blood salvage system, should be available. Use of a drain is advised. McMaster reported wound hematoma in two of his five patients. Anterior spine fusion should be approached with more caution, especially in type I EDS. The retroperitoneal vessels, especially the veins, are friable and at risk for tear during dissection. They can be very difficult to repair and might require vascular consultation or ligation. Vogel and Lubicky reported a patient who experienced avulsion of two segmental arteries from the aorta despite careful handling. This required repair with a pericardial patch. Anterior approaches should be carried out only when deemed essential, and the posterior approach should be used whenever it can effectively be done. During posterior exposure, the presence of thin, ectatic dura increases the risk of CSF leak.
- Neurologic deficits during spinal deformity correction might be more common in EDS. Two patients were reported with paraplegia and one with a partial but permanent neurologic injury. The frequency of this complication cannot be assessed; however, it is likely to be greater than that in the general population. Several factors are hypothesized to account for the neurologic deficits. The ligamentous laxity, vascular fragility, and large, focal deformities that are sometimes seen in this syndrome are undoubtedly risk factors. It is recommended that patients with EDS undergo preoperative magnetic resonance imaging to look for dural ectasia or focal cord distortion. Motor and sensory monitoring of the spinal cord should be done if possible.

Illustrative Case Presentations

CASE 1. Severe Kyphoscoliosis in a 16-Year-Old Male with Marfan Syndrome

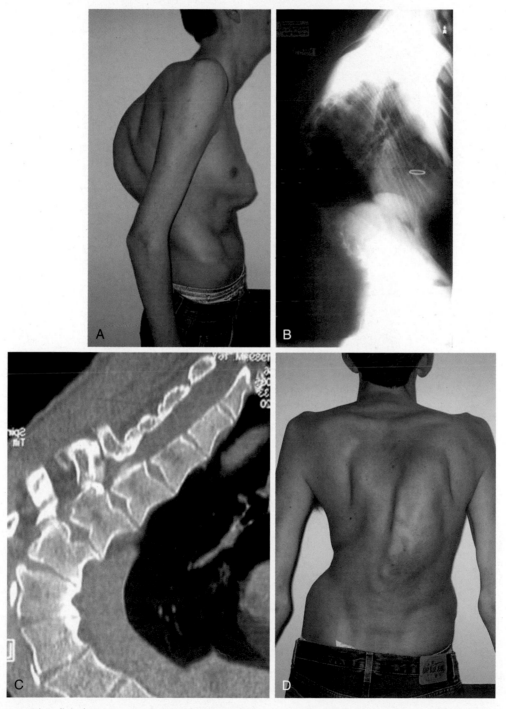

Figure 12-5. A, Preoperative clinical appearance. **B,** Lateral radiograph shows a 95-degree scoliosis. **C,** Computed tomography shows bridging of vertebrae. **D,** Clinical coronal appearance.

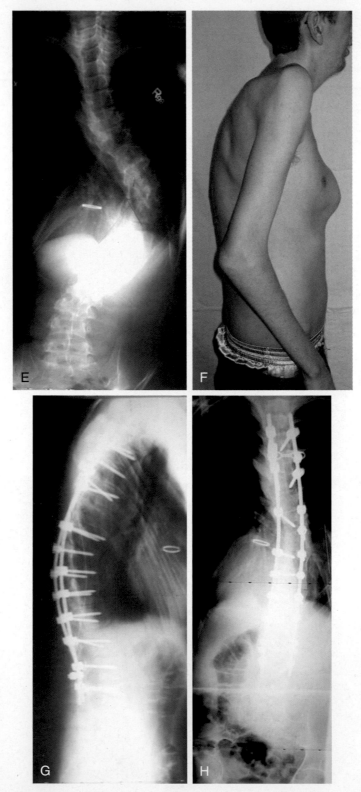

Figure 12-5, cont'd. E, Coronal film showing a 75-degree curve. The patient underwent apical wedge resections and fusions from a posterior approach. **F,** Postoperative sagittal appearance. Postoperative lateral (**G**) and coronal (**H**) radiographs.

CASE 2. A 13-Year-Old Male with Ehlers-Danlos Syndrome and Severe, Progressive Kyphoscoliosis

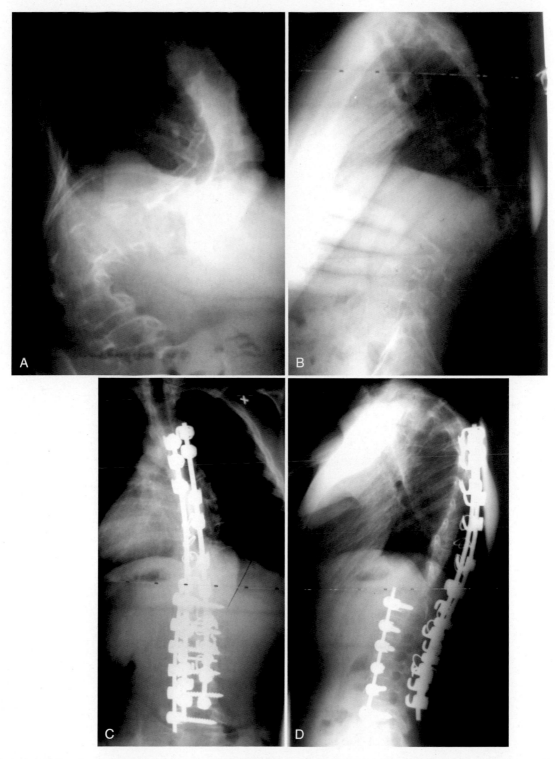

Figure 12-6. A and **B,** Anterior and posterior fusion was performed but was complicated by disintegration of the iliac vein, requiring ligation. The patient tolerated this with development of collateral circulation. Note the development of postoperative proximal junctional kyphosis (**C** and **D**) due to ligamentous laxity.

CASE 3. Scoliosis in a 10-Year-Old with Osteogenesis Imperfecta Treated Surgically

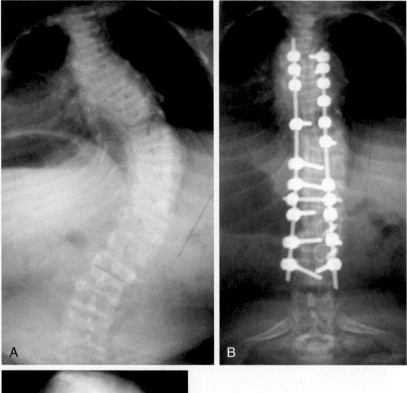

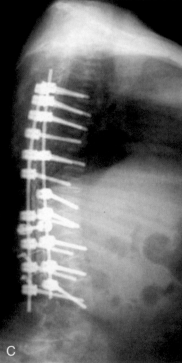

Figure 12-7. A, Preoperatively, the curve measured 66 degrees. **B** and **C,** Use of multiple pedicle screws and flexible rods allowed load sharing and correction, which was maintained at the 2-year follow-up.

REFERENCES

Beighton P, DePaepe A, Steinman B: Ehlers-Danlos syndromes: Revised nosology, Villefranche, 1997. Ehlers-Danlos National Foundation (USA) and Ehlers-Danlos Support Group (UK). Am J Med Genet 1998;77:31–37.

Fattori R, Nienaber CA, Descovich B, et al: Importance of dural ectasia in phenotypic assessment of Marfan's syndrome. Lancet 1999;354:910–913.

Herzka A, Sponseller PD, Pyeritz RE: Atlantoaxial rotatory subluxation in patients with Marfan syndrome. A report of three cases. Spine 2000;25:524–526.

Keane MG, Pyeritz RE: Medical management of Marfan syndrome. Circulation 2008;117:2802–2813.

McMaster MJ: Management of scoliosis. J R Soc Med 1982;75:685–688.

McMaster MJ: Spinal deformity in Ehlers-Danlos syndrome. Five patients treated by spinal fusion. J Bone Joint Surg Br 1994;76:773–777.

Villeirs GM, VanTongerloo AJ, Verstraete KL, et al: Widening of the spinal canal and dural ectasia in Marfan's syndrome: Assessment by CT. Neuroradiology 1999;41:850–854.

SUGGESTED READINGS

Ahn NU, Sponseller PD, Ahn UM, et al: Dural ectasia in the Marfan syndrome: MR and CT findings and criteria. Genet Med 2000;2:173–179.

This study focuses on using magnetic resonance imaging and computed tomography to diagnose dural ectasia with high specificity and sensitivity. According to the authors, their criteria accurately diagnose dural ectasia in adult Marfan patients.

Carter N, Duncan E, Wordsworth P: Bone mineral density in adults with Marfan syndrome. Rheumatology 2000;39:307–309.

This study proves that axial bone mineral density is lower than normal in Marfan adults. This reduction could contribute to fractures seen in the Marfan population.

De Paepe A, Devereux RB, Dietz HC, et al: Revised diagnostic criteria for the Marfan syndrome. Am J Med Genet 1996;62:417–426.

This is a revision of diagnostic criteria for Marfan syndrome and related conditions. Emphasis is placed on skeletal involvement as a major criterion if at least four of eight typical skeletal manifestations are present. It mentions potential contribution of molecular analysis to the diagnosis of Marfan syndrome.

Halko GJ, Cobb R, Abeles M: Patients with type IV Ehlers-Danlos syndrome may be predisposed to atlantoaxial subluxation. J Rheumatol 1995;22:2152–2155.

This study proves that atlantoaxial subluxation could be a more common finding in people with type IV EDS than was previously thought. Examination of the cervical spine radiographically should be considered before general anesthesia is administered to these patients.

Hanscom DA, Winter RB, Lutter L, et al: Osteogenesis imperfecta: Radiographic classification, natural history, and treatment of spinal deformities. J Bone Joint Surg 1992;4-A:598–616.

This is a radiographic study that focuses on classifying the presentations of the different types of osteogenesis imperfecta on the basis of shape, dimensions, and appearance of the long bones; the presence of a trefoil pelvis and protrusio acetabuli; and the shape of the vertebrae.

Hobbs WR, Sponseller PD, Weiss AP, Pyeritz RE: The cervical spine in Marfan syndrome. Spine 1997;22:983–989.

This study focuses on determining cervical spine abnormalities that are present in the Marfan population compared with those seen in the general population. It concludes that on the basis of the increased prevalence of several cervical bony and ligamentous abnormalities, patients with Marfan syndrome were recommended to avoid sports with risks of high-impact loading of the cervical spine.

Letts M, Kabir A, Davidson D: The spinal manifestations of Stickler's syndrome. Spine 1999;24:1260–1264.

This is a complete review of current knowledge, clinical publications, and recent concepts of the causes of Stickler's syndrome correlated with a clinical overall review of the condition.

Rose PS, Ahn NU, Levy HP, et al: Thoracolumbar spinal abnormalities in Stickler syndrome. Spine 2001;26:403–409.

This study states that spinal abnormalities are nearly uniformly observed in Stickler syndrome, progress with age, and are associated with back pain. Although common, scoliosis is generally self-limited (only one patient needed surgical treatment). Recognition of Stickler syndrome allows accurate prognosis for skeletal abnormalities and anticipation of potential surgical complications.

Sponseller PD, Ahn NU, Ahn UM, et al: Osseous anatomy of the lumbosacral spine in Marfan syndrome. Spine 2000;25:2797–2802.

This article focuses on lumbar pedicle width and laminar thickness and the fact that these are significantly reduced in Marfan individuals. Those with dural ectasia demonstrate increased bony erosion of anterior and posterior elements of lumbosacral spine.

Sponseller PD, Hobbs W, Riley LH 3rd, Pyeritz RE: The thoracolumbar spine in Marfan syndrome. J Bone Joint Surg Am 1995;77:867–876.

This study analyzes 113 patients who had Marfan syndrome, 82 of whom were skeletally immature, to characterize the alignment and function of their spines.

Stanitski DF, Nadjarian R, Stanitski CL, et al: Orthopaedic manifestations of Ehlers-Danlos syndrome. Clin Orthop 2000;376:213–221.

This study analyzes the clinical and genetic characteristics of the different types of Ehlers-Danlos. It shows that type III Ehlers-Danlos syndrome is the most debilitating form with respect to musculoskeletal function, compared to the other types.

Tallroth K, Malmivaara A, Laitinen ML, et al: Lumbar spine in Marfan syndrome. Skel Radiol 1995;24:337–340.

Spine radiographs of 28 patients with Marfan syndrome were evaluated for scoliosis and morphologic changes of the L2, L3, and L4 vertebrae. Marfan patients showed a high incidence of scoliosis (64%). The incidence of lumbosacral transitional vertebra was also high (18%). The study describes specific vertebral changes associated with Marfan.

Vogel LC, Lubicky JP: Neurologic and vascular complications of scoliosis surgery in patients with Ehlers-Danlos syndrome: A case report. Spine 1996;21:2508–2514.

This is a series of case reports that concludes that patients with Ehlers-Danlos syndrome could be at high risk for neurologic and vascular complications consequent to scoliosis surgery, necessitating careful perioperative evaluation and management.

CHAPTER 13

Pediatric Infections of the Spine

JOSHUA D. AUERBACH *and* JOHN P. DORMANS

Spinal infections in children are rare but potentially devastating conditions that have the possibility for long-term sequelae. Children differ from adults with respect to bony, developmental, and vascular anatomy of the spine; ability to communicate effectively; potential sources of bacteremia; treatment options; and prognosis following infection. Therefore, an understanding of the anatomic, developmental, clinical, and radiographic features that are unique to pediatric spine infections forms the basis for prompt diagnosis and treatment.

Although *discitis* and *vertebral osteomyelitis* are the terms that are most commonly utilized to describe spinal infections in children, previous descriptions in the literature have used the terms *acute osteitis of the spine, nonspecific spondylitis, narrowing of the intervertebral disc space, intervertebral disc space inflammation, nontuberculous spondylodiscitis,* and *pyogenic infectious spondylitis*. The variable descriptions of these disorders reflect our poor understanding and emphasize the current controversies surrounding the exact etiology of pediatric spinal infections. However, advances in imaging and improved understanding of the pediatric vertebral body and disc space vascular anatomy and development demonstrate that discitis and osteomyelitis are likely separate clinical manifestations of a similar underlying pathophysiologic process. In this chapter, we will describe classic discitis and osteomyelitis as separate clinical entities; however, many patients will likely share characteristics of both and fall somewhere in between the two along the spectrum of disease.

DISCITIS AND OSTEOMYELITIS

Pathophysiology

There is not universal agreement that discitis reflects an underlying infectious etiology. Some authors have cited the absence of positive biopsy and culture results in up to 40% of cases, nonspecific tissue changes, the mild clinical picture, and the resolution of symptoms often without administration of antibiotics as evidence to support an inflammatory or traumatic process.

Most authors, however, propose that an infectious etiology is the most likely cause of disease. It is proposed that children are more predisposed to disc space infections from a hematogenous source than are adults because of the unique vascular supply to the vertebral body and disc space in children (Figs. 13-1 to 13-3). Similar to a long bone, the developing vertebral body contains a growth cartilage, proximal and distal apophyses, and a metaphyseal region that, unlike the adult vertebra, receives a rich vascular supply. In children, blood flow enters the vertebral body posteriorly and is carried proximally and distally, traversing the vertebral end plate via cartilaginous channels, thereby allowing communication with the intervertebral disc (see Figs. 13-1 and 13-2). Infection can arise when a bacterial focus from a distant source is deposited via the rich metaphyseal blood supply through these cartilaginous channels and into the disc space to cause classic discitis. The infectious (and possibly inflammatory) process can spread further into the adjacent vertebral body, causing reactive changes in the opposite end plate, thus providing the bone-disc-bone pattern that is commonly seen in discitis (Fig. 13-4). The abundant vascular supply in young children could also explain the typical good recovery and lack of long-term destruction that are seen in comparison with discitis in adults.

After birth, however, the cartilage end plates become thinner, and the canals are obliterated by approximately age 7 years (see Fig. 13-3). Therefore, in younger patients in whom the cartilaginous channels are patent, discitis is a more common manifestation of the infectious process, although vertebral osteomyelitis has also been described. In older children, in whom the vascular connection with the disc space has been destroyed, vertebral osteomyelitis is more commonly seen (Fig. 13-5). In osteomyelitis, as in discitis, bacteria arise from the end plate, where they can multiply, but instead of traversing the disc space through patent cartilaginous channels, the bacteria spread throughout the vertebral body (see Fig. 13-3). In addition to differences with respect to vascular anatomy, there are other factors that distinguish between spinal infections in children and in adults. The initial source of bacteremia in

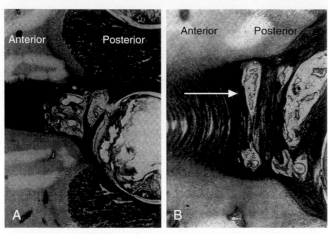

Figure 13-1. A, Posterior thoracic disc from immature human spine. **B,** Posterior lumbar disc region from immature human spine. In both specimens, there is vascular continuity between the posterior vertebral plexus as it courses across the foraminal region and peripheral disc vasculature. Note the contiguous cartilage canals (*arrow*) and proximity of some of the physeal and metaphyseal tissues to the disc. *(From Song KS, Ogden JA, Ganey T, Guidera KJ: Contiguous diskitis and osteomyelitis in children. J Pediatr Orthop 1997;17:470–477.)*

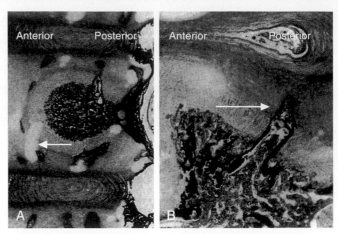

Figure 13-2. A, Human vertebral centrum development (1 year). Note the vascular cartilage canals throughout the nonossified centrum (*arrow*). These are comparable to cartilage canals in the epiphyseal cartilage of long-bone epiphyses. A large vessel crosses the transphyseal region of the primary centrum ossification center, traveling toward the superior disc region. **B,** Specimen from a 6-year-old boy who died of traumatic injury. A transphyseal vascular process extends toward the superior disc and its vessels (*arrow*). *(From Song KS, Ogden JA, Ganey T, Guidera KJ: Contiguous diskitis and osteomyelitis in children. J Pediatr Orthop 1997;17:470–477.)*

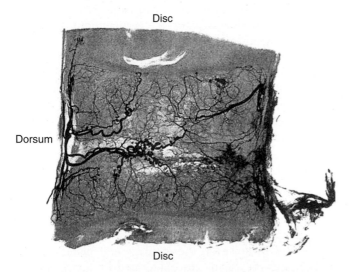

Figure 13-3. Sagittal section through a mature L2 vertebral body, showing the distribution of the nutrient arterioles throughout the body, without vascular communication with the disc space. *(From Wiley AM, Trueta J: The vascular anatomy of the spine and its relationship to pyogenic vertebral osteomyelitis. J Bone Joint Surg 1959;41B:796–809. Reproduced with permission and copyright © of the British Editorial Society of Bone and Joint Surgery.)*

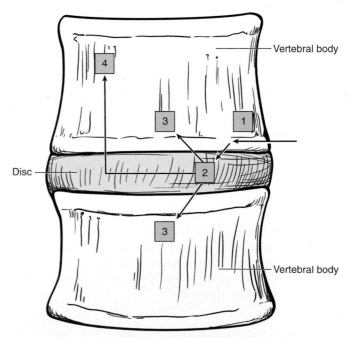

Figure 13-4. Proposed sequence of intervertebral disc infection and evolution to osteomyelitis: (*1*) microabscess in "metaphysis" (adjacent to end plate), (*2*) disc colonized and infected, (*3*) reactive process (or low-grade infection of opposite end plate). (*4*) If diagnosis and treatment are delayed, the infection can develop into vertebral osteomyelitis. *(Redrawn from Wenger DR, Ring D, Hah GV: Pyogenic infectious spondylitis in children. In Weinstein SL [ed]: The Pediatric Spine: Principles and Practice, 2nd ed. Philadelphia: Lippincott Williams & Wilkins, 2001, pp 619–633.)*

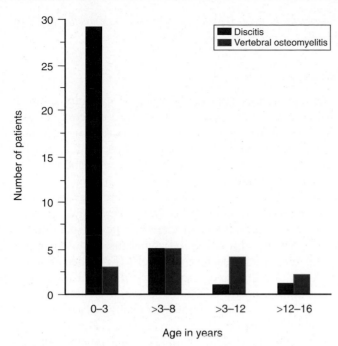

Figure 13-5. Distinct age distribution of children with discitis and vertebral osteomyelitis. *(Redrawn from Fernandez M, Carrol CL, Baker CJ: Diskitis and vertebral osteomyelitis in children: An 18-year review. Pediatrics 2000;105:1299–1304.)*

TABLE 13-1. Clinical Features of Discitis in the Toddler

Symptom	% Affected	Sign	% Affected
Limp, hip or leg pain (refusal to walk)	63	Coin test*	50
		Loss of lordosis	40
		Paraspinal muscle spasm	20
Back pain	27		
Pain-free limb weakness	9	Gibbus	18
		Neurologic signs	9
Fever	0	No classical signs	27
Abdominal pain	0		

*The coin test demonstrates an inability to flex the lower back, assessed by placing an object, such as a coin (or a sweet), on the floor and asking the child to pick it up.

Modified from Brown R, Hussain M, McHugh K, et al: Discitis in young children. J Bone Joint Surg Br 2001;83B:106–111. Reproduced with permission and copyright © of the British Editorial Society of Bone and Joint Surgery.

children is commonly from minor cuts, scrapes, or upper respiratory infections; in adults, infection arises commonly in the elderly and in more serious systemic disorders such as diabetes mellitus, chronic alcoholism, liver cirrhosis, and intravenous drug use. In the classic article by Bonfiglio in which 53 patients with pyogenic vertebral osteomyelitis and concomitant disc space infection are described, 52% of spinal infections in children were preceded by a wound or an infection, and a history of trauma was elicited in 24%. In adults, however, 41% had a remote source of infection (most commonly respiratory or genitourinary), and 55% had diabetes.

Clinical Presentation

Discitis

Children with classic discitis are typically young, usually between 3 and 5 years old, but may be as young as neonates (see Fig. 13-5). As one might expect, the young child who is incapable of verbal communication typically presents with irritability, refusal to walk or bend, with or without limping, or inability to maintain a seated position, whereas older children commonly complain of back or abdominal pain. One of the less common manifestations of early discitis seen in young children may be the Gower sign, or use of the hands to assist in rising, presumably implemented by children to avoid painful motion of the lumbar spine. More common clinical findings in discitis are presented in Table 13-1. Children with discitis may also assume a

position of lumbar extension with resistance to flexion. In a recent study of 57 children with discitis or vertebral osteomyelitis, only 28% of children with discitis presented with a fever greater than 100.3 degrees, and in only 8% did the fever exceed 101.5 degrees. None of these patients had an underlying illness. Another recent study of 11 young children with discitis showed that the average duration of symptoms prior to diagnosis of discitis was 24 days (range: 7 to 56 days) and that the initial diagnosis was incorrect in 54% of cases. Incorrect initial diagnoses included spinal cord abnormalities, irritable hip, osteomyelitis, and tumor. Patients who underwent magnetic resonance imaging (MRI) as part of the diagnostic workup had a statistically shorter time to diagnosis compared to those who did not undergo MRI. Abdominal pain and back pain are more commonly encountered initial presenting complaints in older children and in adolescents, thought to represent retroperitoneal irritation resulting from a psoas abscess.

Osteomyelitis

Children with osteomyelitis are usually older, with an age range of approximately 6 to 12 years at diagnosis. In their series of osteomyelitis and discitis patients over an 18-year period, Fernandez and colleagues reported that 57% of children with osteomyelitis complained of back pain, while other complaints included neck, shoulder, rib, and abdominal pain and one case each of prolonged fever and incontinence. Involvement of the upper cervical spine can cause a child to present with torticollis. In contrast to children with discitis, 78% of children with osteomyelitis had a history of fever, each of which exceeded 102 degrees. The duration of symptoms was also longer in children with osteomyelitis compared with those with discitis (33 days versus 22 days). Although children with osteomyelitis are typically older, vertebral osteomyelitis in infants has been reported and, in contrast to discitis, should be suspected in a child who is systemically ill. Such children have a predilection for recurrent infections and can require extended periods of antibiotic therapy. Physical examination might reveal similar findings in children with discitis, including positive straight leg testing, hamstring tightness, paraspinal muscle spasm, neurologic deficits, and tenderness over the affected region.

Laboratory Findings

The laboratory workup for children who present with the constellation of symptoms that suggest infection, as described above, should include complete blood count with differential and peripheral smear, erythrocyte sedimentation rate (ESR), C-reactive protein (CRP), and blood cultures. Although highly nonspecific, elevated serum markers for infection can help to determine whether or not an infectious etiology is present. An elevated white cell count is typically present in fewer than half of patients with biopsy-proven discitis or osteomyelitis and in even fewer in the setting of chronic infection. Although both CRP and ESR are nonspecific markers for infection and inflammation, CRP is thought to be a more rapid marker in the detection of infection (within 6 hours) and declines after appropriate treatment has been initiated faster than ESR does. The sensitivities of both CRP and ESR have been reported to be as high as 90%, although CRP might be more specific. Another study revealed that in children with discitis, a sterile blood culture was yielded in 88% of cases, compared with 46% of cases of osteomyelitis. Biopsy results will be discussed separately below.

Pathogens

Blood Cultures

In all suspected spinal infections, blood cultures should be drawn, in addition to the aforementioned lab panel, because an infectious organism might be identified without the need for a formal biopsy. A recent review of the literature reported that successful identification of a causative infectious organism was made in approximately 60% of cases (range: 27% to 88%), including blood cultures and biopsy. However, in contrast to other bone and joint space infections in children, the need to accurately identify a specific infectious agent in spinal infections remains controversial. In most cases, a thorough history, physical examination, and evaluation of inflammation markers and imaging studies can lead one to a presumptive diagnosis of discitis or osteomyelitis and the initiation of empiric antibiotic therapy. In the large series reported by Fernandez, blood cultures yielded an organism in 12% of discitis cases and in 57% of osteomyelitis cases. *Staphylococcus aureus* is the most common organism identified, but other organisms identified have included *S. epidermidis*, *Streptococcus* species,

Bartonella henselae (cat-scratch fever), *Salmonella*, and *Propionibacterium acnes* and gram-negative rods.

Biopsy

The role of biopsy in the evaluation of spinal infections in children remains controversial. If the infection persists despite an initial course of antibiotic therapy, it is common to proceed to biopsy to attempt to identify a causative agent. Other instances in which biopsy may be indicated include an immunocompromised host, neurologic deficit, progression of disease despite antibiotic therapy, or any other atypical situation. Other researchers, however, argue that a biopsy should be considered in the initial evaluation of the patient with suspected spinal infection, citing evidence that computed tomography (CT)-guided biopsy is rapid, is cost-effective, may reduce the need for general anesthesia (although conscious sedation carries its own set of risks), and has been shown to change management in up to 35% of cases. In most instances, CT-guided biopsy has largely replaced open biopsy when possible, but the latter might be necessary if CT-guided biopsy yields no organism (Fig. 13-6). The two main objectives in obtaining a frozen section during the biopsy procedure are to ensure that (1) lesional tissue is obtained and (2) harvested tissue is sufficient to determine whether the lesion is infectious in nature or neoplastic (i.e., Ewing sarcoma). The literature reports a diagnostic yield from biopsy ranging from 58% to 91%, slightly better results being found with open biopsy.

In the thoracic spine, surgical options for open biopsy include thoracotomy used for standard anterior thoracic

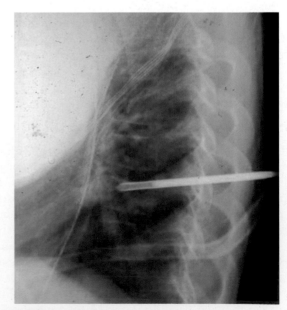

Figure 13-6. Lateral radiograph demonstrating an in-progress spinal biopsy. Thoracic spinal biopsy can be performed by using CT-guided imaging or intraoperative fluoroscopy.

spinal procedures, video-assisted thoracoscopic surgery, and other minimally invasive systems (recently described as an alternative to these larger, potentially more morbid approaches). Similarly, in the cervical and lumbar spine, minimally invasive approaches are becoming viable alternatives to standard open approaches to obtain tissue for suspected infection.

Differential Diagnosis

In addition to discitis and vertebral osteomyelitis, a child who presents with a clinical picture of infection should also warrant consideration of the following other diagnoses: Scheuermann's kyphosis, spinal epidural abscess (usually seen in association with discitis or vertebral osteomyelitis), psoas abscess, sacroiliac infection, osteoid osteoma, osteoblastoma, eosinophilic granuloma, Langerhans cell histiocytosis, and primary malignancy. Consideration should also be given to intervertebral disc calcification and other infectious etiologies, including tuberculous spondylitis, pyomyositis, and fungal infections, some of which are briefly discussed below.

Radiographic Features

Roentgenography

Imaging in the workup for spinal infection should initially include plain radiographs to evaluate for gross vertebral abnormalities and bone destruction, sagittal or coronal plane deformities, and obvious loss of disc height. Such changes, however, rarely manifest prior to 2 weeks of the onset of disease. A recent study of 33 discitis patients revealed that 76% had abnormal radiographs, most commonly loss of disc height and adjacent end plate erosions suggestive of multiple vertebral involvement but also abnormal prevertebral soft tissue contours (Fig. 13-7). Late sequelae include kyphosis, fracture, and vertebral body collapse. In contrast, a recent review of 13 vertebral osteomyelitis patients revealed that plain-film radiographic changes occurred in only 46% of patients with osteomyelitis. Because early identification and treatment have been shown to correlate with improved outcome, advanced imaging is typically warranted to make the diagnosis.

Computed Tomography

The majority of bony changes that are detectable by CT, including end plate destruction, soft tissue masses, and epidural masses, are in most cases also visualized by MRI, which provides additional characterization of the disc and soft tissues. For these reasons, CT is less commonly utilized as a second diagnostic tool after plain radiographs. Another disadvantage of CT is that intravenous contrast (usually metrizamide) is typically required to distinguish between soft tissue masses. However, one remaining role

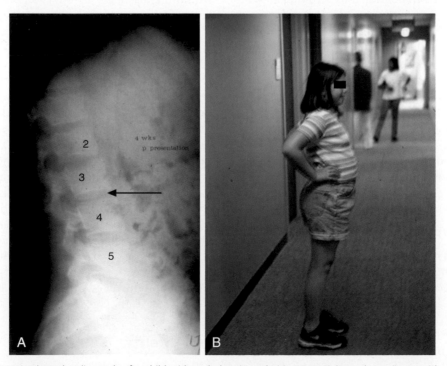

Figure 13-7. A, Representative lateral radiograph of a child with end plate irregularities at L3-4 (*arrow*) consistent with discitis. **B,** Common clinical presentation of a child with discitis; notice posture with hyperextension and resistance to flexion.

for CT in the evaluation of spinal infections in children is CT-guided biopsy.

Bone Scanning

Especially in young children who either are incapable of verbal communication or do not have the ability to localize pain, technetium-99m MDP (methylene diphosphonate) bone scanning remains a good first-line diagnostic tool. If positive, subsequent evaluation with CT or MRI may be better localized to more comprehensively evaluate the disc spaces, vertebral bodies, and surrounding soft tissues. Bone scanning is also effective in the early stages, prior to radiographic evidence of disc space collapse or vertebral end plate changes. The sensitivity of technetium bone scans is reported to be as high as 90%. This sensitivity can be improved to 87% to 98% with the use of three-phase bone scan. One limitation, however, is that the bone scan might be falsely negative if there is insufficient blood supply to the affected region due to bone loss, tumor, space-occupying lesion, and so on. A recent study in young children reported a sensitivity of only one in four using bone scanning, which raises doubts about the sensitivity of bone scan in the detection of discitis in the young children, compared with MRI, which had a reported sensitivity of 100%.

Single-Photon Emission Computed Tomography

Single-photon emission computed tomography (SPECT) has been shown to be more sensitive than planar scintigraphy, allowing for three-dimensional localization and improved contrast. A recent study compared the efficacy of bone and gallium-67 SPECT with MRI to detect spinal osteomyelitis and found that gallium-67 SPECT scan was accurate in the detection of spinal osteomyelitis and accompanying soft tissue infections. The authors recommend this technique as an alternative diagnostic tool if MRI is not available or to augment the diagnostic workup in uncertain cases. Another potential advantage of gallium-67 SPECT is its utility in following infections, since they become negative when the infectious process has resolved, compared with technetium bone scans, which stay positive for months.

Positron Emission Tomography

Recent advances have made positron emission tomography (PET) scanning a potentially useful diagnostic tool in the workup of spinal infections. Specifically, fluorine-18 fluorodeoxyglucose PET (FDG-PET) is useful in following spinal tumors and in the detection of spinal infections. A recent study reported a 100% sensitivity of detection of histopathologically confirmed spinal infections. Another study reported that FDG-PET was the test of choice when compared to MRI, gallium-67 SPECT, and technetium bone scanning in the detection of spinal infections, most notably in patients with low-grade infections, soft tissue infections, and bony degeneration. The main disadvantage of FDG-PET at this point is its inability to reliably distinguish between infection and neoplasm. PET scan has also shown promise in the detection of infection in the postoperative spine. One recent paper reported a negative predictive value of 100% and accuracy of 86%, although the authors acknowledge that PET scan currently is not particularly specific. Future studies will explore this potentially useful adjunct to current diagnostic modalities.

Magnetic Resonance Imaging

Most authors would agree that magnetic resonance imaging (MRI) remains the gold standard diagnostic tool for advanced imaging in the detection of spinal infections. Its improved sensitivity, lack of radiation, and ability to more easily discern among different types of infection and distinguish infection from neoplasm make this modality more useful than CT, which traditionally has been an excellent tool to evaluate bony involvement and, to a lesser extent, surrounding soft tissue abscesses. To successfully perform MRI in young children, it is usually necessary to utilize either general anesthesia or conscious sedation. Typical MRI findings include bone marrow edema (early), which is best detected as decreased signal on T1 or increased signal on T2; diminished distinction of the disc space; adjacent vertebral body end plate involvement; paravertebral soft tissue involvement; erosion of the vertebral end plates; reduced disc height; and increased signal uptake within the disc (Fig. 13-8). While the typical findings are present in approximately 95% of cases, atypical MRI findings have been reported and include increased signal on T1, reduced signal on T2, and involvement of only one vertebral body without involvement of the disc, thought to represent an early stage of disease progression. One series reported sensitivity of 96% and accuracy of 94% in detecting vertebral osteomyelitis, while identification of a soft tissue mass involving the epidural space has a reported sensitivity of 98% for infection. In the earliest suspected cases of vertebral osteomyelitis, post-contrast fat-suppressed T1-weighted MRI is recommended. Postcontrast (Gd-DTPA) MRI is also useful in distinguishing between epidural abscess and solid granulation tissue and more readily determines abscess size compared with noncontrast imaging. In the workup for suspected spinal epidural abscess (i.e., pus under pressure), which often constitutes a surgical emergency requiring urgent decompression, gadolinium-enhanced MRI is the imaging modality of choice.

Treatment

Although most authors currently would agree that discitis represents an infectious etiology and should be treated

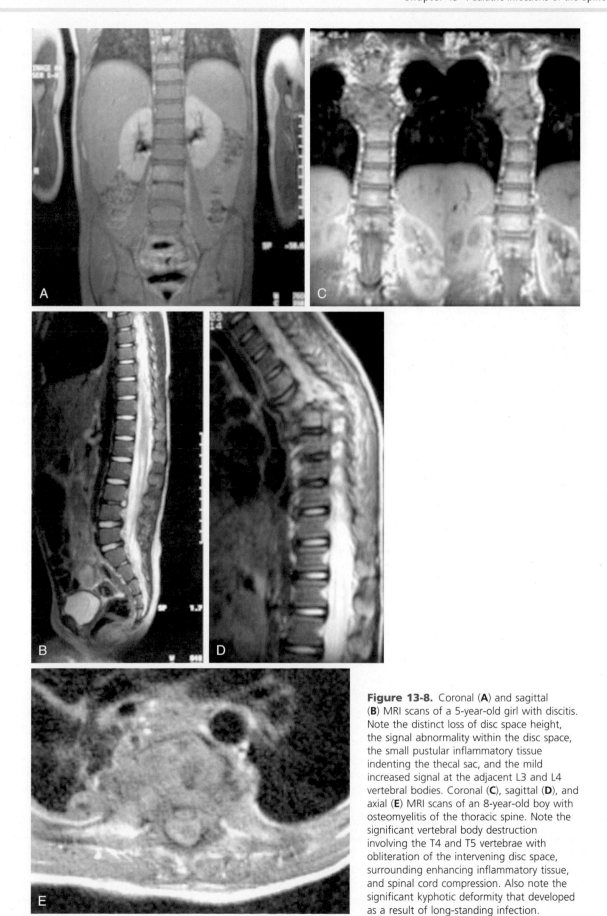

Figure 13-8. Coronal (**A**) and sagittal (**B**) MRI scans of a 5-year-old girl with discitis. Note the distinct loss of disc space height, the signal abnormality within the disc space, the small pustular inflammatory tissue indenting the thecal sac, and the mild increased signal at the adjacent L3 and L4 vertebral bodies. Coronal (**C**), sagittal (**D**), and axial (**E**) MRI scans of an 8-year-old boy with osteomyelitis of the thoracic spine. Note the significant vertebral body destruction involving the T4 and T5 vertebrae with obliteration of the intervening disc space, surrounding enhancing inflammatory tissue, and spinal cord compression. Also note the significant kyphotic deformity that developed as a result of long-standing infection.

with antibiotics for some period of time, previous series in the literature have questioned this infectious etiology. One study of 18 children with nonspecific discitis (without confirmed antimicrobial cause) followed up to 9 years demonstrated no differences between those patients treated with either bed rest and antibiotics or bed rest alone. Other similar reports with small numbers have demonstrated that discitis is self-limiting in most cases, whether or not antibiotics are used in the treatment protocol. Many of these small series, however, are insufficiently powered to be able to claim no difference between the treatment groups and are limited by the use of highly variable treatment regimens. Further, many patients in these studies who failed to improve with immobilization were subsequently begun on antimicrobial therapy and improved rapidly. More recently, it has become more accepted that discitis is infectious in origin, like vertebral osteomyelitis, and should be treated with antibiotics initially. Ring and colleagues recently studied discitis in 47 children who were treated with variable antimicrobial and immobilization regimens. The authors found that among the children who were treated without immobilization, the rate of recurrence or prolonged symptoms was 67% when no antibiotics were administered. In contrast, 18% of children who received intravenous antibiotics and 50% who received oral antibiotics had prolonged or recurrent symptoms. Several recent authors have agreed on the initial use of intravenous antibiotics to minimize the risk of recurrence and to optimize chances for a rapid recovery.

Once the diagnosis has been made on the basis of clinical presentation, lab values, and imaging studies, empiric intravenous antibiotics are begun, usually a first-generation cephalosporin, along with some form of immobilization or bed rest. There is currently no universally agreed-upon duration of therapy, but intravenous antibiotics are typically administered for a period of 1 to 2 weeks, followed by oral antibiotics for a minimum of 2 to 4 weeks, for a total of 4 to 6 weeks of antibiotics. If a specific organism has been identified through blood culture or biopsy (discussed in detail above), then antibiotic therapy is tailored accordingly. During this time, the child is carefully observed for clinical signs of improvement and a normalization in lab values, the most important being the CRP level, which is a more sensitive marker of disease onset (and resolution of disease) than the ESR is.

If symptoms persist despite an appropriate length of empiric antibiotic administration, one option is to obtain a CT-guided, percutaneous or open biopsy in hopes of identifying an organism and modifying the antibiotic regimen for another bout of nonoperative therapy (discussed above). Indications to proceed directly to surgical intervention include failure to improve despite a known organism, rapid clinical worsening consistent with sepsis, neurologic deterioration, progressive deformity, or an abscess that is causing neurologic compromise or is not responsive to antibiotic therapy. In these rare instances, surgical drainage with or without spinal stabilization may be necessary. In most cases, since the pathology is usually located in the anterior elements, an anterior approach is utilized to access the affected vertebral bodies and perform the bony debridement or drainage. The treatment of choice for a neurologic deficit caused by an epidural abscess is prompt surgical decompression, usually posteriorly, with or without fusion. However, an anterior approach can be contemplated if significant anterior column destruction is also identified. Chronic osteomyelitis might require surgery when a biomechanically unstable spine results from progressive deformity in the coronal or sagittal plane, or both. In some instances with severe deformity, a combined anterior-posterior or two-staged procedure using autogenous anterior strut bone grafting could be necessary to initially eradicate infection anteriorly, followed by spinal stabilization via posterior spinal fusion with instrumentation.

Outcomes

A remarkable number of patients with discitis and vertebral osteomyelitis respond appropriately to antibiotics, have a complete resolution of symptoms, and resume normal childhood activities. The rate of recurrence has been shown to be minimized with prompt recognition and initiation of antibiotics but has been shown to range from 0% to 25%. One recent paper reported that 90% of patients were free of pain with a satisfactory functional outcome. Occasionally, patients with cervical involvement may experience limited range of motion (by one third) following spontaneous cervical fusion. Overall, it has been reported that spontaneous fusion following vertebral osteomyelitis is approximately 50% but may be as high as 74% and is most notable in the cervical and upper thoracic spine. Although some restoration of disc space height is common following resolution of infection, most authors have reported varying amounts of disc height restoration, none being restored fully. Two studies found that children with persistent radiographic changes were more likely to experience back pain. Infants with vertebral osteomyelitis have a propensity toward recurrence and might therefore warrant an extended duration of antibiotics to minimize this risk. Long-term outcome in these patients revealed a radiographic appearance similar to that of congenital kyphosis with either anterior failure of segmentation or posterior hemivertebrae. Other late sequelae of spinal infections, although rare, include scoliosis, loss of lordosis, kyphosis, and persistent loss of signal intensity on T2-weighted MRI, possibly reflecting a loss of disc hydration due to disc fibrosis.

TUBERCULOSIS

Thought to be under control in the mid-1980s, tuberculosis (TB) remains an important source of spinal infection in both developed and underdeveloped countries. The rise in number of diagnosed cases in the United States is partly attributable to increased immigration from third-world countries, the AIDS epidemic, intravenous drug use, homelessness, the aging population, and poverty. It has been suggested that the prevalence of TB is inversely proportional to the socioeconomic status of a particular region. Specific challenges that face physicians treating children with TB include drug resistance in some areas of endemic disease, controversy surrounding the indications for operative treatment, and the complex nature of the spinal deformities resulting from long-standing untreated disease that affect many children. Although TB remains less common than discitis and vertebral osteomyelitis, it must be considered in the child with suspected spinal infection who fails to improve with empiric intravenous antibiotic therapy or any child with the aforementioned risk factors.

Spinal involvement of *Mycobacterium tuberculosis* is usually the result of spread from a primary lung or genitourinary source, often quiescent, that spreads via the lymphatic system. In contrast to pyogenic spinal infections that cause damage via direct action of proteolytic enzymes, a delayed hypersensitivity reaction occurs in TB, characterized by low bacterial counts within the lesion. The most common location of spinal involvement in children is the thoracolumbar junction and surrounding segments, while the posterior elements are often spared. Abscess formation is common and indicates active disease. With increasing abscess size, the protective periosteal layer becomes stripped, which can result in devascularization of the vertebral body and an aneurysmal-type defect within the body. Resultant propagation of the abscess into surrounding visceral organs occurs frequently and can cause related pulmonary and visceral complaints.

Clinical Presentation

In milder forms of disease, children may present with weight loss, anorexia, back pain, and fatigue, but rarely fever. Later stages of the disease process can produce pulmonary symptoms that may result either from bronchial compression due to ruptured high thoracic paraspinal abscess into the surrounding lung, which may present as stridor, chest pain, or abdominal pain, or from primary TB involvement of the lung. Other manifestations of late-stage disease include complications from paraspinal abscess formation, draining sinus tract formation, gait disturbance as a result of psoas abscess, scoliosis or kyphosis, spasticity from infection spread into the meninges, and Pott's paraplegia. With cervical spine or occipital involvement, children may present with atlantoaxial rotatory instability, atlantoaxial rotatory fixation, torticollis, dysphagia, and cervical kyphosis.

Making the diagnosis of spinal TB can be difficult in the young child. The utility of the Tine skin test is poor in areas where TB is endemic; however, it remains an important first-line test in suspected cases. A chest radiograph is essential to identify a potential pulmonary lesion. A recent study from Malaysia revealed that ESR may be an important factor in identifying infection and in predicting evolution of paraplegia in spinal tuberculosis, while sputum samples and bacterial culture are less helpful. A positive bacterial culture remains the gold standard diagnostic test but can be difficult to confirm in chronic cases, because of the lower bacterial counts of mycobacteria in bone compared with those of visceral organs.

Imaging

Plain radiographs of the spine typically demonstrate destruction of one or more vertebral bodies with sparing of the disc space in the early phases of the disease. A recent study in adults found that this classic pattern was present in only approximately 50% of cases. The remaining patients demonstrated patterns that were typical of discitis and osteomyelitis with involvement of the disc space and adjacent vertebral bodies. The thoracic spine is more commonly affected than is either the lumbar or cervical spine. Meningeal involvement strongly suggests TB. Four patterns of vertebral involvement have been described: (1) paradiscal (more common in adults) lesions adjacent to the disc with disc space narrowing; (2) anterior subperiosteal lesion, which facilitates propagation of infection under the anterior longitudinal ligament into contiguous vertebral bodies; (3) central lesions (more common in children), which involve the entire vertebral body and are prone to collapse, vertebra plana, and kyphosis; and (4) posterior element disease. The degree of kyphotic deformity is related to the number of involved vertebrae and is most common in the thoracolumbar region. Paraspinal abscesses are common and, in some cases, may track through fascial planes into the mediastinum and lung.

The most salient differences on MRI between tuberculous spondylitis and pyogenic spondylitis are highlighted in Box 13-1. Similarly, a recent study examined the main

---

BOX 13-1 Magnetic Resonance Appearances and Likely Pathogen: Tuberculous Versus Bacterial Spondylitis

MRI Findings Indicating Tuberculous Spondylitis as the More Likely Cause	MRI Findings Indicating Bacterial Spondylitis as the More Likely Cause
Well-defined paraspinal abnormal signal	Ill-defined paraspinal abnormal signal
Thin, smooth abscess wall	Thick, irregular abscess wall
Subligamentous spread to three or more vertebral levels	No subligamentous spread or spread to fewer than three levels
Involvement of multiple vertebral bodies	Involvement of two or fewer vertebral bodies
Rim enhancement around an intraosseous abscess	Absence of intraosseous or paraspinal abscess

From James SL, Davies AM: Imaging of infectious spinal disorders in children and adults. Eur J Radiol 2006;58:27–40.

differences between tuberculous spondylitis and pyogenic spondylitis in adults and concluded that (1) contrast-enhanced studies are important to distinguish between the two, (2) tuberculous spondylitis exhibits a heterogeneous and focal pattern of enhancement, (3) the disc is preserved in TB, (4) TB exhibits a well-defined paraspinal abnormal signal, and (5) TB demonstrates intraosseous abscess with rim enhancement of the vertebral body. Recently, a potential role for FDG-PET has been proposed in the detection of cold tuberculous abscesses.

Treatment

The current recommended first-line chemotherapeutic regimen consists of streptomycin, isoniazid, and rifampin. In some instances (i.e., in poor responders or cases of antibiotic resistance), second-line antibiotic agents ethambutol and pyrazinamide are added. Chemotherapy is recommended for a minimum of 6 months in most cases.

It is unclear whether or not surgical debridement, with or without spinal stabilization, is required in every case of spinal TB. A recent study from the Cochrane review in adults questioned the recommendation for routine surgery for spinal TB. In analyzing 331 patients from two randomized controlled trials in Japan and Korea, the authors concluded that routine surgery cannot be recommended unless it is within the context of a large, randomized controlled trial. In the healthy patient who is diagnosed early with a small abscess and minimal bone destruction, it is reasonable to attempt a trial of nonoperative management. For most others, however, routine surgical intervention is indicated.

When surgery is indicated, it is often performed via an anterior approach, since the vast majority of the pathology in TB of the spine rests in the anterior elements. Access to the anterior elements provides an opportunity to perform an aggressive debridement of the involved soft tissue and bony elements, as well as placement of an anterior strut graft for structural stabilization. The classic Hong Kong operation includes debridement and placement of either autogenous rib or iliac crest between the two prepared end plates while holding the deformity correction. Alternatively, anterior arthrodesis in the treatment of spinal TB has also been proposed with the use of interbody titanium cages. Anterior spinal fusion also facilitates the simultaneous correction of kyphotic deformity by using an oversized graft. Aside from the rare occasion when there is posterior element involvement, posterior spinal fusion alone is generally not recommended. In young children with posterior growth remaining, posterior spinal fusion, in conjunction with anterior debridement and fusion, can prevent progression of kyphosis. A combined anterior-posterior procedure is also potentially indicated for additional spinal stability in the face of a large kyphotic deformity or one that involves multiple levels. With the use of the Hong Kong and other surgical techniques, neurologic decompression and spinal debridement can be achieved while avoiding complications such as late recurrence and progressive spinal deformity.

DISC SPACE CALCIFICATION

In contrast to adults, disc calcification in children is most commonly seen in the cervical spine. Of unknown etiology, disc calcification is often a painful, self-limited process that is occasionally preceded by a traumatic event but may also be secondary to an inflammatory process or upper respiratory infection. It is most commonly seen in males around age 7 to 8 years. Patients usually have one-level involvement, but in some cases, multiple disc spaces may be involved. Sometimes following a preceding history of infection or trauma, children may present with cervical spine involvement manifesting as neck pain, torticollis, stiffness, and spasm, with neurologic involvement in up to 29% of patients. Laboratory values may show a leukocytosis, an elevated CRP or elevated ESR, thus mimicking infection. Lateral cervical spine radiographs reveal dense, oval-shaped disc calcification involving the majority of the disc space. MRI typically reveals low signal intensity on T1-weighted images and high signal intensity on T2-weighted images (see Fig. 13-11 later in the chapter). No correlation has been shown between radiographic findings and severity of symptoms.

The treatment for disc space calcification is almost universally nonoperative. Conservative management consists of pain control, rest, traction, and possibly use of a cervical collar until symptoms abate. Antibiotics are not routinely prescribed. The prognosis for this condition is excellent; a recent report demonstrated that all patients had complete resolution of symptoms at an average of 34 days and resolution of radiographic findings at 15 months. Rarely, surgical intervention is required for cord compression and myelopathy.

PYOMYOSITIS

Pyomyositis is a bacterial infection of muscle that occurs more commonly in tropical regions. Affected children can present with back pain, neck pain, and restricted trunk or neck motion. Pyomyositis must be considered in the differential diagnosis of a child who appears septic. Concomitant abscess formation is common, with some reports as high as 90%. Abscesses may be singular or multiple, and in the back, they commonly involve the multifidus muscle. Although the etiology remains unknown, antecedent trauma that can localize skin flora, most notably staphylococci, into damaged muscle has been proposed. The diagnosis can be made with CT or with MRI, which will reveal abscess formation within the muscle but might also demonstrate coexistent bony changes that could represent either reactive inflammatory changes or early osteomyelitis. An initial attempt can be made at percutaneous drainage of abscesses. Failure to respond to incision and drainage and antibiotic therapy should raise suspicion for a second abscess that was not detected initially.

PEARLS & PITFALLS

PEARLS

■ Although autologous fibula and rib strut grafts are not routinely used for spinal reconstructive surgeries, they remain an excellent option for procedures that require long strut grafts, including anterior thoracic spinal reconstruction for tuberculous or pyogenic spondylitis. These long strut autografts can also be useful in spinal reconstructions following infection for progressive kyphosis or kyphoscoliosis that require multilevel cervical corpectomies, posterior cervical reconstruction, and posterior occipitocervical fusion. For posterior occipitocervical fusions in children, the rib is uniquely shaped to permit maximal graft-recipient bed contact. In children, the rib is also an abundant source of graft material and rapidly regenerates, compared with iliac crest bone graft. If the shape or amount of material of autologous strut graft is improperly matched to the host, then iliac crest bone graft can be used to augment the strut graft.

■ In performing complex spinal reconstruction procedures for infection or other deformities, we recommend the routine use of intraoperative neuromonitoring with combined transcranial motor and somatosensory evoked potential monitoring. By using this combined modality, both the dorsal sensory and ventral motor tracts of the spinal cord can be monitored essentially in real time to facilitate constant evaluation of the cord, as it is susceptible to injury from hypoperfusion, provocative maneuvers, and placement of instrumentation. In cases requiring a reduction of kyphosis or kyphoscoliosis, we recommend a careful, slow reduction with frequent spinal cord stimulation to monitor the vascular status of the cord as it becomes distracted and straightened out from its initial position. By using these aggressive monitoring measures, an impending neurologic injury can be identified while it is still transient, and an appropriate team response can be instituted. This may include some combination of the following steps: correction of hypotension, administration of steroids, reduction of correction, or removal of hardware. If pedicle screw placement in the thoracic spine is anticipated, we recommend the routine use of spontaneous and stimulated electromyelographic monitoring to minimize the likelihood of sustaining a permanent nerve root injury.

■ Surveillance imaging of the spine is particularly important to track spinal tumors and infection. At our institution, it is common to perform posterior spinal fusion with instrumentation at the time of spinal cord tumor excision and decompression, as we have shown significantly reduced rates of deformity progression using this technique. Occasionally, spinal infections also render the spine unstable, thus warranting an aggressive surgical debridement followed by spinal fusion with instrumentation. Using titanium alloy spinal implants facilitates the continued ability to visualize the spinal elements on MRI. The decreased ferromagnetic properties of the titanium alloy promote less distortion and therefore a better image to monitor the spinal tumor or infection.

PITFALLS

■ In children with intervertebral disc calcification, one must resist the temptation to rush to surgery in all patients with a new-onset or progressive neurologic deficit. The natural history of this disease has recently been studied by Dai and colleagues, who demonstrated that all 17 patients in their series with the disease, including the 5 patients with neurologic deficits that corresponded to the expected anatomic distribution of spinal cord compression, had complete resolution of symptoms without the need for surgical intervention. With the numbers available, there was no difference between age, level of calcification, degree of canal compromise, or severity of symptoms with time to resolution of symptoms or of the calcification.

■ Although the classic MRI appearances of the disc, vertebral body, and end plate in spinal infections described above are present in up to 95% of cases, atypical patterns of MRI findings can be seen and must be recognized to avoid a delay in diagnosis. Variations may include isointense or decreased signal in the disc on T1 and isointense or reduced signal change on T2. Additionally, the disc might remain isointense, but the surrounding soft tissues will provide clues to the diagnosis by the presence of fluid or a paravertebral soft tissue abscess. Likewise, an infection is occasionally indicated by vertebral body involvement only and no disc involvement; however, this latter situation might also reflect a Brodie's abscess or chronic infection. In these atypical situations, in which MRI fails to reliably make the diagnosis, especially in a child with these radiologic findings and suspected infection who fails to respond to empiric antibiotic therapy, the treating physician should have a low threshold to proceed to CT-guided biopsy to obtain tissue for more directed antibiotic therapy or to rule out a neoplastic process.

Illustrative Case Presentations

CASE 1. Discitis

E.W. is a 13-year-old female with a chief complaint of low back pain for 3 months that had become more severe over the past 3 weeks. There was no radiation into her lower extremities. Her pain at its worst rated 9/10 and frequently woke her from sleep. The patient reported low-grade fevers over the past 2 weeks but none surpassing 101.0 degrees. Anti-inflammatory medications helped to abate the pain but never completely relieved it. She was never immobilized for any period of time. Evaluation and treatment by her chiropractor did not help. On examination, the patient had 5/5 strength in upper and lower motor examination, sensation was intact in all dermatomes, and reflexes were present and symmetrical. There was focal tenderness over the L3-4 region, and the patient had an antalgic gait. She was more comfortable on her side, with her legs drawn up in a flexed position.

Laboratory values revealed no abnormalities on peripheral WBC count, ESR, or CRP.

Plain-film radiography revealed mild disc space narrowing of approximately 50% with some straightening of the lumbar spine. Bone scan revealed notable uptake in the L3-4 disc space. MRI revealed some loss of disc height and loss of signal at the L3-4 level (Fig. 13-9). There was no abnormal collection or compression on the dural sac or neural elements.

The patient underwent a period of bracing for 2 weeks, along with oral antibiotics for a period of 6 weeks. At the 6-week follow-up, the patient reported complete resolution of symptoms. Repeat MRI revealed persistent loss of disc height and no signal abnormalities in the adjacent vertebral bodies.

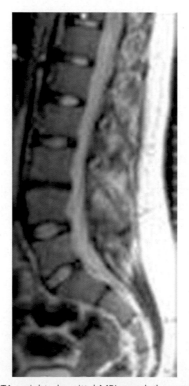

Figure 13-9. T1-weighted sagittal MRI revealed some loss of disc height, loss of signal at the L3-4 level, and loss of distinction between the nucleus pulposus and the annulus fibrosus. There was no abnormal collection or compression on the dural sac or neural elements.

CASE 2. Tuberculosis

J.R. is a 9-year-old male who was seen in a Bhutanese refugee camp in the eastern jungles near Bangladesh. The patient's family had noticed a slight "hump" over his back for several years. This prompted evaluation by a physician, who diagnosed the patient with spinal tuberculosis. The patient then received a 6-month course of antituberculosis chemotherapy at around age 6, but he never had any intervention regarding the developing kyphotic deformity. The kyphus progressed insidiously, and over the past 6 to 12 months prior to arrival in the clinic, the patient showed signs of a progressive paraparesis that rendered him wheelchair bound. There were no known fevers. Physical examination revealed global lower-extremity weakness, diminished sensation in all dermatomes, absent perianal sensation, and absent reflexes bilaterally. There was clonus and a positive Babinski's sign.

Clinical presentation, roentgenography, and MRI (Fig. 13-10) revealed a significant kyphotic deformity with chronic vertebral body destruction. MRI was performed to determine whether this was a recurrent case of tuberculosis or "healed disease," which has a different prognosis. The paraparesis of healed disease, seen months to years following treatment, usually involves chronic compression as the cord drapes over the gibbus, compounded by compression from fibrotic bands and chronic granulation tissue. The surgical procedure of choice to decompress the cord in these cases of healed disease is an internal kyphectomy, which carries a significant neurologic risk.

Another course of antibiotic therapy was undertaken, and within a period of months, the paraparesis had slowly partially resolved, and the patient was able to take a few steps with assistance. Although significantly disabled and living in an area of limited resources, it was recommended that the patient undergo surgical correction, which included anterior débridement and bone grafting followed by posterior instrumentation and fusion to correct and stabilize the significant kyphoscoliotic deformity. The parents, however, refused surgical intervention. Unfortunately, the patient was lost to follow-up.

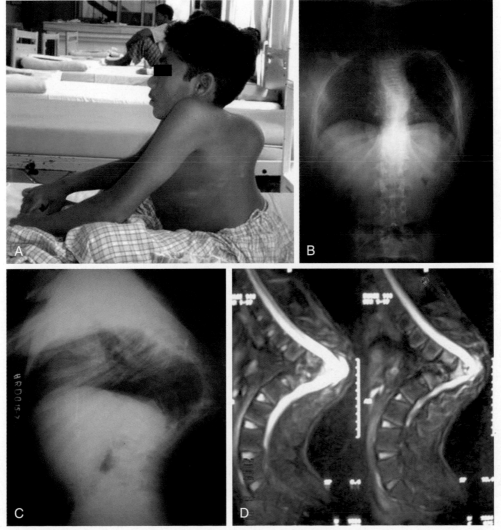

Figure 13-10. A, Clinical picture of an 8-year-old boy with long-standing spinal tuberculosis with prominent kyphotic deformity (gibbus). **B** and **C,** AP and lateral radiographs showing severe kyphoscoliotic deformity. **D,** MRI demonstrating vertebral body destruction, complete obliteration of disc space, draping of spinal cord over sharp angular deformity, and significant kyphosis. *(Courtesy of Dr. David A. Spiegel, MD.)*

CASE 3. Intervertebral Disc Calcification

T.M. is a 9-year-old male who presented with neck pain and torticollis but without neurologic signs or symptoms. The patient was prescribed nighttime cervical traction for several weeks. The pain eventually diminished, and the patient achieved increased range of motion (Fig. 13-11A). At 1 month follow-up, the patient no longer experienced neck pain and had achieved 90% of normal neck range of motion. Plain radiographs revealed disc calcification at the C5-6 level. Lateral and posteroanterior plain radiographs (Fig. 13-11B and 13-11C) show flattening of multiple vertebral bodies. Calcification (arrow) is visible in the intervertebral discs. Axial MRI (Fig. 13-11D) reveals abnormalities of the cervical disc of C4-5. Sagittal MRI (Fig. 13-11E) reveals abnormalities of C2-3, C3-4, and C4-5. Cervical end plates are intact, and there is no evidence of tumor or an infectious process. The patient currently remains free of symptoms.

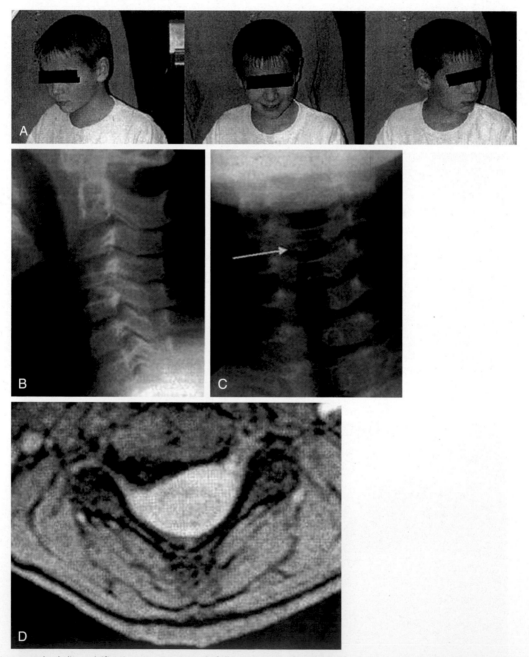

Figure 13-11. Intervertebral disc calcification. **A,** One month following cervical orthosis (daytime) and cervical traction (nighttime), neck range of motion is 90% restored. Lateral (**B**) and posteroanterior (**C**) plain radiographs show flattening of multiple vertebral bodies. Calcification (*arrow*) is visible in the intervertebral discs. **D,** Axial MRI reveals abnormalities of the cervical disc of C4-5. *(From Flynn JM, Dormans JP: Diskitis, osteomyelitis, and intervertebral disc calcification in children. In Cervical Spine Research Society Editorial Committee [eds]: The Cervical Spine, 4th ed. Philadelphia: Lippincott Williams & Wilkins, 2005, pp 537–550.)*

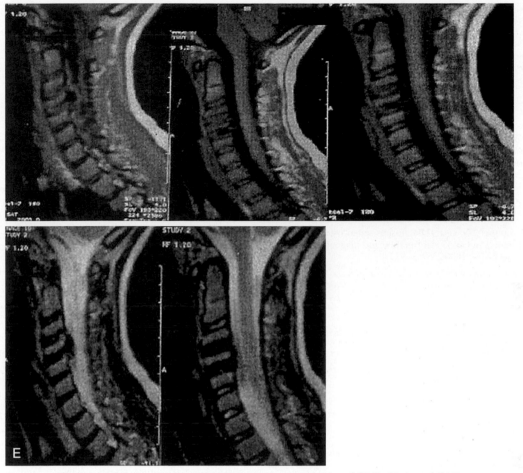

Figure 13-11, cont'd. E, Sagittal MRI reveals abnormalities of C2-3, C3-4, and C4-5.

REFERENCES

Boston HC Jr, Bianco AJ Jr, Rhodes KH: Disk space infections in children. Orthop Clin North Am 1975;6:953–964.

Crawford AH, Kucharzyk DW, Ruda R, Smitherman HC Jr: Diskitis in children. Clin Orthop Relat Res 1991;(266):70–79.

Grünebaum M, Horodniceanu C, Mukamel M, et al: The imaging diagnosis of nonpyogenic discitis in children. Pediatr Radiol 1982;12: 133–137.

Menelaus MB: Discitis. An inflammation affecting the intervertebral discs in children. J Bone Joint Surg Br 1964;46:16–23.

Ryöppy S, Jääskeläinen J, Rapola J, Alberty A: Nonspecific diskitis in children. A nonmicrobial disease? Clin Orthop Relat Res 1993;(297): 95–99.

SUGGESTED READINGS

Bonfiglio M, Lange TA, Kim YM: Pyogenic vertebral osteomyelitis. Disk space infections. Clin Orthop Relat Res 1973;234–247.

Classic article on vertebral osteomyelitis with secondary disc space infection. The authors attempt to clarify the pathogenesis of disc space infection and highlight problems associated with diagnosis and treatment.

Dai LY, Ye H, Qian QR: The natural history of cervical disc calcification in children. J Bone Joint Surg Am 2004;86-A:1467–1472.

Seventeen children with calcified cervical intervertebral discs were evaluated and followed for a mean of 5 years. All patients underwent conservative treatment including analgesia, traction, and/or a cervical collar until symptoms abated. All patients had a complete resolution of symptoms and calcification at an average of 34 days (symptoms) and 15 months (calcification).

Eismont FJ, Bohlman HH, Soni PL, et al: Vertebral osteomyelitis in infants. J Bone Joint Surg Br 1982;64:32–35.

Retrospective cases series of four patients with vertebral osteomyelitis that highlighted the more severe nature of this disease compared with discitis and the potential need for long-term antibiotics in this population to prevent recurrence.

Fernandez M, Carrol CL, Baker CJ: Diskitis and vertebral osteomyelitis in children: An 18-year review. Pediatrics 2000;105:1299–1304.

Single-institution experience over 18 years in treating vertebral osteomyelitis and discitis in children. The authors report the clinical, radiographic, diagnostic, and treatment differences between discitis and osteomyelitis.

Flynn JM, Dormans JP: Discitis, osteomyelitis, and intervertebral disc calcification in children. In Clark C (ed): The Cervical Spine, 4th ed. Philadelphia: Lippincott Williams & Wilkins, 2005, pp 537–550.

Review chapter highlighting etiology, pathogenesis, diagnosis, and treatment for intervertebral disc calcification, osteomyelitis, discitis, and tuberculosis of the cervical spine.

James SL, Davies AM: Imaging of infectious spinal disorders in children and adults. Eur J Radiol 2006;58:27–40.

Review article highlighting key updates on established and novel imaging techniques used to diagnose and follow infectious spinal conditions in adults and children.

Jutte PC, Loenhout-Rooyackers JH: Routine surgery in addition to chemotherapy for treating spinal tuberculosis. Cochrane Database Syst Rev 2006;CD004532.

The authors reviewed randomized controlled trials with a minimum of 1 year follow up that compared surgery with chemotherapy versus chemotherapy alone to evaluate the role of surgery in addition to chemotherapy in spinal tuberculosis. They concluded that insufficient evidence existed to support the routine recommendation for surgery, although the review was limited by number of patients available.

Klockner C, Valencia R: Sagittal alignment after anterior debridement and fusion with or without additional posterior instrumentation in the treatment of pyogenic and tuberculous spondylodiskitis. Spine 2003;28:1036–1042.

Retrospective clinical study comparing 49 patients with pyogenic and tuberculous spondylodiscitis treated with anterior débridement and bone grafting with 22 patients who also received posterior instrumentation. The authors concluded that in single-level spondylodiscitis without major structural loss, anterior surgery alone is adequate, but additional posterior instrumentation may be warranted in patients with multiple-level involvement or kyphotic deformity, or both.

Love C, Patel M, Lonner BS, et al: Diagnosing spinal osteomyelitis: A comparison of bone and Ga-67 scintigraphy and magnetic resonance imaging. Clin Nucl Med 2000;25:963–977.

This study compared the accuracy of bone and Ga-67 scintigraphy and MRI in the detection of vertebral osteomyelitis. The authors concluded that SPECT Ga-67 was a reliable alternative if MRI was unable to be performed, or an adjunct to MRI in unclear cases.

Luk KDK, Leong JCY, Ho EKW: Tuberculosis of the spine. In Weinstein SL (ed): The Pediatric Spine: Principles and Practice, 2nd ed. Philadelphia: Lippincott Williams & Wilkins, 2001, pp 635–648.

Review chapter on epidemiology, pathology, clinical presentation, treatment, and prognosis for children with tuberculosis of the spine.

Ring D, Johnston CE, Wenger DR: Pyogenic infectious spondylitis in children: The convergence of diskitis and vertebral osteomyelitis. J Pediatr Orthop 1995;15:652–660.

Retrospective review of 47 patients with presumed pyogenic infectious spondylitis (discitis) were followed for an average of 4 years. The authors concluded that immobilization and treatment with intravenous antibiotics lead to a more rapid recovery and decreased likelihood of recurrence.

Song KS, Ogden JA, Ganey T, Guidera KJ: Contiguous diskitis and osteomyelitis in children. J Pediatr Orthop 1997;17:470–477.

The authors report on 16 patients with contiguous discitis and vertebral osteomyelitis. Histologic specimens from immature vertebral bodies clearly demonstrate patent vascular channels providing direct communication between the disc and the vertebral body.

Spiegel PG, Kengla KW, Isaacson AS, Wilson JC Jr: Intervertebral discspace inflammation in children. J Bone Joint Surg Am 1972;54:284–296.

Classic article that reviewed the clinical presentation, pathology, and long-term clinical and radiographic outcomes of 45 children with pyogenic spondylitis.

Spiegel DA, Meyer JS, Dormans JP, et al: Pyomyositis in children and adolescents: Report of 12 cases and review of the literature. J Pediatr Orthop 1999;19:143–150.

In this retrospective review of 12 children with pyomyositis, the authors conclude that MRI with gadolinium may help differentiate between early and late infection and may identify coexistent bone changes in up to 58% of patients. Percutaneous drainage may be successful and should be considered as an alternative to formal incision and drainage.

Sponseller PD: Inflammatory and Infectious Disorders of the Child's Spine. In DeWald RL, Arlet V, Carl AL, O'Brien M (eds): Spinal Deformities: The Comprehensive Text. New York: Thieme, 2003, pp 694–700.

Comprehensive review of the literature on infectious disorder afflicting the pediatric spine, including diskitis, ostetomyelitis, tuberculosis, and fungal infections.

Torpey BM, Dormans JP, Drummond DS: The use of MRI-compatible titanium segmental spinal instrumentation in pediatric patients with intraspinal tumor. J Spinal Disord 1995;8:76–81.

The authors demonstrate that using titanium alloy implants for spinal instrumentation results in less scatter and distorted images on MRI. This allows periodic surveillance of the spine without the need for removal of spinal hardware to more comprehensively follow up patients with spinal tumors.

Wenger DR, Ring D, Hah GV: Pyogenic infectious spondylitis in children. In Weinstein SL (ed): The Pediatric Spine: Principles and Practice, 2nd ed. Philadelphia: Lippincott Williams & Wilkins, 2001, pp 619–633.

Thorough review of pyogenic infectious spondylitis in children.

CHAPTER 14

Pediatric Neoplasms of the Spine

JOHN P. DORMANS *and* SHEILA CONWAY ADAMS

EPIDEMIOLOGY OF SPINE TUMORS

Spinal tumors in pediatric patients, while rare, should always be considered in the differential diagnosis of back symptoms in children. Primary tumors of the spine represent between 2% and 8% of skeletal tumors, benign bone lesions predominating in children and young adults. As a broad generality with exceptions, benign tumors tend to occur in the posterior spinal elements in younger patients, while malignant tumors occur in the vertebral bodies of adolescents and adults. Of the lymphoid tumors, acute leukemia is the most common childhood cancer, acute lymphoblastic leukemia being most likely to present with bone involvement. Understanding the epidemiology of childhood cancer allows the clinician to form a broad differential, and establishing the correct diagnosis requires a thorough history, physical examination, radiographic evaluation, and often advanced imaging and biopsy. This chapter discusses the approach to the child who has a suspected spinal neoplasm and reviews the most common primary benign and malignant bone tumors of the spine in the pediatric population.

GENERAL APPROACH TO DIAGNOSIS

Though the differential diagnosis of a child with back pain is long (Box 14-1), a thorough history and physical examination can help to rule out many etiologies and suggest a diagnosis. The most common presentation of a child with a spinal tumor is gradual onset of pain, as either back or radicular pain. Other signs and symptoms may include local tenderness, neurologic changes, gait abnormalities, or spinal deformity. Neurologic deficits occur in up to one third of patients, highlighting the importance of a comprehensive neuromuscular examination. Because of the deep location of the spine, a mass is seldom the presenting finding of a spinal tumor. In fact, these tumors may be incidental findings on imaging acquired for other diagnostic reasons.

Radiographic evaluation should include high quality plain radiography of the spinal segments involved. In deformity cases, standing 3-foot posterior to anterior (PA)

and lateral scoliosis films should be obtained. Depending on the suspected lesion, computed tomography (CT), magnetic resonance imaging (MRI), or bone scan may also be indicated. Since infection is often in the differential, laboratory evaluation with a complete blood count, sedimentation rate, and C-reactive protein may be useful.

Once a spinal tumor has been identified, treatment should be aimed at the specific etiology. A multidisciplinary team approach is strongly advocated for patients with a spinal sarcoma, leukemia, and spinal Langerhans cell histiocytosis. This team ideally includes the surgeon, oncologist, radiologist, and surgical pathologist. Such an approach offers fewer delays in diagnosis, increased survival in patients with malignant neoplasms, and fewer complications. If these resources are not available to the surgeon, early referral to a tertiary center should be considered.

CLASSIFICATION

Classification of Benign and Malignant Tumors

On diagnosis of a spine tumor or tumor-like process, the lesion should be classified as benign or malignant, and the Enneking classification systems are commonly utilized (Table 14-1). Benign tumors are categorized as latent, active, and locally aggressive. Stage 1 benign tumors (latent) are intracapsular, do not metastasize, and are often incidental findings on radiography with dense surrounding reactive bone. These lesions are usually asymptomatic and resolve without intervention. Stage 2 benign tumors (active) are likewise intracapsular and rarely metastasize. However, unlike Stage 1 lesions, these are actively growing and consequently are more likely to produce local symptoms. On radiography, these may appear destructive with usually only a thin rim of reactive bone. Stage 3 benign lesions (aggressive) have the most destructive appearance on radiography and are often expansile with soft-tissue extensions. They typically grow at a rapid rate and are subsequently more likely to cause local signs and symptoms. Rarely, these tumors can metastasize.

BOX 14–1 Differential Diagnosis of Back Pain in Children

Common	Less Common	Uncommon
Muscular strain	Infection (discitis/	Herniated nucleus pulposus
Spondylolysis	osteomyelitis)	Ankylosing spondylitis
Spondylolisthesis	Scheuermann's kyphosis	Juvenile rheumatoid arthritis
		Spinal cord tumor
		Bone/soft-tissue tumors
		Psychogenic/secondary gain

Table 14-1. Enneking Staging for Benign and Malignant Musculoskeletal Lesions

Stage	Grade	Site	Metastasis
1	G_0	T_1	M_0
2	G_0	T_1	M_0
3	G_0	T_{1-2}	M_{0-1}
IA	G_1	T_1	M_0
IB	G_1	T_2	M_0
IIA	G_2	T_1	M_0
IIB	G_2	T_2	M_0
IIIA	G_1 or G_2	T_1	M_1
IIIB	G_1 or G_2	T_2	M_1

G_0, benign; G_1, low-grade malignant; G_2, high-grade malignant; T_1, intracompartmental; T_2, extracompartmental; M_0, none; M_1, present.

Table 14-2. Treatment-Based Classification for Pediatric Tumors of the Spine

Classification	Examples
Benign, favorable natural history	Langerhans cell histiocytosis
	Osteoid osteoma
	Osteochondroma
Benign, locally aggressive	Aneurysmal bone cyst
	Giant cell tumor
	Osteoblastoma
Malignant	Ewing sarcoma
	Osteosarcoma
	Leukemia
	Lymphoma
	Metastatic disease

The Enneking classification for malignant neoplasms is based on grade, site, and the presence or absence of metastasis. These three variables are used to classify malignant tumors into various stages, as indicated in Table 14-1. This staging system is useful in guiding not only surgical options but also the need for chemotherapy or radiation therapy.

We advocate a treatment-based approach to the pediatric spine in which lesions are grouped into three categories: benign lesions with favorable natural history (Enneking stage 1), benign active or aggressive lesions (Enneking stage 2 and 3), and malignant lesions (Table 14-2). Benign lesions with a favorable natural history usually do not require biopsy or surgical excision. Nonoperative treatment is appropriate, as many lesions resolve without surgical intervention. Benign but locally aggressive tumors require biopsy and excision, owing to their locally destructive behavior and tendency for recurrence. Localized malignant sarcomas of the spine require biopsy, surgical excision when possible, and adjuvant therapy, depending on the specific tumor. The next section will review the most common pediatric spinal neoplasms in each of these categories.

Benign Tumors with a Favorable Natural History

Osteochondroma

Osteochondroma is a common benign tumor of bone, making up 30% to 40% of all benign bone tumors. These lesions have an affinity for the long bones and occur most commonly in the second or third decade of life. Osteochondromas are thought to arise from a laterally displaced area of the developing physis; growth after physeal closure is not expected. Osteochondromas occur in the solitary form or in a multifocal syndrome called multiple hereditary exostosis (MHE), an autosomal dominant disease with variable penetrance.

Spinal osteochondromas represent about 1% of solitary osteochondromas and occur in 7% to 9% of patients with MHE, with a predilection for the posterior elements. The distribution within the spine is as follows: cervical spine (50% to 60%) and thoracic and below (40%). Though typically asymptomatic, these lesions can cause nerve or cord compression in up to 1% of cases, necessitating a thorough neurologic examination with specific evaluation for spasticity and long-tract signs in all patients with MHE. Patients with cervical osteochondromas may present with Horner syndrome (due to compression of the paravertebral sympathetic centers), dysphagia, hoarseness, and vascular compression. Patients with spinal osteochondromas associated with MHE are more likely to present with neurologic sequelae and at a younger age.

On plain radiography, osteochondromas usually appear as a sessile or pedunculated bony exostosis, with cortex and spongiosa contiguous with the underlying bone. Calcifications may be present within the otherwise radiolucent cartilaginous cap. When osteochondromas are difficult to visualize on plain radiography, CT scan is the preferred study to visualize the bony architecture (Fig. 14-1). MRI or CT myelogram is a useful study to define the relationship of the osteochondroma to the neural elements, especially in cases with neurologic symptoms.

When the diagnosis is unclear, biopsy with intra-operative frozen section should be performed for definitive diagnosis. Excisional biopsy is recommended in some cases, as incisional biopsy can provide insufficient material to differentiate between osteochondroma and low-grade chondrosarcoma. Though uncommon, incomplete excision can lead to local recurrence. Pathology and histology of an

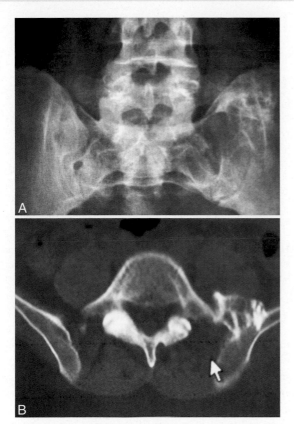

Figure 14-1. Plain radiograph (**A**) and CT scan (**B**) demonstrating a symptomatic osteochondroma of the left pelvis in a 22-year-old female with MHE who presented with left-sided low back pain.

osteochondroma will reveal a cap of benign hyaline cartilage resembling a disorganized growth plate, covered peripherally by perichondrium.

Osteochondromas require treatment only in the event of mechanical or neurologic symptoms; most symptoms resolve with surgical excision. Indications for stabilization depend on the amount of instability following surgical excision.

Malignant transformation has been reported in fewer than 1% of solitary lesions and up to 10% of patients with multifocal lesions. A rapidly enlarging mass, new onset pain, growth after skeletal maturity, and recurrence are suspicious for malignant change. If sarcomatous degeneration is suspected, CT scan or MRI can be helpful to assess the size of the cartilaginous cap. In a skeletally mature child, a cap greater than 1 centimeter is worrisome for malignancy; however, this criterion is not applicable to younger children with open physes.

Langerhans Cell Histiocytosis

Langerhans cell histiocytosis (LCH), also known as eosinophilic granuloma, is a self-limited proliferative disorder. LCH affects the spine in 6% to 15% of cases, and multicentric and extraspinal lesions are common. Patients with LCH present with a wide range of signs and symptoms,

including pain, stiffness, torticollis, kyphosis, and scoliosis. Neurologic symptoms, though not classically associated with LCH, are present in fewer than 15% of patients.

Three variants of this disease process exist. The most severe form, Letterer-Siwe disease, is a life-threatening condition of infants and young children characterized by multiorgan involvement. Hand-Schuller-Christian disease is a less fulminant multifocal variant with a classic triad (though not always present) of skull lesions, exophthalmos, and diabetes insipidus. The most common variant is solitary or multifocal eosinophilic granuloma of bone without visceral involvement.

The pathogenesis of LCH is unknown, though environmental, infectious, immunologic, and genetic etiologies have been suggested. Studies have demonstrated evidence of human herpesvirus type 6 (HHV-6) in tissue from children with LCH lesions. However, a recent real-time polymerase chain reaction analysis demonstrated no difference in the prevalence of HHV-6 in the tissues of LCH patients compared with tissues from patients without the disease.

The classic appearance of spinal LCH on plain radiography has been termed *vertebrae plana*, which is complete collapse of the vertebral body with preservation of disc space (Fig. 14-2). It should be noted that vertebrae plana is not pathopneumonic for LCH, as this radiographic appearance has been noted in both benign and malignant pediatric tumors. Alternatively, LCH may present in the vertebral body with only partial collapse or in the posterior elements. Lesions are relatively evenly distributed throughout the spine, with a slight predilection for the cervical spine, and multiple spinal and extraspinal lesions may exist.

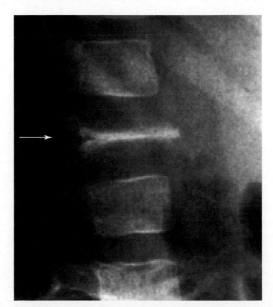

Figure 14-2. Plain radiograph of an eosinophilic granuloma of the lumbar spine demonstrating the classic appearance of vertebrae plana. (*Adapted with permission from Garg S, Dormans JP: Tumors and tumor-like conditions of the spine in children. J Am Acad Orthop Surg 2005;13:372–381.*)

Mild scoliosis or kyphosis with LCH is unusual and is not always associated with asymmetric vertebral body collapse. Bone scan or skeletal survey should be routinely obtained to evaluate for multiple sites of disease, which occur in up to 50% of cases. Skeletal survey is preferable, owing to the improved sensitivity over bone scan in detecting multiple bony lesions in LCH. MRI is particularly useful in identifying the presence or absence of an associated soft-tissue mass and for identifying the most representative and accessible area for biopsy.

Histology of the lesional tissue reveals three different predominant cell types: (1) sheets of histiocytes with a longitudinally oriented nuclear groove (aka "coffee-bean" nuclei), (2) giant Langerhans cells, and (3) frequent eosinophils (accounting for the term *eosinophilic granuloma*). Other cell populations may include lymphocytes, plasma cells, leukocytes, and lipid-laden macrophages. Electron microscopy of the histiocytes characteristically reveals cytoplasmic tennis racket–shaped bodies, termed *Birbeck granules*. Positive immunohistochemistry staining with CD-1 and S-100 protein can assist in the diagnosis of LCH and can help to differentiate this entity from other small, round blue cell tumors.

Conservative treatment of LCH is usually recommended owing to the benign natural history of these lesions. Full or partial reconstitution of vertebral height is common, with greater potential for reconstitution existing in younger patients, independent of treatment modality. However, biopsy might be required to establish definitive diagnosis, owing to the variable radiographic appearance of these lesions and wide differential diagnosis. Supportive treatment with pain medication, short durations of bed rest, and external immobilization is often appropriate. Rarely, surgical intervention is required for lesions associated with neural compression or instability. Radiation therapy as an alternative to surgical intervention has lost favor, owing to its questionable effectiveness and associated risks. Chemotherapy has a demonstrated role in cases with visceral involvement but might not affect the natural history of bony lesions.

Osteoid Osteoma

Osteoid osteomas are benign, radiodense lesions with a central radiolucent nidus that often arise in the second decade of life, approximately 10% of lesions occurring in the spine. The classic presentation is a painful lesion, often with increased pain at night, relieved by salicylates or non-steroidal anti-inflammatory agents (NSAIDs). Frequently, back pain precedes radiographic findings. As many as 77% of patients with spinal osteoid osteomas are reported to have a deformity at the time of diagnosis, making osteoid osteoma the most common cause of painful scoliosis. The typically eccentric lesion of the posterior elements is usually on the concave side of the curve near the apex and is associated with rapid curve onset. Neurologic symptoms

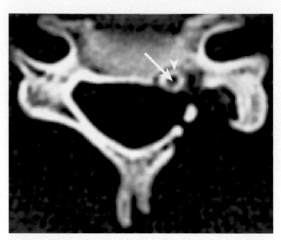

Figure 14-3. CT scan of an osteoid osteoma of the cervical spine with well-circumscribed nidus. *(Adapted with permission from Garg S, Dormans JP: Tumors and tumor-like conditions of the spine in children. J Am Acad Orthop Surg 2005;13:372–381.)*

are rare and occur with much less frequency than with osteoblastoma, a similar but more aggressive lesion.

On plain radiographs, osteoid osteoma is a sclerotic, eccentric lesion that typically arises in the posterior elements of the spine. The lumbar spine is the most common location, followed by cervical, thoracic, and sacral spinal regions. The relatively radiolucent nidus, which is the highly vascular region of bone formation, is usually defined as 1.5 to 2 centimeters or less (Fig. 14-3). Lesions larger than 2 centimeters are typically considered osteoblastomas. When the nidus is difficult to identify on plain radiography, a fine-cut CT scan (2- or 3-mm cuts) is recommended. Bone scan is highly sensitive for osteoid osteoma and can help to localize a suspected lesion prior to CT scan. Care should be taken in evaluating patients with osteoid osteoma by MRI, as extensive surrounding edema can lead to the misdiagnosis of an aggressive tumor.

A classic appearance on radiography and CT scan is often diagnostic for osteoid osteoma. In questionable cases, biopsy with intraoperative frozen section should be obtained for definitive diagnosis. The histology of the nidus consists of irregular woven bone trabeculae embedded in benign fibrovascular stroma and is clearly demarcated from the surrounding reactive, sclerotic lamellar bone. These histologic findings should differentiate this lesion from a Brodie's abscess of bone, which is frequently in the differential diagnosis.

Osteoid osteomas are self-limited, but the patient might require treatment for pain, deformity, or neurologic symptoms. Treatment options include prolonged medical management, CT-guided ablation techniques, and surgical removal of the nidus. Medical management with salicylates or NSAIDs is a viable and effective treatment option for painful lesions without neurologic deficit or associated deformity. However, Kneisl and colleagues found that the average duration of NSAID treatment was 33 months, and this might not be acceptable to many patients and families, given the pain intensity and risks associated with long-term NSAID use.

CT-guided radiofrequency ablation and percutaneous removal techniques are established treatment modalities for extraspinal osteoid osteoma; however, far fewer cases of such successful treatment exist for the spine. Therefore, surgical excision of symptomatic spinal lesions is our recommended treatment for cases that are refractory to medical management. Removal of the lesion alleviates the tumor pain within hours to days, and failure of pain resolution is likely indicative of incomplete removal of the nidus. Surgical treatment of associated scoliosis at the time of resection is controversial and will be discussed later in the chapter.

In our experience, the previously discussed benign tumors with favorable natural histories require biopsy when the diagnosis is questionable or unclear. Surgical treatment should be reserved for cases that fail medical management or cause persistent pain, neurologic symptoms, spinal instability, or significant deformity. In the next section, the most common benign but locally aggressive tumors of the pediatric spine will be discussed.

Benign But Locally Aggressive Tumors

Aneurysmal Bone Cyst

Aneurysmal bone cysts (ABCs) are benign bone lesions representing approximately 1% of primary bone tumors and approximately 15% of primary spine tumors occurring in all ages. These lesions frequently present in the pediatric population, with the majority of patients under the age of twenty. Lesions of the lumbar vertebrae are most common; however, ABCs can present at any vertebral level. Pain, as back pain with or without radiculopathy, is the most common presenting symptom. While neurologic symptoms are usually rare and mild, severe neurologic involvement secondary to cord and/or nerve root compression can occur. Other signs and symptoms include stiffness, kyphosis, and scoliosis. In addition to the variability of presenting symptoms, the natural history of ABCs is variable, some lesions behaving in an indolent manner and others behaving in a locally aggressive manner.

On plain radiography, the lesion is expansile and radiolucent with a thin rim of reactive bone. ABCs almost always arise from the posterior elements of the spine. However, it is not uncommon for the vertebral body to be involved, and when it is, it is likely an intraosseous extension from the posterior elements. Pathologic microfractures and vertebrae plana associated with complete collapse, though rare, are also reported in the literature. Kyphosis or scoliosis can occur secondary to the lesion, and these deformities can be reactive or structural. CT scan is useful to evaluate the extent of bony destruction, while MRI better delineates the lack of associated soft-tissue mass with ABCs, degree of expansion, and neural canal compromise and classically reveals fluid/fluid levels and septation (Fig. 14-4).

Confirmation of the diagnosis with biopsy and intraoperative frozen section characteristically reveals blood-filled cysts with fibrous septa. Giant cells often line the cysts and can be quite abundant. The absence of malignant cells producing osteoid helps to differentiate this entity from telangiectatic osteosarcoma. Of note, ABCs can be secondary to other benign or malignant tumors, and the pathologic specimen should be thoroughly evaluated with this in mind.

Following intraoperative frozen section for confirmation, we recommend surgical excision of ABCs with a four-step approach: (1) intralesional curettage, (2) high-speed burring, (3) careful electrocauterization of remaining cyst wall, and (4) the selective use of phenol for aggressive or recurrent ABCs (with care to avoid contact with the dura or great vessels). Additionally, bone grafting might be indicated when significant bony defects exist. Spinal titanium instrumentation at the time of excision should be considered, especially in the face of significant posterior destabilization, structural scoliosis, or kyphosis.

As an alternative to surgery, selective arterial embolization of ABCs has been suggested, with a few reports of successful treatment in spinal ABCs. However, given the limited data on this as a primary treatment modality in the spine, we view this as a reasonable option in more indolent cases or when the morbidity of surgical resection is unacceptably high. However, as an adjunct to surgery, preoperative selective arterial embolization could be effective at decreasing intraoperative blood loss. Irradiation as a treatment option has fallen out of favor, owing to its questionable efficacy and multitude of side effects.

Though most recurrences of ABCs occur within the first year, radiographic follow-up should continue for at least 2 years. Any patient receiving radiation therapy should be followed indefinitely, owing to the risk of secondary sarcomas.

Osteoblastoma

Osteoblastoma is a benign but locally aggressive bone-forming lesion of children and young adults with a predilection for the posterior elements of the spine. Often grouped with osteoid osteoma, owing to similarities in histology, it is differentiated by its larger size (>2 cm) and more aggressive behavior. Osteoblastomas represent fewer than 1% of primary bone tumors but approximately 10% of spinal tumors. In fact, 30% to 40% of all osteoblastomas occur in the spine.

Similar to osteoid osteoma, patients with this lesion frequently present with back pain, stiffness, and tenderness. Night pain is likewise common but with a more variable response to NSAIDs. Neurologic symptoms are

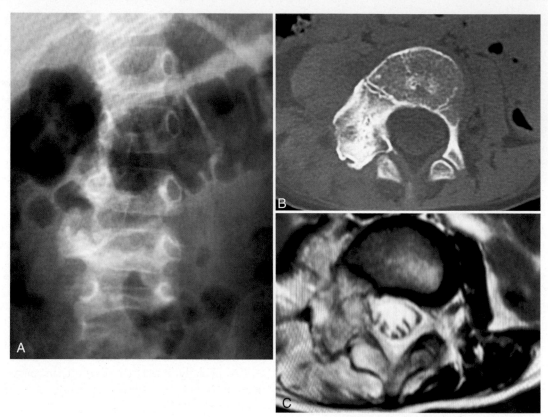

Figure 14-4. Plain radiograph (**A**), CT scan (**B**), and MRI (**C**) demonstrating an osteoblastoma with concurrent ABC features of the right L4 pedicle in a 3-year-old male with back pain and swelling.

frequent with osteoblastoma given their larger size and more aggressive biology. Painful scoliosis is a common presentation, typically with an eccentric thoracic or lumbar lesion of the posterior elements located on the concave aspect of the apex of the main curve. Cervical lesions are more likely to present with torticollis.

On plain radiography, osteoblastomas are usually expansile, radiodense lesions of the posterior spinal elements; however, the vertebral body may be affected as well (see Figs. 14-7A and 14-7B, later in the chapter). Multiple levels of the spine can be involved, and the thoracic and lumbar spinal regions are most frequently affected, followed by the cervical spine and the sacrum. Bone scan is a reliable screening tool for the localization of occult osteoblastomas. When plain radiography is not diagnostic, CT scan will best define bony architecture, while MRI is more useful to characterize soft-tissue extension or edema.

Owing to the aggressive nature of these lesions, biopsy with intraoperative frozen section and resection are necessary. They are usually done at the same surgical setting as definitive resection. The histology is similar to that of osteoid osteoma, with a rich fibrovascular stroma, irregular spicules of woven bone, and osteoblastic rimming. These osteoblasts have abundant cytoplasm and prominent, regular nuclei. Additionally, multinucleated giant cells may be

present in variable numbers, frequently leading to a misdiagnosis of giant cell tumor.

"Aggressive osteoblastoma" is recognized by some clinicians as an entity that is separate from typical osteoblastoma with more aggressive histology, characterized by large hypertrophic osteoblasts with pleomorphic nuclei and numerous giant cells. "Malignant osteoblastoma" is an additional variant, described by Schajowicz and colleagues as a tumor of low-grade malignancy with an even more aggressive natural history. Certainly, there is a continuum of histologic variants, with the most aggressive variant resembling osteosarcoma. The absence of sarcomatous spindle cells, anaplastic giant cells, and intense cellular atypia helps to differentiate osteoblastoma from malignant osteosarcoma.

Treatment for osteoblastoma of the spine is extended intralesional surgical excision versus en bloc resection, when possible. Stabilization with titanium instrumentation is frequently indicated, owing to the large amount of bony involvement, location in the posterior elements, expansile nature, and associated spinal deformity. Because of the hypervascularity of ABCs, consideration can be given to preoperative selective arterial embolization. Radiation therapy should be avoided, owing to the significant risks associated with radiation in children and young adults.

In our experience, many benign tumors of the pediatric spine with aggressive natural histories require surgical treatment. We recommend open biopsy with intraoperative frozen section usually followed by same-anesthesia excision of the lesion. Surgical stabilization might be necessary, owing to associated deformity or spinal instability. Preoperative selective arterial embolization can be beneficial in reducing intraoperative blood loss with more vascular tumors.

Malignant Tumors

Ewing Sarcoma

Ewing sarcoma is a malignant tumor of neuroectodermal origin that was initially described as "diffuse endothelioma of bone" by James Ewing in 1921. Ewing sarcoma commonly occurs in the second decade of life and is infrequent in children younger than 5 years of age. Representing 10% of primary malignant bone tumors, approximately only 3% to 10% of primary Ewing lesions occur in the spine. However, the spinal column is a common site of metastatic disease, spinal metastasis being a frequent preterminal event in patients with relapsing disease. In addition to primary and metastatic Ewing sarcoma of the bone, extraosseous epidural spinal Ewing sarcoma can occur and should be in the differential diagnosis of a malignant spinal lesion in a child.

Ewing sarcoma of the spine classically presents with local and/or radicular pain, up to two thirds of cases having neurologic deficits, including bowel and bladder dysfunction. Additional common symptoms, including fever and weight loss, might lead to a misdiagnosis of osteomyelitis. Laboratory findings such as leukocytosis and an elevated erythrocyte sedimentation rate can further complicate this important differentiation.

Radiographic findings are extremely variable in patients with Ewing sarcoma. Plain radiography typically reveals irregular destruction of the vertebral body with occasional vertebral collapse. While the majority of lesions are lytic with a permeative or moth-eaten pattern, Ewing sarcoma can also be blastic or mixed in appearance. Although the anterior vertebrae are more classically involved, destruction of the posterior elements does occur. Of primary vertebral lesions, the sacrum is most frequently affected, followed by the lumbar and thoracic regions. Patients with Ewing sarcoma usually present with a large soft-tissue mass, which is best evaluated with MRI (Fig. 14-5). This soft-tissue mass is a key element in differentiating Ewing sarcoma from other benign spinal tumors in the differential diagnosis. Staging should include a comprehensive history and physical, CT scan of the chest (to evaluate for pulmonary metastasis), technetium total body bone scan (to evaluate for additional bone lesions), and bone marrow aspirate (to evaluate for intramedullary involvement).

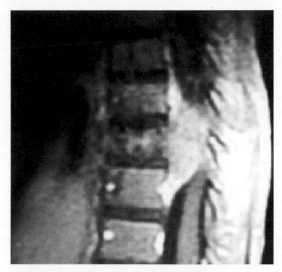

Figure 14-5. Magnetic resonance image of Ewing sarcoma demonstrating a soft-tissue mass with cord compression. *(Adapted with permission from Garg S, Dormans JP: Tumors and tumor-like conditions of the spine in children. J Am Acad Orthop Surg 2005;13:372–381.)*

Open biopsy with intraoperative frozen section of Ewing sarcoma of the spine is usually recommended to ensure adequate and representative specimen for diagnosis. Alternatively, CT-guided biopsy can be used in cases in which Ewing sarcoma is highly probable, as in the biopsy of a suspected metastatic site in a patient with known Ewing sarcoma. When a soft-tissue component is present, this is the preferable biopsy source, as it can be more representative of the malignancy. With osteomyelitis often in the differential diagnosis, gram stain and cultures at the time of biopsy are advised.

The histopathologic diagnosis of Ewing sarcoma relies on a combination of light microscopy, immunohistochemistry, and molecular and genetic studies. On the basis of histology alone, Ewing sarcoma can be difficult to differentiate from other small blue cell lesions such as lymphoma of bone, osteomyelitis, neuroblastoma, and rhabdomyosarcoma. On light microscopy, lesional tissue from a patient with Ewing sarcoma classically appears as sheets of poorly differentiated small blue cells with little stroma. Periodic acid Schiff staining, which detects the presence of intracellular glycogen, is present in 80% to 90% of Ewing sarcoma specimens. Classic findings on immunohistochemistry include positive reactivity for MIC2 (CD99), neuron-specific enolase, and vimentin with negative staining on muscle, epithelial, and hematopoietic markers. With real-time polymerase chain reaction genetic testing, a translocation between chromosome 11 and chromosome 22 (t11,22) and the subsequent chimeric protein (EWS-FL1) are highly specific for Ewing sarcoma.

Ewing sarcoma is a very aggressive tumor with a high rate of local recurrence and metastatic disease requiring chemotherapy, surgery, and/or radiation. Multiagent preoperative and postoperative chemotherapy for patients with resectable localized Ewing disease has increased the 5-year survival rate from 5% to approximately 70%; however, the 5-year survival rate in patients with primary Ewing sarcoma of the spine is less than 50%. This could be due to the fact that patients with spinal Ewing sarcoma often present late, with advanced or metastatic disease, owing to the deep location of the tumor. Neoadjuvant chemotherapy, however, can decrease the size of the soft-tissue component, making local control attainable. Frequently utilized chemotherapeutics include vincristine, cyclophosphamide, doxorubicin, actinomycin D, ifosfamide, and etoposide.

Surgical resection can be appropriately attempted in patients with nonmetastatic Ewing sarcoma because complete surgical excision has been demonstrated to improve local control and disease-free survival rates. Successful surgical stabilization after resection can be more readily accomplished with sophisticated spinal instrumentation such as pedicle screw fixation and vertebral body endoprostheses.

Radiation may have a role in local treatment of patients with Ewing sarcoma of spine as a primary treatment modality or as an adjunct to surgical intervention. However, radiation in a child has significant risks, including radiation-induced malignancy, local recurrence, growth disturbance, fracture, neuritis, vasculitis, and spinal cord injury. Furthermore, radiation treatment of primary Ewing sarcoma of the spine has been associated with a high local recurrence rate, most relapses occurring within the field of radiation. Consequently, radiation in children is currently advised for unresectable primary tumors or for cases with positive surgical margins.

Poor prognostic indicators in Ewing sarcoma include large tumor volume and metastatic disease at diagnosis. Some studies have shown sacral location to be an additional poor prognostic indicator; however, others have found no change in outcomes in patients with primary sacral lesions compared to other spinal locations. Elevated sedimentation rate and lactate dehydrogenase levels have also been described as being associated with a worse prognosis. Histologic response to chemotherapy, or chemotherapy-induced tumor necrosis, is an additional prognostic factor, high degrees of necrosis (>90%) correlating with better disease-free survival. Relapse of Ewing sarcoma has a very poor prognosis, early relapse (less than 2 years after initial treatment) having a worse outcome than late relapse.

Osteosarcoma

Osteosarcoma is a primary malignant tumor of bone, representing 20% of primary bone tumors. Osteosarcoma occurs most frequently in the second decade, at sites of greatest bone growth, while secondary osteosarcomas and pagetoid osteosarcomas occur more frequently in older populations. Spinal osteosarcoma represents up to 14% of primary spinal tumors and 1% to 4% of all osteosarcomas. Within the spine, the thoracolumbar and sacral regions are the most common locations, cervical lesions being the least common. As with many spinal tumors, pain is the most common presenting symptom. Neurologic deficits with a wide range of severity are encountered in up to 70% of cases. Laboratory values are variable; however, an elevated alkaline phosphatase level is frequently noted at initial presentation.

Multicentric osteosarcoma (also known as osteosarcomatosis) is considered by some to be a disease variant characterized by a synchronous appearance of multiple skeletal tumors, representing 1% to 5% of all osteosarcomas. Alternatively, these multifocal cases might represent early metastatic disease, as supported by the high incidence of pulmonary metastasis at diagnosis.

The most common appearance of spinal osteosarcoma on plain radiography is osteoblastic; however, osteolytic and mixed radiographic appearances do occur. Most osteosarcomas originate in the vertebral body and extend toward the posterior elements. Paravertebral and adjacent vertebrae involvement are common. CT scan of the lesion may be useful in delineating the extent of bony involvement, while MRI will best define the soft-tissue component.

Radiographic staging of osteosarcoma should include high-quality standing PA and lateral spinal radiographs with cone-down views, a chest CT scan, and a whole-body bone scan. Early metastasis is common in patients with spinal osteosarcoma, with pulmonary metastasis as the most frequent site.

The classic histologic pattern of patients with osteosarcoma is production of immature osteoid by malignant osteoblasts (spindle cell malignant stroma). Multiple histologic variants exist, including chondroblastic, fibroblastic, telangiectatic, and small cell patterns. It is critical and frequently challenging to distinguish osteosarcoma from benign osteoblastoma. The keys to correct diagnosis are complete analysis of a presumed osteoblastoma specimen for even small areas of atypia, increased cellularity, and nuclear pleomorphism. These findings plus areas of necrosis, absence of osteoblastic rimming, and abundant mitotic activity suggest a diagnosis of osteosarcoma.

Current multimodality treatment for patients with spinal osteosarcoma includes neoadjuvant chemotherapy, surgery, and radiation. Prior to neoadjuvant chemotherapy, the prognosis for patients with osteosarcoma was dismal, with an overall 10-year survival rate of approximately 5%, with most patients with spinal osteosarcoma dying within the first year. The addition of chemotherapy has dramatically improved the prognosis for patients with localized disease of the extremity, with current 5-year continuous disease-free survival rates greater than 60%.

Recommendations for neoadjuvant therapy in spinal osteosarcoma are largely based on the data for osteosarcoma of the extremity; however, small series on spinal osteosarcomas show less dramatic improvements in patient survival. This has generally been attributed to the difficulty in obtaining a wide resection for local control in patients with spinal osteosarcoma, compared with those with osteosarcoma of the extremity. The fact that most treatment failures in spinal osteosarcoma are local recurrences supports this argument. Therefore, current treatment recommendations include preoperative chemotherapy, followed by complete surgical resection with wide margins and subsequent adaptations in neoadjuvant chemotherapy. When tumor invades the spinal canal, the acquisition of negative surgical margins may be difficult and necessitate sacrifice of neural elements. However, the best chance for long-term survival exists with en bloc vertebral column resection with wide margins, which can lead to permanent neurologic deficits in some patients with spinal osteosarcoma.

Chemotherapeutic agents that are utilized include methotrexate, adriamycin, vincristine, ifosfamide, etoposide, cisplatin, bleomycin, cyclophosphamide, and dactinomycin. Following preoperative chemotherapy, the patient should be restaged with radiographs and MRI of the lesion followed by surgical resection.

Radiation therapy may be advised if the tumor is unresectable, if positive margins exist after surgical excision, or in cases of metastatic disease. However, osteosarcoma is not considered a particularly radiosensitive tumor, and surgical resection with neoadjuvant chemotherapy offers the best chance of local control and survival.

Patients should be followed for a minimum of 5 years after completion of treatment. Pulmonary metastasis and local recurrence are the most common sites of relapse in osteosarcoma of the spine. Poor prognostic indicators include sacral location, metastasis, large tumor size, and poor histologic response to chemotherapy.

In our experience, primary malignant tumors of the pediatric spine are optimally treated with neoadjuvant chemotherapy and surgical resection with wide margins. Surgical stabilization with titanium instrumentation is frequently necessary to treat spinal instability, and this will be discussed in further detail in the sections below.

TREATMENT

Surgical Treatment

Surgical treatment of tumors of the spine is indicated in patients with aggressive and malignant tumors for local control. Patients with benign tumors frequently require surgical excision for pain relief or because of neurologic signs or symptoms. Thorough multidisciplinary preoperative planning is essential for the successful treatment of pediatric spine tumors, with critical aspects of surgical planning including approach, surgical margins, determination of spinal stability, deformity correction, and spinal stabilization.

Surgical Approach

The surgical approach to the spine is dictated by the location of the tumor, goals of surgery, and concerns for subsequent deformity. A posterior approach is indicated in tumors of the posterior elements, as is the case with most benign tumors. As this approach can put the young child at risk for subsequent kyphosis, fusion and spinal instrumentation should be considered.

An anterior approach is better suited for tumors of the vertebral body and when anterior decompression is required, as is often the case for malignant tumors such as Ewing sarcoma and osteosarcoma. Occasionally, a combined anterior and posterior approach with instrumentation is also needed for adequate spinal stabilization. In such cases, a staged or simultaneous anterior and posterior surgical procedure may be employed. En bloc spondylectomy can be performed from a combined anterior-posterior approach. This technique is preferable to a piecemeal intralesional excision in malignant tumors and can be successfully performed with negative margins.

As an alternative to a staged anterior-posterior approach, the senior author uses a "sloppy lateral" position for some very young patients, which allows simultaneous exposure of the anterior and posterior spine from the same surgical field. This is feasible in select pediatric patients, owing to their smaller body habitus, which eases mild intraoperative repositioning.

Stabilization

The decision to stabilize the spine with instrumentation can be made preoperatively if instability is present or intraoperatively if subsequent resection introduces instability. Reconstruction should be aimed at supporting the resected vertebral column. In the case of a vertebrectomy, an anterior femoral ring allograft with or without a vertebral spacer or endoprosthesis and augmentation with posterior instrumentation is recommended for reconstruction. Lateral mass plates, posterior wiring, and screw and rod constructs with autologous bone graft and halo immobilization are effective methods of posterior stabilization after cervical tumor resection. If only the posterior elements of the spine have been violated, posterior instrumentation alone should suffice. Failure to identify and address instability intraoperatively can lead to late deformity, especially in young children. This will be addressed in greater detail in the "Pearls and Pitfalls."

The method and timing of surgical stabilization are especially important in the treatment of spinal tumors.

Historically, segmental spinal instrumentation involved the use of conventional stainless steel implants. However, owing to the ferromagnetic properties of these implants, the accuracy of postoperative spinal CT and MRI is often compromised by scatter distortion. This is problematic in the treatment of patients with spinal tumors, as they frequently require postoperative imaging to assess the adequacy of spinal decompression and to monitor for tumor recurrence. The senior author initially described the use of MRI-compatible titanium segmental spinal instrumentation in the treatment of pediatric patients with spinal tumors when surgical stabilization is indicated and close postoperative image follow-up is required. This allows for instrumentation at the time of primary tumor resection while not precluding adequate postoperative imaging. Cases have been described in which information gained from postoperative MRI following titanium segmental spinal instrumentation has significantly altered or affected patient care.

Surgical Treatment of Deformity

Deformity in association with spinal lesions is a common finding and may be the initial presenting complaint. Scoliosis, kyphosis, and torticollis have all been associated with neoplastic spinal lesions. Rapid onset of the spinal curvature or a painful curve is suggestive of a pathologic lesion. The etiology of the deformity may be secondary to pain, spasm, or a deforming force from the tumor itself. Lesions are typically asymmetric and located on the concave side at the apex of the main curve. Severity of the curvature is related to the age of onset and the duration of symptoms prior to treatment.

Recommendations on the treatment of patients with deformity are largely based on data from osteoid osteomas and osteoblastomas, as these lesions account for the majority of deformity cases. If spontaneous correction of the deformity is expected with excision of the lesion, as is often the case with adolescents who develop mild deformity near skeletal maturity, treatment of the lesion will be the solitary goal of surgery. In the growing child, young age of onset and long duration of symptoms are risk factors for curve progression or advanced deformity and might necessitate surgical stabilization at the index procedure. In addition, if instability will be introduced via removal of the lesion, the curve is at higher risk for progression and should be stabilized. This is more likely the case in malignant or aggressive lesions requiring a large resection of the posterior elements.

Complications of Surgery

The surgical treatment of spinal tumors comes with a number of significant potential complications. The most serious of these include death, recurrent tumor, neurologic deficit, spinal deformity, and dural tears. Other common surgical complications are excessive blood loss, pseudarthrosis (symptomatic and asymptomatic), instrumentation failure, infection, and other wound problems. Many of these issues are compounded by radiation and chemotherapy in the oncology patient.

Chemotherapy

Modern effective treatment of malignant bone tumors includes neoadjuvant chemotherapy. The goals of preoperative chemotherapy include early treatment of micrometastasis, reduction in primary tumor bulk prior to resection, and selection of high-risk groups requiring alternative chemotherapeutic regimens.

Chemotherapeutic agents have a multitude of side effects, varying with each particular agent. Common side effects and toxicities include alopecia, cardiac toxicity, cystitis, diarrhea, hepatic toxicity, hypersensitivity reactions, pulmonary toxicity, myelosuppression, mucositis, neurotoxicity, renal toxicity, ototoxicity, syndrome of inappropriate antidiuretic hormone, and secondary leukemia. Though the medical oncologist usually manages these medications and their side effects, the surgeon must be aware of these effects, as they can dramatically affect surgical recovery and patient outcomes. In addition to the above-listed side effects, chemotherapeutics (especially alkylating agents) have been shown to augment the carcinogenic risk of radiation.

In the treatment of patients with Ewing sarcoma and osteosarcoma, a higher percentage of tumor necrosis (>90%) in response to chemotherapy has been shown to correlate with better disease-free survival. MRI findings, such as reduction in soft-tissue mass and a change in tumor volume and signal intensity, can be used to assess response to chemotherapy and guide medical and surgical treatment. This information can also be used as a prognostic indicator and can guide selection of appropriate postoperative chemotherapy regimens.

Radiation Therapy

The role of radiation in the treatment of pediatric neoplasia has changed with improvements in chemotherapy and surgical techniques and with a better understanding of the long-term sequelae of radiation therapy. Wide surgical excision, when attainable, has become the preferred treatment for local control of primary malignant spinal sarcomas. However, radiation is frequently utilized for unresectable malignant tumors, positive margins, metastatic lesions, and local recurrence.

Radiation has a multitude of side effects, including telangiectasis, fibrosis, tissue atrophy, endarteritis obliterans, flexion deformities, skin changes, growth disturbance, fracture, spinal cord injury, and organ-specific complications. These side effects are related to total radiation dose, technique, and dosage rate.

One of the most concerning complications associated with radiation therapy is the risk of secondary malignancy. Radiation-induced sarcomas occur within the field of radiation and may arise from normal bone or pathologic bone. The latent period between radiation exposure and secondary sarcoma is variable, ranging from 5 to 42 years. Risk increases with radiation dose and with younger age at exposure.

PEARLS & PITFALLS

- Diagnostic errors occur in the field of oncology because of the relative rarity of these disease processes and the great variability of patient presentation. Delay in proper diagnosis, inaccurate diagnosis, and improper and inadequate staging are errors that can lead to delayed or inappropriate treatment. A meticulous history and physical examination, high-quality radiographic evaluation, and proper biopsy technique are the keys to accurate diagnosis and successful treatment.

- The biopsy of bone tumors is a critical procedure, owing to its profound implications for diagnosis, treatment, and patient outcome. Different methods of biopsy exist, and the ideal method is guided by the location of the tumor, tumor characteristics, surgeon preference, and institutional capabilities.

- Percutaneous biopsy methods are less invasive methods of obtaining pathologic tissue and include fine-needle aspiration and Tru-cut (Baxter Health Care Corporation) needle biopsy techniques. These methods are often performed under CT localization and are indicated for bone tumors with an accessible soft-tissue component. Limitations include small tissue sample size, difficulty establishing tissue grade, and a lower diagnostic accuracy than is the case in open biopsy. Though frequently utilized in the appendicular skeleton, the application of percutaneous biopsy in the spine is more limited, owing to the close proximity of the tumor to critical neural elements. Ideal candidates for percutaneous biopsy in primary spinal tumors are patients who require only a diagnostic biopsy (e.g., eosinophilic granuloma), patients with recurrent tumors, or patients with tumors for which definitive treatment may be radiation or chemotherapy (e.g., lymphoma). Complications can include bleeding, infection, pneumothorax, and neurologic injury.

- Open biopsy is the gold standard for the biopsy of bone and soft-tissue tumors and is the most frequently utilized technique in the spine. The accuracy of open biopsy is approximately 91% to 96%, with failure resulting from sampling errors. Principles of proper technique include meticulous hemostasis, longitudinal incisions, and avoidance of intermuscular or internervous planes. Placement of the biopsy incision should allow its full excision if further surgical resection of the tumor is required. Biopsy from the soft-tissue component with the least amount of mineralization is preferable to biopsy of the bone itself, as intraoperative frozen sections can technically be completed only on the soft-tissue component. Because infection is frequently part of the differential diagnosis, aerobic, anaerobic, fungal, and acid-fast bacillus cultures are advised. Closure of the wound in multiple layers will minimize and localize any undesired hematoma. Drains, if necessary, should be placed in line with the biopsy incision so that future excision of both the drain site and biopsy path is possible.

- Errors at the time of biopsy are common and can adversely affect patient treatment options and patient outcomes. Mankin and colleagues demonstrated that biopsy-related problems with malignant bone and soft-tissue tumors are five times more likely when biopsy is performed at a referring institution rather than at the treating institution. Such problems include wound breakdown, hemorrhage, infection, and fracture. Additionally, difficulty with the initial biopsy altered treatment in 18.2% of patients, 75% of these biopsies occurring at the referring institution. In 8.5% of cases, errors in biopsy adversely affected patient prognosis and outcome, with 4.5% undergoing unnecessary amputation. These data highlight the importance of meticulous biopsy technique and preoperative planning. Referral to a tertiary treating institution is advised prior to biopsy if the surgeon or institution cannot perform this critical diagnostic procedure accurately.

- Postlaminectomy kyphosis is a complication of posterior surgery of the spine, especially in children. The etiology of iatrogenic kyphosis is attributed to facet resection and compression of the cartilaginous end plates. Risk factors include multiple-level decompressions and/or laminectomy, facet resection, preoperative sagittal instability, anterior pseudarthrosis, skeletal immaturity, and preoperative kyphosis.

- Postlaminectomy kyphosis frequently presents as progressive symptoms after a period of postoperative improvement. Signs and symptoms may include pain, instability, deformity, and myelomalacia; treatment should be aimed at correction of the deformity and stabilization. If the decision is made not to instrument the spine after primary resection of posterior elements, close postoperative clinical and radiographic evaluation is necessary.

Illustrative Case Presentations

CASE 1. L4 Aneurysmal Bone Cyst with Reactive Scoliosis

T.T. is a 9-year-old boy with spinal asymmetry, back pain, and occasional night pain. On examination, he has tenderness to palpation along the L4 vertebral body, pain with forward flexion, and no neurologic deficits. Plain radiography demonstrates an 11-degree left lumbar scoliosis with radiolucent changes in the L4 body and erosion of the pedicle. CT scan demonstrates an expansile lytic lesion of the L4 vertebral body, with asymmetric vertebral collapse (Figs. 14-6A and B). MRI demonstrates fluid-fluid levels in the L4 vertebral body, compression, and retropulsion onto the thecal sac with no soft-tissue mass.

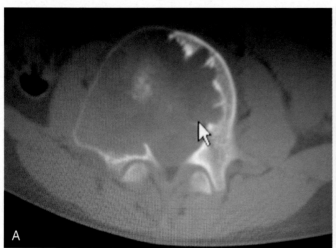

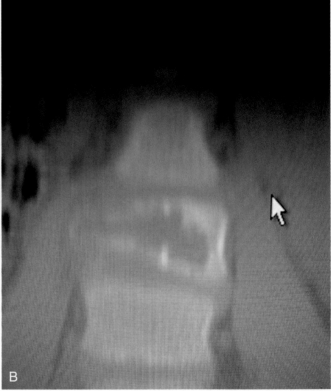

Figure 14-6. A and **B,** CT images demonstrating an aneurysmal bone cyst of L4 in a 9-year-old male patient presenting with low back pain.

The patient underwent preoperative selective arterial embolization. In the operative room, he was placed in a "sloppy lateral" position to allow simultaneous anterior and posterior approaches to the spine from one surgically prepped field. An open biopsy with intraoperative frozen section was carried out through a posterior approach. Histology was reviewed by the operating surgeon and pathologist, confirming a diagnosis of aneurysmal bone cyst without evidence of malignancy. Through a right-sided retroperitoneal exposure, the tumor was removed by using a four-step approach to the treatment of aneurysmal bone cysts: (1) curettage, (2) cauterization of remaining cyst wall, (3) high-speed burring, and (4) careful phenolization. An expandable titanium cage with local autologous and allogenic bone graft was used for vertical reconstruction. The posterior resection and decompression were completed through the extended midline longitudinal biopsy incision. A titanium pedicle screw and rod fixation were used to stabilize the spine from L3 to L5 (Figs. 14-6C and D). At the most recent follow-up, the patient was without tumor recurrence, neurologic sequelae, pain, or spinal deformity.

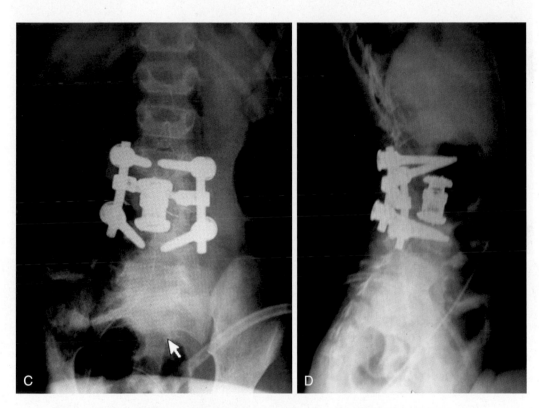

Figure 14-6, cont'd. C and **D,** Postoperative images showing L35 titanium instrumentation.

CASE 2. T4 Osteoblastoma with Structural Scoliosis

J.G. is a 13-year-old female who was referred for evaluation of rapid-onset scoliosis. Radiography reveals an unbalanced curve, with a 35-degree left thoracic curve and a 28-degree compensatory lumbar curve (Fig. 14-7A). On CT scan, a well-contained posterior T4 vertebral lesion and fourth rib lesion were identified (Fig. 14-7B). Open biopsy with intraoperative frozen section confirmed a diagnosis of osteoblastoma.

Utilizing a posterior approach, surgery involved a partial vertebral corpectomy at T4 and a posterior spinal fusion from T2 to L1 with titanium instrumentation, supplemented with local autograft and allograft (Figs. 14-7C and D). At the most recent follow-up, the patient was without pain, tumor recurrence, neurologic sequelae, or recurrent spinal deformity.

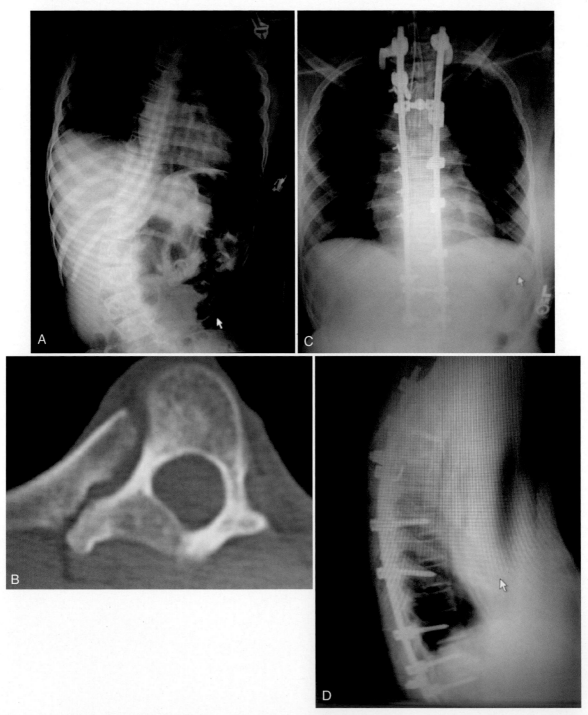

Figure 14-7. Plain radiograph (**A**) and CT scan (**B**) of a 13-year-old female patient with a rapid-onset, painful scoliosis associated with an osteoblastoma of T4. **C** and **D,** Postoperative images following resection of T4 osteoblastoma and T2 to L1 titanium instrumentation.

REFERENCES

Kneisl JS, Simon MA: Medical management compared with operative treatment for osteoid-osteoma. J Bone Joint Surg Am 1992;74:179–185.

Schajowicz F, Lemos C: Malignant osteoblastoma. J Bone Joint Surg Br 1976;58:202–211.

SUGGESTED READINGS

Albrecht S, Crutchfield JS, SeGall GK: On spinal osteochondromas. J Neurosurg 1992;77:247–252.

A report of 5 cases and review of 130 cases of osteochondroma of the spine with analysis of epidemiology, clinical and radiographic features, distribution, and treatment results.

Campanacci M, Cervellati G: Osteosarcoma: A review of 345 cases. Ital J Orthop Traumatol 1975;1:5–22.

A review of 345 cases of osteosarcoma with analysis of epidemiology, anatomic distribution of lesions, symptomotology, radiographic and histologic features, and treatment outcomes.

Cottalorda J, Kohler R, Sales de Gauzy J, et al: Epidemiology of aneurysmal bone cyst in children: A multicenter study and literature review. J Pediatr Orthop B 2004;13:389–394.

Retrospective multicenter review of aneurysmal bone cysts in children (including 161 cases in the mobile spine) with analysis of epidemiology and distribution of lesions.

Cotterill SJ, Ahrens S, Paulussen M, et al: Prognostic factors in Ewing tumor of bone: Analysis of 975 patients from the European Intergroup Cooperative Ewing Sarcoma Study Group. J Clin Oncol 2000;18:3108–3114.

A retrospective analysis of 975 patients with Ewing sarcoma of bone identifying metastasis at diagnosis, with primary site and age as adverse prognostic factors. Treatment with surgery, alone or in addition to radiation, was superior to radiotherapy alone in regard to local relapse rates.

Enneking WF: A system of staging musculoskeletal neoplasms. Clin Orthop Relat Res 1986;304:9–24.

Classic article with description of a system for staging benign and malignant musculoskeletal lesions.

Ewing J: Classics in oncology: Diffuse endothelioma of bone. James Ewing. Proceedings of the New York Pathological Society, 1921. CA Cancer J Clin 1972;22:95–98.

Classic article with the original radiographic and histologic description of Ewing sarcoma.

Garg S, Dormans JP: Tumors and tumor-like conditions of the spine in children. J Am Acad Orthop Surg 2005;13:372–381.

A comprehensive review of tumors of the spine in children and presentation of a classification scheme based on the natural history.

Garg S, Mehta S, Dormans JP: Langerhans cell histiocytosis of the spine in children: Long-term follow-up. J Bone Joint Surg Am 2004;86-A:1740–1750.

Analysis of 26 children with LCH of the spine with description of epidemiology, distribution of lesions, radiographic findings, associated deformity, and natural history.

Hopper KD, Moser RP Jr, Haseman DB, et al: Osteosarcomatosis. Radiology 1990;175:233–239.

Analysis of a subset of 690 osteosarcoma cases characterized by multiple skeletal sites of disease ("osteosarcomatosis") focusing on epidemiology, location and distribution of lesions, and prevalence of pulmonary metastasis.

Ilaslan H, Sundaram M, Unni KK, Shives TC: Primary vertebral osteosarcoma: Imaging findings. Radiology 2004;230:697–702.

Retrospective review of 198 cases of primary vertebral osteosarcoma with analysis of epidemiology, tumor location, radiographic features, and histologic variations.

Kuttesch JF Jr, Wexler LH, Marcus RB, et al: Second malignancies after Ewing sarcoma: Radiation dose-dependency of secondary sarcomas. J Clin Oncol 1996;14:2818–2825.

Analysis of 266 survivors of Ewing sarcoma demonstrating a radiation dose-dependant risk for secondary sarcoma with a mean latency period of 7.6 years.

Mankin HJ, Lange TA, Spanier SS: The hazards of biopsy in patients with malignant primary bone and soft-tissue tumors. J Bone Joint Surg Am 1982;64:1121–1127.

A multicenter analysis of biopsies of malignant bone and soft-tissue tumors comparing outcomes when biopsy was completed at a referring institution versus a treating center. Diagnostic errors, biopsy complications, and reduction in treatment options correlated with the biopsies performed at referring institutions.

Papagelopoulos PJ, Currier BL, Shaughnessy WJ, et al: Aneurysmal bone cyst of the spine: Management and outcome. Spine 1998;23:621–628.

Retrospective analysis of 52 cases of aneurysmal bone cysts of the spine leading to treatment recommendation of preoperative selective arterial embolization, excision, bone graft, and selective fusion.

Ruggieri P, McLeod RA, Unni KK, Sim FH: Osteoblastoma. Orthopedics 1996;19:621–624.

A retrospective review of 306 cases of osteoblastoma with analysis of clinical and pathologic characteristics and differentiating features from osteosarcoma.

Saifuddin A, White J, Sherazi Z, et al: Osteoid osteoma and osteoblastoma of the spine: Factors associated with the presence of scoliosis. Spine 1998;23:47–53.

A retrospective study and meta-analysis of 465 cases of osteoid osteoma and osteoblastoma of the spine with analysis of patterns of scoliosis in relation to location of pathologic lesions.

Schuck A, Ahrens S, von Schorlemer I, et al: Radiotherapy in Ewing tumors of the vertebrae: Treatment results and local relapse analysis of the CESS 81/86 and EICESS 92 trials. Int J Radiat Oncol Biol Phys 2005;63:1562–1567.

Retrospective analysis of 116 patients with primary vertebral Ewing sarcoma demonstrating a 22.6% local relapse rate in patients treated with definitive radiotherapy, most relapses occurring in the radiation field.

Tucker MA, D'Angio GJ, Boice JD Jr, et al: Bone sarcomas linked to radiotherapy and chemotherapy in children. N Engl J Med 1987;317:588–593.

An analysis of 9170 childhood cancer survivors demonstrating a 2.7-fold increased risk of developing a bone sarcoma in those patients who received radiation therapy compared to matched controls. Treatment with alkylating agents was also linked to development of bone cancer in this population, risk increasing with cumulative drug exposure.

Weinstein JN, McLain RF: Primary tumors of the spine. Spine 1987;12:843–851.

An analysis of 103 patients with primary tumors of the spine with description of symptomatology, epidemiology, pathology, and tumor distribution.

Wilkins RM, Pritchard DJ, Burgert EO Jr, Unni KK: Ewing sarcoma of bone: Experience with 140 patients. Cancer 1986;58: 2551–2555.

Retrospective review of 140 patients with Ewing sarcoma of bone demonstrating improved 5-year survival rates for patient undergoing complete surgical resection (74%) compared with those who did not (34%).

CHAPTER 15

Neurofibromatosis

DIANE VON STEIN *and* ALVIN H. CRAWFORD

The neurofibromatoses are a spectrum of diseases that present with a wide range of clinical manifestations. Four distinctive forms of neurofibromatosis are recognized, although variant forms probably exist:

1. Neurofibromatosis-1 (NF-1), von Recklinghausen's disease or peripheral neurofibromatosis, is an autosomal dominant disorder. The entity is common and affects 1 in 3500 individuals. It is the most common single-gene disorder in humans. The gene locus of neurofibromatosis in humans has been identified and localized to the long arm of chromosome 17.

2. Neurofibromatosis-2 (NF-2), or central neurofibromatosis, is also an autosomal dominant disorder, estimated to affect 1 in 50,000 individuals. Characteristically, there is a schwannoma of the eighth cranial nerve.

3. Segmental neurofibromatosis is characterized by café-au-lait macules dispersed in bands on the skin and limited to one or a few body segments.

4. Schwannomatosis involves multiple deep and painful schwannomas. Although there is overlap with NF-2 in presentation and phenotype, schwannomatosis is clinically and molecularly distinct.

This chapter focuses on NF-1 (von Recklinghausen's disease), the most common form of neurofibromatosis and the most likely to be encountered by the spinal surgeon.

Neurofibromatosis is the most common single-gene disorder known to humans. About 50% of all NF-1 cases are spontaneous mutations. The manifestations of NF-1 may vary, but each individual who carries the gene eventually shows some clinical features of the disease. The Consensus Development Conference at the National Institute of Health in 1987 concluded that the diagnosis of NF-1 could be assigned to a person with two or more of the following criteria:

1. The presence of more than six café-au-lait spots measuring at least 15 mm in diameter in adults or five café-au-lait spots of 5 mm in children

2. Two or more neurofibromas of any type or at least one plexiform neurofibroma

3. Freckling in the axillary or inguinal region

4. Optic glioma

5. Two or more Lisch nodules (iris hamartomas)

6. A distinctive bony lesion (anatomic dysplasia or sphenoid wing distortion)

7. A first-degree relative with NF-1 by the above criteria

Comprehensive genetic testing for NF-1 has recently become available on a clinical basis. Direct sequencing is now able to detect the causative mutation in 95% of individuals with NF-1. Testing can now be offered to confirm or rule out the diagnosis in uncertain cases, such as young children with café-au-lait spots only, and for prenatal diagnosis.

The above clinical criteria are useful even in young children. There seems to be two peaks in the occurrence of severe clinical problems for NF-1 patients: one from 5 to 10 years of age and the second from 36 to 50 years of age. At the second peak, 75% of the clinical problems are related to malignancy. There is extreme variability in features and complications of NF-1 among affected individuals. Approximately one third of patients with NF-1 will suffer serious medical and cosmetic complications over their lifetime; the remaining two thirds will have mild to moderate involvement. The orthopedic complications usually present early and include spinal deformities of scoliosis and kyphoscoliosis. Other orthopedic complications include bony dysplasia with congenital bowing and pseudarthrosis of the tibia and the forearm (usually ulna), overgrowth phenomenon of the extremity, and soft-tissue tumors.

Scoliosis is the most common osseous abnormality associated with NF-1. It may vary from a mild, nonprogressive form to severe curvature that is considered to be dystrophic (Table 15-1). The cause of spinal deformity is unknown, but it might be secondary to osteomalacia, a localized neurofibroma that erodes bone, an endocrine disturbance, or mesodermal dysplasia. The exact prevalence of spinal deformities is unknown but is reported to be between 10% and 60%. We have reservations about estimating the incidence on the basis of the occurrence in populations in tertiary referral institutions that have a primary interest in the disease or spinal deformity. At our institution, it is 23%. Spinal changes may occur throughout and are usually divided into soft-tissue and bony

TABLE 15-1. The Radiographic Characteristics of Dystrophic Spinal Deformities

Dystrophic Feature	Percentage
Rib penciling	62
Vertebral rotation	51
Posterior vertebral scalloping	31
Vertebral wedging	36
Spindling of transverse processes	31
Anterior vertebral scalloping	31
Widened interpediculate distance	29
Enlarged intervertebral foramina	25
Lateral vertebral scalloping	13

pathology of the entire vertebral column. Some of the complications of treatment of spine problems reflect the treating physician's lack of understanding of the disease process and potential pitfalls with surgery. Other complications are inherent in the disease process itself. The goal is to prevent problems from occurring by understanding the unusual and unique characteristics of spinal problems in NF-1. It is imperative that the patient understands the importance of careful follow-up observation because of the very real tendency for progression of spinal neuropathology that may continue throughout life.

CERVICAL SPINE DEFORMITIES

The cervical spine in NF-1 patients has not received enough attention in the literature and should be evaluated at the initial scoliosis investigation. There may be early evidence of dystrophic changes on lateral radiographs. Cervical abnormalities occur more frequently when scoliosis or kyphoscoliosis is present in the thoracolumbar region, which distracts the examiner's attention to the more obvious deformity. The most common cervical abnormality is kyphosis. Often, the cervical lesion is asymptomatic. When it is symptomatic, pain is the most common presenting symptom.

The most common abnormality is a severe cervical kyphosis, most often seen following surgery, which itself is highly suggestive of the disorder (Fig. 15-1). Ogilvie reported on the surgical treatment of cervical kyphosis by anterior fusion with iliac crest or fibular bone graft or both. He considered halo traction a useful prelude if the kyphosis is greater than 45 degrees. When progressive cervical kyphosis is the presenting deformity, preoperative halo traction of flexible deformities followed by posterior fusion is the treatment of choice. If the deformity is rigid, then anterior soft tissue release followed by traction is thought to be safer. If sufficient bone stock is present, internal fixation with rods, wires, screws, or hooks may be used posteriorly. Sublaminar wire fixation may be difficult secondary to dural ectasia and osseous fragility. If there is osteolysis with poor bone stock of the vertebral body, anterior and posterior fusion is needed. Postoperative halo vest immo-

bilization is recommended. Of Yong-Hing and coworkers' 56 patients with NF-1, 17 were found to have cervical abnormalities. Of these, 7 patients were asymptomatic, whereas the rest had either limited motion or pain in the neck and 4 had neurologic deficits, which probably could be attributed to cervical instability. Four of the 17 patients required fusion of the cervical spine. Curtis and associates describe 8 patients with paraplegia and NF-1. Four cases were due to cervical spine instability or intraspinal pathology in the cervical spine.

Attention should also be paid to C1-2. Isu and colleagues describe three patients with NF-1 who had C1-2 dislocation with neurologic deficit, and all improved after decompression and/or fusion. It is worthwhile to note that in none of these patients were any bony changes in the C1-2 relation seen on flexion/extension. Therefore, relying only on these views to detect instability is unwise. Most of the problems that we have seen in the cervical spine are those that occur after excision of tumors, which included resection of the laminae and posterior elements (Fig. 15-2). Postoperatively, the spine is unstable and tends to develop progressive kyphosis. Therefore, one must be aware of the NF-1 patient who presents with a scar in and about the neck and gives a history of having a mass removed in the past. We have recently noted patients who have undergone extensive soft-tissue (tumor) excision who have also developed significant kyphosis. It is possible that removal of the ligamentum nuchae and interspinous ligament could predispose to kyphosis.

All patients with NF-1 who (1) undergo surgery, (2) require endotracheal anesthesia, (3) require cranial traction, or (4) present with neck tumors should have a cervical spine roentgenogram. Widening of the neuroforamina on oblique views may be represented by dumbbell lesions characteristic of neurofibromas exiting the spinal canal. If there is any suspicion of instability, computed tomography (CT) or flexion/extension magnetic resonance imaging (MRI) is appropriate. Other reasons for obtaining cervical spine roentgenograms in the NF-1 patient include torticollis and dysphagia. Always obtain skull roentgenograms prior to applying a halo or Gardner-Wells pins.

THORACOLUMBAR DEFORMITIES
Nondystrophic Curves

Peculiar to NF-1 is the concept of dystrophic and nondystrophic spinal changes. Nondystrophic scoliosis is the most common spinal deformity in NF-1. The findings, treatment, and complications are similar to those of a normal idiopathic curve, with the following exceptions:
1. NF patients present earlier than their idiopathic counterparts do.
2. A somewhat worse prognosis can be anticipated for progression.

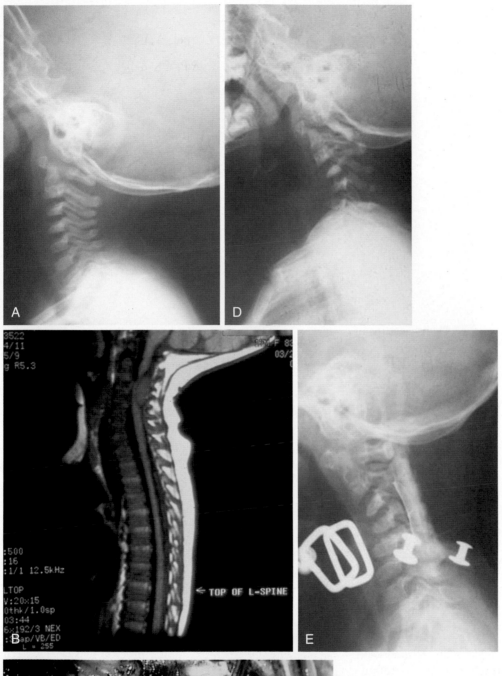

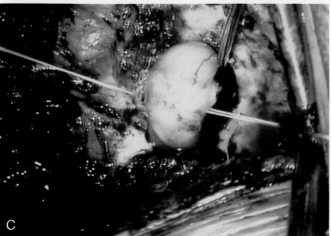

Figure 15-1. Spinal instability following laminectomy in a very young child who complained of neck pain and decreased range of motion. A posterior spinal fusion was performed by using fibular allograft. **A,** Presenting lateral cervical spine radiograph with slightly decreased lordosis. **B,** Magnetic resonance image illustrating extra dural neurofibroma at C3 to C4 with spinal cord indentation. **C,** Operative view of neurofibroma excision. **D,** Lateral cervical spine radiographs 6 months after laminectomy and neurofibroma excision illustrating significant kyphosis of the entire cervical spine and a dystrophic appearance of the midapical vertebra. **E,** Lateral view following posterior spinal fusion with fibular allograft.

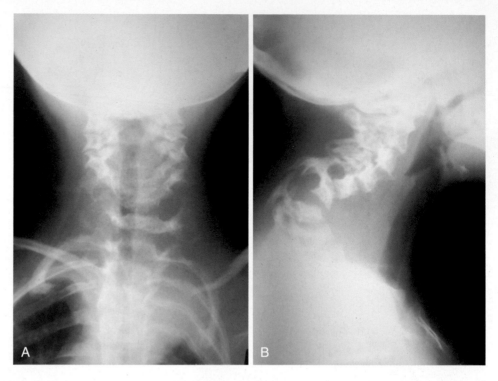

Figure 15-2. This child underwent multiple laminectomies for decompression of a large neurofibroma at the C5-6 level. He subsequently presented with a severe kyphosis of the mid-lower cervical spine. **A,** Frontal view showing enlargement of the neuroforamina at the C7-8 junction. **B,** Lateral view illustrating severe kyphosis at the C6-7 level following laminectomy. The loss of the posterior (tension) supporting structures has allowed each involved facet joint surface to slide and subluxate on its opposing surface, producing increased compressive force on the anterior portion of the vertebral bodies. There has been an unhinging of the posterior articular facets, resulting in complete disengagement.

3. There is a higher pseudarthrosis rate after spinal fusion.

This might be due to a process termed *modulation* (see "Nondystrophic Curves") in which a nondystrophic curve takes on the characteristics of a dystrophic curve.

Treatment of Nondystrophic Curves

If the patient has a curve of 20 to 25 degrees and fewer than three of the dystrophic characteristics, the patient is simply observed (Figs. 15-3A to D). Bracing is used when progression has been demonstrated or the patient presents with a curve greater than 25 degrees and is skeletally immature. Deformities that exceed 40 degrees need posterior spinal fusion with segmental instrumentation. Curves that are greater than 55 to 60 degrees are treated with anterior release with bone grafting, followed by instrumented posterior spinal fusion. This is necessary because the curve is usually more rigid than a similar-size curve would be in idiopathic scoliosis; also, the loss of correction and failure of fusion are more common in patients with NF-1. The authors recommend postoperative orthotic immobilization, although other clinicians have treated these patients without postoperative bracing with good early results.

Dystrophic Curves

The concept of dystrophic curves is based on roentgenographic findings that can be detected as early as age 3 years (Figs. 15-3E to I). The patient may present with a true scoliosis, with a normal kyphosis of less than 50 degrees, or frequently with a kyphoscoliosis, with severe kyphotic curvature of more than 50 degrees.

A dystrophic curve is characterized by a short-segment (usually involving four to six vertebrae) sharply angulated deformity, usually in the upper part of the thoracic spine (Fig. 15-4). The nine radiographic characteristics of dystrophic spinal deformities are identified in Table 15-1. These include scalloping of the vertebral bodies, sharpening of the vertebral margins, severe rotation of the apical vertebra, widening of the spinal canal or the intervertebral foramina, penciling of the ribs, spindling appearance of the transverse process, and a paravertebral mass. Apical vertebral rotation can become so severe that it rotates out of the support axis such that the vertebrae are approximated against one another in a complex three-dimensional pattern (Fig. 15-5). Findings on plain roentgenograms may occasionally be interpreted as a congenital deformity. Rib penciling is present when the width of the rib is less than that of the narrowest portion of the second rib. Vertebral scalloping is present when the depth of scalloping is more than 3 mm in the thoracic spine or more than 4 mm in the lumbar spine. Although scalloping is found in all locations, posterior scalloping is most consistent with the diagnosis of NF-1. The causes of these changes are in some cases intraspinal pathology, such as tumors, meningoceles, or dural ectasia, but the changes may also occur with entirely normal intraspinal contents. In these cases, the dystrophic changes are explained by a primary bone dysplasia. Although all of these various features have been associated with dystrophic deformity, a universally accepted diagnos-

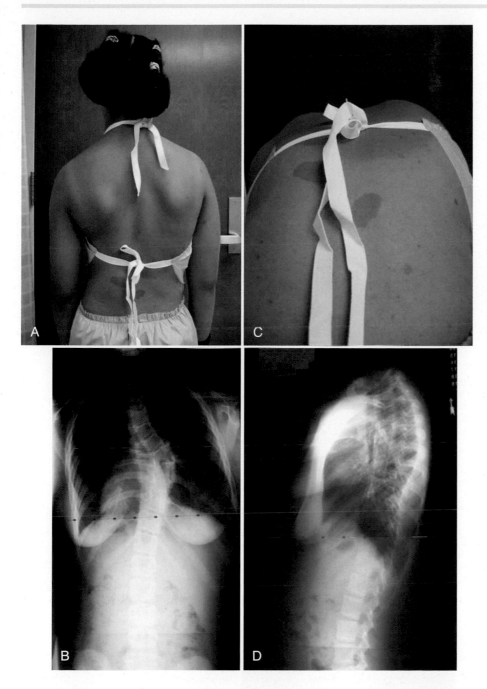

Figure 15-3. Two children with neurofibromatosis type I and scoliosis. One has the nondystrophic type of scoliosis, and the second has the characteristic dystrophic scoliosis that is thought to be associated with neurofibromatosis type I. **A,** Clinical photograph of child who presented with multiple café-au-lait spots, referred by her pediatrician because of a positive Adams forward-bending scoliosis test. This is a nondystrophic idiopathic-appearing curvature. She had a 45-degree curvature and was recommended to have corrective surgery. **B,** Standing posteroanterior thoracolumbar radiograph. The curvature cannot be distinguished from idiopathic scoliosis. **C,** Clinical photograph of Adams forward-bending test from behind shows a minor rib hump, but note the multiple café-au-lait spots. **D,** Lateral thoracolumbar roentgenogram showing curvature that is indistinguishable from idiopathic scoliosis.

Continued

tic criterion does not exist. It is important to detect patients who have a dystrophic curve because these curves are characterized by a rapid course of progression and a higher rate of pseudarthrosis following fusion.

Spinal deformity being followed as idiopathic (nondystrophic) may subsequently show dystrophic changes, a condition called *modulation* (Fig. 15-6). Modulation refers to the ability of a spinal deformity to transform by acquiring various dystrophic morphologic features. A nondystrophic curve can become dystrophic, and a dystrophic curve can acquire further dystrophic changes. This is unique to spinal deformities in NF-1. These dystrophic changes may

evolve slowly or aggressively. Progressively increasing dystrophic changes in a spinal deformity can, at a certain point, alter the behavior of the spinal curve and herald a course of rapid curve progression (Fig. 15-7). Whole-spine MRI should be employed to clarify the classification of curve type at presentation in patients with NF-1 and spinal deformities. In a recently reported study, 4 of 11 patients who were classified initially as having idiopathic-like curves on plain roentgenograms were found to have dystrophic features on MRI. In retrospect, some of these findings could be found on reevaluation of their radiographs.

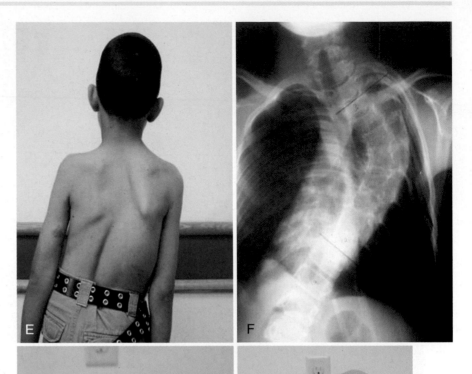

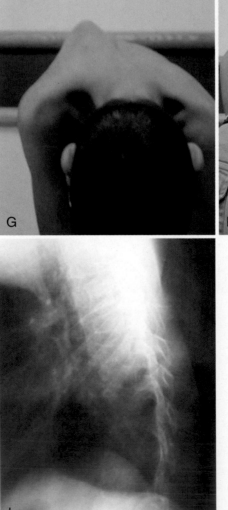

Figure 15-3, cont'd. E, Clinical photograph of a 13-year-old boy with dystrophic scoliosis. There is truncal imbalance to the right. Note the multiple café-au-lait spots. **F,** Posteroanterior roentgenogram showing short, segmented, sharply angulated curvature of the cervicothoracic region with significant rotation. **G,** Clinical photograph of Adams forward-bending test seen from the head down. Note the sharp angulation of the right rib cage. **H,** Clinical photograph of Adams bend test seen from behind, illustrating the sharp rotation of the rib cage as well multiple café-au-lait spots. **I,** Lateral thoracolumbar sacral spine roentgenogram showing thoracic lordosis.

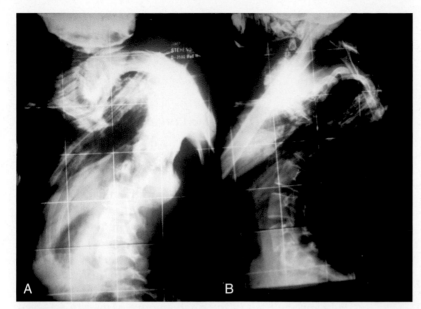

Figure 15-4. Radiographs of a 21-year-old scoliosis patient with severe rotation and angulation. **A,** Coronal plane radiograph showing significant hairpin coronal plane curvatures, which is more than likely a manifestation of the significant kyphosis and rotatory deformity that the child has. **B,** Sagittal plane radiograph showing the striking kyphosis. *(Courtesy of Dr. Klaus Zielke, Badwildengen, Germany.)*

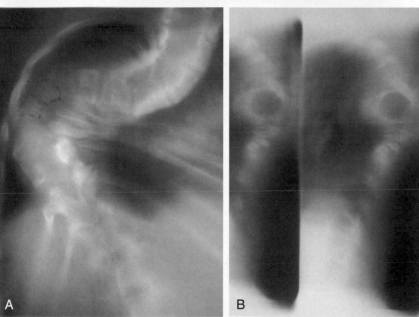

Figure 15-5. This 16-year-old child underwent polycycloidal tomography of what was considered to be a short-segment sharply angulated curvature. **A,** The anterior view shows the upper limb of the curvature to be presenting horizontally. **B,** The two lateral plain polytomography views illustrate the horizontal alignment of the curvature by virtue of the fact that one sees an axial view of the spinal canal. Even more impressive is the enlargement of the spinal canal secondary to dural ectasia. One might note the inverse ratio of the widened canal and the anterior-posterior dimension of the vertebral body reversed from its normal relationships. The anteroposterior diameter of the body is usually twice that of the spinal canal.

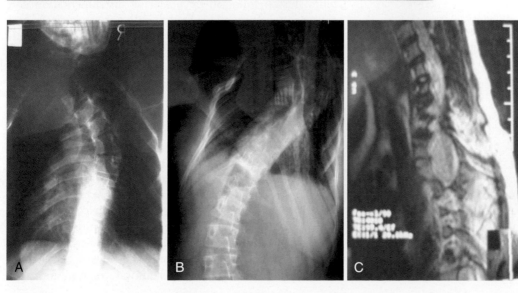

Figure 15-6. Progressive scoliosis followed over 4 years. It was thought on the initial radiograph that the child had a nondystrophic scoliosis, but 4 years later, it has obviously modulated into a dystrophic deformity. MRI confirms widening of the spinal canal secondary to dural ectasia. **A,** Initial radiograph showing moderate spinal deformity with no dystrophic characteristics. **B,** Follow-up radiograph 4 years later showing a significant dystrophic curvature. **C,** MRI illustrating widening of the spinal canal and the thecal sac secondary to dural ectasia.

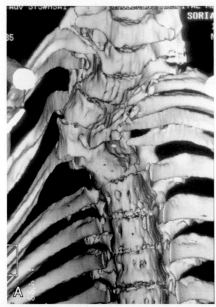

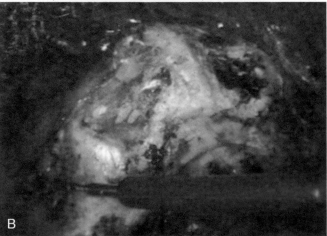

Figure 15-7. A 12-year-old child with dystrophic thoracic scoliosis who underwent anterior release and fusion by video-assisted thoracoscopic surgery. **A,** Three-dimensional reconstructed computed tomogram illustrating significant rotation of the upper thoracic vertebra. **B,** Thoracoscopic view of the anterior apical vertebra. The anterior longitudinal ligament has rotated completely posteriorly on the concave side and is attached to the concave rib heads. The vertebral body appears to have spun around toward the convex side.

With the large number of characteristics found in dystrophic curves, it would be beneficial to the patient and clinician to determine whether one or more of these findings may be more predictive of the curves that are at greatest risk for progression. Risk factors for substantial progression are an early age of onset, a high Cobb angle at the first examination, an abnormal kyphosis, vertebral scalloping, severe rotation at the apex of the curve, location of the apex of the curve in the middle to caudal thoracic area, penciling of one rib or more on the concave side or on both sides of the curve, and penciling of four ribs or more. Based on 91 patients, a recent study made the following observations: (1) Spinal deformity that develops before 7 years of age should be followed closely for evolving dystrophic features (modulation). (2) When a curve acquires either three penciled ribs or a combination of three dystrophic features, clinical progression is almost a certainty.

Treatment of Dystrophic Curves

There is no justification to observe the dystrophic curve in NF-1 because it always progresses. Studies have shown that curves that are treated with a Milwaukee brace progress at a rate similar to that of untreated curves. Early fusion is the best treatment. Fusion in the young individual stunts the growth of the truncal height only minimally because the curve is usually short with a poor growth potential in the involved vertebrae. In theory, the use of subcutaneous growing rods would allow for further growth, although Mineiro and Weinstein, in 2002, questioned its value on the basis of the small amount of growth achieved and the number of procedures required. However, only one of their patients had neurofibromatosis. More recent technological designs of universal instrumentation and localized fusion of anchor sites of growing rods may improve these results.

In spite of meticulous planning and treatment, major complications can occur with surgical treatment. Even in patients who have no neurologic deficit, it is necessary to evaluate the contents of the spinal canal to minimize the possibility of neurologic injury during correction. High-volume myelography or MRI can be used for identifying space-occupying lesions in the spinal canal.

The authors recommend that curves that are less than 20 degrees be observed for progression at 6-month intervals. Curves that are between 20 degrees and 40 degrees should be fused posteriorly and instrumented from the neutral vertebra above to the neutral vertebra below. If the curve is more than 40 degrees or kyphosis is greater than 50 degrees, anterior surgery with discectomy and intervertebral fusion followed by posterior instrumentation and fusion is recommended. Endoscopic anterior release and fusion in either the prone or lateral decubitus position has been found to be effective in managing these cases.

Preoperative traction in severe curves with a flexible kyphosis can improve pulmonary function and minor neurologic deficits and can diminish the curve before fusion (Fig. 15-8). In 2002, Halmai and associates reported their protocol for treating dystrophic curves that were greater than 60 degrees using an average of 3 weeks of preoperative halo vest traction, the rationale for traction being the potential to decrease intraoperative neurologic complications by gradual correction of curvature preoperatively. Careful neurologic monitoring of not just the patient's ability to move the extremity but also motor strength should be documented during periods of traction. The current authors recommend anterior release, nasojejunal tube alimentation, and craniofemoral traction for rigid

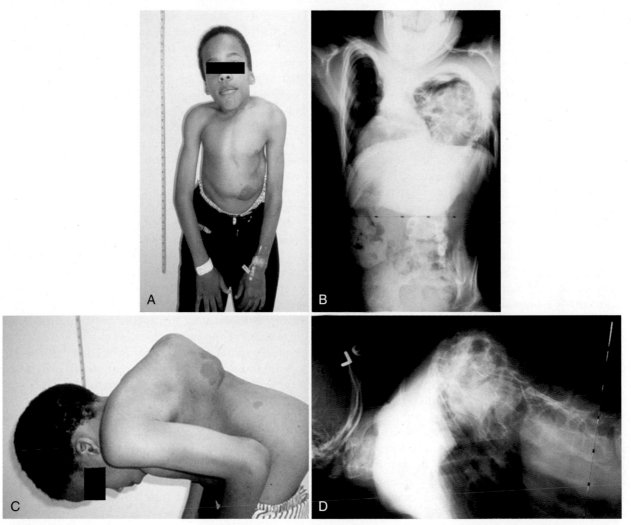

Figure 15-8. This 11-year-old child was referred with mild paraplegia after undergoing seven surgical procedures of the spine. The previous procedures were done with subcutaneous growing rods, which had been removed. **A,** Frontal clinical view of the child showing significant café-au-lait spots as well as a plexiform neurofibroma over the left inferior-anterior rib cage. **B,** Posteroanterior view of the thoracolumbar spine showing significant angular deformity in a hairpin turn of more than 200 degrees. **C,** A lateral clinical photograph of the patient bending over, illustrating the clinically significant kyphosis of the midthoracic spine. In addition, there is a very large plexiform neurofibroma at the base of the kyphosis. **D,** A standing lateral thoracolumbar sacral film (rotated 90 degrees counter clockwise to compare directly with the clinical bending of the patient) illustrating the severe kyphosis in this child. Note that in the midapical region, there is a lucency of the spinal canal, as one sees a cephalocaudal view. This confirms the fact that the severe rotation has caused the middle portion of the spine to be horizontally positioned on this view.

curves that are greater than 90 degrees. For curves that are greater than 100 degrees in any plane, anterior and posterior release is followed by tube alimentation and craniofemoral traction.

When posterior exposure is performed, careful decortication must be undertaken because erosion of the lamina is frequently seen, owing to dural ectasia. We dissect with electrocautery because of the potential of plunging an elevator through thin, weakened lamina. Dural ectasia with an expansion of the thecal sac due to an increase in hydrostatic pressure occurs quite frequently with dystrophic curves. This phenomenon causes spinal canal expansion, erosion, and ligamentous instability to the spinal canal and costovertebral complex. Meticulous fusion after decortication must be carried out by using abundant bone graft over a broad area. Care should be taken to remove all soft tissue

from interposition in the area of the bone graft. Autologous bone graft is preferred to allograft. Instrumentation should be used when possible, but dystrophic vertebrae are not always good recipients for hooks because of osteoporosis and deformation of the posterior elements. Hook dislocation is therefore not infrequent. Pedicle screw anchors provide the best foundation. Patients with dystrophic curves should undergo CT imaging to best appreciate the often distorted anatomy prior to considering pedicle screw insertion. Often, the pedicles have been eroded away by either neurofibroma or dural ectasia and might not support the implant. Hooks, screws, wires, or cable anchors should be used if at all possible to stabilize these cases for fusion. In situ fusion and immobilization in a brace or cast are rarely necessary and represent a poor alternative. Anecdotal reports of off-label use of bone morphogenic proteins to assist in bony union of fusion mass have not been confirmed.

If kyphoscoliosis (kyphosis of more than 50 degrees) is present, anterior and posterior fusion should always be performed. When anterior fusion is performed, thorough intervertebral disc space exposure is extremely important. The disc and end plate should be completely removed. Fusion must be as long as possible, with the addition of strut grafting in the curve concavity for severe angular deformity. One should attempt to get the strut graft into the vertical weight-bearing axis of the spine. The recipient area should be well exposed (which is technically difficult because of severe apical rotation), and the strut graft that is inserted should be in contact with bone. Graft material that is surrounded by neurofibromatous soft tissue has a tendency to resorb. Multiple strut grafts should be used, and the fibula, being the strongest, should be placed most anteriorly. A rib graft that is swung on the vascular pedicle might also be helpful. The exposure is occasionally extremely difficult from the concave side, however, and the apical vertebra often may be subluxated or so severely rotated that it is not in alignment with the rest of the spine. Such malalignment makes it difficult to place anterior strut graft in the concavity of the kyphosis. Shufflebarger believes that the anterior procedure should be undertaken from the concave side with multiple strut grafts and that a convex discectomy would destabilize the spine. We have not had a problem with the convex approach and continue to recommend it for release and fusion but not for strut grafting. Since initiation of anterior and posterior release followed by craniofemoral traction for no fewer than 10 days in curvatures greater than 100 degrees, the difficulty of obtaining correction has diminished, and structural segmental intervertebral grafts are used in addition to struts. Because of the ability to gain more correction with extensive release and traction, we are more aggressive with anterior interventional segmental fusion than with strong strut grafts, especially when it is reinforced with posterior fusion.

In spite of rigid instrumentation, postoperative bracing in NF-1 patients is recommended in an effort to prevent pseudarthrosis. The external support should be maintained until a fusion mass with trabecular pattern is seen. Despite well-done surgery, pseudarthrosis with loss of correction is frequent, even in the hands of experienced spine surgeons. The reason for failure of the surgery is usually inadequate anterior procedure. Crawford reported a 15% incidence of pseudarthrosis in 46 patients, and Sirois and Drennan reported a 31% incidence. The integrity of the fusion mass can be evaluated by bone scanning, tomography, MRI, or second-look surgery about 6 months after the initial surgery, although most often this is not necessary with the use of current generation implants and adequate fusion technique.

Another complication during surgery can be bleeding. Soft-tissue manifestations of NF-1 may complicate an otherwise well-planned surgery. Excessive plexiform venous channels are described around the vertebral bodies, making it difficult to access the vertebra. Careful subperiosteal dissection using monopolar and bipolar cautery is essential. The authors strongly recommend the use of local hemostatic topical agents. Bleeding can be intense enough to require packing off of the wound in one location and proceeding with dissection at another level temporarily. The anesthesiologist should be made aware of the potential for bleeding in operating on this deformity. Soft-tissue tumors from NF-1 can be highly vascular, so postoperative hematoma is not uncommon. Therefore, meticulous hemostasis must be carried out during surgery, and a wound drain must be placed. Postoperative epidural hematoma causing paraplegia has been described.

Sirois and Drennan reported complications that required additional surgery in 9 of 23 patients who underwent treatment of dystrophic curves. These included four reexplorations and augmentations 6 months postoperatively, two revisions for instrumentation dislocation, two extensions of the fusion mass for curve extension, and one multiple spinal osteotomy for increasing deformity despite a solid fusion mass for curve extension. In patients who are still growing, if anterior and posterior fusion is not done, there is an increased incidence of progression of the curve and the crankshaft phenomenon. Additional reported and not infrequent complications include urinary tract infection, dural leak, and thrombophlebitis. After anterior surgery, pulmonary problems with pneumonia, atelectasis, and hemothorax may be seen. Ileus is observed especially during the period of time between staged anterior and posterior surgery if the patient is kept in traction. The current authors strongly recommend nasojejunal intubation and hyperalimentation for all patients who undergo staged anterior posterior surgery.

Kyphoscoliosis

Kyphoscoliosis is defined as scoliosis associated with kyphosis of 50 degrees or greater. If kyphosis is present, appropriate dynamic roentgenograms (i.e., hyperextension lateral over a bolster to evaluate the flexibility of the curve) should be obtained. Paraplegia is not uncommon in patients with severe kyphosis. If a flexible kyphosis is causing paraplegia, the treatment should be halo-assisted traction (but with extreme caution), with close neurologic or evoked potential monitoring during the course of the traction. CT or MRI to rule out rib protrusion into the spinal canal is mandatory in all NF-1 patients with paraplegia.

We have found the trapdoor procedure extremely beneficial to surgically approach the anterior cervicothoracic junction in patients whose curve apex is in this region. This approach between the sternocleidomastoid, manubrium, and fourth thoracic interspace permits intervertebral disc excision, bone grafting by either intradiscal structural support, or rib/fibular bridge grafting (Fig. 15-9).

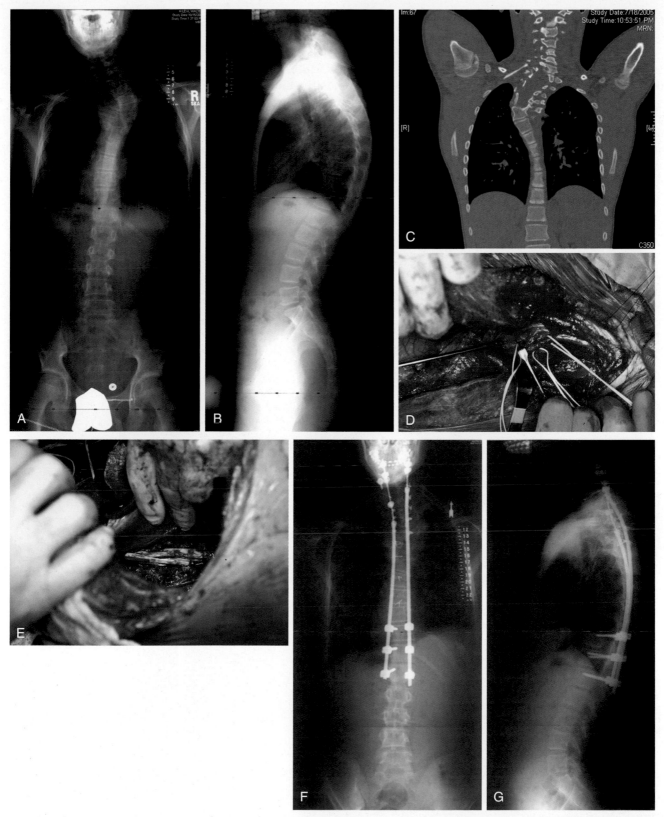

Figure 15-9. This 14-year-old male presented with a progressive dystrophic curve at the cervicothoracic junction. He underwent anterior release and fusion from C5 to T5 followed by posterior instrumentation and fusion from C5 to L1. A trapdoor approach was used to facilitate the anterior surgery. **A,** Standing posteroanterior thoracolumbar sacral spine film. Note the obliquity and rotation of the first, second, and third ribs on the right side. **B,** On the lateral radiograph, the cervicothoracic kyphosis is obscured by the shoulders. **C,** This MRI illustrates the extreme widening of the spinal canal secondary to dural ectasia at the cervicothoracic junction. **D,** The head is to the right, and the foot is to the left. The hand is retracting the right sternum. Loops have been placed around the vessels for safety. **E,** The head is to the left, the mediastinum is being retracted, and fibula strut grafts have been placed across the cervicothoracic junction. Note the vessel loops at 11 o'clock in this illustration. **F,** Standing postoperative posteroanterior view showing multiple anchors of wires, rods, and screws to fuse the cervicothoracic spine. **G,** Standing postoperative lateral view illustrating rod contouring with pedicle screw anchors at the cephalad and caudal fused area.

If the kyphosis is flexible, traction will correct some of the kyphosis and will also reduce cord compression and possibly improve the neurologic deficit (Fig. 15-10). Following traction, anterior spinal cord decompression and strut-assisted fusion should be performed, followed by a posterior fusion. Deep drainage is necessary in all patients who undergo anterior reconstructive surgery because of significant bleeding that can occur once the patient is normotensive. These patients should be observed carefully afterward for the development of pseudarthrosis. Augmentation of the fusion mass should be performed at 6 months if pseudarthrosis (no evidence of trabeculae) is suspected or there is loss of correction.

If the kyphosis is rigid, traction should not be used. Traction in these cases stretches the mobile spinal segments above and below the kyphosis, increasing the tension and point compression on the midapical spinal cord, which can cause further damage. Therefore, a combination of

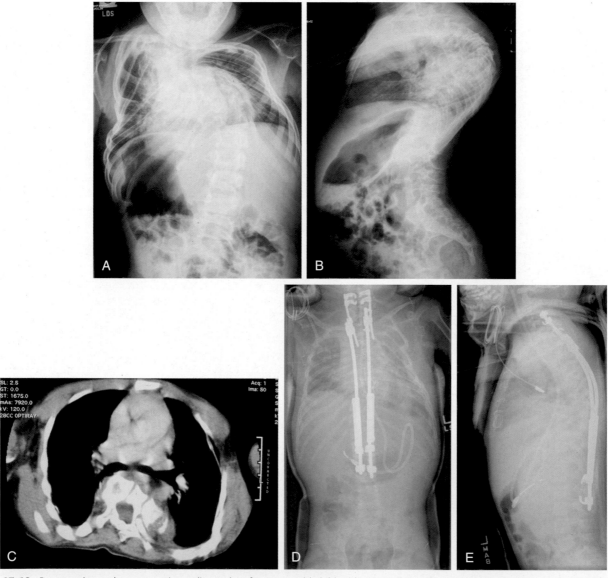

Figure 15-10. Preoperative and postoperative radiographs of a 5-year-old child with severe dystrophic kyphoscoliosis. This child underwent bilateral open trapdoor procedures of the anterior cervicothoracic region, posterior soft tissue release, and craniofemoral traction to achieve correction of her severe deformity. A posterior cervical thoracic fusion using pediatric Isola growing rods was performed following 2 weeks of traction. **A,** Frontal view illustrating the severe left cervical thoracic kyphoscoliosis. There was dural ectasia with widening of the thoracic canal and penetration of three ribs into the spinal canal. **B,** Standing preoperative lateral cervical thoracolumbar sacral radiograph illustrating the severe kyphotic deformity in this child. **C,** Axial MRI of thoracic spine at midapical region illustrating severity of deformity with three horizontal vertebrae (lateral projection) and head of a rib in the spinal canal. **D,** Postoperative posterior-anterior cervical thoracolumbar spine radiograph revealing the instrumentation construct, as well as the nasojejunal tube used to provide hyperalimentation for this child. **E,** Standing lateral cervical/thoracolumbar radiograph illustrating the instrumentation construct. Note the stainless steel wire closures of the sternum following the trapdoor procedure, the nasojejunal tube for hyperalimentation, and a Medipore. The child was placed in a Minerva cast for immobilization.

direct anterior release, disc excision, and intervertebral fusion followed by 7 to 10 days of traction and then posterior spine fusion is recommended. We have successfully used traction of up to 35% body weight with no permanent neurologic sequelae. The vertebral bodies are occasionally extremely porotic and will tend to bleed freely from the cancellous surfaces. The end plate is the strongest element, and bleeding can be minimized with a meticulous annulus and discal release. Plenty of bone graft should be utilized.

Because of the association between paraplegia and kyphoscoliosis, there is a tendency to perform laminectomies to relieve pressure from the cord. Laminectomy only for cord compression and kyphoscoliosis is contraindicated, however. Occasionally, a neurologic improvement may be seen after a posterior approach with incision of the dura because this can release pressure on the cord. Laminectomy does not decompress the neural elements because the compression is anterior and removal of bone posteriorly destabilizes the spine, potentially increasing the kyphosis. Laminectomy alone also removes valuable bone stock required for a posterior spinal fusion. Occasionally, paraplegia is related to protrusion of a rib into the spinal canal. This will usually be evident on CT or MRI. Removal of this protrusion should prevent neurologic deterioration. The use of pedicle screw anchors is required in situations in which posterior decompression has been carried out. Remember to get a CT scan prior to surgery when instrumentation is planned in order to assess pedicle and vertebral morphology and size.

Paraplegia

Paraplegia is not an infrequent complication of spinal deformities in NF-1. The neurologic compromise may be related to spinal deformity, instability of the costovertebral complex causing direct protrusion of a rib into the spinal cord, vertebral angulation, tumor, or dural ectasia. Paraplegia that presents in a younger age group is frequently caused by spinal deformity, and paraplegia in the older age group is often a result of tumor. Paraplegia after corrective surgery is often due to the compression exerted on the spinal cord by unrecognized neurofibroma or rib head the intraspinal space. Rarely reported is the patient who presents with paraparesis due to rib displacement. This may have an insidious onset or can occur after a trauma. Bony dysplasia, intervertebral foraminal enlargement, and rotation of vertebral bodies all can contribute mechanically to allow the heads of the ribs to displace in the canal.

In the spinal deformity group, kyphosis is the most frequent cause of paraplegia. Increased kyphosis leads to excessive axial tension on the spinal cord and especially on the posterior dura, which compresses the spinal cord against the anterior vertebral body. Paraplegia is rare in a pure scoliotic curve; if it is present, a workup for intraspinal pathology should be done. If paraplegia is present, MRI or CT with myelography is appropriate to find the cause of paraplegia. With a severe deformity, interpretation of these images can be confusing, however, and often inconclusive.

Radicular symptoms have been reported as well, due to vertebral arteriovenous fistulas. The most common form is a dural arteriovenous fistula sited in the sleeve of the thoracolumbar nerve root. Kähärä and colleagues reported recently on a posttraumatic arteriovenous fistula that caused radicular symptoms due to a mass effect of the dilated epidural venous space.

Prior to surgery, the source of paraparesis, paraplegia, or radiculopathy needs to be thoroughly investigated so that the surgeon is prepared to perform the necessary surgery and to have the appropriate assistance available.

Spondylolisthesis

Spondylolisthesis in patients with NF-1 is rare. Spondylolisthesis is usually secondary to increased anteroposterior diameter of the spinal canal, with elongation and thinning of the pedicles, causing a pathologic forward progression of the anterior elements of the spinal column. The causes of pathologic instability are frequently dural ectasia, meningocele, and neurofibroma. MRI or CT with contrast is absolutely necessary for preoperative evaluation. The treatment in severe slips is anterior and posterior spinal fusion. Fusion is difficult to obtain because of the mechanical alignment of the lumbosacral region and poor bone formation. The authors recommend at least an L4 to sacrum anterior and posterior fusion with lumbosacral instrumentation. If iliosacral anchors are used to protect the sacral screws, they should be removed once the lumbosacral fusion is solid. Postoperative orthotic immobilization is strongly recommended.

SPINAL CANAL PATHOLOGY
Dural Ectasia and Intrathoracic Meningocele

A unique finding in NF-1 and Marfan syndrome is dural ectasia. This is an expansion of the dural sac from an unknown etiology. MRI or high-volume CT-myelography can distinguish dural ectasia from tumors (Fig. 15-11). The expanding dura can cause erosion of the vertebral body and pedicle and later, destabilization of the spine, with possible spontaneous dislocation (Fig. 15-12). Dural ectasia can in some cases be so expansive to the spinal canal that the spinal cord is not injured, even if extreme tortuosity or spine dislocation has developed. The treatment is traction followed by fusion.

Meningocele is a protrusion of the spinal meninges through the intervertebral foramen or through an erosion of the vertebral body. It contains a subarachnoidal space filled with cerebrospinal fluid and causes a paravertebral cystic swelling. It is usually located in the thoracic spine.

Figure 15-11. A three-dimensional reconstructed view at the midthoracic level as well as a CT, both illustrating significant spinal deformity, protrusion of the rib head into the vertebral canal, and widening of the canal secondary to dural ectasia. **A,** The rib head has protruded into the very widened spinal canal, which has been expanded secondary to dural ectasia. **B,** Several axial CT images showing the erosive effects of dural ectasia. There is significant widening of the spinal canal; and erosion of the lamina, transverse processes, and pedicle on the right has permitted displacement of a rib into the canal. (**A,** *Contributed by Stephen Tredwell, MD.*)

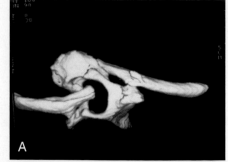

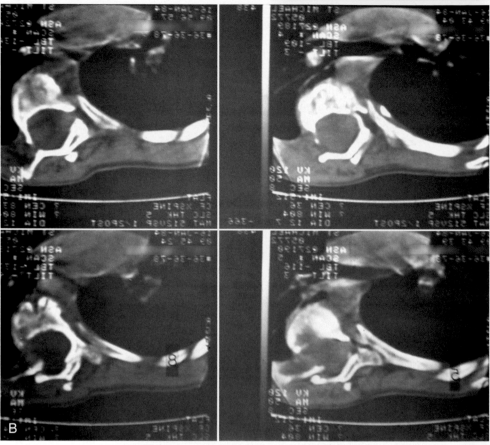

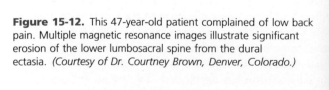

Figure 15-12. This 47-year-old patient complained of low back pain. Multiple magnetic resonance images illustrate significant erosion of the lower lumbosacral spine from the dural ectasia. *(Courtesy of Dr. Courtney Brown, Denver, Colorado.)*

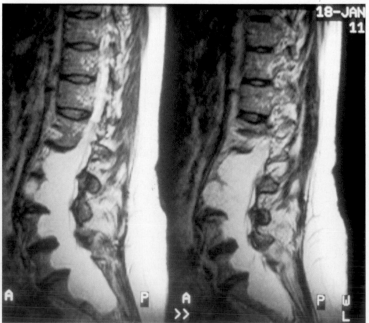

Meningocele and dural ectasia are variations of the same phenomenon, meningocele being more localized. Meningocele can often be an incidental finding on chest radiograph, or symptoms such as pain or neurologic compromise might be seen. If an intrathoracic meningocele expands, causing pressure on adjacent structures, it can cause coughing or dyspnea. If the symptomatic meningocele is massive or symptomatic, it should be approached and removed.

Dumbbell Lesion

A dumbbell lesion is a solitary neurofibroma that is constricted as it exits the neural foramen. The constriction gives the neurofibroma the appearance of a weightlifter's dumbbell (Fig. 15-13). With continued growth, erosion and widening of the intervertebral foramen occur. Erosion can, however, also be caused by meningocele, and MRI can be helpful to distinguish between the two. Spinal canal neurofibromas may be intradural or extradural and are most commonly seen in the cervical and thoracic regions. We recommend early fusion in patients who had a laminectomy for resection of a spinal canal tumor to prevent spinal column instability, usually kyphosis. Pedicle screw anchors are effective for instrumentation but the spine must be imaged prior to implantation. Other tumors can come from the nerve sheath or from the nerve itself, presenting as interstitial hypertrophy, in which case the nerve is the tumor and the tumor is the nerve. The neurofibroma is usually benign but it may cause complications by its local growth. The intraspinal portion of the tumor may cause cord compression and root failure. The peripheral tumor can create compression of blood vessels, nerves, lung, and pleura. Resection of the tumor originating from the nerve can result in a neurologic loss. Patients need to be advised of this possible neurologic deficit prior to surgery.

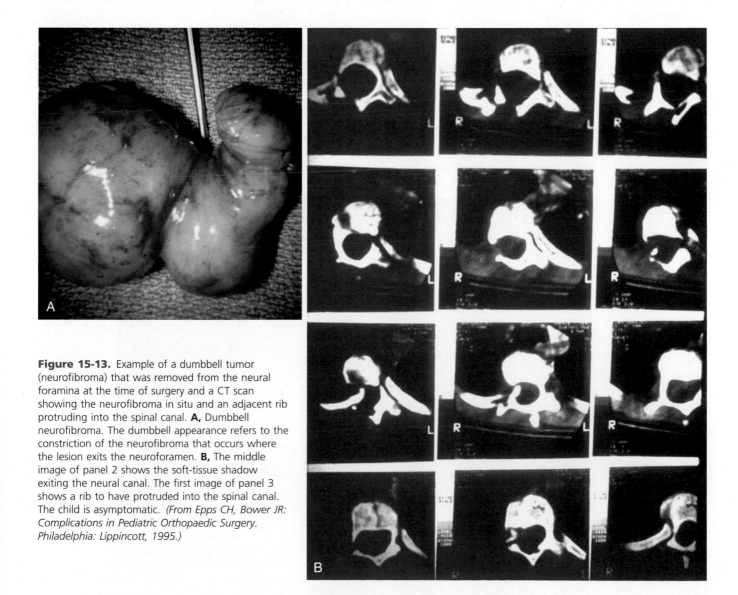

Figure 15-13. Example of a dumbbell tumor (neurofibroma) that was removed from the neural foramina at the time of surgery and a CT scan showing the neurofibroma in situ and an adjacent rib protruding into the spinal canal. **A,** Dumbbell neurofibroma. The dumbbell appearance refers to the constriction of the neurofibroma that occurs where the lesion exits the neuroforamen. **B,** The middle image of panel 2 shows the soft-tissue shadow exiting the neural canal. The first image of panel 3 shows a rib to have protruded into the spinal canal. The child is asymptomatic. *(From Epps CH, Bower JR: Complications in Pediatric Orthopaedic Surgery. Philadelphia: Lippincott, 1995.)*

- Scoliosis is the most common osseous abnormality associated with neurofibromatosis type 1 (NF-1) and is found in 20% to 30% of patients.
- The cervical spine must be imaged once the diagnosis of thoracic scoliosis has been confirmed. Subtle deformities may exist that would make anesthesia or traction problematic. Patients who are considered for cranial traction should also have a skull radiograph to rule out occasionally seen erosive lucent defects.
- All curvatures that show dystrophic characteristics (see Table 15-1) should undergo MRI or contrast CT.
- Severe deformities should be observed for pedicle morphology that may be eroded away by neurofibroma. On occasion, costovertebral dissociation occurs, and the head of the rib displaces into the spinal canal with or without accompanying neuropathy.
- Patients under 7 years old who show more than three dystrophic characteristics usually develop progressive deformities.
- Progressive early-onset scoliosis in young children does not respond to bracing, and growing rods should be considered to control the deformity prior to skeletal maturity.
- All progressive dystrophic curves should be treated aggressively with anterior and posterior stabilization.
- Dural ectasia, a progressive expansion of the dural sac, can cause progressive widening of the spinal canal. Severe curvatures can exist without neuropathy because of the increased space available for the spinal cord. Dural ectasia is ubiquitous and can continue to erode the vertebral column after solid spinal fusion.
- Spondylolisthesis occurs as a result of thinning and instability of the pedicles from the dural ectasia and neurofibroma exiting the neuroforamina. The sacrum and pelvis might not be secure enough to support screws. Be proactive, and stabilize the deformity early.
- Excision of the smallest tumor requiring partial or complete laminectomy and interspinous ligament release should be followed by spinal fusion to prevent instability into kyphosis.

Illustrative Case Presentations

CASE 1. A 5-Year-Old Female with a History of Multiple Neurofibromas

This child's pediatrician initially noted a lumbar scoliosis, which became progressive (Fig. 15-14). The patient had no complaints referable to the curvature. On physical examination, she was noted to have some small subcutaneous neurofibromas and numerous café-au-lait spots (Fig. 15-15). Neurologic examination was normal.

Figure 15-16 shows the neurofibromas on CT scan. Figures 15-17 to 15-19 show long-term follow-up.

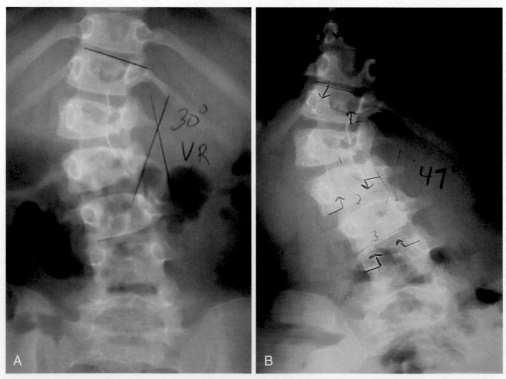

Figure 15-14. A, A 30-degree curve 13 months prior to surgery. **B,** Progression to 47 degrees at the time of surgery.

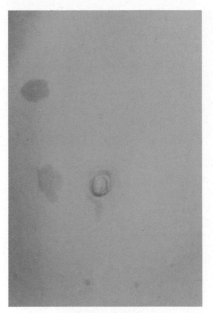

Figure 15-15. Café-au-lait spots on the abdomen.

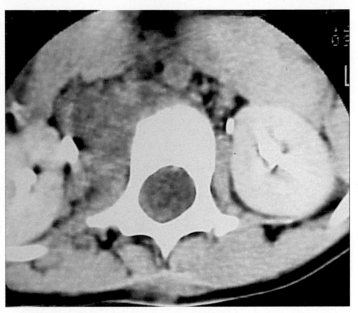

Figure 15-16. CT scan of retroperitoneal neurofibromas.

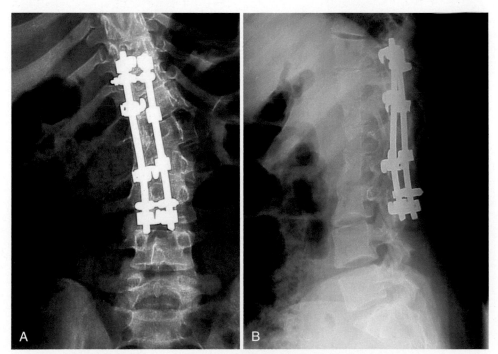

Figure 15-17. A and **B,** Long-term follow-up roentgenograms at 10 years.

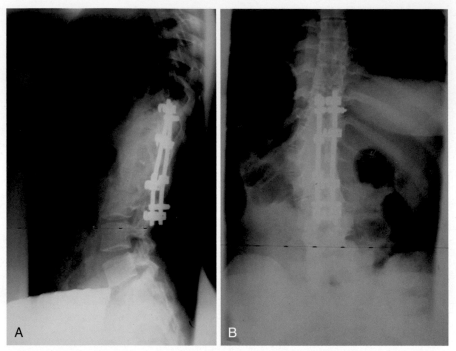

Figure 15-18. **A** and **B,** Follow-up roentgenograms 17 years later, showing slight disc height loss at the level below the fusion.

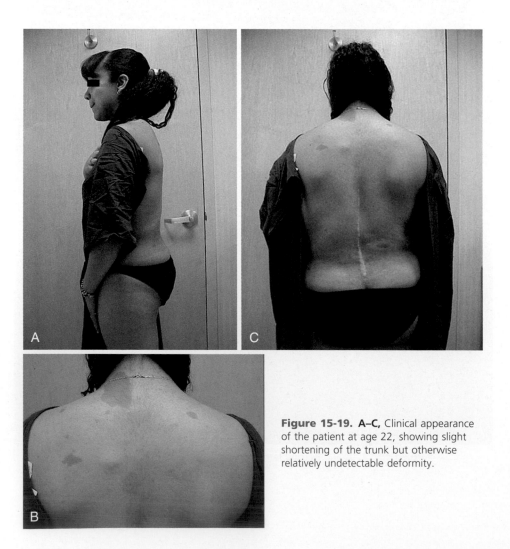

Figure 15-19. A–C, Clinical appearance of the patient at age 22, showing slight shortening of the trunk but otherwise relatively undetectable deformity.

CASE 2. A 13-Year-Old Female with Neurofibromatosis

This 13-year-old female with NF-1 (Fig. 15-20) presented with a 114-degree thoracic scoliosis. She had been noted to have a cervicothoracoabdominal mass biopsy diagnosed as benign plexiform neurofibroma. She underwent a posterior spinal fusion and multiple costoplasties to diminish her rib hump. She will be in a brace for 6 weeks as a result of the costoplasties.

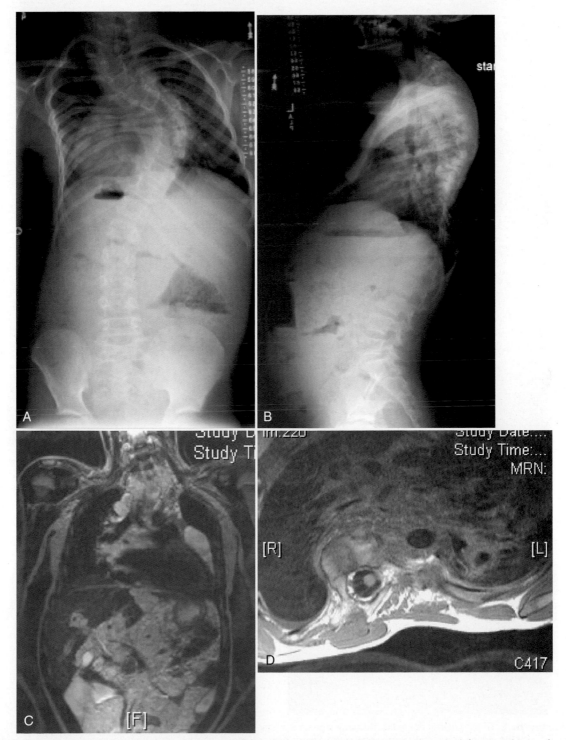

Figure 15-20. A, Posteroanterior (PA) thoracolumbar spine radiograph showing a 114-degree main thoracic deformity. This is a focal short segment severe deformity with apical concave rib penciling and rotation. **B,** Lateral thoracolumbar spine radiograph showing a severe thoracic lordosis and prominent rib hump. **C,** Coronal magnetic resonance image (MRI) showing a visible mediastinal mass encircling the great vessels and a tracheobronchial tree extending and infiltrating into the abdomen and surrounding abdominal organs. **D,** Axial MRI illustrating a paratracheal tumor mass in the chest completely surrounding the mediastinal contents, compressing the carina, and almost encircling the spinal column with encroachment of the vertebral bodies and pedicles.

Continued

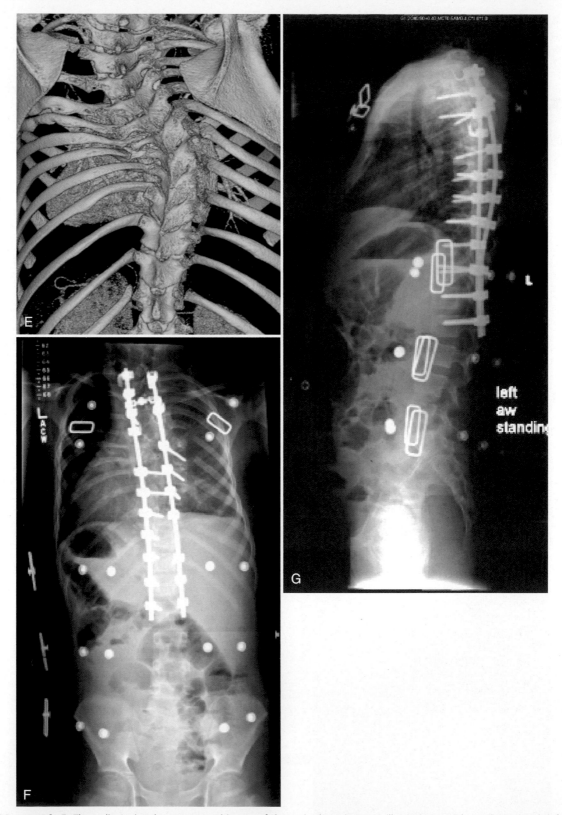

Figure 15-20, cont'd. E, Three-dimensional reconstructed image of the main thoracic curve, illustrating angular and rotational deformity as well as erosive changes over the lamina and ribs. **F,** Postoperative PA thoracolumbar spine radiograph illustrating correction of the deformity. Note the rib segment defects from costoplasty. The costoplasty is protected with bracing for 6 weeks. **G,** Lateral thoracolumbar spine radiograph illustrating some correction of thoracic lordosis and decrease in rib hump.

ACKNOWLEDGMENT

Kind appreciation is extended to Elizabeth Schorry, MD, and Sherry Powell for their contributions during the preparation of this manuscript.

REFERENCES

Crawford, AH: Neurofibromatosis. In Weinstein SL (ed): The Pediatric Spine: Principles and Practice. New York: Raven Press, 1994, pp 619–649.

Crawford AH: Neurofibromatosis in children. Acta Orthop Scand Suppl 1986;218:1–60.

Curtis BH, Fisher RL, Butterfield WL, Saunders FP: Neurofibromatosis with paraplegia: Report of eight cases. J Bone Joint Surg Am 1969;51:843–861.

Jacobsen DS, Crawford AH: Complications in neurofibromatosis. In Epps CH Jr, Bowen JR (eds): Complications in Pediatric Orthopaedic Surgery. Philadelphia: JB Lippincott, 1995, pp 649–683.

Kähärä V, Lehto U, Ryymin P, Helén P: Vertebral epidural arteriovenous fistula and radicular pain in neurofibromatosis type I. Acta Neurochir (Wien) 2002;144:493–496.

Kumar K, Crawford AH: Role of "Bovie" in spinal surgery: Historical and analytical perspective. Spine 2002;27:1000–1006.

Listernick R, Charrow J: Neurofibromatosis type 1 in childhood. J Pediatr 1990;116:845–853.

Messiaen LM, Callens T, Mortier G, et al: Exhaustive mutation analysis of the Nf1 gene allows identification of 95% of mutations and reveals a high frequency of unusual splicing defects. Hum Mutat 2000;1:541–555.

Mineiro J, Weinstein SL: Subcutaneous rodding for progressive spinal curvatures: Early results. J Pediatr Orthop 2002;22:290–295.

Ogilvie J: Neurofibromatosis. In Bradford DS, Winter RB, Lonstein JE (eds): Moe's Textbook of Scoliosis and Other Spinal Deformities, 3rd ed. Philadelphia: WB Saunders, 1995, pp 338–347.

Rezaian SM: The incidence of scoliosis due to neurofibromatosis. Acta Orthop Scand 1976;47:534–539.

Riccardi VM, Kleine B: Neurofibromatosis: A neoplastic birth defect with two age peaks of severe problems. Birth Defects Orig Artic Ser 1877;13:131–138.

Savini R, Parisini P, Cervellati S, Gualdrini G: Surgical treatment of vertebral deformities in neurofibromatosis. Ital J Orthop Traumatol 1983;9:13–24.

SUGGESTED READINGS

Akbarnia BA, Gabriel KR, Beckman E, Chalk D: Prevalence of scoliosis in neurofibromatosis. Spine 1992;17(suppl):S244–S248.

Experience in a comprehensive, multispecialty neurofibromatosis clinic leads the authors to suggest that the association of spinal deformity with neurofibromatosis is less frequent than is usually assumed. Previously reported statistics can be partly attributed to preselection of patients seen by spinal surgeons and to the predominant referral of patients who have severe manifestations of neurofibromatosis. The authors believe that 10% is representative of the true prevalence of spinal deformity in an otherwise unselected cross section of neurofibromatosis patients.

Durrani AA, Crawford AH, Choudhury SN, et al: Modulation of spinal deformities in patients with neurofibromatosis type 1. Spine 2000;25:69–75.

Spinal deformities in patients with neurofibromatosis 1 should be regarded as deformities in evolution. One should resist assigning these evolving deformities to either the dystrophic or nondystrophic end of the spectrum without considering the possibility of modulation across the spectrum. A spinal deformity that develops before 7 years of age should be followed closely for evolving dystrophic features (i.e., modulation). When a curve acquires either three penciled ribs or a combination of three dystrophic features, clinical progression is almost a certainty.

Funasaki H, Winter RB, Lonstein JB, Denis F: Pathophysiology of spinal deformities in neurofibromatosis: An analysis of seventy-one patients who had curves associated with dystrophic changes. J Bone Joint Surg Am 1994;76:692–700.

The findings in 71 patients who had previously untreated spinal deformities associated with dystrophic changes and who had neurofibromatosis were reviewed to identify the risk factors for progression of the curve as well as the natural history of the dystrophic changes and curve patterns.

Halmai V, Doman I, de Jonge T, Illes T: Surgical treatment of spinal deformities associated with neurofibromatosis type 1: Report of 12 cases. J Neurosurg 2002;97:310–316.

In this study, the surgical treatment of dystrophic curves always included 360 degrees fusion and the use of a tibial corticocancellous graft, which must be placed on the concave side of the curve in the frontal plane, the graft thereby providing biomechanical support.

Isu T, Miyasaka K, Abe H, et al: Atlantoaxial dislocation associated with neurofibromatosis: Report of three cases. J Neurosurg 1983;58:451–453.

In this case report, atlantoaxial dislocation was found in three patients with neurofibromatosis. Roentgenographic findings included marked reduction of sagittal diameter at the C-1 vertebral level, and cervical spine abnormalities associated with mesodermal dysplasia, such as posterior scalloping of the cervical spinal bodies with dural ectasia and vertebral body deformity (vertebral body dysplasia). The pathogenesis of atlantoaxial dislocation associated with neurofibromatosis is discussed.

Ramachandran M, Tsirikos AI, Lee J, Saifuddin A: Whole-spine magnetic resonance imaging in patients with neurofibromatosis type 1 and spinal deformity. J Spinal Disord Tech 2004;17:483–491.

In a mixed population of pediatric and adult patients with NF-1, normal neurologic function, and spinal deformity, MRI of the whole spine proved useful in the identification of occult vertebral dysplasia and in demonstration of intraspinal and paraspinal neoplasms.

Shufflebarger HL: Cotrel-Dubousset instrumentation in neurofibromatosis spinal problems. Clin Orthop Relat Res 1989;245:24–28.

In this study, Cotrel-Dubousset instrumentation was employed in 12 patients with neurofibromatosis with spinal deformity. The author concluded that Cotrel-Dubousset instrumentation is effective in the surgical management of neurofibromatous spinal abnormalities.

Sirois JL 3rd, Drennan JC: Dystrophic spinal deformity in neurofibromatosis. J Pediatr Orthop 1990;10:522–526.

A retrospective review was performed to investigate patterns of spinal deformity associated with neurofibromatosis and the incidence of pseudarthrosis and curve progression after spinal fusion. Twenty-three of the 32 patients (72%) with spinal deformity had dystrophic curve patterns. The incidence of pseudarthrosis was 38% for the dystrophic group undergoing isolated posterior fusion. Their average curve progression was 12.7 degrees, and they required an average of 1.7 procedures to achieve solid posterior fusion. Kyphoscoliotic curves should be treated with combined anterior/posterior fusion.

Winter RB, Moe JH, Bradford DS, et al: Spine deformity in neurofibromatosis: A review of one hundred and two patients. J Bone Joint Surg Am 1979;61:677–694.

The natural history, associated anomalies, and response to operative and nonoperative treatment were reviewed in 102 patients with neurofibromatosis and spine deformity. Eighty patients were found to have curvatures associated with dystrophic changes in the vertebrae and ribs. The presence of dystrophic changes such as rib penciling, spindling of the transverse processes, vertebral scalloping, severe apical vertebral rotation, foraminal enlargement, and adjacent soft-tissue neurofibromas was found to be highly significant in prognosis and management.

Yong-Hing K, Kalamchi A, MacEwen GD: Cervical spine abnormalities in neurofibromatosis. J Bone Joint Surg Am 1979;61:695–699.

Fifty-six patients with neurofibromatosis were examined for abnormalities of the cervical spine, and 17 of them had demonstrated lesions there. Of the 34 patients who had scoliosis or kyphoscoliosis, 15 (44%) had cervical lesions. Many of the patients with those lesions were asymptomatic. To avoid the complications that are attributable to the cervical spine, the authors recommend roentgenographic examination in all neurofibromatosis patients who are about to have general anesthesia or skull traction for treatment of scoliosis.

CHAPTER 16

Spinal Deformity in Skeletal Dysplasia

GILBERT CHAN *and* WILLIAM G. MACKENZIE

OVERVIEW

Skeletal dysplasias are a heterogeneous group of disorders that affect bone and cartilage formation. The abnormality results from a specific genetic defect that results in a wide variety of clinical manifestations, among which disproportionate short stature is a common presentation.

Spinal deformity is a common occurrence in skeletal dysplasia. The deformities and the degree of severity vary with the diagnosis. An early and precise diagnosis is important because the natural history of many of these disorders is known and can aid in the evaluation and management. In achondroplasia, foramen magnum stenosis is common early in life and is potentially life threatening, while lumbar and cervical stenosis in this condition usually develops later in life, in the second and third decades.

Another factor to consider in treating these conditions is the anatomic structure of the spine in each dysplasia. Some of these disorders, such as achondroplasia, have spinal stenosis, making it dangerous to use fixation in the spinal canal. In diastrophic dysplasia, cervical kyphosis is common. Surgical management can be complicated by the high incidence of cervical spina bifida. Careful delineation of the spinal anatomy is an important part of the preoperative evaluation.

The more common conditions that are prone to development of spinal deformities are discussed in this chapter and are summarized in Table 16-1.

EVALUATION

Evaluation of a child with skeletal dysplasia should be tailored to each specific condition, which requires knowledge of the deformities that are common to the dysplasia and its natural history. A detailed history and physical examination will often reveal clues to any abnormality that might be present. Questions directed at respiratory function, sleep habits, and motor development and control often provide clues to the presence of any neurologic abnormalities. A history of respiratory symptoms or sleep distur-

bance can point to involvement of the cervical spine or foramen magnum. Other pertinent questions to consider include endurance, gait abnormalities, and bladder and bowel habits.

A detailed neurologic examination is required at each visit; the examination should include motor strength, sensation, and reflexes. Any pathologic reflex should be identified and recorded; any residual primitive reflex should also be recorded. The examination may be difficult to conduct in the younger child, but clues as to the degree of motor involvement can be observed by letting the child play and perform simple tasks such as walking, running, going up and down the steps, or holding onto or playing with simple toys such as blocks. In the very young child or infant, hypotonia and weakness might be manifested by an inability to extend the head or extremities against gravity. Any symptom or sign that points to possible neurologic involvement warrants a more detailed examination aimed at identifying the cause and determining whether these signs or symptoms are secondary to spinal cord compression.

CLASSIFICATION

Achondroplasia

Achondroplasia is the most common of the heritable short-limbed dysplasias. Inheritance is autosomal dominant, although as many as seven eighths of new cases arise from a new mutation. The disorder is caused by a mutation in the *fibroblast growth factor receptor 3 (FGFR-3)* gene located on 4p16.3. The typical mutation leads to overactivity of the FGFR-3 receptor; this, in turn, leads to growth inhibition in bones that are formed by enchondral ossification. From birth, these children are beset by a myriad of problems, most of which are due to abnormal enchondral ossification. Among the early problems that this population encounters is foramen magnum stenosis in as many as 60% of individuals. At birth, the foramen magnum is small. This is due to a defect in enchondral ossification and a premature fusion of the synchondroses. The defect in

TABLE 16-1. Conditions That Are Prone to Involve Development of Spinal Deformities

Condition	Inheritance Pattern	Chromosome Locus	Gene	Spinal Deformity
Achondroplasia	AD	4p16.3	FGFR3	Foramen magnum stenosis Thoracolumbar kyphosis Spinal stenosis
Hypochondroplasia	AD	4p16.3	FGFR3	Increased lumbar lordosis
Thanatophoric dysplasia	AD	4p16.3	FGFR3	Foramen magnum stenosis Kyphoscoliosis Restrictive lung disease
Pseudoachondroplasia	AD	19q12-13.1	COMP	Cervical instability Thoracolumbar kyphosis Lumbar hyperlordosis Scoliosis
Multiple epiphyseal dysplasia	AD	19p13.1	COMP	Atlantoaxial instability
Metatropic dysplasia	AD/AR	Unknown	Unknown	Odontoid hypoplasia Cervical instability Cervical stenosis Kyphoscoliosis/scoliosis Severe platyspondyly
Diastrophic dysplasia	AR	5q32-33	DTDST	Cervical kyphosis Scoliosis Spinal stenosis
Spondyloepiphyseal dysplasia congenita	AD	12q31.1-q13.3	Col2A1	Cervical instability Odontoid hypoplasia Scoliosis Platyspondyly Kyphosis Lumbar hyperlordosis
Kniest dysplasia	AD	12q31.1-q13.3	Col2A1	Cervical instability Kyphoscoliosis
Spondyloepimetaphyseal dysplasia	AD	12q31.1-q13.3	Col2A1	Cervical instability Scoliosis Kyphosis Lumbar lordosis
Spondyloepiphyseal dysplasia tarda	XLR	Xp22.2-p22.1	SEDL	Platyspondyly C1 to C2 instability
MPS IV				
Morquio syndrome A	AR	16q24.3	GALNS	Odontoid hypoplasia
Morquio syndrome B	AR	3p21.33	GLB1	Cervical instability Platyspondyly Kyphosis Spinal stenosis
MPS I Hurler syndrome	AR	4p16.3	IDA	Atlantoaxial instability Lumbar kyphosis Spinal stenosis
MPS II Hunter syndrome	AR	Xq27.3-q28	IDS	Cervical stenosis secondary to retro odontoid soft-tissue thickening
Cleidocranial dysostosis	AD	6p21	CBFA1	Basilar impression Scoliosis
Camptomelic dysplasia	AD	17q24.3-q25.1	SOX9	Kyphoscoliosis
Chondrodysplasia punctata	AD, XLR, XLD, maternal ingestion	6q22-q24 Xp22.3 Xp11.23-p11.22	EBP PEX7 Arylsulfatase	Kyphoscoliosis
Spondylothoracic dysplasia	AR	2q32.1	Unknown	Congenital scoliosis with symmetric deformity of the thorax
Spondylocostal dysostosis	AR	19q13	DLL3	Congenital scoliosis with asymmetric deformity of the thorax

AD, autosomal dominant; AR, autosomal recessive; XLD, X-linked dominant; XLR, X-linked recessive.

enchondral ossification causes a decrease in the size of the petrous portion of the temporal bone, the sphenoid, and the ethmoid bone, leading to a reduced size of the structures that form the base of the skull. The fourth component that makes up the base of the skull is the occiput, a part of the calvarium, which grows by intramembranous ossification and is unaffected. Foramen magnum stenosis can lead to a potentially life-threatening situation; it has been implicated as a cause of sudden infant death in this population and can cause significant neurologic injury secondary to cervicomedullary compression. Many of these children present with frank neurologic findings such as hypotonia, weakness, and hyperreflexia or with apnea and other respiratory symptoms such as cyanosis and respiratory distress. Since these children are also more prone to develop respiratory tract infection due to midface hypoplasia and the relatively small chest cavity, these causes must be ruled out. A detailed history and examination of the infant might not be enough to distinguish etiologies that are primarily neurogenic from those that are primarily pulmonary in origin. Pauli and colleagues reviewed 13 children with achondroplasia who were previously thought to have expired from sudden infant death syndrome and showed that the probable cause was brain stem or cervical cord compression; as a result, they recommended routine polysomnographic and apnea monitoring. Imaging techniques such as computed tomography (CT) scans and magnetic resonance imaging (MRI) have greatly enhanced diagnostic potential by allowing a more detailed view of the compression. Individuals with achondroplasia typically display a diamond-shaped foramen magnum, in contrast to the round shape seen in normal individuals. Hecht and colleagues showed that the foramen magnum in children with achondroplasia who are at risk for developing neurologic compromise had CT measurements in the transverse plane and sagittal plane that were 5 standard deviations and 4 standard deviations below the norm, respectively. An MRI study done on children with achondroplasia reflected similar values. Somatosensory evoked potential tests and sleep studies can be helpful in identifying neurologic abnormalities. Current recommendations by the American Academy of Pediatrics, not universally accepted, advocate performing CT, MRI, flexion/extension radiographs, and polysomnography in the neonatal period, repeat examinations being performed as indicated. There is no evidence that primary upper cervical instability occurs in children with achondroplasia; hence flexion/extension radiographs are of little use. MRI demonstrates the stenosis and cord compression. An early MRI examination, as early as 2 weeks, may be used to demonstrate and identify infants who are at risk for developing cervicomedullary compression. Children who have documented foramen magnum stenosis without any neurologic signs or symptoms should be followed closely. Current indications for surgical decompression include a symptomatic child with docu-

mented foramen magnum stenosis. If hydrocephalus is present, then shunting should alleviate the symptoms. Surgical decompression is safe and effective in treating symptomatic patients. There is no need for a fusion. Good results have been shown after surgical intervention, most patients experiencing improvement. Delay in decompression can lead to irreversible neurologic damage and death. Complications include neurologic injury, cerebrospinal fluid leaks, pseudomeningocele, and death.

Spinal column abnormalities frequently occur in achondroplasia. Thoracolumbar kyphosis is well documented. This deformity develops as the child begins to sit and can be seen in up to 50% to 95% of children in early infancy. The majority, up to 90%, of these deformities will resolve once the child begins to ambulate. The factors that influence progression are unclear. There have been reports that prolonged propped sitting might result in progression of kyphosis. Other researchers have reported that anterior wedging of the apical vertebrae could result in persistence of the kyphosis. Persistent kyphosis, especially when combined with an excessive lumbar lordosis below, could aggravate an already small spinal canal and cause neurologic symptoms. The onset of neurologic symptoms is usually progressive and insidious. The role of bracing in the treatment of the kyphosis remains controversial. Pauli and colleagues recommend prohibition of propped sitting and bracing in children in whom the kyphosis persists after independent sitting. Whether bracing truly alters the natural history of the condition is still in question. Currently, spinal fusion is the treatment of choice for progressive kyphosis. Indications for treatment are variable in the literature. Some clinicians would recommend a fusion if the kyphosis has not resolved by 5 or 6 years of age in children in whom the kyphosis measures greater than 40 degrees accompanied by the presence of a single wedged apical vertebra. Others would recommend fusion if the curve reached 60 to 70 degrees. In our institution, nonprogressive kyphosis without significant wedging in children younger than 2 years of age is observed and expected to resolve spontaneously. Bracing is reserved for children older than 2 years with a kyphosis of greater than 50 degrees and when apical wedging is present. In patients older than 6 years of age with persistent or progressive kyphosis of greater than 50 degrees with signs of neurologic compromise and evidence of spinal cord compression, a spinal fusion and decompression are indicated. Anterior release and fusion with posterior decompression, instrumentation, and fusion constitute the classic treatment. A posterior-only approach with pedicle screw instrumentation could be sufficient to treat the condition.

The spinal canal is small in achondroplasia and has been attributed to failure of longitudinal growth at the neurocentral synchondroses. It has been shown to be one third to one half the size of normal. The interpedicular distance is narrower, accounting for a smaller transverse diameter;

the AP diameter is smaller, but the posterior portion of the vertebral body shows scalloping. The pedicles are shortened and thickened. These morphologic changes in the spine are initially asymptomatic, but symptoms of canal stenosis are usually present around the third to fourth decade of life. Up to 30% of cases are reported to present as early as the second decade of life. The stenotic segments are more common over the cervical and lumbar regions. Aside from the relatively smaller size of the canal, the facet joints tend to hypertrophy and, combined with a shortened and thickened pedicle, lead to a narrowing of the foramina in these patients. The lumbar stenosis may further be aggravated by the lumbar lordosis, which usually manifests itself once these children begin to ambulate. Children with both lower lumbar hyperlordosis and thoracolumbar kyphosis are at a higher risk for neurologic compromise. Symptoms may be mild, manifesting as back pain to severe neurogenic claudication, paraplegia, and paresthesia. Imaging techniques such as MRI and CT can be used to demonstrate stenosis and compression. A myelogram can be used to demonstrate compression and aid in surgical planning; however, the relative stenosis of the spine accompanied by degenerative changes in older age groups make standard myelographic techniques difficult. To overcome this, a lateral C1-2 approach can be utilized. Careful assessment of the entire spine is recommended, and once the neurologic symptoms can be attributed to stenotic segments, an early decompression is advised. Depending on the number of stenosed segments, a multilevel laminectomy might be required to decompress the spine in the child; however, in the older individual, laminectomies alone might not suffice, owing to degenerative changes, and are often combined with foraminotomies. Another treatment option to consider is interapophyseolaminar decompression, a technique described by Thomeer and colleagues in which a decompression is performed without a laminectomy. The microsurgical technique consists of removing the caudal portion of the vertebral lamina, leaving the ligmantum flavum intact; bilaterally reducing the medial portion of the inferior articular process; and continuing undercutting through the lamina and facet joint, keeping the lamina intact. Thomeer and van Dijk showed relief of symptoms in 71% of their cases. This technique involved undercutting the lamina and facets from within the canal after removal of the caudal spinous process and ligamentum flavum. It carries the advantage of causing less destabilization of the spine. In cases in which thoracolumbar kyphosis is noted with the stenosis, a posterior spinal fusion is also indicated, since progression of the kyphosis has been reported following laminectomy. Ain and colleagues reported a 100% incidence of postlaminectomy kyphosis in skeletally immature children with achondroplasia who had undergone multilevel laminectomies. They recommend a concomitant fusion for all skeletally immature individuals who undergo a multilevel laminectomy of at least five levels.

Scoliosis also occurs in achondroplasia but is generally uncommon. It is usually mild and follows a benign course. Other spinal disorders such as cervical instability and spinal dysraphism have been reported in this population but are rare.

Diastrophic Dysplasia

Diastrophic dysplasia is a recessive condition caused by mutations in the *SLC26A2* (also known as DTDST) gene located on 5q32-q33.1. This transmembrane glycoprotein is critical in cartilage for sulfation of proteoglycans and matrix organization. The resulting cartilage is abnormally weak with a poor loading response, resulting in the various skeletal deformities associated with this condition.

Cervical kyphosis is very common in diastrophic dysplasia. The general incidence has been reported to be 24% to 33% with a higher incidence before 18 months of age (96%). It has been identified in neonates, suggesting that it might develop in utero and might be secondary to the hyperflexed position of the fetus. The natural history of this disorder is that it tends to improve spontaneously with age. In the majority of cases, the kyphosis resolved by a mean of 7.1 years of age. Improvement in neck extensor strength could be a factor associated with resolution, allowing for ossification of the previously hypoplastic vertebra. Initial kyphosis greater than 60 degrees with severely hypoplastic vertebrae can result in progressive kyphosis. The cervical spinal canal in diastrophic dysplasia is narrowed in comparison to the normal population, which places the individual at increased risk for neurologic compromise with progressive kyphosis.

A cervical spine radiograph is always warranted during the first evaluation, especially in the younger child. Regular follow-up radiographs every 6 months will be needed to observe for progression of the kyphosis. The role of conservative management, such as bracing, in these patients is not clear and has not been well documented. There are no published guidelines of precise surgical indications; however, a progressive kyphosis with documented spinal cord compression and symptoms of neurologic compromise will require decompression and fusion. Posterior fusion with interspinous wiring is satisfactory for moderate kyphosis with no spinal cord compression. Lateral mass and cervical pedicle screw fixation can be utilized as allowed by the anatomy, using current generation implant systems. In severe deformity with spinal cord compression, anterior decompression and fusion with posterior fusion are required. Care should be taken in approaching the cervical spine posteriorly, as there is a high incidence of spina bifida occulta associated with diastrophic dysplasia.

Scoliosis is common in diastrophic dysplasia with an incidence between 37% and 88%. Scoliosis usually develops during the second decade of life. The presentation of scoliosis may vary from mild scoliosis to rapidly progressive types. The severity of the deformity is age related. In one study, patients who presented with scoliosis earlier than 3 years of age tended to have more progressive curves than did those who presented later than 15 years of age. With regard to pulmonary function, the severity of the curve was also found to be inversely related to lung volume. It is important to identify the children who are at high risk for progression, as neglected cases afford little correction, and early treatment has been advocated. Bracing has not been documented to be of any value, although it might be worthwhile to brace flexible curves in the younger child to delay fusion and allow for pulmonary development. Growing rod systems have been used in younger children and may be performed for progressive curves in this group. In the older child, anterior and posterior fusion has provided the best results.

The thoracic and lumbar spinal canal is narrower at all levels in comparison to that in the normal population. This is important to document preoperatively to plan the instrumentation technique. The spine also demonstrates decreased mobility, which may be due to rapid degeneration of the facet joints and discs. This can predispose these patients to symptomatic spinal stenosis later in life. Vertebral anomalies and atlantoaxial instability have been reported in the literature but are relatively rare.

These patients are born with normal-appearing vertebrae, which deform in areas of spinal deformity, as the cartilage has an abnormal response to loading. It is our opinion that this is developmental secondary to abnormal bone growth and pressure response.

Metatropic Dysplasia

Metatropic dysplasia is a rare form of rhizomelic dwarfism that is characterized at birth by a long trunk and short limbs, but rapid development of kyphoscoliosis results in a shortened trunk. There are three described forms of the condition: a nonlethal autosomal recessive form, a nonlethal autosomal dominant form, and a lethal form that is possibly autosomal recessive. It has been attributed to an uncoupling of enchondral and perichondral growth. The exact gene defect and chromosome locus have yet to be identified. This disorder can be identified by the characteristic platyspondyly that is found during infancy. This can resolve to an almost normal-looking vertebra at a later age and, if present, might denote the autosomal dominant form.

Odontoid hypoplasia is very common in this patient population. Shohat and colleagues confirmed the presence of odontoid hypoplasia in all 12 of their cases, with some cases severe enough to have subluxation even in neutral position. Odontoid hypoplasia can lead to atlantoaxial instability, causing severe neurologic compromise. Cervical stenosis has also been documented in metatropic dysplasia. The stenotic segment may occur throughout the entire cervical spine with or without symptoms of myelopathy. Activity modification and regular follow-up should

be advised, as patients are at high risk for developing atlantoaxial instability. All of these children require lateral flexion/extension cervical spine radiographs early in life and on a yearly basis thereafter. Instability with an atlantodens interval greater than 5 mm or space available for the cord of less than 13 mm should be evaluated with a flexion/extension MRI. Significant instability without cord compression or myelopathic signs and symptoms usually requires a posterior fusion. If there is significant stenosis with cord compression in neutral position, a decompression and fusion procedure is required. Fusion often has to be extended to the occiput. Instrumentation options in these young children include posterior wiring and transarticular screws; rarely is there space for plates, although current screw-rod implants may be considered. A halo vest can be applied to stabilize the patients postoperatively depending on the stability of spinal fixation.

Kyphoscoliosis occurs early, often in the first year of life, in metatropic dysplasia and is rapidly progressive. A left thoracolumbar curve is the most common pattern observed. These children have short ribs, and often the thoracic cage is stiff, resulting in severe restrictive lung disease. Progressive thoracic deformity aggravates the lung disease. Bracing has not been effective in controlling curve progression. Spinal stenosis is common, and severe cord compression may occur, resulting in paraparesis or quadriparesis. Surgical decompression and stabilization are indicated for patients with progressive deformity and neurologic compromise. The use of instrumentation can be challenging because of the significant deformity, spinal stenosis, severe platyspondyly, and poor mineralization. Standard growing rod systems can be difficult to use. Hybrid VEPTR (Synthes Spine, West Chester, PA) devices extending from the pelvis to the upper ribs are an option, but a severe kyphosis makes this technique difficult.

Spondyloepiphyseal Dysplasia

Spondyloepiphyseal dysplasia congenita is an autosomal dominant condition caused by a mutation in the *collagen II, alpha I (COL2A1)* gene located on 12q13. The alpha I chain forms a homotrimer, which composes the fibrillar collagen II. This protein plays a critical structural role in the vitreous of the eye. Several different skeletal dysplasias can result from *COL2A1* abnormalities, depending on the location of the mutation.

Atlantoaxial instability frequently develops and results from odontoid hypoplasia and ligamentous laxity. Myelopathic symptoms can be seen in 33% to 65% of involved patients. Respiratory symptoms, hypotonia, delay in motor milestones, and gait abnormalities should raise the suspicion of atlantoaxial instability. Minor trauma or simply flexing the cervical spine can be enough to cause neurologic compromise. Each child should have a detailed examination of the cervical spine. Nakamura and colleagues reviewed 16 cases of spondyloepiphyseal dysplasia congenita and found that 10 mm was the critical value for the space available for the cord; they also showed that patients with marked short stature of less than 7 standard deviations below the norm with severe coxa vara were at significant risk for development of myelopathic symptoms. Posterior fusion is the treatment of choice and should be done even in asymptomatic patients with demonstrable atlantoaxial instability. Miyoshi and colleagues recommended evaluating the sagittal canal diameter prior to reduction and recommended a C1 laminectomy for patients with a small sag-ittal canal diameter. In children younger than 5 years of age, the arch of C1 might not be sufficiently ossified, and it might be necessary to extend the fusion from the occiput to C2. Svennson and colleagues recommended that fusion without instrumentation stabilized postoperatively with a halo vest might be all that is required, but the series from our institution showed a 50% pseudarthrosis rate from this technique. The need for a halo vest postoperatively can be avoided by using transarticular screws or plates.

Scoliosis develops relatively early and is usually present before 10 years of age. The pattern of progression is variable, ranging from nonprogressive to rapidly progressive curves that require immediate treatment. In the younger child, the scoliosis is often flexible and can be managed by bracing. Some authors advocate performing a spinal fusion for curves greater than 35 degrees in the growing child. The spinal canal is not stenotic, and spinal instrumentation can usually be accommodated. Growing rod instrumentation can be used in the younger child; studies have shown that it effectively controls curve progression while allowing for growth. In the older child, segmental instrumentation with hooks or pedicle screws can be used. Kyphosis and excessive lumbar lordosis are also seen in this condition. The lumbar lordosis is frequently accompanied by a shortened psoas and coxa vara. Correcting the lordosis is better achieved through the pelvis or the hip.

The tarda form of the disorder is secondary to a mutation in the *SEDL* gene, which encodes for a 140-amino-acid protein named sedlin and is X-linked recessive. This disorder manifests later, usually at 10 to 14 years of age. Back pain usually presents at puberty, and radiographs show platyspondyly with a mild kyphosis. Upper cervical instability and scoliosis occur in this type of spondyloepiphyseal dysplasia.

Pseudoachondroplasia

Psuedoachondroplasia is an autosomal dominant condition caused by a mutation in the cartilage oligomeric matrix protein located on 19q13. Cartilage oligomeric matrix protein is an extracellular matrix protein, and mutations in it cause abnormal matrix protein trafficking with the chondrocytes. The alteration in cartilage structure produces an abnormal response to stress.

Thoracolumbar kyphosis and lumbar lordosis are commonly present. The vertebral bodies on lateral view show a biconvex shape, some showing an anterior tongue. These often resolve, and the patient exhibits normal-looking vertebrae at adulthood; one third of patients will continue to develop persistent platyspondyly. Interpedicular distance is normal. Scoliosis is associated with pelvic obliquity in most cases and is relatively mild. These curves are often flexible and appear not to progress beyond skeletal maturity. The incidence of scoliosis has been reported to be as high as 48%, with 24% of those who have scoliosis requiring operative intervention. The majority of these can be managed with bracing. The truly structural curves, not associated with pelvic obliquity, appear to be milder. The spinal canal is typically not narrowed in pseudoachondroplasia, making it possible to use hooks that enter the canal.

Odontoid abnormalities and cervical spine instability occur commonly. Spinal fusion is indicated for documented instability with evidence of cord compression.

Mucopolysaccharidosis

The mucopolysaccharidoses (MPSs) are a group of lysosomal storage diseases characterized by an inability to degrade glycosaminoglycans secondary to an enzyme deficiency. Although not true skeletal dysplasias, these disorders usually result in disproportionate short stature.

MPS type I (Hurler syndrome) is an autosomal recessive condition caused by mutations in the *alpha-L-iduronidase (IDUA)* gene located on chromosome 4p16.3. The *IDUA* gene encodes a lysosomal enzyme that is required for degradation of the glycosaminoglycans dermatan sulfate and heparan sulfate. Mutations in this gene lead to the accumulation of these compounds throughout the body. In the skeleton, the pattern of dysostosis multiplex is seen. Hypoplasia of the odontoid has been shown to occur in MPS I. This can resolve spontaneously with age or lead to atlantoaxial instability. MRI examination of the cervical spine in these children might show soft-tissue thickening around the tip of the odontoid, which can aggravate cord compression due to instability. High lumbar kyphosis with anterior vertebral wedging is the most common spinal deformity seen in these patients. The progression of the kyphosis is variable; it can progress very rapidly even at an early age and cause cord compression. Nonoperative management with bracing can be instituted initially to slow progression. If the curve continues to progress beyond 40 degrees, then posterior spinal fusion should be performed. Scoliosis and short-segment kyphosis in the thoracic spine have also been reported. Spinal stenosis is common.

Mucopolysaccharidosis type II (Hunter syndrome) is an autosomal recessive condition caused by a mutation in the *iduronate 2-sulfatase (IDS)* gene located on chromosome Xq28. The resulting defective enzyme (IDS) fails to degrade the glycosamino-glycans dermatan sulfate and heparan sulfate, similar to but at a different location of action from MPS type I. Consequently, mutations in this gene lead to the accumulation of these compounds throughout the body. In the skeleton, the pattern of dysostosis multiplex is seen. Soft-tissue thickening behind the odontoid peg, dural thickening, and thickened meninges have all been reported to cause myelopathy in MPS type II. Cervical decompression with duraplasty is the treatment of choice.

Mucopolysaccharidosis type IV (Morquio syndrome) is an autosomal recessive condition in either the *N-acetyl-galactosamine-6-sulfatase (GALNS)* gene on chromosome 16q24.3 or the *beta-galactosidase (GLB1)* gene on chromosome 3p21.33. Although they are clinically indistinguishable, Morquio syndrome caused by GALSNS deficiency is termed type A, and Morquio syndrome caused by GLB1 deficiency is termed type B. Both the GALNS and GLB1 enzymes are required for the degradation of the glycosaminoglycans keratan sulfate and chondroitin 6-sulfate. Mutations in either of these genes lead to an accumulation of these compounds throughout the body. In the skeleton, the pattern of dysostosis multiplex is again seen. The spine in MPS type IV exhibits platyspondyly, which on lateral radiographs demonstrates the flame-shaped vertebrae that are characteristic of the condition. Kyphosis and scoliosis may occur to a moderate degree. Spinal cord compression may occur secondary to thoracolumbar kyphosis or focal stenosis. Manifestations as severe as paraparesis have been reported. However, these tend to occur more commonly in older children and in the adult population. Thoracolumbar kyphosis can be treated initially by bracing. Surgical indications include progression of kyphosis despite brace treatment and neurologic deterioration. Treatment is by anterior decompression and posterior spinal fusion, although one can achieve the anterior decompression via a posterior-based corpectomy. Dalvie and colleagues reported good results in four cases that were treated with correction, decompression, and fusion with instrumentation, all performed anteriorly.

Odontoid dysplasia with atlantoaxial instability is a frequent occurrence in MPS IV. This deformity results from odontoid hypoplasia and ligamentous laxity. The hypoplastic odontoid may be a result of excessive movement at the time of ossification. Blaw and Langer reviewed eight cases of MPS IV and found odontoid abnormalities with atlantoaxial subluxation and dislocation present in all cases in their series, 50% of patients showing signs of cervical cord compression. Lipson reviewed 11 cases with odontoid dysplasia, all of whom had atlantoaxial instability, and found that all were at increased risk for neurologic compromise. Nelson and colleagues found odontoid dysplasia in all 12 of their cases and suggested that this was present in all cases of MPS IV. Decreased endurance can be the first sign of myelopathy and might be incorrectly attributed to lower-extremity deformity. Quadriparesis and respiratory arrest have also been reported secondary to atlantoaxial instability. Another factor to consider in determining the etiology of myelopathic symptoms is soft-tissue thickening. Stevens and colleagues examined 13 cases using flexion/extension cervical myelograms and found that severe spinal cord compression was due to extradural soft-tissue thickening that was not relieved by flexion or extension. They also found that the soft tissue resolves spontaneously after posterior spinal fusion similar to rheumatoid pannus. These children should be screened at an early age, as myelopathic symptoms typically manifest by 4 to 6 years of age. Any evidence of cervical cord compromise is an indication for posterior spinal fusion and decompression if required. Ransford and colleagues showed that early surgical intervention is associated with better results, while patients with chronic myelopathic symptoms showed little to no recovery. Blaw and Langer showed that there may be persistence of corticospinal tract signs and the presence of residual neurologic deficits after surgical decompression. Lipson likewise demonstrated that once quadriparesis has been established, functional recovery is limited even after surgical intervention.

Thanatophoric Dysplasia

Previously confused with achondroplasia, thanatophoric dysplasia is a rare lethal skeletal dysplasia that results from a mutation in the *FGFR-3* gene located on 4p16.3. Like achondroplasia, the mutation leads to overactivity of the FGFR-3 receptor, and this in turn leads to growth inhibition in the enchondrally formed bones. The degree of receptor overactivity is much more extreme than that in achondroplasia, and the resultant bone formation defects are far more severe. Thanatophoric dysplasia has an incidence of 1 in every 20,000 births, making it the most common of the lethal chondrodystrophies. Thanatophoric dysplasia can be classified into two types based on the shape of the femur. Type I is associated with a curved, short femora with or without a cloverleaf skull; type II is associated with straight femora and a severe cloverleaf skull. Foramen magnum stenosis is common and may result in severe cord compression, leading to death. The interpedicular space is narrowed distally. Platyspondyly has been demonstrated to occur in utero, and the severity of the vertebral body change is more severe when compared with achondroplasia. Respiratory failure is a common cause of death in this population, and the majority of patients die after birth, although prolonged survival has been reported. It still remains questionable whether early intervention for neurologic problems provides any benefit.

Kniest Dysplasia

Kniest dysplasia is an autosomal dominant condition that is caused by a mutation in the *collagen II alpha I (Col2A1)* gene located on 12q13. The alpha I chain forms a homotrimer that composes the fibrillar collagen II. This protein plays a critical structural role in the vitreous of the eye. Several different skeletal dysplasias can result from COL2A1 abnormalities, depending on the location of the mutation. The cartilage in Kniest dysplasia is abnormally soft and results in the characteristic histologic Swiss cheese appearance. Cervical spine instability has been reported and can be effectively treated with an occipito-C2 fusion. The odontoid is usually widened. Vertebral body abnormalities are common, including anisospondyly (different abnormal shapes of the vertebral bodies), platyspondyly (flattened vertebral body shape with reduced distance between the end plates), and wedging of the vertebrae. The lower lumbar vertebrae have a pear-shaped appearance, with the posterior body taller than the anterior portion. Kyphoscoliosis occurs at an early age but is generally mild. Lumbar lordosis and fixed hip flexion contractures are common findings.

Camptomelic Dysplasia

Camptomelic dysplasia is an autosomal dominant condition caused by a mutation in the sex-determining region *Y-box-9 (SOX-9)* gene located on chromosome 17q24.3-q25.1. This gene encodes for a DNA transcription factor that plays an important role in both chondrocyte differentiation and genital development. On occasion, female patients with camptomelic dysplasia have been shown to have XY karyotypes.

Hypoplasia of the thoracic pedicles is commonly seen in the disorder. Abnormalities of the cervical spine are a frequent occurrence, including kyphosis, hypoplastic or absent vertebrae, congenital anomalies, and fusion. Kyphoscoliosis is also a frequent occurrence. The severity of scoliosis is variable, ranging from mild to severe forms. Bracing is ineffective in halting the progression of the larger curves. The progressive curves may compromise respiratory function, and aggressive management is recommended. Anterior and posterior fusion has been the treatment of choice for progressive kyphoscoliosis. Preoperatively, spinal anatomy must be evaluated radiographically to determine whether instrumentation can be used. If it is not possible to use instrumentation, a halo vest will provide stability. Postoperative complications include pseudarthrosis and neurologic compromise.

Chondrodysplasia Punctata

Chondrodysplasia punctata describes a heterogeneous group of conditions with multiple genetic causes. There are autosomal dominant and recessive forms, X-linked dominant and recessive forms, and a form that can result from in utero exposure to warfarin. These conditions are characterized by short stature and stippled epiphyses. Scoliosis is common, occurs early in life, and is of two types: a more progressive dysplastic type and a nondysplastic type that follows a more benign course. Bracing may be started at an early age; however, definitive management is with

spinal fusion. Best results are achieved with anterior strut grafting and posterior fusion. Complications include pseudarthrosis and progression after fusion. Instrumentation may be used in the older age groups.

Cervical stenosis has been described and can result in cord compression and paraplegia. Early recognition can aid in preventing serious complications. Cervical spine instability has been reported in this condition. Afshani and colleagues reported the occurrence of atlantoaxial instability in two siblings. Separation of the dentocentral synchondrosis at C2 was the cause of cervical instability in the series published by Mason and colleagues. This can be treated by performing an occiput to C2 fusion.

Spondylocostal Dysostosis and Spondylothoracic Dysplasia

These rare disorders are characterized by a short trunk with rib and vertebral anomalies. The chest deformities are often severe enough to cause restrictive lung disease. There has been great confusion surrounding these two conditions. Solomon and colleagues divided the two groups based on the distribution of defects. Those with bilateral fusion of the ribs at the costovertebral joints with segmentation and formation defects of the vertebrae were classified as spondylothoracic dysostosis, and those with intrinsic rib anomalies with no symmetric rib fusions were classified as spondylocostal dysostosis. Both conditions are associated with multiple anomalies of the various organ systems, such as cardiac defects, urinary tract anomalies, and renal and gastrointestinal tract abnormalities.

Spondylothoracic dysplasia is an autosomal recessive condition that has been mapped to chromosome 2q32.1. The gene that is responsible for this condition is still unknown. The condition is characterized by multiple segmental and formation defects in the spine as well as bilateral rib fusions and multiple anomalies of the various organ systems. The thorax manifests with the characteristic fanlike configuration. Cornier and colleagues report a 56% survival rate at 6 months of age; the majority of deaths were caused by pulmonary failure secondary to restrictive lung disease.

Spondylocostal dysplasia is secondary to a mutation in the *Delta-like 3* gene (DLL3) that has been mapped to chromosome 19q13. This gene encodes for a ligand in the notch gene signal pathway that plays an important role in patterning of the axial skeleton. Multiple vertebral malformations are also seen, along with rib defects. The thoracic malformation is asymmetric, which might act as a tether and lead to a progressive scoliosis. The restrictive lung disease in this group is not as severe, owing to the asymmetry of the deformity.

Treatment is aimed at arresting curve progression and addressing the restrictive lung disease at the same time. This can be achieved by addressing the thoracic insufficiency by performing multiple expansion thoracoplasties with VEPTR instrumentation (Synthes).

DIAGNOSTIC PROCEDURES

On the initial clinic visit, screening radiographs should be requested for the specific spinal deformity that can occur with the condition. Standing anteroposterior and lateral views of the spine are standard views to be requested for patients who are at risk of developing kyphosis or scoliosis. Anteroposterior and lateral radiographs with lateral flexion/extension views of the cervical spine are requested for those who are at risk of developing cervical instability. Lateral flexion/extension radiographs taken in the maximum range provide the most useful information. Concerns of iatrogenic neurologic injury during positioning are valid. In the conscious patient, the risks are often minimal; however, the physician may be requested to be present if there is serious concern about the risks involved. Measured parameters on cervical flexion/extension radiographs should include space available for the cord at stenotic levels, the anterior atlantodens interval and the posterior atlantodens interval. The space available for the cord in an average-statured infant at the level of C2 is 13 mm; in a 3- to 6-year-old child, the space available for the cord measures 17.9 ± 1.3 mm; at 7 to 10 years, it is 18.8 ± 1 mm; and at 11 to 14 years, it is 19.4 ± 1.1 mm. Once documented, any deformity should be followed closely, and repeat radiographs should be taken to document any progression of the deformity. This is usually done every 6 months. Anterior atlantodens interval measurements of 4 mm, pseudosubluxation at the level of C2 and C3, and mild kyphosis in flexion can all occur in normal children.

CT is useful in demonstrating a more detailed view of the osseous structures of the spine. It is used best in surgical planning, in which it helps in determining the extent of the deformity, whether the spine may be instrumented, and the type of instrumentation that is most appropriate. CT can also be used in the young child for determination of lung volumes, especially in children who are predisposed to pulmonary complications owing to thoracic insufficiency and restrictive lung disease. MRI examination is lengthy and has the disadvantage of requiring sedation in young children. It is very accurate in demonstrating cord compression and intrinsic abnormalities of the spinal cord. Flexion/extension views are useful for demonstrating dynamic spinal cord compression. When the child is lying down in most situations, the size of the head normally places the cervical spine in a flexed position. When the external auditory meatus is in line with the shoulder, the cervical spine is in neutral position. Neutral position is achieved by placing a recess for the occiput or raising the trunk with padding or blankets. Placing additional padding underneath the thorax allows for extension of the cervical spine. At present, the protocol at the authors' institution involves taking the neutral and extension views of the cervical spine initially. When no compression is noted, the flexion view may be taken. Other uses for the MRI include evaluation of cerebrospinal fluid flow to document cord compression and magnetic resonance angiography to evaluate cranial blood flow. CT myelography can also be used to demonstrate spinal cord compression and stenosis but has the disadvantage of being an invasive procedure.

Other methods are useful to delineate whether symptoms are neurogenic in origin. These include sleep studies and urodynamics. Other procedures, such as somatosensory and motor evoked potentials, are useful in assessing myelopathy and the degree of cord compromise by performing flexion and extension maneuvers under anesthesia.

Ultrasound may be used in the younger child to demonstrate the spinal canal and its contents. This can be achieved adequately until 6 months of age. It has the advantage of being economical and noninvasive. It provides a useful evaluation of spinal cord tethering, lipomeningocele, syringomyelia, and other congenital anomalies. It has the disadvantage that it cannot be used once ossification of the posterior vertebral elements has taken place.

SUMMARY

The natural history of the spinal deformity associated with a skeletal dysplasia will greatly influence the treatment. The anatomy and structure of the spine in each condition are crucial in planning treatment. These children are prone to two potentially life-threatening conditions that must be addressed when present: stenosis and instability of the cervical spine and severe restrictive lung disease. In the presence of neurologic signs and symptoms, early intervention is mandatory. Although some of the deformities may be severe and complex, careful preoperative planning with adequate preparation can obviate most complications and achieve optimal treatment.

PEARLS & PITFALLS

- Each skeletal dysplasia has its own unique set of spinal deformities requiring specific evaluation and management.
- In the young child, hypotonia and weakness may be manifested by an inability to extend the head or extremities against gravity; this might indicate spinal cord compression.
- Up to 60% of children with achondroplasia present with foramen magnum stenosis, which must be addressed early to prevent neurologic injury secondary to cervical medullary spinal cord compression.
- Thoracolumbar decompression for spinal stenosis in skeletally immature children with achondroplasia requires posterior spinal fusion and instrumentation to prevent progressive postlaminectomy kyphosis.
- Cervical kyphosis is common in diastrophic dysplasia and resolves spontaneously in the majority of children.

- Radiographic evaluation of the spinal canal should be routine prior to considering spinal instrumentation because stenosis is common in many different diagnoses.
- All children, possibly with the exception of those with achondroplasia, should be considered to be at risk for upper cervical instability and stenosis, and flexion/extension lateral cervical spine radiographs should be routine.

- Late subaxial instability can be seen after successful upper cervical fusion.
- Restrictive lung disease is common in children with skeletal dysplasia, and the management of spinal deformities should allow growth of the thoracic cage and spine if at all possible.

Illustrative Case Presentations

CASE 1. A 15-Year-Old Male with Achondroplasia Who Developed Reduced Walking Tolerance, Lower-Extremity Weakness, and Sensory Changes in the Lower Extremities with Activity That Were Relieved by Rest

Neurologic examination showed normal motor strength, no sensory loss, and grade 2 reflexes with no clonus. A posterior decompression was performed with removal of the posterior elements of L1-4 and undercutting of L5. Smith-Peterson osteotomies were performed to achieve the desired sagittal balance, followed by a posterior fusion stabilized by pedicle screw instrumentation (Fig. 16-1).

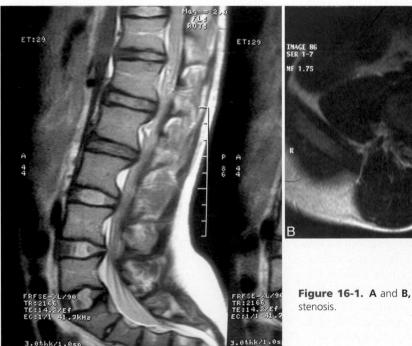

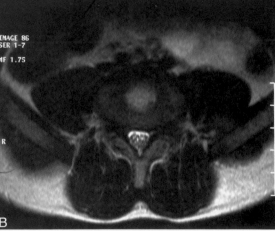

Figure 16-1. A and **B,** MRI revealing moderate lumbar stenosis.

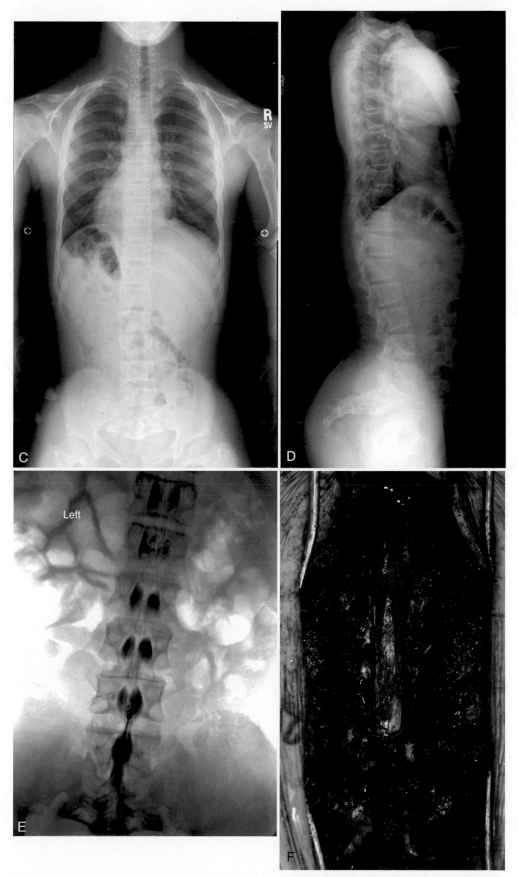

Figure 16-1, cont'd. C and **D,** Preoperative anteroposterior and lateral spine radiographs showing no scoliosis and thoracolumbar kyphosis with anterior wedging at L1. **E,** Preoperative myelogram showing significant lumbar stenosis with sparing of L5-S1 levels. **F,** A posterior decompression was performed with removal of the posterior elements of L1-L4 and undercutting of L5.

Continued

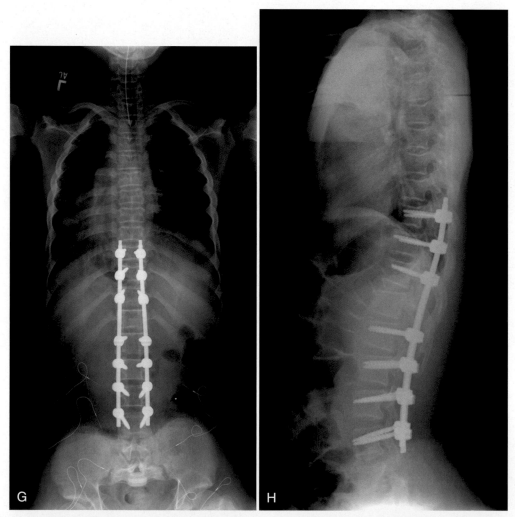

Figure 16-1, cont'd. G and **H,** Smith-Peterson osteotomies were performed to achieve the desired sagittal balance, followed by a posterior fusion stabilized by pedicle screw instrumentation.

CASE 2. A 17-Year-Old Female Diagnosed with Achondroplasia

At 4 months of age, the patient had apneic episodes secondary to foramen magnum stenosis, which was decompressed. At 8 years of age, she underwent decompression of her thoracolumbosacral spine for spinal stenosis. At age 10, she underwent posterior spinal fusion for progressive kyphosis. Instrumentation failed at the L2-3 level and was revised with an anterior plate. At 16 years of age, she began to experience low back pain that would radiate to both her lower extremities and urinary urgency and frequency. There was 5/5 strength on both lower extremities, and no sensory deficit was noted. Asymmetric deep tendon reflexes were elicited left greater than right with clonus at the left ankle. She had continuous progression of the kyphosis due to a pseudarthrosis. Subsequent to myelography, she underwent operative management consisting of a two-stage procedure. In the first stage, a posterior decompression was performed, and pedicle screws were inserted. Two days later, she underwent an anterior release and osteotomies, decompression, and fusion. Anterior cages and bone graft were used at L2-3 and L3-4 interspaces. The posterior incision was then opened, and the posterior rods were inserted while doing simultaneous anterior and posterior correction (Fig. 16-2). On latest follow-up, 3 years postoperatively, she has normal strength, no back pain, and no residual neurologic symptoms.

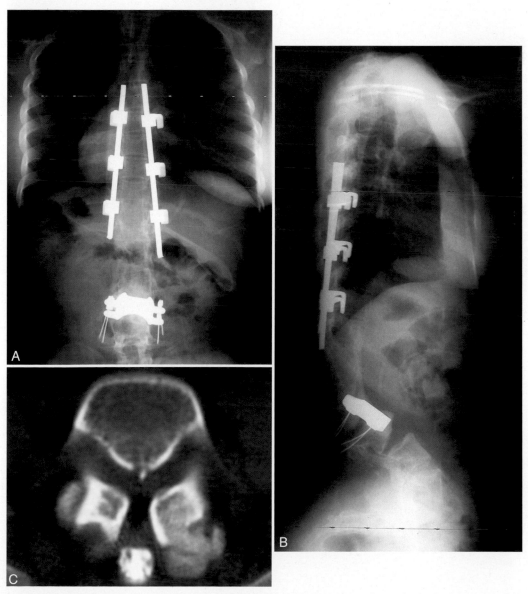

Figure 16-2. A and **B,** Preoperative anteroposterior and lateral radiographs demonstrate a 90-degree kyphosis. **C,** Preoperative myelogram revealed facet hypertrophy and lateral recess stenosis.

Continued

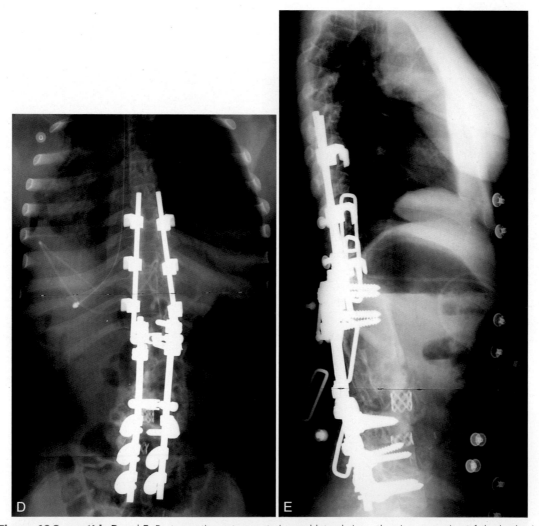

Figure 16-2, cont'd. D and **E**, Postoperative anteroposterior and lateral views showing correction of the kyphosis.

CASE 3. A 2-Year-Old Male Diagnosed with Diastrophic Dysplasia

Initial radiographs showed a 68-degree cervical kyphosis, a 34-degree thoracolumbar kyphosis with anterior wedging at L1, and a 52-degree right thoracic scoliosis. A staged procedure was performed. The first stage consisted of an application of a halo vest and two-level posterior spinal fusion and a growing rod. The hooks at the superior end of the construct were placed at the level of T2-3, and the inferior end was placed at the levels of T12 and L2, spanning the thoracolumbar kyphosis. This was followed a week later with posterior cervical fusion. Spina bifida was seen from C3 to C6. The wires were placed through the posterior element of C2 superiorly and sublaminarly at C6 (Fig. 16-3).

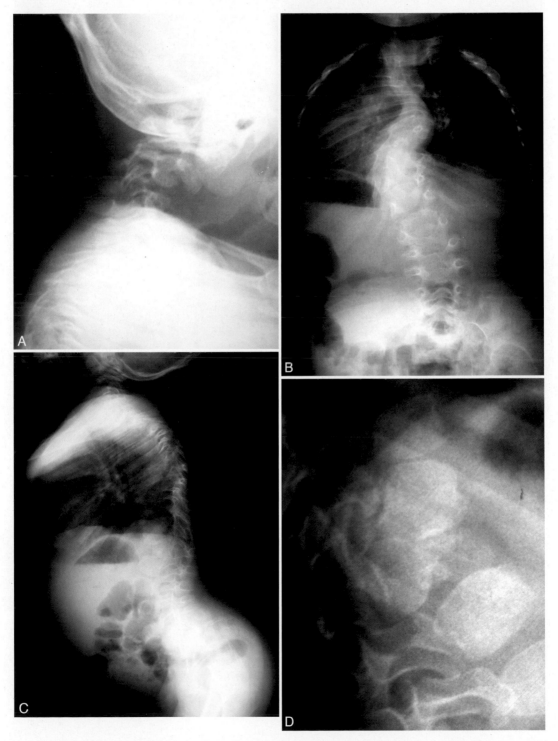

Figure 16-3. A, On 1-year follow-up, a lateral spine radiograph showed a cervical kyphosis of 74 degrees, while (**B**) anteroposterior and (**C**) lateral standing spine radiographs showed progression of the right thoracic curve to 73 degrees. **D,** The thoracolumbar kyphosis remained at 34 degrees with a dysplastic L1 vertebra seen at the apex of the kyphosis. The patient's neurologic examination was normal.

Continued

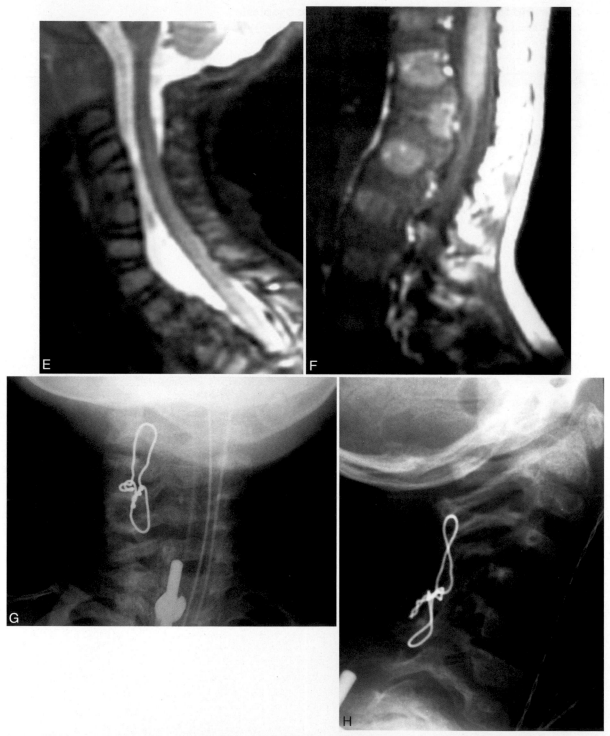

Figure 16-3, cont'd. E, MRI showed no cord compression at the level of the midcervical spine. **F,** However, flattening of the clonus was noted at the level of the thoracolumbar kyphosis. The canal was also noted to be large at this level. A staged procedure was performed. **G** and **H,** The first stage consisted of an application of a halo vest and two-level posterior spinal fusion and a growing rod. The hooks at the superior end of the construct were placed at the level of T2-3, and the inferior end was placed at the levels of T12 and L2, spanning the thoracolumbar kyphosis. This was followed a week later with posterior cervical fusion. Spina bifida was seen from C3 to C6.

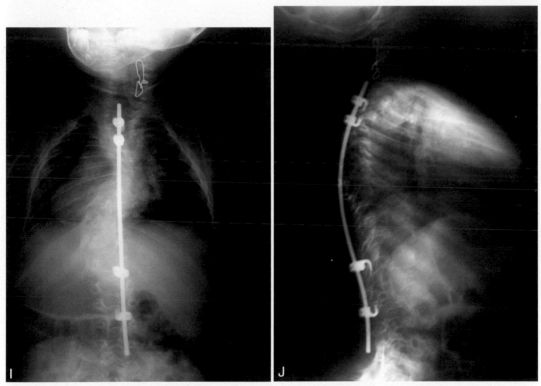

Figure 16-3, cont'd. I and **J,** The wires were placed through the posterior element of C2 superiorly and sublaminarly at C6.

CASE 4. A 5-Year-Old Girl Diagnosed with Morquio Syndrome

At $4^1/_2$ years of age, the patient presented with decreased endurance, easy fatigability, and weakness in her hands. On examination, her upper extremities showed a motor strength of 4+/5 on both upper extremities. Grip strength was weaker, with a 4–/5 grade on the left hand and a 3/5 grade on the right hand. Motor strength was 5/5 on both lower extremities. Deep tendon reflexes were ++ on all extremities, with a positive Babinski sign noted on the right. She underwent C1-2 posterior decompression and fusion with transarticular screws. The procedure was followed by a posterior decompression and fusion of C7 to T4. At 3-year follow-up, she shows complete resolution of neurologic symptoms, and radiographs show a stable fusion mass without loss of fixation (Fig. 16-4).

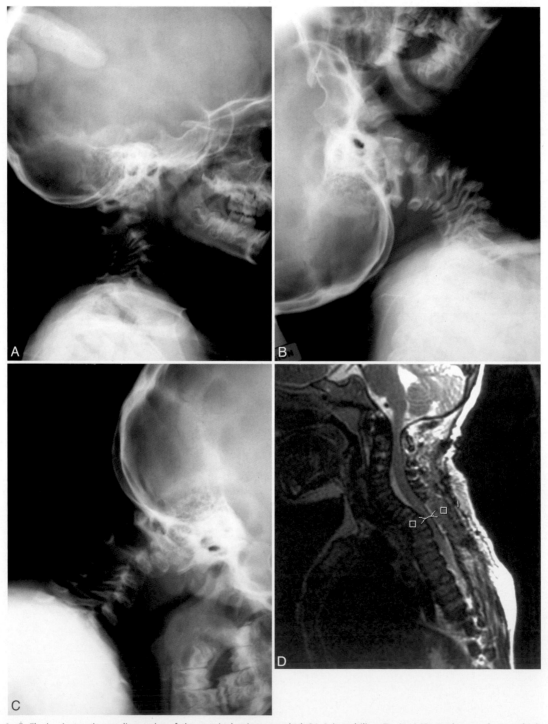

Figure 16-4. A–C, Flexion/extension radiographs of the cervical spine revealed C1-2 instability. **D,** An MRI study was done, which showed stenosis and cord compression at the level of the cervicothoracic junction and stenosis and narrowing of the cord at C2.

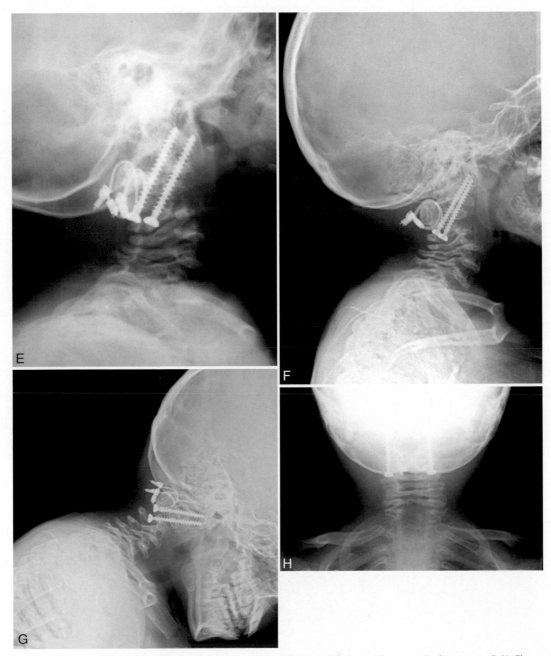

Figure 16-4, cont'd. E, The patient underwent C1-2 posterior decompression and fusion with transarticular screws. **F–H,** The procedure was followed by a posterior decompression and fusion of C7 to T4. At 3-year follow-up, the patient shows complete resolution of neurologic symptoms, and radiographs show a stable fusion mass without loss of fixation.

CASE 5. A 10-Year-Old Female Diagnosed with Chondrodysplasia Punctata (Conradi Syndrome) Who Presented with Progressive Kyphoscoliosis

The patient had a 69-degree right thoracic curve from T2 to T10 and a 66-degree thoracolumbar curve from T10 to L3. A detethering procedure was done through a partial S3 laminectomy and resection of the filum terminale. Five months after the tethered cord was addressed, she underwent operative stabilization of her kyphoscoliosis. The procedure started with an anterior spinal fusion using rib strut grafts from T9 and L2. The body of T11 consisted mostly of fibrous and hyaline cartilage. Posteriorly, the spine was noted to be abnormal, especially at the apex of the kyphosis. The spinal canal was small, with oblique facets noted in the lumbar spine (Fig. 16-5).

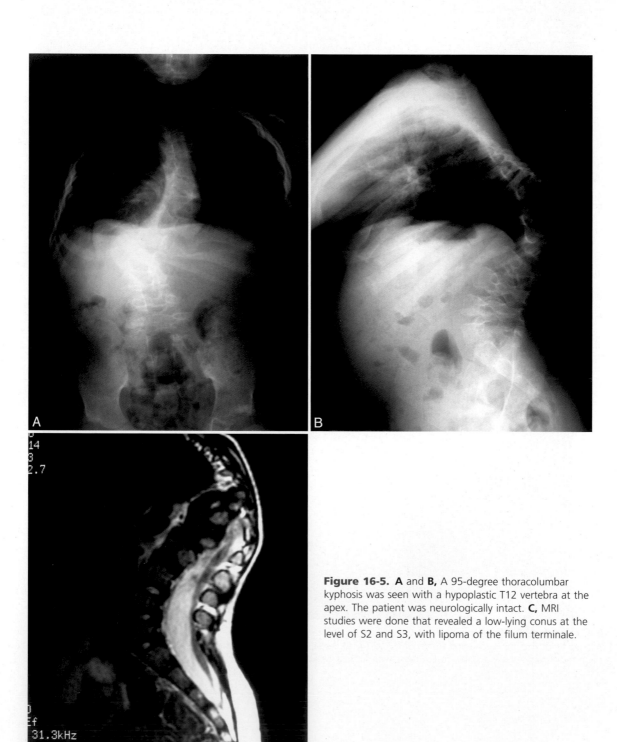

Figure 16-5. A and **B,** A 95-degree thoracolumbar kyphosis was seen with a hypoplastic T12 vertebra at the apex. The patient was neurologically intact. **C,** MRI studies were done that revealed a low-lying conus at the level of S2 and S3, with lipoma of the filum terminale.

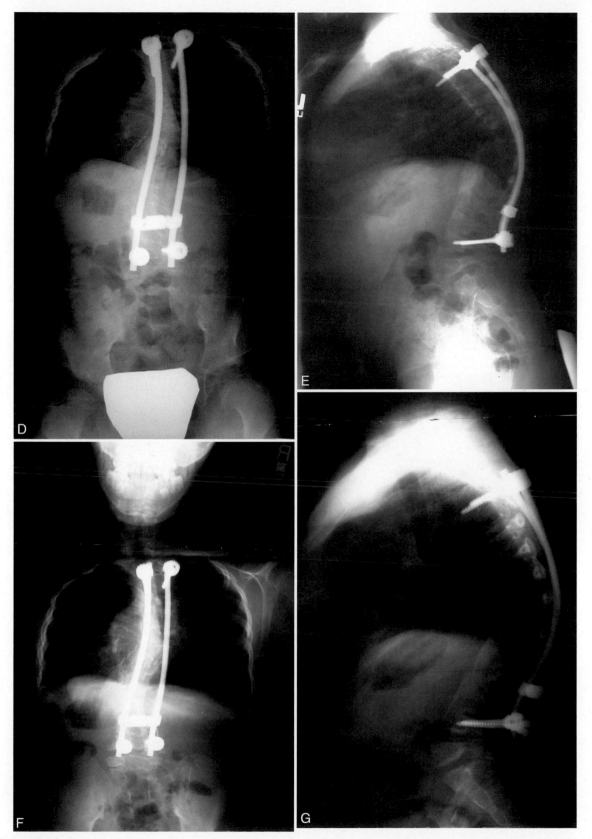

Figure 16-5, cont'd. D and **E,** Pedicle screws were placed at the levels of T4 and L4. **F** and **G,** Two years postoperatively, the patient shows no loss of correction and a solid fusion mass anteriorly.

CASE 6. A 12-Year-Old Male with Spondyloepiphyseal Dysplasia Congenita

The patient's progressive scoliosis was initially managed at another institution with a Milwaukee brace. He presented with a right thoracic curve of 34 degrees and a left thoracolumbar curve of 33 degrees. At 1-year follow-up, curve progression was noted. The patient underwent a posterior spinal fusion with pedicle screw instrumentation (Fig. 16-6).

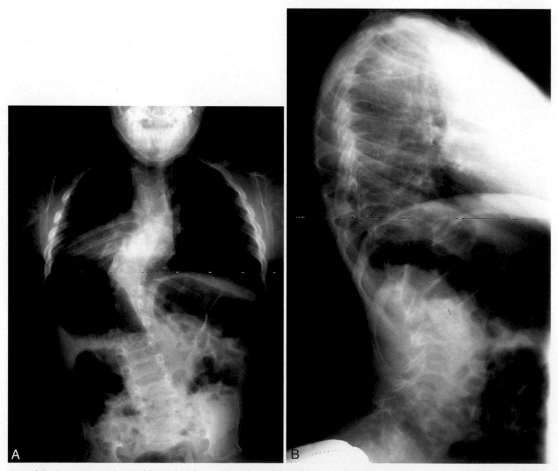

Figure 16-6. A and **B,** Anteroposterior and lateral radiographs taken show the right thoracic curve measuring 48 degrees and the left thoracolumbar curve progressing to 50 degrees. The patient underwent a posterior spinal fusion with pedicle screw instrumentation.

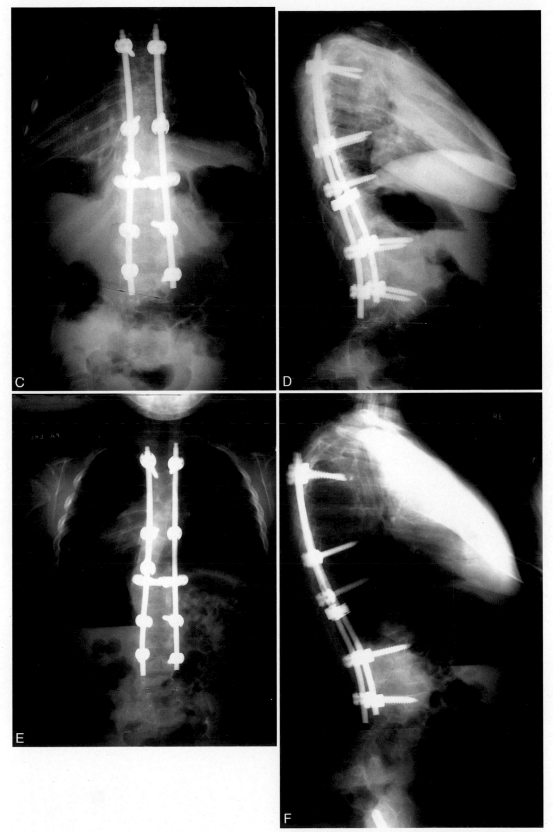

Figure 16-6, cont'd. **C** and **D,** Postoperative anteroposterior and lateral radiographs showing good correction. **E** and **F,** On 1-year follow-up, anteroposterior and lateral radiographs show a fusion with no curve progression.

CASE 7. An 8-Year-Old Female with Chondrodysplasia Punctata and Progressive Restrictive Lung Disease

At 2 years of age, the patient was noted to have a progressive scoliosis that measured 40 degrees from T3 to T8. This was treated with an anterior fusion using an anterior rib strut spanning T4 to T8 and a posterior fusion from T2 to T8. The curve postoperatively measured 42 degrees. The curve was noted to gradually progress and was accompanied by continued deterioration of the patient's pulmonary function. After careful preoperative evaluation, she underwent placement of a hybrid VEPTR device. The superior end was placed on the second and third ribs on the left, and the inferior end was placed on the lamina of L2 (Fig. 16-7).

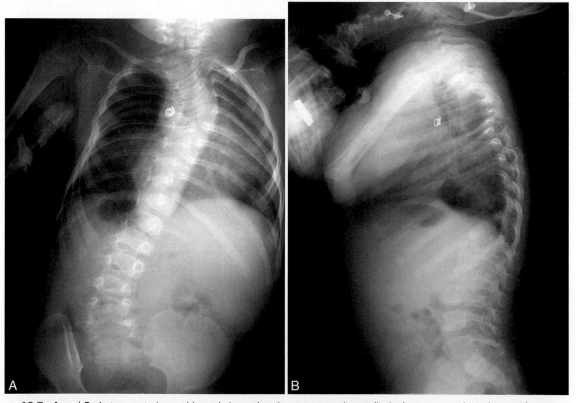

Figure 16-7. A and **B,** Anteroposterior and lateral views showing a progressive scoliosis that measured 40 degrees from T3 to T8.

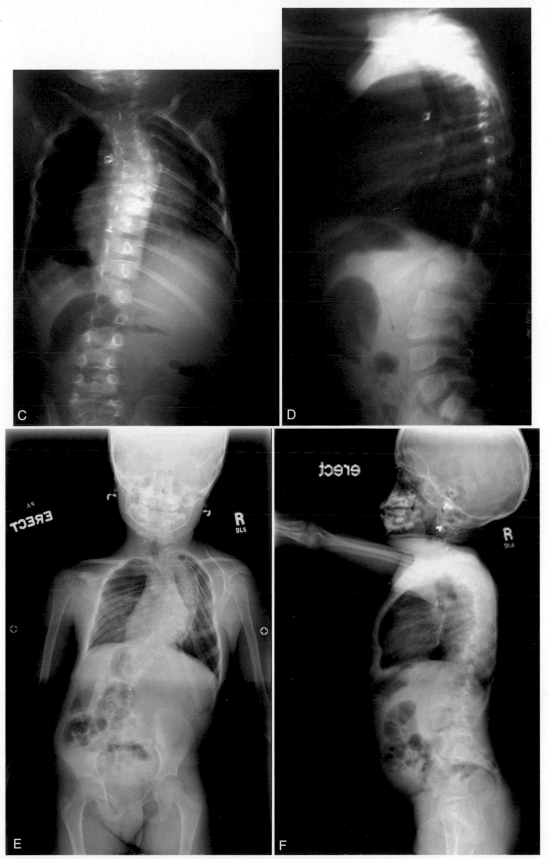

Figure 16-7, cont'd. C and **D,** This was treated with an anterior fusion using an anterior rib strut spanning T4 to T8 and a posterior fusion from T2 to T8. The curve postoperatively measured 42 degrees. The curve was noted to gradually progress and was accompanied by continued deterioration of the patient's pulmonary function. **E** and **F,** Preoperative radiographs taken show an 82-degree right thoracic curve. CT lung volumes were taken that showed the lung volume to be 415 mL on the left and 296 mL on the right. Her total lung volume measured 711 mL, which was below the fifth percentile for children her age.

Continued

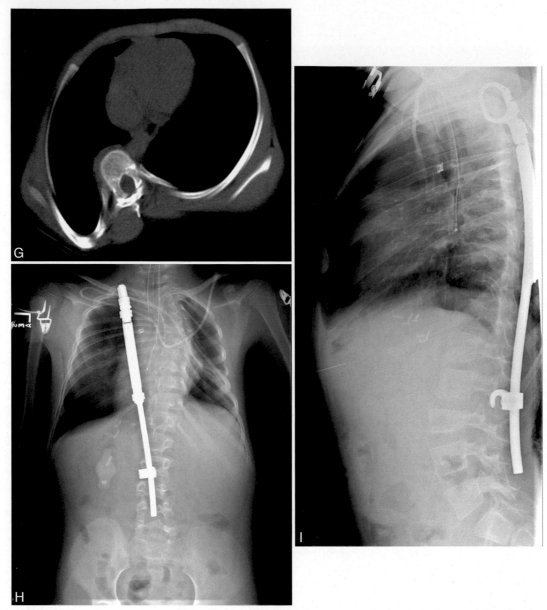

Figure 16-7, cont'd. G, A cross-sectional CT scan through the middle of the thorax shows a diminished right lung volume with rotation of the spine and thorax. **H** and **I,** After careful preoperative evaluation, the patient underwent placement of a hybrid VEPTR device. The superior end was placed on the second and third ribs on the left, and the inferior end was placed on the lamina of L2.

ACKNOWLEDGMENT

The authors would like to thank Dr. Michael B. Bober for his contribution of insight into the genetics of each dysplasia. The authors would also like to thank Aaron G. Littleton for his technical assistance in preparation of this chapter.

REFERENCES

Afshani E, Girdany BR: Atlanto-axial dislocation in chondrodysplasia punctata. Report of the findings in two brothers. Radiology 1972; 102:399–401.

Ain MC, Shirley ED, Pirouzmanesh A, et al: Postlaminectomy kyphosis in the skeletally immature achondroplast. Spine 2006;31:197–201.

Blaw ME, Langer LO: Spinal cord compression in Morquio-Brailsford's disease. J Pediatr 1969;74:593–600.

Cornier AS, Ramirez N, Arroyo S, et al: Phenotype characterization and natural history of spondylothoracic dysplasia syndrome: A series of 27 new cases. Am J Med Genet A 2004;128:120–126.

Dalvie SS, Noordeen MH, Vellodi A: Anterior instrumented fusion for thoracolumbar kyphosis in mucopolysaccharidosis. Spine 2001;26: E539–E541.

Lipson SJ: Dysplasia of the odontoid process in Morquio's syndrome causing quadriparesis. J Bone Joint Surg Am 1977;59:340–344.

Miyoshi K, Nakamura K, Haga N, Mikami Y: Surgical treatment for atlantoaxial subluxation with myelopathy in spondyloepiphyseal dysplasia congenita. Spine 2004;29:E488–E491.

Nakamura K, Miyoshi K, Haga N, Kurokawa T: Risk factors of myelopathy at the atlantoaxial level in spondyloepiphyseal dysplasia congenita. Arch Orthop Trauma Surg 1998;117:468–470.

Nelson J, Thomas PS: Clinical findings in 12 patients with MPS IV A (Morquio's disease). Further evidence for heterogeneity. Part III: Odontoid dysplasia. Clin Genet 1988;33:126–130.

Pauli RM, Breed A, Horton VK, et al: Prevention of fixed, angular kyphosis in achondroplasia. J Pediatr Orthop 1997;17:726–733.

Pauli RM, Scott CI, Wassman ER Jr, et al: Apnea and sudden unexpected death in infants with achondroplasia. J Pediatr 1984;104:342–348.

Ransford AO, Crockard HA, Stevens JM, Modaghegh S: Occipito-atlanto-axial fusion in Morquio-Brailsford syndrome. A ten-year experience. J Bone Joint Surg Br 1996;78:307–313.

Solomon L, Jimenez RB, Reiner L: Spondylothoracic dysostosis: Report of two cases and review of the literature. Arch Pathol Lab Med 1978;102:201–205.

Shohat M, Lachman R, Rimoin DL: Odontoid hypoplasia with vertebral cervical subluxation and ventriculomegaly in metatropic dysplasia. J Pediatr 1989;114:239–243.

Stevens JM, Kendall BE, Crockard HA, Ransford A: The odontoid process in Morquio-Brailsford's disease. The effects of occipitocervical fusion. J Bone Joint Surg Br 1991;73:851–858.

Svensson O, Aaro S: Cervical instability in skeletal dysplasia. Report of 6 surgically fused cases. Acta Orthop Scand 1988;59:66–70.

Thomeer RT, van Dijk JM: Surgical treatment of lumbar stenosis in achondroplasia. J Neurosurg 2002;96:292–297.

Tolo VT: Spinal deformity in short-stature syndromes. Instr Course Lect 1990;39:399–405.

Tolo VT: Surgical treatment of kyphosis in achondroplasia. Basic Life Sci 1988;48:257–259.

SUGGESTED READINGS

Ain MC, Shirley ED: Spinal fusion for kyphosis in achondroplasia. J Pediatr Orthop 2004;24:541–545.

Persistent thoracolumbar kyphosis in patients with achondroplasia is typically prevented with sitting modifications and bracing. When the kyphosis persists and progresses despite bracing, spinal fusion is indicated to prevent further progression and neurologic complications. This study suggests that when nonoperative treatments fail, this procedure for thoracolumbar kyphosis in the achondroplastic patient can be done safely and effectively.

Beighton P, Bathfield CA: Gibbal achondroplasia. J Bone Joint Surg Br 1981;63-B:328–329.

A thoracolumbar gibbus is an uncommon but potentially dangerous feature of achondroplasia. This is a series of unselected South African Negro achondroplasts. They suggest that wedging on the vulnerable vertebral bodies in the Negro achondroplastic infant can probably be prevented by avoiding this custom.

Campbell RM Jr, Hell-Vocke AK: Growth of the thoracic spine in congenital scoliosis after expansion thoracoplasty. J Bone Joint Surg Am 2003;85-A:409–420.

Longitudinal growth of the thoracic spine in a normal child has been estimated to be 0.6 cm/year between the ages of 5 and 9 years. After expansion thoracoplasty, growth of the thoracic spine was approximately 8 mm/year in our series of children with congenital scoliosis and fused ribs. After expansion thoracoplasty, both the concave and the convex sides of the thoracic spine and unilateral unsegmented bars appeared to grow in these patients. When a thorax is already foreshortened by congenital scoliosis, control of spine deformity with expansion thoracoplasty allows growth of the thoracic spine, and it is likely that the longer thorax provides additional volume for growth of the underlying lungs with probable clinical benefit.

Faye-Petersen OM, Knisely AS: Neural arch stenosis and spinal cord injury in thanatophoric dysplasia. Am J Dis Child 1991;145:87–89.

Bony abnormalities caused by thanatophoric dysplasia affect the base of the skull and the vertebrae as well as the ribs and appendicular long bones. This study suggests that the causes of death in patients with thanatophoric dysplasia and other severe forms of osteochondrodysplasia should be sought in neuraxial injury rather than being attributed solely to pulmonary hypoplasia.

Friede H, Matalon R, Harris V, Rosenthal IM: Craniofacial and mucopolysaccharide abnormalities in Kniest dysplasia. J Craniofac Genet Dev Biol 1985;5:267–276.

Serial roentgenoephalograms of a male patient with Kniest dysplasia were obtained between 1 7/12 and 11 3/12 years of age and were analyzed and compared to cephalometric normative data. This study suggests that the diagnosis of Kniest dysplasia can usually be made from roentgenograms of the extremities, the spine, and the pelvis. However, the morphologic characteristics of the head, as shown by cephalometric analysis, and the increased urinary excretion of keratan sulfate add confirmatory evidence that is useful in differential diagnosis.

Gollogly S, Smith JT, White SK, et al: The volume of lung parenchyma as a function of age: A review of 1050 normal CT scans of the chest with three-dimensional volumetric reconstruction of the pulmonary system. Spine 2004;29:2061–2066.

A review of 3400 sequential CT scans of the thorax obtained at a single institution over a 3-year period from 2000 to 2003 was performed. Normal values for the volume of lung parenchyma as a function of age and sex increase the clinical utility of a standard CT scan of the thorax in evaluating children with complex spinal deformities. They are a useful adjunct to pulmonary function testing. These data can be used in the preoperative and postoperative evaluation of patients who are at risk of thoracic insufficiency syndrome, particularly in patients younger than 5 years of age, when standard pulmonary function testing cannot be accomplished.

Hecht JT, Nelson FW, Butler IJ, et al: Computerized tomography of the foramen magnum: Achondroplastic values compared to normal standards. Am J Med Genet 1985;20:355–360.

Computerized tomographic dimensions of the foramen magnum of 63 achondroplastic individuals were compared to standards established for nonachondroplastic individuals. The size of the foramen magnum in patients with achondroplasia was small at all ages, particularly in patients with serious neurologic problems. The study suggests that measurement of the foramen magnum could identify achondroplastic individuals who are at high risk of developing neurologic complications.

Keiper GL Jr, Koch B, Crone KR: Achondroplasia and cervicomedullary compression: Prospective evaluation and surgical treatment. Pediatr Neurosurg 1999;31:78–83.

The association between sudden death and cervicomedullary compression in infants with achondroplasia has been well described. The results of this prospective study confirm that early clinical and MRI evaluations are necessary to determine whether infants with achondroplasia have cervicomedullary compression. With early recognition, an immediate decompression can be performed safely to avoid serious complications associated with cervicomedullary compression, including sudden death.

Mason DE, Sanders JO, MacKenzie WG, et al: Spinal deformity in chondrodysplasia punctata. Spine 2002;27:1995–2002.

Three types of spinal deformities were identified in children with chondrodysplasia punctata in this study, including cervical bony disruption, a slowly progressive, nondysplastic scoliosis that responds well to standard fusion techniques, and a dysplastic kyphoscoliosis, which is rapidly progressive and resistant to fusion. The best results in dysplastic curves are obtained with an anterior strut graft and a posterior fusion. The patients must be observed long-term for further vertebral dysplasia and progressive kyphoscoliosis.

Morgan DF, Young RF: Spinal neurological complications of achondroplasia: Results of surgical treatment. J Neurosurg 1980;52:463–472.

Spinal neurologic complications caused the admission of 17 patients with achondroplasia to the UCLA-affiliated hospitals between 1955 and 1979. These patients constituted 41% of all achondroplastic patients admitted during that period. The spinal stenotic syndromes could be divided into three groups: Group I, thoracolumbar stenosis (ten patients); Group II, foramen magnum and upper cervical stenosis (five patients); and Group III, generalized spinal stenosis (two patients). Early recognition, prompt clinical evaluation, and safe and accurate radiologic analysis of spinal neurologic complications of achondroplasia will allow appropriate decompressive surgical procedures to be performed.

Orioli IM, Castilla EE, Barbosa-Neto JG: The birth prevalence rates for the skeletal dysplasias. J Med Genet 1986;23:328–332.

This study was undertaken to establish the prevalence rates at birth of the skeletal dysplasias that can be recognised in the perinatal period, using the database of the Latin-American Collaborative Study of Congenital Malformations (ECLAMC) for the years 1978 to 1983 on 349,470 births (live and stillbirths). The most frequent types of skeletal dysplasia were achondroplasia, with a prevalence rate between 0.5 and 1.5 per 10,000 births; the thanatophoric dysplasia/achondrogenesis group (0.2 and 0.5 per 10,000 births); and osteogenesis imperfecta (0.4 per 10,000 births).

Poussa M, Merikanto J, Ryoppy S, et al: The spine in diastrophic dysplasia. Spine 1991;16:881–887.

Diastrophic dysplasia is an autosomal recessive disorder of the skeleton, characterized by disproportionate short stature, generalized joint deformities, clubfeet, deformed ear pinnae, and, frequently, spinal deformity and cleft palate. Diastrophic dysplasia is more common in Finland than elsewhere. The authors studied 101 patients with an age range from newborns to 79 years to determine the frequency and type of spinal deformities and the early signs of progressive cases and to follow the natural history of the disease.

Rimoin DL, Siggers DC, Lachman RS, Silberberg R: Metatropic dwarfism, the Kniest syndrome and the pseudoachondroplastic dysplasias. Clin Orthop Relat Res 1976;114:70–82.

Metatropic dwarfism, the Kniest syndrome, and pseudoachondroplastic dysplasia are specific chondrodystrophic disorders that have in common dysplasia of the metaphyses, epiphyses, and vertebrae. Metatropic dwarfism and the Kniest syndrome have been confused with Morquio's disease and with each other in the past but can be easily distinguished on the basis of radiographic features, clinical features, and cartilage pathology.

Ruiz-Garcia M, Tovar-Baudin A, Del Castillo-Ruiz V, et al: Early detection of neurological manifestations in achondroplasia. Childs Nerv Syst 1997;13:208–123.

Achondroplasia is the most frequent bone dysplasia. The mode of inheritance is autosomal dominant. The incidence of neurologic complications ranges between 20% and 47%; frequently, the symptoms are subtle but are due to such serious conditions as cervicomedullary compressive syndromes, syringomyelia, or hydrocephalus; therefore, the early identification of this disorder is very important. The authors concluded that the neurologic manifestations of pediatric patients with achondroplasia are frequent and very important, demanding comprehensive clinical evaluation even in asymptomatic patients, especially those with severe hypotonia or SSER alterations.

Thomas SL, Childress MH, Quinton B: Hypoplasia of the odontoid with atlanto-axial subluxation in Hurler's syndrome. Pediatr Radiol 1985;15:353–354.

There appears to be an increased incidence of hypoplasia of the odontoid in Hurler's syndrome. As this predisposes to atlantoaxial subluxation, it should be sought in this mucopolysaccharidosis as well as in Morquio's syndrome.

CHAPTER 17

Isthmic and Dysplastic Spondylolisthesis

EDWARD W. SONG, BARON S. LONNER, *and* THOMAS J. ERRICO

Spondylolisthesis is defined as a nonphysiologic translation of a vertebra on its caudal segment. It typically refers to a forward slippage (anterolisthesis) but may be manifest as retrolisthesis or lateral listhesis (which is often combined with a rotational component). The most widely utilized classification of spondylolisthesis is that of Newman and Wiltse, in which five types are described based on their etiology. These types are I, dysplastic or congenital; II, isthmic; III, degenerative; IV, traumatic; and V, pathologic. A sixth subtype is often discussed and is termed iatrogenic. Isthmic and dysplastic spondylolistheses are the most common types presenting in childhood and will be the focus of this chapter (Fig. 17-1).

A brief description of types III through VI follows. Degenerative spondylolisthesis occurs secondary to disc degeneration and subsequent collapse and hypermobility, resulting in facet subluxation and segmental slippage. Patients may present with symptoms of neurogenic claudication due to the resulting spinal stenosis. The level that is most commonly affected is the L4-5 level, where the facets are oriented sagittally, allowing anterolisthesis with intact but degenerate anatomy. Traumatic spondylolisthesis is the result of an acute fracture occurring in any part of the vertebrae excluding the pars interarticularis and most commonly results from disruption of the facet complex. The pathologic type is related to a loss of the structural integrity of a vertebra due to a disease process such as a localized lesion, for example, infection or neoplasm or a more generalized disease such as osteopenia. Finally, iatrogenic spondylolisthesis is related to a surgical intervention, typically a decompressive laminectomy in which the integrity of the facet joints and other posterior supporting structures is compromised.

Dysplastic spondylolisthesis is the result of a congenital deficiency in the L5-S1 facet joints. The facets are hypoplastic or even vestigial in nature and are often sagittally oriented, making them less able to resist shear stresses and the natural tendency for anterior translation of the L5 vertebra based on these forces. Less commonly, lumbosacral kyphosis and spondylolisthesis may result from a failure of anterior vertebral body formation at the affected level. Associated spina bifida occulta is also often present at the L5 or S1 level or both.

Isthmic spondylolisthesis is the result of a defect in the pars interarticularis. This is further subdivided into three subtypes: A, B, and C. Type A is defined as a lytic stress fracture that arises from repetitive stress to the region of the pars interarticularis. Type B is characterized by an elongated pars interarticularis due to stretching of the region like taffy from shear stresses as repeated injuries to the area attempt to heal. The third subtype is an acute fracture to the pars interarticularis.

The distinction between isthmic and dysplastic spondylolisthesis might not always be clear; for example, when a spondylolisthesis with dysplastic features increases in severity, a defect may develop in the region of the pars interarticularis, giving it the appearance of an isthmic spondylolisthesis. The Marchetti-Bartolozzi classification divides spondylolisthesis into two major subgroups: developmental and acquired (Box 17-1). This division is defined by the presence or absence of abnormal tissue development (dysplasia) at the level of spondylolisthesis. Some of the dysplastic changes that may be seen include facet tropism, deficient L5 and S1 lamina, elongation of the pars interarticularis, rounding of the dome of the sacrum, and a trapezoidal-shaped L5 vertebra. This differentiation allows for recognition of the differing natural histories of these two etiologies and consequently more specific treatment strategies. The Marchetti-Bartolozzi system also allows for the classification of postsurgical, pathologic, and degenerative forms of spondylolisthesis.

EPIDEMIOLOGY AND BIOMECHANICS

The most common cause of significant back pain in the child is spondylolysis with or without spondylolisthesis. The incidence of spondylolysis and spondylolisthesis is elevated in certain populations and appears to be related to predisposing activities and genetic and racial factors. From 19% to 70% of first-degree relatives of individuals

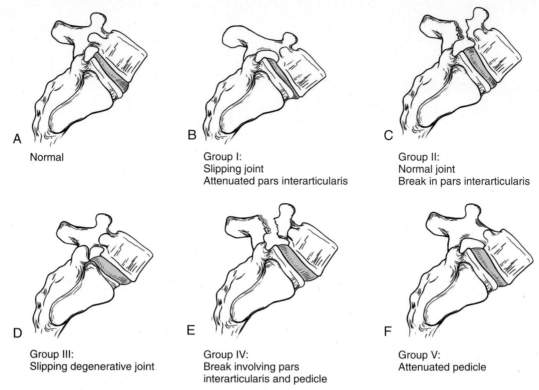

Figure 17-1. The five different pathologies described by the Wiltse classification: **A,** Normal. **B,** I: Slipping joint, attenuated pars interarticularis. **C,** II: Normal joint, break in pars interarticularis. **D,** III: Slipping degenerative joint. **E,** IV: Break involving parts interarticularis and pedicle. **F,** V: Attenuated pedicle.

BOX 17-1 Marchetti-Bartolozzi Classification for Spondylolisthesis

Acquired

Traumatic
Acute fracture
Stress fracture

Postsurgical
Direct
Indirect

Pathologic
Local
Systemic

Degenerative
Primary
Secondary

Developmental

High Dysplastic
With lysis
With elongation

Low Dysplastic
With lysis
With elongation

---

with type I or II spondylolisthesis are similarly affected. There is a 2:1 female to male predominance for dysplastic type spondylolisthesis.

Isthmic spondylolisthesis has not been documented at birth, and the incidence increases with age. Spondylolysis has been found in 3% to 4% of 5- to 7-year-olds and reaches 6% in the 6- to 18-year-old age group and in adults. The defect is found in 6.4% of white males compared to 2.8% of black males. It occurs in 2.3% versus 1.1% of white and black females, respectively. The incidence has been reported to be as high as 50% in the Inuit population.

In addition to hereditary and racial factors, environmental or biomechanical factors play an important role in the incidence and course of the disorder. Athletes in sports that involve repetitive hyperextension of the lumbosacral spine are predisposed to developing isthmic spondylolisthesis. Eleven percent of female adolescent gymnasts have been found to have bilateral spondylolysis. Divers, weight lifters, swimmers engaged in the butterfly stroke, and offensive linemen in football are also predisposed. Spina bifida occulta at L5 or S1 may also predispose to stress fracture in the pars interarticularis.

Healing of spondylolysis is complicated by the fact that the center of gravity in the upright individual is anterior to the sacrum, and the force vector tends to displace the L5 body forward on the sacrum. As a result of shear forces, incompetence of the subjacent disc can occur, resulting in gradual slippage of the involved vertebrae. Owing to shear and tension forces on the posterior elements, nonunion or healing and remodeling in an elongated position can occur. Incomplete healing of the fracture generally produces a fibrocartilaginous tissue response that may be exuberant and can result in symptomatic compression of the underlying nerve root (i.e., L5 in the case of L5 spondylolysis).

A number of factors predispose to slip progression, including female gender, skeletal immaturity at diagnosis, and a high-grade slip (>50%) on presentation. Also, lumbosacral kyphosis denoted radiographically by the slip angle increases the likelihood of slip progression. Overall, progression occurs in only approximately 5% of children and adolescents. Progression is unlikely in early adulthood, but late progression is associated with degenerative disc disease. Spondylolisthesis of greater than 25% at L4-5 has been associated with an increased likelihood of early degenerative disc disease.

CLINICAL PRESENTATION AND NATURAL HISTORY

Most commonly, the patient with isthmic or dysplastic spondylolisthesis presents with back pain. Pain is often referred to the buttocks, groin, and proximal thigh. Patients may complain of pain radiating below the knee to the foot. This may be associated with numbness or weakness in the great toe in cases of L5-S1 involvement. Spondylolysis is the most common cause of back pain in the adolescent and preadolescent population. Suspicion of this problem is raised in individuals engaged in high-risk sports. Urinary stress incontinence, new onset of bed wetting, urinary retention, or bowel abnormalities can occur, particularly in cases of severe dysplastic spondylolisthesis in which the posterior arch remains intact. In these cases, slippage of more than 50% results in cauda equina stretch and compression, which may be symptomatic. In cases of isthmic spondylolisthesis, cauda equina compression is less likely, since the posterior arch remains in place as the vertebra slips anteriorly. Urinary symptoms often go unreported, so it is imperative that the examiner query the patient about this and consider sending the patient for urometric evaluation. It is not uncommon for affected individuals to be asymptomatic. A low-grade spondylolisthesis might be discovered incidentally on a lateral radiograph that was obtained for a scoliosis evaluation.

Asymptomatic patients may have a paucity of physical findings. Contrarily, patients may present with back spasms and restricted thoracolumbar motion. In high-grade slips, patients may have a characteristic Phalen-Dickson sign consisting of hip and knee flexion contractures with a crouched, stiff-legged gait as a result of flexion of the pelvis and tight hamstrings (Fig. 17-2). A palpable step-off may be noted in the lumbosacral region, along with a local kyphosis and a secondary compensatory lordosis that may extend up to the thoracic region. Trunk shortening may be seen, as well as rib cage impingement on the iliac crests. Isolated hamstring tightness, which is commonly found, may be a result of nerve root irritation or stretch. Neurologic testing may reveal weakness of the extensor hallucis

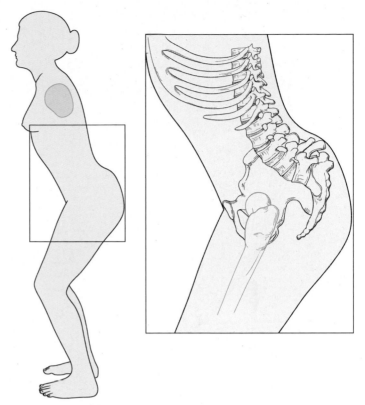

Figure 17-2. Phalen-Dickson sign. *(Redrawn from Skinner HB: Current Diagnosis and Treatment in Orthopedics, 4th ed. New York: McGraw-Hill, 2006, with permission.)*

longus, L5 dermatome sensory loss, and positive nerve root tension signs, such as straight leg raising.

IMAGING

Standard radiographic evaluation should include standing anteroposterior (AP), lateral, and oblique views of the lumbar spine. The percentage of slippage (Fig. 17-3) and etiology of the slip can be determined with these studies. Full-length standing AP and lateral roentgenograms of the spine provide information on coronal and sagittal balance and the presence of scoliosis. Scoliosis may be idiopathic and unrelated to the spondylolisthesis, or it may be what is termed an olisthetic scoliosis that emanates from the level of the spondylolisthesis as a result of rotation associated with the translation. Oblique radiographs may reveal a fracture of the pars interarticularis, seen as a so-called collar sign on the "Scottie dog" view (Fig. 17-4). Alternatively, an elongation of the pars, seen as a so-called greyhound sign, or sclerosis from a healing response may be noted. In cases of high-grade slippage, the Napoleon's hat sign may be noted on the AP radiograph in which an appearance of an inverted hat is found. A Ferguson view in which the X-ray beam is directed parallel to the lumbosacral disc may reveal findings such as spina bifida occulta, facet hypoplasia, or sagitally oriented facet joints.

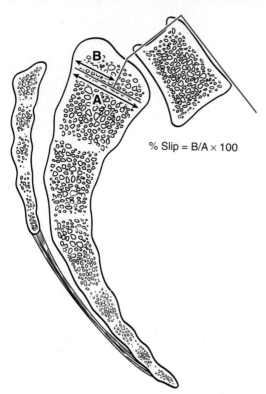

% Slip = B/A × 100

Figure 17-3. Percentage of slippage.

In cases in which spondylolysis is suspected despite a lack of a conclusive finding on roentgenographs, single- photon emission CT (SPECT) scanning is often diagnostic. The study utilizes radionuclide tracers like a bone scan but provides sectional and multiplanar computer formatted

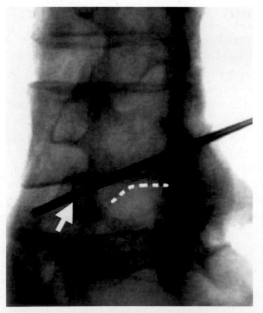

Figure 17-4. Lumbar oblique radiograph of "Scottie dog." *(From Phillips FM, Ho E, Cunningham BW: Radiographic criteria for placement of translaminar facet screws. Technical Report. Spine J 2004;4:465–467.)*

imaging to reveal increased bone activity in an area of injury. In addition, the images provide more anatomic detail and are able to provide spatial separation of bony structures. An old injury that is not actively in the healing stage might not be revealed with this modality, though. In this situation, magnetic resonance imaging (MRI) or CT scanning can be diagnostic. The MRI adds additional information on the integrity of the intervertebral disc of the involved motion segment as well as that of adjacent segments.

Various radiographic analyses can be performed, including percentage of the slip (see Fig. 17-3), Meyerding classification (grade 1 to 4), slip angle, lordosis, sagittal balance (C7 sagittal plumbline), and pelvic incidence, among other parameters. The Meyerding classification of spondylolisthesis grade is based on the percentage of slip evaluated on a standing lateral radiograph. Anterior translation of one vertebra on the subjacent vertebrae of 0% to 25% is a grade I slip, 26% to 50% is a grade II slip, 51% to 75% is a grade III slip, and 76% to 100% is a grade IV slip. A grade V slip has been defined as one exceeding 100%. The term *spondyloptosis* refers to a 100% slip in which the cephalad vertebra has dropped below the level of the superior end plate of the caudad vertebra (typically the sacrum). Grade I and II slips have traditionally been termed *low-grade slips*, and grade III, IV, and V slips have been termed *high-grade slips.*

The lumbosacral disc is typically the most lordotic of all the discs. In some cases of spondylolisthesis, the alignment is reversed in the sagittal plane and the involved segment becomes kyphotic. This can be quantified by the slip angle (Fig. 17-5). This angle is defined by the line drawn parallel to the superior end plate of L5 and its intersection with the perpendicular to a line drawn along the posterior aspect of the S1 vertebra. This value should normally be negative, denoting lordosis, as opposed to positive for kyphosis. In cases of long-standing and high-grade slips, secondary changes are often noted in the sacrum, which becomes rounded and often beaked at its anterior aspect and in the L5 vertebra in which the posterior inferior corner resorbs and becomes wedged.

Among other parameters, pelvic incidence has been found to have an association with slip progression (Fig. 17-6). The higher the pelvic incidence, the greater is the extent of slip that has been found. Pelvic incidence is a quantification of sacral position within the pelvis. It is measured by taking the angle from a line drawn perpendicular to the midpoint of the superior end plate of the sacrum with a line drawn from the center of the bifemoral head axis to the midpoint of the sacrum.

NONOPERATIVE MANAGEMENT

Asymptomatic patients with grade I or II slips are treated by observation at 6-month intervals. Patients may be advised to avoid hyperextension activities, although individuals who are involved in high-level athletics such as

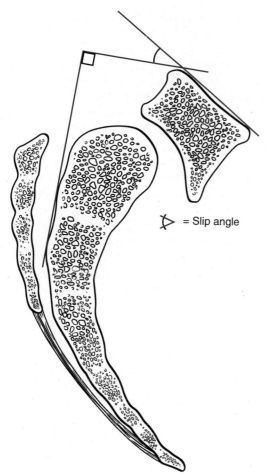

= Slip angle

Figure 17-5. Slip angle.

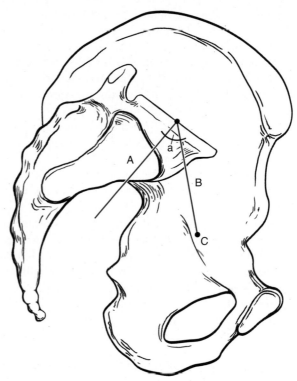

Figure 17-6. Pelvic incidence. **A** is the line drawn perpendicular to the midpoint of the superior endplate of the sacrum. **B** is the line drawn from the center of the bifemoral head axis to the midpoint of the sacrum. **C** is the center of the bifemoral head axis.

gymnastics are often reluctant to stop practicing the sport. They should be counseled about the repetitive injury being incurred and the possibility of the onset of symptoms and slip progression with continuance of their sport. Generally, patients with a grade III or IV slip are treated operatively, particularly if they are skeletally immature. If they have reached the end of growth and are asymptomatic, they may be closely observed.

In symptomatic patients with grade I isthmic spondylolisthesis, in which the fragments of the pars interarticularis are in close apposition, an attempt can be made to heal the defect with a 3- to 6-month course of bracing. An antilordotic brace is utilized to unstress the region. The patient should be instructed to wear the brace full time and to refrain from sports. Pelvic tilts for abdominal strengthening can be done with the brace on. Healing might not be possible in individuals with a chronic defect, particularly if a SPECT scan is not active in the region of the pars interarticularis.

The symptomatic patient with grade I or II isthmic or dysplastic spondylolisthesis should refrain from sports for a period of 2 to 3 months. Acetaminophen may be used as an analgesic. Nonsteroidal anti-inflammatory medication should be avoided in patients in whom healing of a spon-

dylolytic defect is the goal, owing to its potential deleterious effect on fracture healing. Physical therapy can be useful, with emphasis on hamstring stretching and abdominal strengthening. Bracing may be instituted in patients in whom activity modification has not been beneficial and is most often effective in mitigating or eliminating symptoms. The athlete may resume noncontact sports in a brace if they have become pain-free and can then be weaned from the brace gradually.

In a patient with significant radiculopathy, a selective nerve root block of the involved nerve root(s) may be attempted. If relief has not been achieved after 2 to 3 injections, surgery should be contemplated. Finally, injection of the spondylolytic defect itself with local anesthetic combined with corticosteroid can provide relief of back pain. If the relief is temporary, this proves diagnostic for the defect to be considered the pain generator and has implications for surgical treatment. Success of nonoperative treatment might depend on the degree of slippage.

OPERATIVE MANAGEMENT

In the patient with low-grade spondylolisthesis that has failed nonoperative treatment, in the skeletally immature individual who presents with a grade III or IV slip or spondyloptosis, and in the mature patient with a high-grade slip that has failed nonsurgical modalities, operative management is indicated. A number of different approaches have been advocated, from direct repair of the pars interarticularis to in situ posterolateral arthrodesis with or without instrumentation, anterior-posterior arthrodesis, decompression and posterior interbody fusion with transvertebral strut grafting from a posterior or anterior approach, posterior reduction or combined anterior-posterior reduction of high-grade slips, and finally vertebrectomy for spondyloptosis. All of these techniques may potentially be useful. The choice of the approach is often dictated by the surgeon's experience with various approaches and the techniques that have provided the best results in the individual's hands.

Repair of a spondylolytic defect may be considered in cases in which slippage is absent or minimal. This offers the advantage of preserving the motion segment. The subjacent disc must be intact on MRI. A diagnostic block of the defect is helpful to determine prognosis; that is, if a block provides temporary relief, the patient may be a good candidate for repair. The technique can be done with wiring around the transverse process and spinous process, direct screw fixation of the fracture, pedicle screw lamina hook connected by a short rod under compression, or combination of pedicle screw and wiring. The fracture is first debrided of fibrocartilage to bleeding bony surfaces, and autogenous iliac crest grafting is performed. The authors favor the hook-rod construct. Healing of the defect is most predictable in patients 25 years of age or younger with slips of less than 2 mm and for lesions of L1-4. Repair of L5 fractures has been less reliable.

Posterolateral fusion in situ has been the gold standard treatment for operatively managed spondylolisthesis. The results are most predictable when the technique is applied to low-grade slips. The addition of transpedicular instrumentation increases the arthrodesis rate. The pseudarthrosis rate and risk of postoperative slip progression are increased in treating slips of greater than 50%, particularly with slip angles of more than 50 degrees. The risk of pseudarthrosis is also increased in patients with dysplastic L5 transverse processes with small surface area even when the fusion is extended one level proximal (i.e., L4). Progression of slip in patients with high-grade slips even in the face of solid arthrodesis often occurs due to shear forces and tension on the fusion mass, particularly in cases of significant lumbosacral kyphosis. For this reason, partial reduction of the slip and circumferential fusion should be considered.

Clinical results have been good in patients in whom sagittal balance is maintained or restored after successful posterolateral fusion. Hamstring tightness often resolves, as does radiculopathy. Olisthetic scoliosis often partially resolves with stabilization and arthrodesis of the spondylolisthesis. In cases of persistent hamstring tightness or leg pain, pseudarthrosis and/or residual nerve root compression should be suspected. Decompressive laminectomy without arthrodesis (Gill procedure) has been advocated

in the past but has been met with predictably poor results. It is contraindicated in the pediatric population. Central decompression and/or foraminotomy combined with fusion is indicated, however, in cases of significant foraminal stenosis and marked central stenosis associated with severe dysplastic spondylolisthesis.

High rates of solid arthrodesis and resolution of symptoms have been reported with posterior decompression, partial resection of the dysplastic dome of the sacrum (sacroplasty), and interbody fusion combined with transvertebral fibula strut grafting. This typically results in a partial reduction of lumbosacral kyphosis and translation (Fig. 17-7).

Reduction of high-grade spondylolisthesis has been somewhat controversial, in part owing to its association with a significant incidence of nerve root injury, although the majority have resolved. The rationale for this approach is to restore sagittal balance, to decrease the likelihood of postoperative slip progression and pseudarthrosis, and to improve cosmesis. Furthermore, it has been shown that the incidence of postoperative cauda equina syndrome is lessened by reduction of high-grade spondylolisthesis in comparison to in situ fusion. It has been postulated, although not proven, that adjacent segment degeneration over the long term may be mitigated by restoring anatomic alignment. It is probably most appropriately utilized in individuals with significant lumbosacral kyphosis and in those with sagittal imbalance, with or without preoperative neurologic deficits.

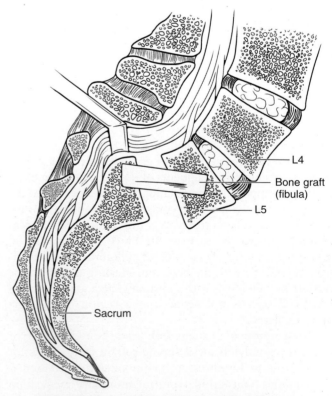

Figure 17-7. Sacroplasty with transvertebral fibula strut.

Instrumented reduction makes the L5 nerve root vulnerable to traction injuries. A cadaveric study has shown increases in L5 tension with reductions of anteroposterior translation of the L5 vertebral body of greater than 50%. However, some clinicians have found that decompression and spinal column shortening by sacral dome resection has helped in limiting L5 complications. Others have noted high rates of L5 nerve root complications despite using these techniques in conjunction with reduction. The incidence of postoperative cauda equina syndrome has been found to be significantly less with reduction and decompression than with in situ fusion.

Techniques for reduction include anterior release, sacral dome resection, and reduction with interbody fusion followed by posterior instrumented fusion of one or two segments and posterior decompression, sacroplasty, transforaminal interbody fusion with monosegmental or bisegmental transpedicular instrumentation and fusion. More important than the amount of translational correction achieved is the reduction in lumbosacral kyphosis. Again, stretching of the L5 nerve root has been shown to increase significantly after reduction of greater than 50% of AP translation. This may be lessened by resecting the sacral dome, which effectively shortens the spine. Regardless of the technique that is utilized, the patient's family must be informed of the significant risk of temporary or permanent nerve root injury that may be manifested by footdrop.

Complete vertebrectomy has been advocated for the patient with spondyloptosis of the L5 vertebra. This procedure is a shortening operation that would, in theory, minimize the risk of nerve root stretch and injury. It involves an anterior corpectomy of the fifth lumbar vertebra followed in a staged fashion by removal of the corresponding posterior elements and transpedicular fixation from L4 to the sacrum with the L4 body resting directly on the sacrum. Despite the shortening effect, a high rate of temporary nerve root injuries and some permanent footdrops have been reported. Nevertheless, this remains an important option for the patient with this difficult problem.

Isthmic or dysplastic spondylolisthesis can often be managed nonoperatively. Treatment options for low-grade slips include activity modification, physical therapy, and bracing. Patients who have failed to respond to nonoperative modalities and those with grade III to V slips are surgical candidates. Repair of the spondylolytic defect may be beneficial in individuals with isthmic spondylolisthesis with minimal translation, an intact subjacent intervertebral disc, age under 25, and defects proximal to L5. Posterior in situ arthrodesis with or without instrumentation is indicated for low-grade slips. Reduction either from a combined anterior-posterior approach or from an all-posterior approach with sacroplasty and circumferential fusion is indicated for individuals with significant lumbosacral kyphosis or sagittal imbalance, with or without preoperative neurologic deficits, but is associated with a significant risk of nerve root traction injury. Finally, vertebrectomy is an option for the individual with spondyloptosis.

PEARLS & PITFALLS

PEARLS

- Symptomatic patients diagnosed with grade I and II isthmic or dysplastic spondylolisthesis should refrain from sports for 2 to 3 months.
- Symptomatic patients with grade I isthmic spondylolisthesis, close apposition of the pars interarticularis, and activity on SPECT scanning may heal with antilordic bracing.
- Physical therapy may be useful, with emphasis on hamstring stretching and abdominal strengthening.
- Operative treatment is indicated in:
  - Low-grade spondylolisthesis that has failed nonoperative treatment.
  - Skeletally immature individuals who present with grade III or IV slippage or spondyloptosis.
  - Skeletally mature patients with high-grade slippage that have failed nonsurgical modalities.
- The addition of transpedicular instrumentation increases the rate of arthrodesis.
- In high-grade spondylolisthesis:
  - Partial reduction of the slip
  - Circumferential fusion
- Olisthetic scoliosis often partially resolves with stabilization and arthrodesis of the spondylolisthesis.
- Repair of a spondylolytic defect may be considered in cases of absent or minimal slippage and offers the advantage of preserving the motion segment. The authors favor the hook-rod construct.

PITFALLS

- NSAIDs should be avoided in patients who are candidates for healing of a spondylolytic defect.
- Surgical repair of a defect is less predictable in patients older than 25 years of age, with slips of more than 2 mm, and lesions at L5.
- The risk of pseudarthrosis and postoperative slip progression is increased when treating slips of greater than 50% and with a slip angle greater than 50 degrees.
- The risk of pseudarthrosis is increased in patients with dysplastic L5 transverse processes with small surface area.
- Decompressive laminectomy without arthrodesis (Gill procedure) has had poor results.
- L5 nerve root stretch has been shown to increase significantly after reduction of greater than 50% of AP translation.

Illustrative Case Presentations

CASE 1. High-Grade Isthmic Spondylolisthesis

The patient is a 12-year-old female who presented with back and leg pain, stress incontinence, and gait abnormalities. On examination, she had a crouched gait, stood with hips and knees flexed, and had a hyperlordotic lumbar spine (Figs. 17-8A and B). Adams test showed a right thoracic rib hump. Neurologic examination showed 4/5 extensor hallucis longus weakness on the right. Radiographic imaging revealed dysplastic L5-S1 spondylolisthesis with 67% slip and a 44-degree slip angle (see Figs. 17-8A and B). A right thoracic scoliosis of 57 degrees was noted. MRI showed severe stenosis at the level of the slip.

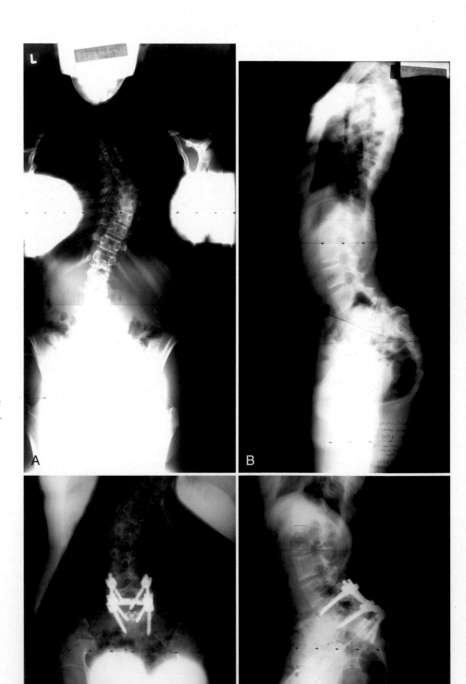

Figure 17-8. A, Preoperative anteroposterior view. **B,** Preoperative lateral view. **C,** Postoperative anteroposterior view. **D,** Postoperative lateral view.

The patient was treated by posterior reduction, sacral dome osteotomy, and circumferential fusion, all from a posterior approach. AP translation was corrected from 67% to 0% (Fig. 17-8C). Slip angle was reduced from 44 degrees to 13 degrees. Sagittal balance improved. Partial resolution of the scoliosis was noted initially, but further surgical treatment was required (Figs. 17-8E and F).

Postoperatively, the patient's course was complicated by left foot (L5) dysesthesia, which was treated with gabapentin and oral corticosteroids. Her symptoms resolved within 4 weeks postoperatively. EHL weakness completely resolved by 6 months postoperatively.

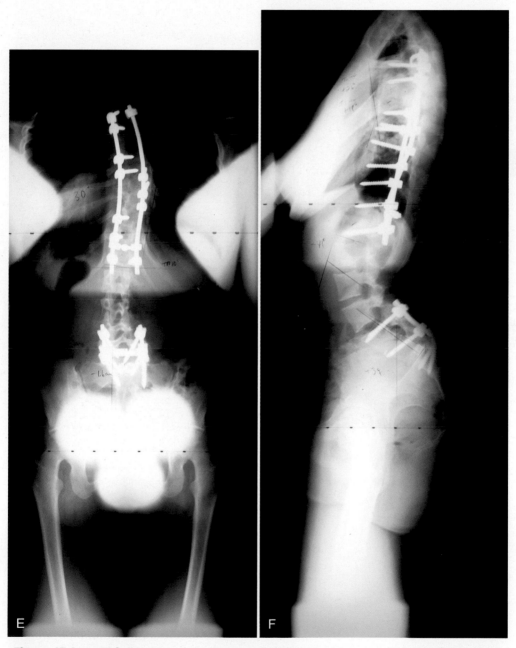

Figure 17-8, cont'd. E, Post–second surgery anteroposterior view. **F**, Post–second surgery lateral view.

CASE 2. High Grade Spondylolisthesis and Olisthetic Scoliosis
The patient is a 12-year-old female who presents with history of progressive scoliosis. Notable is that she has no complaints of back or lower extremity pain. Radiographs showed significant right thoracic curve but also high grade isthmic spondylolisthesis. She had a normal neurologic examination. The remaining exam showed right thoracic curve and lumbosacral prominence consistent with high-grade slip.

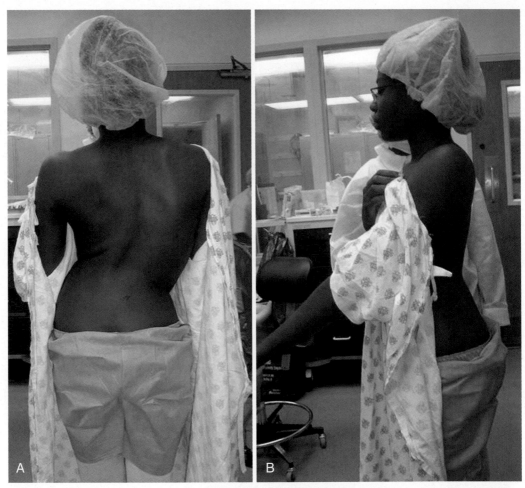

Figure 17-9. Preoperative views. **A** and **B,** Clinical appearance.

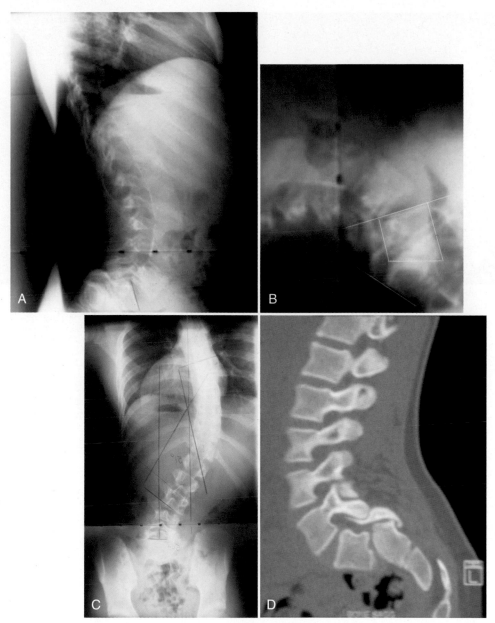

Figure 17-10. **A** and **B,** Lateral roentgenographic views of high-grade L5-S1 isthmic slip. **C,** Anteroposterior view. **D,** Sagittal CT image of the deformity.

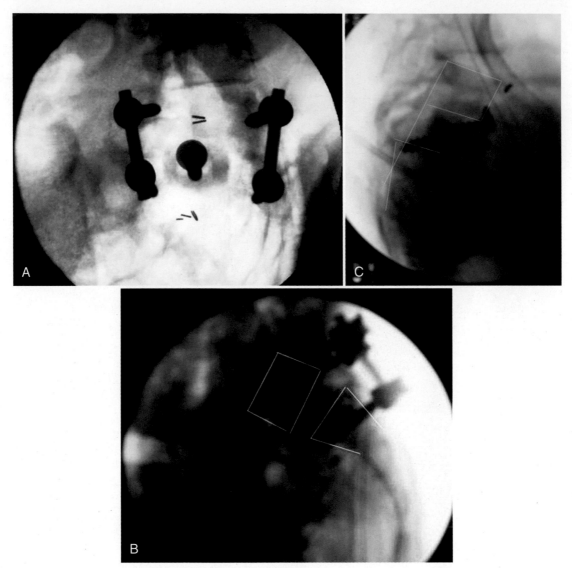

Figure 17-11 A, Postoperative anteroposterior view. **B,** Postoperative lateral view. **C,** Intraoperative lateral view after anterior graft insertion but before pedicle screw insertion.

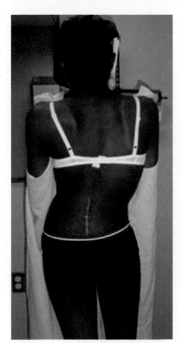

Figure 17-12. Postoperative clinical view at 6 weeks showing early improvement of scoliosis.

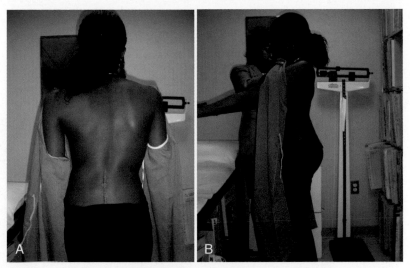

Figure 17-13. **A** and **B,** Clinical appearance at 4 months.

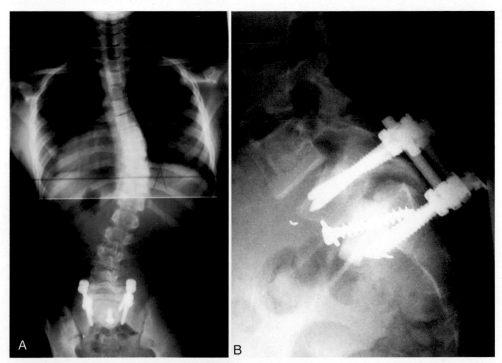

Figure 17-14. **A** and **B,** Anteroposterior and lateral radiographic views at 4 months.

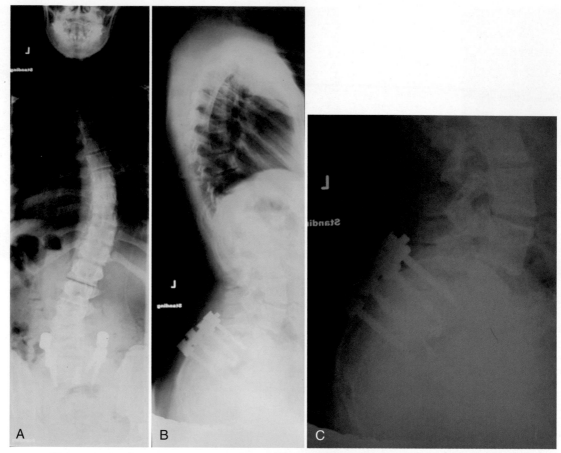

Figure 17-15. A–C, Anteroposterior, lateral, and close-up lateral roentgenographic views at 2 years.

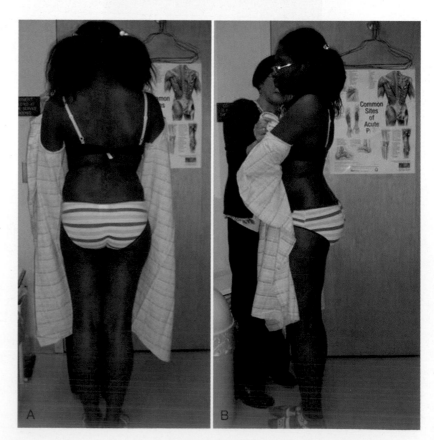

Figure 17-16. A and **B,** Clinical appearance at 2 years.

REFERENCES

Bell DF, Ehrlich MG, Zaleske DJ: Brace treatment for symptomatic spondylolisthesis. Clin Orthop 1988;236:192-198.

Boos N, Marchesi D, Zuber K, Aebi M: Treatment of severe spondylolisthesis by reduction and pedicular fixation. Spine 1993;12:1655–1661.

Bradford DS, Boachie-Adjei O: Treatment of severe spondylolisthesis by anterior and posterior reduction and stabilization. J Bone Joint Surg 1990;72-A:1060–65.

Gaines RW, Nichols WK: Treatment of spondyloptosis by two stage L5 vertebrectomy and reduction of L4 onto S1. Spine 1985;10:650–686.

Hansen DS, Bridwell KH, Rhee JM, Lenke LG: Dowel fibular strut grafts for high-grade dysplastic isthmic spondylolisthesis. Spine 2002;27:1982–1988.

Labelle H, Roussouly P, Berthonnaud E, et al: Spondylolisthesis, pelvic incidence, and sacropelvic balance. Spine 2004;29:2049–2054.

Lonstein JE: Spondylolisthesis in children. Spine 1999;24:2640–2648.

Matthiass HH, Heine J: The surgical reduction of spondylolisthesis. Clin Orthop 1986;203:34–44.

Pizzutillo PD, Hummer CD: Nonoperative treatment for painful adolescent spondylolysis or spondylolisthesis. J Pediatr Orthop 1989;9:538–540.

Pizzutillo PD, Mirenda W, MacEwen GD: Posterolateral fusion for spondylolisthesis in adolescence. J Pediatr Orthop 1986;6:311–316.

Shufflebarger HL: High grade isthmic spondylolisthesis: Monosegmental surgical treatment. Paper presented at SRS Annual Meeting, New York, 1998.

Smith MD, Bohlman HH: Spondylolisthesis treated by a single-staged operation combining decompression with in situ posterolateral and anterior fusion. J Bone Joint Surg Am 1990;72:415–420.

Tonino A, van der Werf G: Direct repair of lumbar spondylolysis: 10-year follow-up of 12 previously reported cases. Acta Orthop Scand 1994;65:91–93.

SUGGESTED READINGS

Antoniades SB, Hammerberg KW, DeWald RL: Sagittal plane configuration of the sacrum in spondylolisthesis. Spine 2000;25:1085–1091.

This is a retrospective radiographic study of sagittal lumbopelvic alignment. Lateral radiographs of the lumbar spine and pelvis were examined for 214 patients with spondylolisthesis and compared to those of 160 controls. This was done with dedicated software and analyzed the following parameters: pelvic incidence (PI), sacral slope (SS), pelvic tilt (PT), lumbar lordosis (LL), thoracic kyphosis (TK), and grade of spondylolisthesis. They found that PI, SS, PT, and LL are significantly greater (P < 0.01) in subjects with spondylolisthesis, while TK is significantly decreased. The PI showed a direct linear correlation with SS, PT, and LL. Furthermore, the differences between the two populations increase in a direct linear fashion as the severity of the spondylolisthesis increases. They concluded that pelvic anatomy strongly influences the incidence of spondylolisthesis and may predispose to progression.

Boxall D, Bradford DS, Winter RB, Moe JH: Management of severe spondylolisthesis in children and adolescents. J Bone Joint Surg 1979;61:479–495.

The authors reviewed their results for treatment of 43 patients with L5-S1 spondylolisthesis of 50% or greater treated variously by arthrodesis, decompression and arthrodesis, reduction and arthrodesis, and nonoperatively. They found that the slip angle was as important a measure as the percentage of slip in predicting progression. Hamstring tightness did not correlate with neural deficit. Arthrodesis alone, even in the presence of minor neural deficits or tight hamstrings gave relief of pain and resolution of deficits and tightness. They relate their belief that postoperative extension casting achieves a significant reduction in the percentage of slip and angle. In some cases, progression of spondylolisthesis was found to occur in spite of solid arthrodesis.

DeWald, RL, Faut MM, Taddonio RF, Neuwirth MG: Severe lumbosacral spondylolisthesis in adolescents and children: Reduction and staged circumferential fusion. J Bone Joint Surg Am 1981;63:619–626.

In addition to their description of technique, common pathologic findings of severe spondylolisthesis were described. There was a preponderance of dyspla-

sia, or congenital deficiency of the L5-S1 facet joints. Examples included facets that were hypoplastic or even vestigial in nature or sagittally oriented. Associated spina bifida occulta and, rarely, failure of anterior vertebral body formation were also found.

Frederickson BE, Baker D, McHolick WJ, et al: The natural history of spondylolysis and spondylolisthesis. J Bone Joint Surg Am 1984;66:699–707.

The authors found that progression is unlikely after early adulthood but that degenerative disc disease can result in late progression.

Harris IE, Weinstein SL: Long-term follow-up of patients with grade III and IV spondylolisthesis: Treatment with and without posterior fusion. J Bone Joint Surg Am 1987;69:960–969.

The authors compared nonoperative and in situ intralaminar fusion with 18- and 24-year follow-up. Their results suggest that symptomatic patients with grade III or IV slips be treated operatively, particularly if they are skeletally immature. If they have reached the end of growth and are asymptomatic, they may be closely observed.

Hu SS, Bradford DS, Transfeldt EE, Cohen M: Reduction of high-grade spondylolisthesis using Edwards instrumentation. Spine 1996;21:367–371.

The authors looked at 16 patients with an average preoperative slip of 89% and an average slip angle of 50 degrees. They performed an aggressive reduction using the Edwards Modular Spine system to get a postoperative result with an average slip of 29% and an average slip angle of 24 degrees. Complications included three neurologic injuries and four failures of hardware. They found the technique to be technically demanding.

Lenke LG, Bridwell KH: Evaluation and surgical treatment of high-grade isthmic dysplastic spondylolisthesis. Instr Course Lect 2003;52:525–532.

The authors recommend that high-grade isthmic dysplastic spondylolisthesis be treated surgically by central and foraminal decompression and fusion. They believe that partial reduction aimed at improving the slip angle is effective and reduces the risk of L5 nerve root injury compared to complete reduction. Solid anterior and posterior spinal fusion provided the best long-term results.

Meyerding HW: Spondylolisthesis. Surg Gynecol Obstet 1932;54:371–377.

The Meyerding classification of spondylolisthesis grade is based on the percentage of slip evaluated on a standing lateral radiograph. Anterior translation of one vertebra on the subjacent vertebra of 0% to 25% is a grade I slip, 26 to 50% is a grade II slip, 51% to 75% is a grade III slip, and 76% to 100% is a grade IV slip. A grade V slip has been defined as one exceeding 100%. The term spondyloptosis refers to a 100% slip in which the cephalad vertebra has dropped below the level of the superior end plate of the caudad vertebra (typically the sacrum). Grade I and II slips have traditionally been termed low-grade slips, and grades III, IV, and V slips have been termed high-grade slips.

Molinari RW, Bridwell KH, Lenke FF, et al: Complications in the surgical treatment of pediatric high-grade, isthmic dysplastic spondylolisthesis: A comparison of three surgical approaches. Spine 1996;21:1701–1711.

This is a retrospective review of 32 patients with greater than 50% slip treated with one of three techniques: in situ L4–sacrum posterior fusion, decompression with instrumented posterior fusion, and reduction and circumferential instrumented fusion. The incidence of pseudarthrosis was 45% (5 of 11) in the first group, 29% (2 of 7) in the second group, and 0% (0 of 19) in the third group. All 7 patients who had pseudarthrosis had small L5 transverse process surface area. Only one persistent neurologic deficit was found (unilateral extensor halucis longus weakness). Function, pain, and satisfaction were similar in patients with solid fusions.

Petraco DM, Spivak JM, Cappadona JG, et al: An anatomic evaluation of L5 nerve stretch in spondylolisthesis reduction. Spine 1996;71:594–598.

A cadaveric study showing significant increases in L5 nerve root tension with anteroposterior translation of the L5 vertebral body of greater than 50%.

Saraste H: Long-term clinical and radiological follow-up of spondylolysis and spondylolisthesis. J Pediatr Orthop 1987;7:631–638.

A clinical and radiologic follow-up study with at least 20 years of observation was made of 255 spondylolysis and spondylolisthesis patients for examination of the clinical course and its possible correlation to radiographic findings. The progression of slipping was small and not correlated to age at diagnosis and initial degree of spondylolisthesis. Disc height reduction at the spondylolytic level occurred at an earlier age and was more severe than that in a normal control group. Symptoms were correlated to radiographic pathology. Risk factors for low-back symptoms were greater than 25% slipping, low lumbar index in L5 spondylolysis, spondylolysis at the L4 level, and early disc degeneration.

Schoenecker PL, Cole HO, Herring JA, et al: Cauda equina syndrome after in situ arthrodesis for severe spondylolisthesis at the lumbosacral junction. J Bone Joint Surg Am 1990;72:369–377.

The authors identified 12 patients who had cauda equina syndrome after in situ arthrodesis for grade 3 or 4 spondylolisthesis. Five of the 12 had complete recovery. The authors felt that if preoperative nerve root dysfunction existed, decompression should be performed along with the fusion. They also suggested that if an acute cauda equina syndrome followed an otherwise uneventful in situ arthrodesis, immediate decompression including resection of the posterior rim of the dome of the sacrum and adjacent intervertebral disc. In addition, posterior instrumentation and reduction should be performed.

Stewart TD: The age incidence of neural-arch defects in Alaskan natives, considered from the standpoint of etiology. J Bone Joint Surg Am 1953;35:937–950.

Isthmic spondylolisthesis has not been documented at birth but becomes apparent at about 2 years of age. The incidence of spondylolysis increases with age; it is found in 3% to 4% of 5- to 7-year-olds, reaches 6% in the 6- to 18-year-old age group, and does not increase in adulthood. There appears to be a genetic/ethnic influence, as suggested by the fact that the incidence has been reported to be as high as 50% in the Inuit population.

Wiltse LL, Newman PH, Macnab I: Classification of spondylolysis and spondylolisthesis. Clin Orthop 1976;117:23–29.

The most widely utilized classification of spondylolisthesis. Five types are described based on their etiology: type I, dysplastic or congenital; II, isthmic; III, degenerative; IV, traumatic; and V, pathologic.

Wiltse LL, Rothman LG: Spondylolisthesis: Classification, diagnosis, and natural history. Semin Spine Surg 1993;5:264–280.

An expansion of Wiltse and Newman's classification to include a sixth subtype. termed iatrogenic, which is commonly due to aggressive laminectomy with facet and or to pars resection. The natural history of the various types was reviewed.

CHAPTER 18

Myelomeningocele Spinal Deformities

VINCENT ARLET *and* JEAN OUELLET

The surgical management of spinal deformities caused by myelomeningocele presents challenges relating to satisfactory surgical outcome, avoidance of complications, and need for late revision. Several factors contribute to the difficulty of surgical management:

1. Often, the deformity is of early onset, observed at 2 or 3 years of age, and can be severe by the time the patient reaches 7 years of age. In addition, a significant number of patients with myelomeningocele experience premature puberty. This has a significant impact on the surgical strategy, as one wants to maximize spinal growth if possible.

2. The skin is often of low quality, thin, and adherent to the myelomeningocele underneath. Skin breakdown is common, necessitating multiple skin flaps. A plastic surgeon is often needed to plan surgical incisions or flaps. Decubitus ulcers often develop over the ischia and gibbus of the deformity.

3. Infection represents a major challenge in these patients. The incidence of infection ranges from 10% to almost 50%. Infection is favored by sphincter incontinence, bacteremia from urinary tract infection, and the poor condition of the skin.

4. The myelomeningocele patient's neurosurgical pathology is often complex. When a shunt trajectory is in line with or crosses the incision, it might have to be dissected or even cut and reconnected to allow safe placement of instrumentation. Postoperatively, such shunts can malfunction and might need to be revised. Often, myelomeningocele patients have a tethered cord, and spinal distraction can pose a serious risk to the integrity of the cord. A Chiari decompression might be required before the spinal deformity correction.

5. These patients have also numerous orthopedic problems that might need to be addressed before correction of the spinal deformity. The surgeon must pay careful attention to the status of the hips. Hip flexion contractures might require a release. A lack of hip flexion, on the other hand, can prevent any surgical correction of the spine, as the patient will not be able to sit postoperatively. Self-catheterization, possible on a flexed trunk, might not be possible after spinal surgery and fusion down to the pelvis because the patient might no longer be able to see his or her perineum. Very careful attention must be given to myelomeningocele patients who have some useful mobility in their lower extremities. A significant number of these patients will require lumbosacral mobility to retain the waddling gait they need for ambulation. Extension of fusion to the lower spine might therefore be a contraindication in these patients.

6. Finally, the surgical technique is very demanding and difficult, often requiring two stages to ensure appropriate fusion, with increased risk of infection, pseudarthrosis, neurologic complications, and need for future revision if the procedure is not successful immediately.

EPIDEMIOLOGY

Myelomeningocele is the most common neural tube defect, estimated to occur in 1 of every 800 births. Prenatal triple screening for an elevated alpha-fetoprotein level during the first trimester is diagnostic in 85% of cases. Ultrasound is also very effective in screening for neural tube defects. The cause of myelomeningocele is unknown, but a deficiency in folic acid is believed to have a role in the pathogenesis of these neural tube defects.

In Europe, where prenatal screening is common, the incidence of myelomeningocele has dropped dramatically, as most of these pregnancies are terminated before the end of gestation. In the rest of the world and in places where such screening is not as systematic, neural tube defects are still seen. Religious considerations also play a role in the termination of the pregnancy.

CLASSIFICATION

Spinal deformities in myelomeningocele can be one of three types: congenital kyphosis, scoliosis, and lordosis.

Congenital kyphosis is observed at birth, generally develops in the middle or upper lumbar spine, and usually progresses to approximately 100 degrees. Untreated, it progresses 5 to 12 degrees per year.

Scoliosis has several causes, some occurring together. Flaccid scoliosis is the most classic, with a typical C-shaped curve and a collapsing spine with an element of kyphosis. These curves are most often progressive. Congenital anomalies such as hemivertebrae, congenital bars, and jumbled spine with defect of segmentation or formation are often present at the thoracic or lumbosacral level. An element of spasticity is often present. A tethered cord can also play a role in the pathogenesis of scoliosis. Tethered cord syndrome can result from a lipomeningocele, a diastematomyelia, or a thick filum terminale. It may be associated with pain, decreased neurologic function or change in bladder habit (increased bladder spasticity), and lumbar lordosis. Finally, hydromyelia can account for scoliosis. Screening with magnetic resonance imaging can allow for early treatment (shunting or Chiari decompression), and in mild or moderate scoliosis (less than 30 degrees), treatment of the hydromyelia can stop the progression of the curve.

Scoliosis is common in high-level paraplegia, observed in almost 100% of cases. Scoliosis is observed in 60% of cases of L4 paraplegia, with 40% of patients requiring surgery.

SYMPTOMATOLOGY

Classically, patients are referred to a spina bifida clinic for management of progressive deformity, decubitus ulcers, progressive loss of function, or increased spasticity. In many cases, it is the progression of the deformity on serial roentgenograms that will pose the surgical indication. Patients with myelomeningocele-related spinal deformities should undergo spinal imaging once or twice a year, depending on their age and the evolution of the deformity.

CLINICAL EVALUATION

The general evaluation must include the patient's nutritional status, which can range from malnourishment to obesity. Malnutrition can result from decreased abdominal size and increasing kyphosis or lordosis. In contrast, a significant number of myelomeningocele patients will end up markedly obese as they get older and can become wheelchair bound because of their lack of activity.

Neurosurgical evaluation should include shunt function, upper-extremity strength, and motor skills to assess for possible loss of function that can be observed in tethering of the cord.

The urologic evaluation should include inquiry about catheterization, the frequency of urinary tract infection, and whether the patient has undergone any previous diversion procedures. Diversion procedures (e.g., the Mitro-

fanoff procedure) and cystostomies can interfere with the performance of the anterior stage of the surgical procedure; therefore, it might be preferable to perform anterior surgery before a diversion procedure.

The orthopedic evaluation consists of the following: If the patient can walk, it is essential to determine whether the patient is using the lumbosacral junction to power his or her gait, because a fusion extending to the sacrum can have a detrimental effect on the patient's locomotion. Orthoses can assist these patients in walking. The presence of a leg-length discrepancy, often the consequence of repeated lower-extremity surgeries or fractures, must be assessed carefully. In the presence of a pelvic obliquity, the examiner must determine whether the obliquity is functional, due to leg-length discrepancy; infrapelvic, due to abduction/adduction hip contracture; suprapelvic, due to the spine deformity itself; or intrapelvic, due to an asymmetric and deformed pelvis. To distinguish these different causes of pelvic obliquity, one must use blocks under the feet (if the patient can walk) and a tape measure and must examine the patient sitting and prone with the legs hanging down off the table.

If the patient cannot walk and is in a wheelchair, evaluation of the upper extremities is essential, as they represent the only function for locomotion for these patients. The need for the patient to use the arms for sitting balance might in itself represent an indication for spinal surgery that will free the hands. Checking for increased pressure over the ischium and performing sitting balance pressure mapping before the surgery can be helpful in assessing the sitting balance. Hip flexion contractures should be assessed, as hip surgery might need to be performed before the spinal procedures.

Specific attention should be given to the sagittal balance of these patients. In patients with congenital kyphosis, one must look at the compensatory hyperlordosis of the thoracic and cervical spine; if it is too rigid, it could require an anterior release before posterior correction.

SPECIFIC WORKUP BEFORE SURGERY

Each case of myelomeningocele deformity should be assessed individually.

Usually, plain roentgenograms are required to assess the deformity. They should be obtained with the patient in the sitting or standing position, depending on the functional ability of the patient. Side-bending and traction films or lateral shoot-through films over a sandbag can be helpful to assess the flexibility of the deformity.

Magnetic resonance imaging of the whole spinal cord is mandatory to assess for possible Chiari malformation, cervical syrinx, or tethering of the cord. Untethering of the cord may have a positive outcome on the progression of the scoliosis, especially if the deformity is mild (less than 40 degrees) at the time of the release, as outlined by Pierz and colleagues.

Computed tomography with thin slices and three-dimensional reconstruction is very helpful, especially in the presence of congenital malformations, previous surgery, or failed fusions.

Urinalysis is necessary to identify possible urinary tract infection prior to surgery.

Consultation between the neurosurgeon and a urologist is an important prerequisite of spinal surgery, as urologic function can be affected by the surgery, and urodynamic studies will be required as part of the follow-up.

SPECIFIC TREATMENTS

Congenital Kyphosis

The incidence of congenital kyphosis in patients with myelomeningocele is 8% to 15%. The kyphotic deformity is usually progressive and increases the patient's disability. Progression of deformity causes recurrent skin breakdown over the apex of the kyphosis, impaired sitting balance, necessitating use of the hands for support, and collapse of the lower rib cage onto the anterior thighs, which can ultimately cause respiratory compromise. Conservative treatment with spinal braces does not prevent progression of the deformity and can cause skin breakdown at the apex of the deformity. Crawford and colleagues recommend that kyphectomy be performed at the time of the initial closure. Reporting on 11 patients with an average correction of 77 degrees, they observed long-term recurrence over time but in the form of a more harmonious kyphosis. In the classic technique that is used in newborns, one or two apical vertebrae are decancelled, and nonresorbable sutures or tapes are passed around the pedicles. The deformity is corrected by pushing over the apex and tightening the nonresorbable sutures. Unfortunately, in many instances, the patient is seen at an older age and has a significant kyphotic deformity. Many different techniques have been described for correction and stabilization since the first technique of kyphus resection described by Sharrard and Drennan. Classically, management of rigid congenital kyphosis in myelomeningocele consists of kyphectomy followed by posterior instrumented fusion; however, pseudarthrosis and loss of correction still occur after such procedures, with a rate as high as 50% in some series. We therefore devised a posterior-anterior sequence in which the posterior correction associating kyphectomy and strong lumbopelvic fixation is followed by an anterior spinal fusion using an inlay strut graft to achieve long-term stability of the spinal fusion. In very young patients, only the posterior sequence might be tried in an effort to maximize the growth of the lumbar spine. The surgical technique of our posterior-anterior sequence is shown in Figures 18-1 and 18-2. Using this technique in patients older than 4 to 5 years of age, we have not observed any recurrence of the deformity and have seen only one case of infection in more than 20 cases (see Case 1).

Maintenance of the correction and recurrence of the deformity are the main long-term concerns with all posterior-only techniques described in the literature. Compared with reports of posterior-only techniques in the literature, we have not observed any loss of correction over time with our posterior-anterior technique.

Scoliosis

According to the 25-year prospective study of Bowman and colleagues, 49% of patients with spina bifida will develop scoliosis. Bracing is usually not helpful in these patients, who are often obese and have multiple skin and urologic problems. Classically, bracing is prescribed for progressive and moderate curves of less than 40 degrees in patients younger than 8 years of age. Spinal fusion is more effective after the eighth year and not too detrimental to the overall growth of these patients, who often have premature puberty. However, bracing can be harmful to the rib cage in patients with paralytic curves and can cause pressure sores or even chest deformity and lordosis. The braces that are most commonly used are bivalve polypropylene jackets.

Approximately half of patients with spinal deformities will require surgery, and each case must be tailored to the needs of the patient and the ambulatory and functional status. If the patient is walking, it might be better to avoid a lumbosacral fusion that could hinder gait. On the other hand, if the deformity is severe enough that it hinders sitting or the dynamic balance of the patient when he or she is walking, fusion, even down to the sacrum, might benefit the patient. Curves that are greater than 40 degrees should be considered for surgery. Before surgery, parents should be advised that the child's functional status could deteriorate for the first 12 to 18 months, as described by Schoenmakers and colleagues.

Some patients can lose their capacity to ambulate, which is why in some instances, it is wise to wait until the child spontaneously prefers the use of the wheelchair for his or her daily activities. Often, we see teenagers with L3 or even L4 paraplegia who prefer the use of the wheelchair over the braces and canes they were using at a younger age.

Some curves can be treated by posterior surgery alone if the posterior elements to be included in the fusion are intact. The treatment of such curves follows closely that of idiopathic scoliosis. However, in the ambulatory patient who uses the lumbosacral junction to power gait, avoiding extension of the fusion in the lumbar spine might allow the patient to maintain the same walking capacity as existed preoperatively (see Case 2).

Because of the lack of posterior elements, pseudarthroses and instrumentation-related complications are often encountered. The rate of pseudarthrosis can range from 10% to almost 50%, depending on the series and the surgical technique used (posterior-alone versus circumferential). In

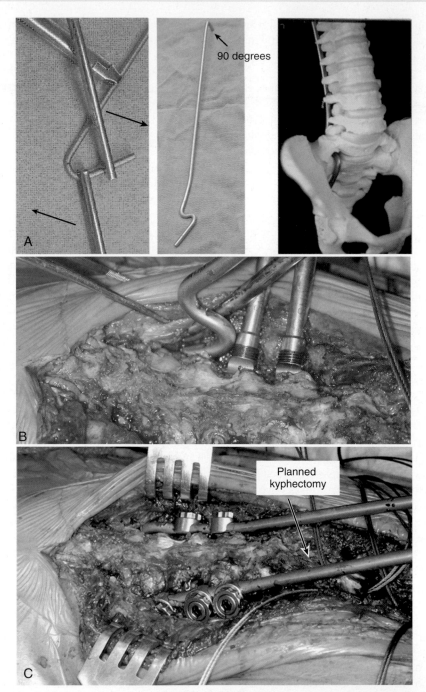

Figure 18-1. Kyphectomy with modified Dunn-McCarthy fixation for congenital kyphosis: Posterior sequence. **A,** Precontouring of the rod to fit the anatomy of the upper sacrum. *Left:* The first bend is made in the rod (*arrows*). *Middle:* The long S-shaped curve with the two bends is formed in the distal portion of the rod (*arrow*). A 90-degree bend is made in the proximal end to control rotation of the rod once it is inserted into the pelvis. *Right:* The rod is inserted into the L5-S1 foramen, buttressing the anterior sacrum. **B,** Operative view of the insertion of the precontoured long S-shaped rod over the sacral ala. The tip of the rod is inserted into the L5-S1 foramen, over the sacral ala, and in front of the sacrum. In the front of the sacrum, the rod is retroperitoneal underneath the bifurcation. **C,** The two rods are inserted into the pelvis and locked into the distal pedicle with screws. They are cross-linked to prevent rotation and to achieve distal stable foundation.

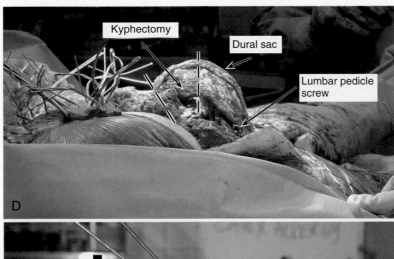

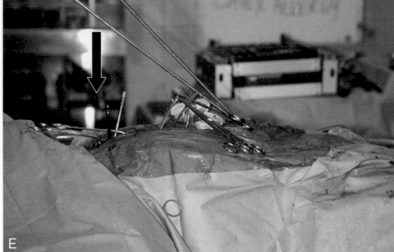

Figure 18-1, cont'd. D, To avoid significant bleeding, the spine is exposed in an extraperiosteal fashion. The dural sac is usually not ligated but is retracted laterally after the nerve roots are cut. Spinal resection is planned to include the more proximal compensatory lordotic deformity *(dashed lines)*. **E,** Once the kyphectomy is done, the correction is achieved by cantilevering the rods that were pointing to the ceiling onto the thoracic implants (cable wires for this patient). *(From Odent T, Arlet V, Ouellet J, Bitan F: Kyphectomy in myelomeningocele with a modified Dunn-McCarthy technique followed by an anterior inlayed strut graft. Eur Spine J 13:2004:206–212, with permission.)*

planning a spinal fusion for these patients, it is recommended that the level where the posterior elements are missing be assessed, as a posterior-only fusion at this level is unlikely to be possible. Computed tomography with three-dimensional reconstruction affords the most accurate assessment of the level of spinal dysraphism. Classically, to decrease the rate of pseudarthrosis, the sequence has been to perform the anterior release and fusion first, followed by the posterior fusion. This has the advantage in stiff curves of loosening up the deformity for better correction posteriorly. However, the disadvantage is that anteriorly, one may use only morcellized bone graft, and the posterior surgery must be performed either at the same time or shortly (a few days) afterward. In Banta's series, the rate of nonunion despite anterior and posterior spinal fusion was more than 10%. Some authors advocate the use of anterior instrumentation first, followed by posterior instrumentation. Another disadvantage of performing the anterior instrumentation first is that this might prevent additional correction posteriorly. With the advent of strong posterior pedicle fixation and sacropelvic fixation techniques such as the MW and modified Dunn-McCarthy techniques, we have found that the classic sequence does not hold true except in very rigid curves. We prefer

in most cases to perform the posterior correction first, achieving the goal of deformity correction (spine balanced in the sagittal and coronal plane over the pelvis). A few weeks or even months later, a complementary anterior fusion is carried out. This sequence has the main advantages of obtaining a very strong anterior fusion with structural or inlay grafts that are locked in the anterior vertebral bodies. The patient may even be discharged between the two stages to recuperate from the posterior surgery. No brace is needed postoperatively if one uses strong segmental pedicle instrumentation and modern pelvic fixation such as MW fixation or the equivalent (see Case 3).

Another subgroup of patients may be considered for anterior-only surgical stabilization. Anterior-only stabilization has the advantage of working in a healthy area of the spine with a decreased chance of infection. We do not hesitate in selected cases (i.e., patients with moderate and flexible curves less than 65 degrees) to perform all the surgery from the anterior even if it has to involve a double thoracotomy to access both curves in the thoracic and lumbar spines. The extent of the anterior fusion can be from T4 to L4 and exceptionally L5. Naturally, such an operation can be done only if the patient is old enough and has enough bone stock anteriorly that the anterior screws

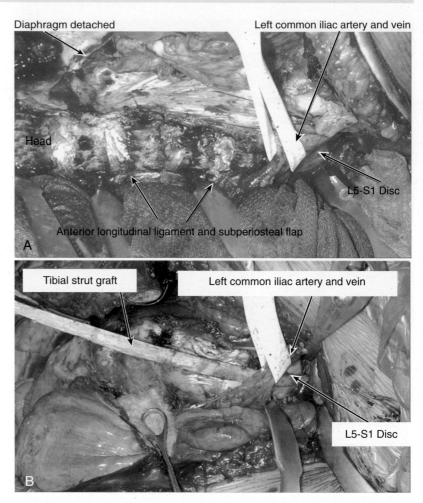

Figure 18-2. Kyphectomy with modified Dunn-McCarthy fixation for congenital kyphosis: anterior sequence. **A,** Exposure of the thoracolumbar spine. The patient's head is on the left; the patient's left side is at the top. The lumbar spine is exposed after the diaphragm is detached. The anterior longitudinal ligament is lifted off as a periosteal flap. The left common iliac artery and vein are isolated on a nonlatex vessel loop. The L5-S1 disc is identified (the tip of the needle is in L5-S1). Discectomies are then performed, and a trough is created in the vertebral bodies to allow the tibial strut graft to be keyed in between the S1 vertebral body and T10. **B,** Preparation of the tibial strut graft (photograph taken prior to the dissection of the osteoperiosteal flap). The tibial graft is passed underneath the bifurcation.

can find adequate purchase. Sponseller and colleagues' experience with anterior-only fusion in myelomeningocele spinal deformity corroborates our own experience. Basobas and coworkers have even advocated the use of short anterior-only fusion in selected cases of myelomeningocele to avoid the complications of the posterior surgery and leave as much of the spine mobile to maintain function. However, in our experience, long-term follow-up of patients with short anterior fusion has been disappointing, with progression of the deformity outside of the instrumented zone and the need for later revision (see Case 4).

Lordosis

Patients with increasing thoracolumbar lordosis present with abdominal crowding, chest restriction, and eventually a fixed deformity. Special attention should always be given to the assessment of the cervical spine, which may be involved with the overall deformity. Patients might have a fixed cervical lordosis with lack of cervical flexion. They adjust their horizontal gaze by hyperflexing around the hip joints and the low lumbar spine. In such cases, a fusion

down to the pelvis can prevent adjustment of the horizontal gaze after the surgery.

In cases of lordosis, one should always rule out a possible tethering of the cord.

Surgical treatment of the lordosis might require anterior wedge resection followed by posterior instrumentation (see Case 5).

Spinal Fusion for Scoliosis with Pelvic Obliquity

The issue of pelvic obliquity correction is still open to debate. In the ambulatory patient, it is almost always preferable not to include the pelvis in the fusion, as this can hinder the gait of the patient. However, in the patient in whom the spinal pelvic obliquity is progressive and represents a major hindrance to maintaining balance and normal hip function, extending the fusion to the pelvis in an ambulatory patient might be the only choice. The patient has to be warned that although sitting balance will be improved, walking capacity could be less or require some assistance (see Case 6).

In the wheelchair-bound patient, the presence of recurrent ischial pressure sores is an indication to correct the pelvic obliquity by fusing the spine, in most instances to the sacropelvis. However, in some rare cases of mild pelvic obliquity, it is possible to stop at L4 or L5 when these vertebrae are not rotated and perfectly parallel to the pelvis (see Case 7). This will have the advantage of leaving some lumbosacral mobility to shift pressure points during sitting. Only moderate pelvic obliquity (less than 15 to 20 degrees) can be improved with such treatment. When doing correction of the pelvic obliquity, how much correction should we aim for? Most authors agree that correcting the pelvic obliquity to less than 15 degrees is adequate. This is the reason why some authors rarely include the sacrum in the correction of pelvic obliquity. However, earlier methods of fixation, such as the Luque-Galveston technique, did not control the lumbosacral junction well enough, and it has been our experience that the pelvic obliquity will recur, often after an extended period of time. The lack of complete correction with the Galveston fixation (no distraction, compression) led us to abandon completely this type of fixation for our preferred MW fixation.

With such a technique, we usually can achieve an almost 100% correction of the pelvic obliquity, which has the advantage of improving the patient's comfort and eliminating the need for an additional wedge built into the cushion. Because of the excellent strength of the construct, it is possible for the patient to sit right away without any kind of brace and, in most cases, to start with the posterior fixation first.

Revision Surgery for Spina Bifida Patients

Because of the complexity of spinal procedures and the continuous growth of the spine, revision surgery is often required to treat pseudarthroses, extend the fusion, or create osteotomies. It is essential to avoid repeating the mistakes of the index surgery. In most cases, a combined anterior and posterior technique will be required.

The goal of revision surgery remains the same: to achieve a solid fusion and a balanced spine. The spine surgeon might have to choose between extending the fusion proximally or distally, performing spinal osteotomies or spinal resection, and doing anterior fusion with possible anterior column support. In the paraplegic patient, it is possible to use an anterior approach on the side opposite the previous anterior surgery, which has the advantage of being easier to dissect and does not carry the neurologic risk of spinal cord devascularization that exists in the non-paraplegic patient (see Case 8).

CONCLUSIONS

Surgical correction of spinal deformity in myelomeningocele remains a surgical challenge and must be tailored for each case. Because of the numerous potential complications, this surgery must be done only in specialized spina bifida centers. Attention to every detail is essential to have a positive outcome. The best outcome will require an extensive understanding of the disease, the functional requirements of the patient with respect to ambulation and urologic needs, the natural history of the disease, and the advanced surgical skills of modern spinal deformity surgery. Most patients will require a circumferential fusion and strong modern fixation with pedicle screws and, when appropriate, strong lumbopelvic fixation. If the indications and the techniques are chosen carefully, patients will benefit from such a challenging surgery.

PEARLS & PITFALLS

PEARLS

- Circumferential spinal fusion is the mainstay of treatment.
- If the spine is flexible, do posterior fusion first and anterior fusion second.
- If the spine is rigid, do anterior release first, followed by posterior fusion.
- Consider anterior surgery alone whenever it is possible: in teenagers, moderate curves.
- Use modern fixation: pedicle screws, iliac screw fixation, MW fixation for pelvic obliquity.
- Use Dunn-McCarthy or modified fixation for correction of congenital kyphosis.
- Use abundant bone graft, allograft, or autograft whenever available.
- Plan surgery with a plastic surgeon for skin incision, flaps, and closure.
- Tell patients what they can realistically expect and explain the risks of surgery (e.g., infection, blood loss).

PITFALLS

- Do not fuse to the pelvis in walkers, as function will decrease.
- Do not neglect other medical problems (e.g., shunt, bladder catheterization).
- Avoid fusing too short in thoracolumbar levels and pelvic obliquity.

Illustrative Case Presentations

CASE 1. An 8-Year-Old Boy with Recurrent Skin Breakdown over the Thoracic Kyphosis and Progression of the Deformity

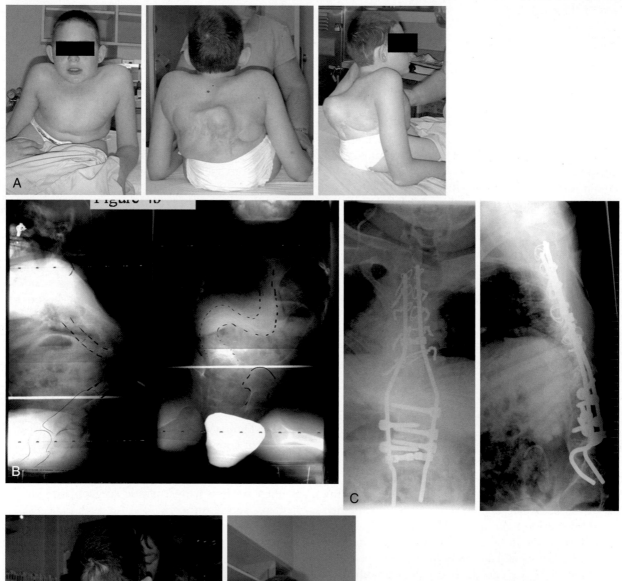

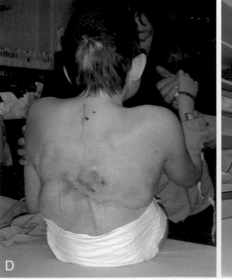

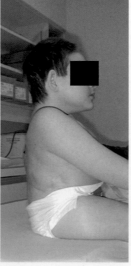

Figure 18-3. A, Preoperative clinical view. Kyphectomy was followed by anterior inlay tibial strut grafting. Radiographic appearance before (**B**) and after (at the 5-year follow-up) (**C**) the two-stage procedure. The lumbar spine shows solid anterior fusion. **D,** Postoperative clinical view.

CASE 2. A 13-Year-Old Girl with L4 Paraplegia Who Walks Using Her Lumbar Spine to Compensate for Her Lack of Gluteal Muscles

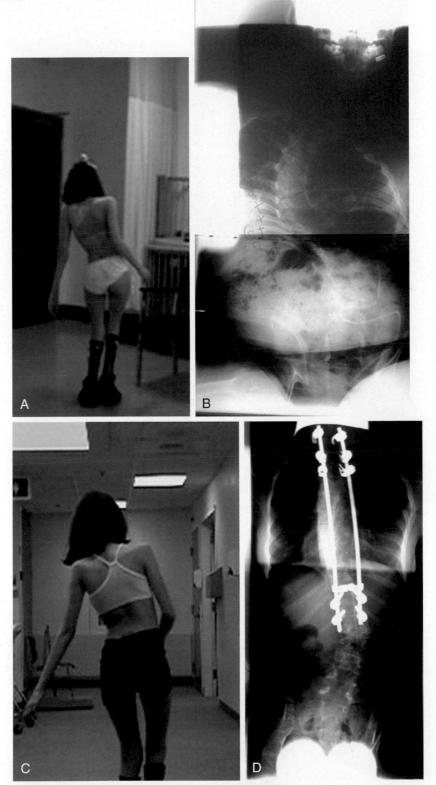

Figure 18-4. A, Clinical photograph taken from a movie of her waddling gait that requires lumbar spine mobility. The accompanying roentgenogram (**B**) is static. **C** and **D,** One year after selective posterior thoracic fusion with little correction to maintain balance, her gait (pattern and speed) is maintained, and she can ambulate as well as she could before the surgery. More correction of the thoracic curve would have led to imbalance. Further extension of the fusion in the lumbar spine would have impeded her walking (pattern and speed). The photo and static roentgenogram were taken from a movie of her gait.

CASE 3. A 16-Year-Old Patient with Progressive Flaccid Kyphoscoliosis and a Thoracolumbar Paraplegic Level

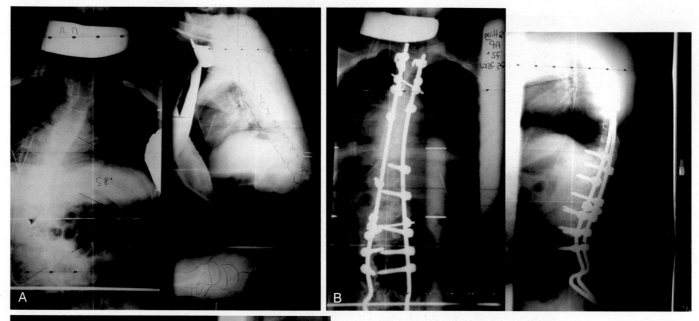

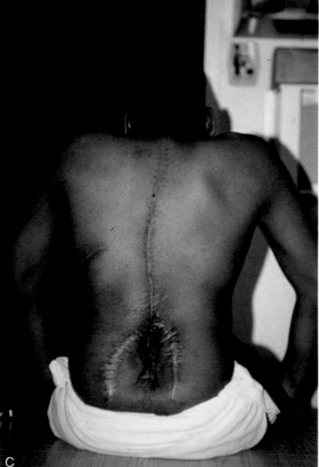

Figure 18-5. A, Roentgenograms showing a clinically flexible deformity. Posterior fixation was performed, followed by anterior fusion. A modified Dunn-McCarthy technique was used because the major deformity was kyphotic. Anterior fusion from T10 to the sacrum with structural and inlay grafting was performed 2 months later. **B,** Clinical view at 2 years' follow-up. **C,** Observe the inverted Y incision used to avoid areas of poor skin.

CASE 4. A 10-Year-Old Boy with Progressive Deformity, Multiple Ventriculoperitoneal Shunt Revisions, and a Tethered Cord

The patient is nonambulatory. Because of the poor skin quality, an anterior-only approach was chosen to treat the two curves. Release of the tethered cord was done initially. Several weeks later the deformity was addressed.

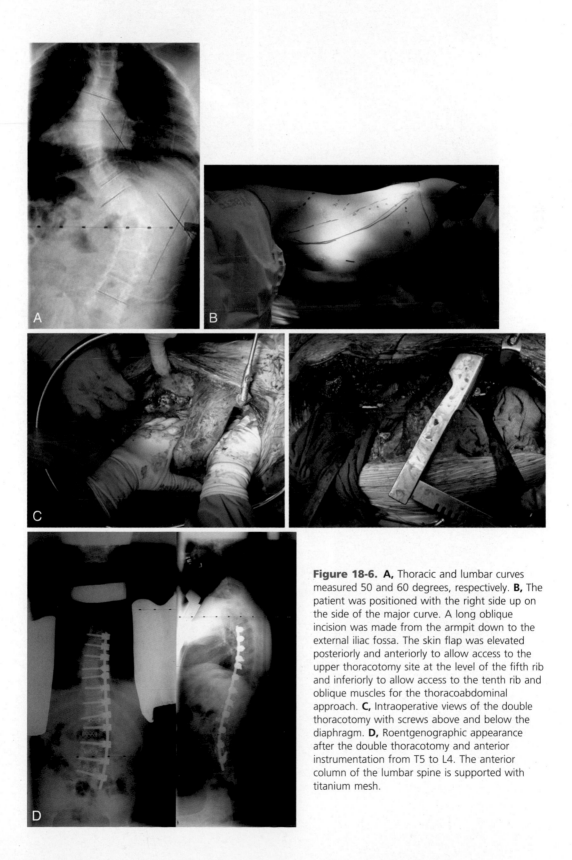

Figure 18-6. A, Thoracic and lumbar curves measured 50 and 60 degrees, respectively. **B,** The patient was positioned with the right side up on the side of the major curve. A long oblique incision was made from the armpit down to the external iliac fossa. The skin flap was elevated posteriorly and anteriorly to allow access to the upper thoracotomy site at the level of the fifth rib and inferiorly to allow access to the tenth rib and oblique muscles for the thoracoabdominal approach. **C,** Intraoperative views of the double thoracotomy with screws above and below the diaphragm. **D,** Roentgenographic appearance after the double thoracotomy and anterior instrumentation from T5 to L4. The anterior column of the lumbar spine is supported with titanium mesh.

CASE 5. An 8-Year-Old Girl with Thoracolumbar Lordosis

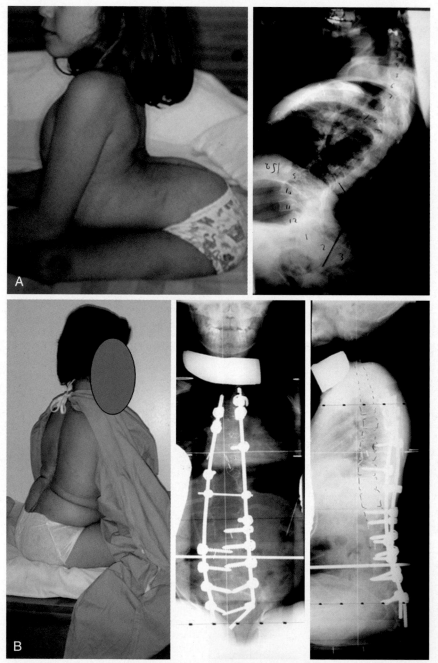

Figure 18-7. A, Preoperative clinical and roentgenographic views. **B,** Postoperative view following anterior wedge resection and posterior segmental instrumentation. The patient began to put on weight after the spinal procedure.

CASE 6. A 16-Year-Old Girl with Progressive Spinal Pelvic Obliquity, Inability to Sit Straight, and Lumbar Pain

The patient was ambulatory (L4 level).

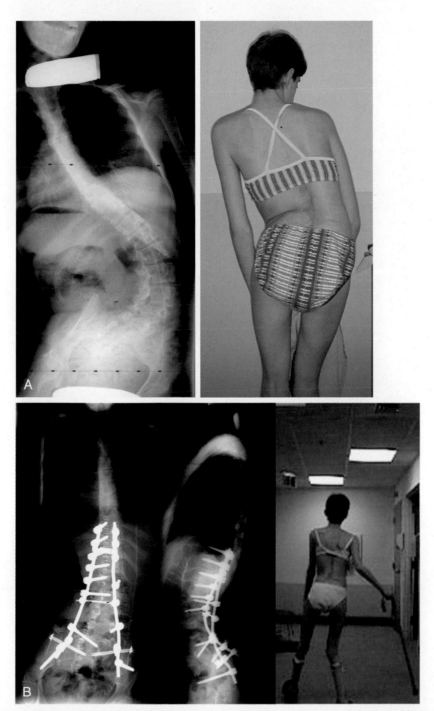

Figure 18-8. A, Preoperative static roentgenographic and clinical views. Her hips do not show any abduction/adduction contracture. **B**, After correction with posterior instrumentation and MW fixation, the patient could sit better but required a cane for balance and walking purposes. Her gait speed was decreased.

CASE 7. A 16-Year-Old Boy with Recurrent Pressure Sores over the Left Ischium and Multiple Past Neurosurgical Procedures

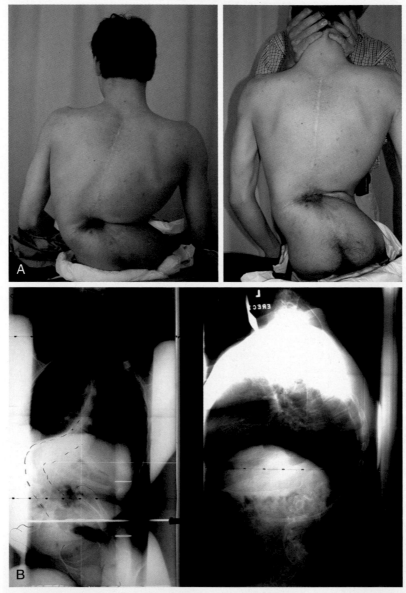

Figure 18-9. A, The pelvic obliquity was very stiff, as observed on the traction view (*right*). Because of the rigidity, an anterior release was performed first. **B,** Roentgenograms confirmed the magnitude of the curve and pelvic obliquity.

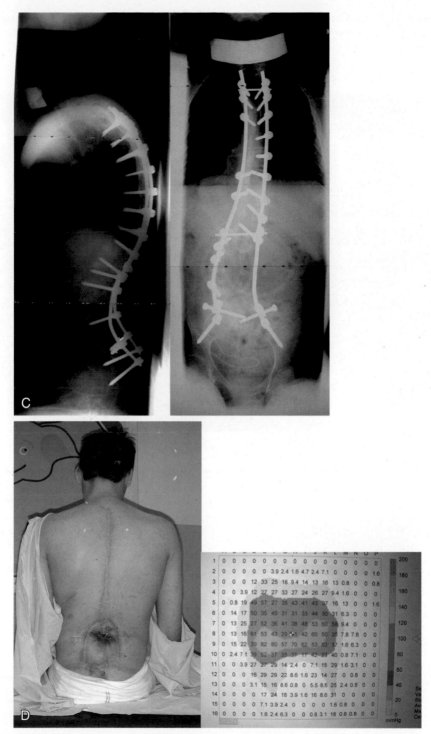

Figure 18-9, cont'd. C, Following anterior release of the thoracolumbar curve. the fusion was extended to the sacrum anteriorly through a tibial inlay graft from L4 to the sacrum. Posteriorly, the correction of the pelvic obliquity was achieved through MW fixation. **D,** Postoperatively, the patient's sitting balance was greatly improved, with a 100% correction of the pelvic obliquity, as shown in the clinical photograph and on the pressure mapping. Observe the reverse-Y incision with smooth edges used to avoid the poor skin area at the lumbosacral junction.

CASE 8. A 16-Year-Old Girl Requiring Revision for Return of Pelvic Obliquity and Pressure Sore

The patient had good quadriceps function on the left side and no strength on the right side. She was treated with spinal column resection at the L3 level and partial removal of the Dwyer instrumentation, followed by a posterior shortening procedure at L3 and long segmental instrumentation. The patient maintained her quadriceps function on the left side.

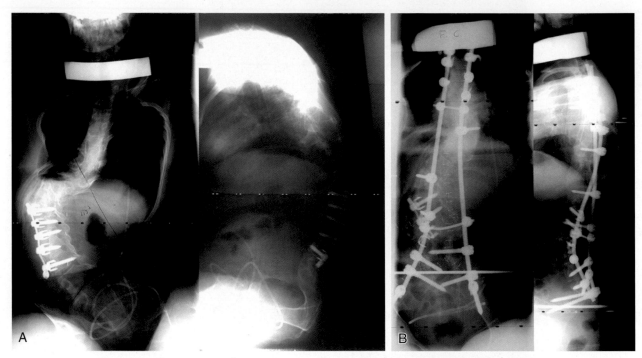

Figure 18-10. A, Preoperative roentgenographic view. **B**, Postoperative roentgenographic view.

REFERENCES

Arlet V, Marchesi D, Papin P, Aebi M: The "MW" sacropelvic construct: An enhanced fixation of the lumbosacral junction in neuromuscular pelvic obliquity. Eur Spine J 1999;8:229–231.

Basobas L, Mardjetko S, Hammerberg K, Lubicky J: Selective anterior fusion and instrumentation for the treatment of neuromuscular scoliosis. Spine 2003;28:S245–S248.

Brown HP: Management of spinal deformity in myelomeningocele. Orthop Clin North Am 1978;9:391–402.

Doers T, Walker JL, van den Brink K, et al: The progression of untreated lumbar kyphosis and the compensatory thoracic lordosis in myelomeningocele. Dev Med Child Neurol 1997;39:326–330.

Heydemann JS, Gillepsie R: Management of myelomeningocele kyphosis in the older child by kyphectomy and segmental spinal instrumentation. Spine 1987;12:37–41.

Hoppenfeld S: Congenital kyphosis in myelomeningocele. J Bone Joint Surg 1967;49:276–280.

Huang TJ, Lubicky JP: Kyphectomy and segmental spinal instrumentation in young children with myelomeningocele kyphosis. J Formos Med Assoc 1994;93:503–508.

Hull WJ, Moe JH, Lai C, Winter RB: The surgical treatment of spinal deformities in myelomeningocele. J Bone Joint Surg 1975;57A:1767.

Lowe GP, Menelaus MB: The surgical management of kyphosis in older children with myelomeningocele. J Bone Joint Surg 1978;60B: 40–45.

Martin J, Kumar SJ, Guille JT, et al: Congenital kyphosis in myelomeningocele: Results following operative and non-operative treatment. J Pediatr Orthop 1994;14:323–328.

Mintz LJ, Sarwak JF, Dias LS, Schafer MF: The natural history of congenital kyphosis in myelomeningocele: A review of 51 children. Spine 1991;16(suppl):348–350.

Nolden MT, Sarwark JF, Vora A, Grayhack JJ: A kyphectomy technique with reduced perioperative morbidity for myelomeningocele kyphosis. Spine 2002;27:1807–1813.

Odent T, Arlet V, Ouellet J, Bitan F: Kyphectomy in myelomeningocele with a modified Dunn-McCarthy technique followed by an anterior inlayed strut graft. Eur Spine J 13:2004:206–212.

Sharrard WJ: Spinal osteotomy for congenital kyphosis in myelomeningocele. J Bone Joint Surg 1968;50B:466–471.

Stella G, Ascani E, Cervellati S, et al: Surgical treatment of scoliosis associated with myelomeningocele. Eur J Pediatr Surg 1998;8(suppl)1: 22–25.

Thomsen M, Lang RD, Carstens C: Results of kyphectomy with the technique of Warmer and Fackler in children with myelodysplasia. J Pediatr Orthop B 2000;9:143–147.

Wild A, Haak H, Kumar M, Krauspe R: Is sacral instrumentation mandatory to address pelvic obliquity in neuromuscular thoracolumbar scoliosis due to myelomeningocele? Spine 2001;26:E325–E329.

SUGGESTED READINGS

Banta JV: Combined anterior and posterior fusion for spinal deformity in myelomeningocele. Spine 1990;15:946–952.

This author describes his surgical experience with 50 children who were treated with a combined anterior and posterior fusion. He concludes that anterior fusion of the dysraphic spine allows greater correction of both spinal deformity and pelvic obliquity in addition to contributing significant strength to the fusion mass. In addition, he determines that segmental spinal instrumentation with sublaminar and pedicular wiring to custom-contoured Luque rods provides excellent correction and immediate postoperative stability.

Bowman RM, McLone DG, Grant JA, et al: Spina bifida outcome: A 25-year prospective. Pediatr Neurosurg 2001;34:114–120.

This report outlines the 20- to 25-year outcomes of an original cohort of patients with a myelomeningocele treated in a nonselective, prospective manner. The authors conclude that at least 75% of children born with a myelomeningocele can be expected to reach their early adult years. Late deterioration is common. One of the greatest challenges in medicine today is establishing a network of care for these adults with spina bifida.

Crawford AH, Strub WM, Lewis R, et al: Neonatal kyphectomy in the patient with myelomeningocele. Spine 2003;28:260–266.

This is a retrospective cohort study that investigated a group of neonates with myelomeningocele who underwent a kyphectomy in conjunction with dural sac closure during the first few days of life. The study concludes that kyphectomy at the time of dural sac closure in the neonate is a safe procedure with excellent initial correction. However, eventual recurrence is expected.

Geiger F, Parsch D, Carstens C: Complications of scoliosis surgery in children with myelomeningocele. Eur Spine J 1999;8:22–26.

This study evaluates whether the high incidence of complications in scoliosis surgery in myelomeningocele could be attributed to the surgical technique and whether improvements are possible. The authors conclude that instrumented anterior and posterior fusion is justified in this group of patients, and they recommend the careful checking of shunt function prior to acute correction of spinal deformity.

Labbé AC, Demers AM, Rodrigues R, et al: Surgical wound infections following spinal fusion: A case-control study in a children's hospital. Infect Control Hosp Epidemiol 2003;24:591–595.

The objectives of this study were to determine the rates of surgical-site infections after spinal surgery and to identify the risk factors associated with infection. The authors conclude that patients with myelodysplasia are at a higher risk for surgical site infections after spinal fusion. Antibiotic prophylaxis may reduce the risk of infection, especially in high-risk patients such as those with myelodysplasia or those undergoing fusion involving the sacral area.

Lindseth RE, Stelzer L: Vertebral excision for kyphosis in children with myelomeningocele. J Bone Joint Surg 1979;61A:699–704.

This study compares three types of operations, all including vertebral-body excision, that were performed to decrease and stabilize the kyphosis in 23 children with myelomeningocele.

Lintner SA, Lindseth RE: Kyphotic deformity in patients who have myelomeningocele. J Bone Joint Surg 1994;76A:1301–1307.

This is a retrospective review of the results of resection of the lordotic segment cephalad to the apical vertebra of a kyphotic deformity in 39 patients who had had a myelomeningocele.

McCall RE: Modified Luque instrumentation after myelomeningocele kyphectomy. Spine 1998;23:1406–1411.

The study's objective was to evaluate long-term results of a vertebral resection with modified Luque fixation for the correction of myelomeningocele kyphotic deformity. It concludes that kyphectomy is an excellent method of correcting rigid kyphotic deformity in patients with myelodysplasia.

McCarthy RE, Bruffet WL, McCullough FL: S-rod fixation to the sacrum in patients with neuromuscular spinal deformities. Clin Orthop 1999;364:26–31.

This article describes a form of pelvic fixation that has been designed for use in patients with neuromuscular spinal deformities to overcome the problems imposed by the Galveston technique. One end of a Luque rod is bent into an S-shaped configuration and placed over the sacral ala, supplying firm fixation across the lumbosacral junction without crossing the sacroiliac joint.

McMaster MJ: The long-term results of kyphectomy and spinal stabilization in children with myelomeningocele. Spine 1998;13:417–424.

This study has a mean follow-up of 7 years and 4 months to skeletal maturity of patients who underwent resection of their kyphus, internal fixation, and spinal fusion. It describes the surgical and nonsurgical complications related to this technique.

Osebold WR, Mayfield JK, Winter RB, Moe JH: Surgical treatment of paralytic scoliosis associated with myelomeningocele. J Bone Joint Surg Am 1982;64:841–856.

This study describes the spines of forty patients with myelomeningocele and paralytic scoliosis that were surgically stabilized at the Twin Cities Scoliosis Center between 1960 and 1979 with a posterior spine fusion and Harrington instrumentation extending to the sacrum, combined with anterior fusion using either Dwyer or Zielke instrumentation.

Pierz K, Banta J, Thomson J, et al: The effect of tethered cord release on scoliosis in myelomeningocele. J Pediatr Orthop 2000;20:362–365.

To better understand the effects of detethering on scoliosis in persons with myelomeningocele, the authors retrospectively reviewed the cases of 21 patients with spinal dysraphism and scoliosis who had undergone a detethering procedure.

Schoenmakers MA, Gulmans VA, Gooskens RH, et al: Spinal fusion in children with spina bifida: Influence on ambulation level and functional abilities. Eur Spine J 2005;14:415–422.

The objective of this study was to determine the influence of spinal fusion on ambulation and functional abilities in children with spina bifida for whom early mobilization was stimulated. This study concludes that within the first 6 months after spinal fusion, more caregiver assistance is needed in self-care and mobility than was the case prior to surgery. It takes about 12 months for abilities to return to the presurgery level, with small improvements after this point.

Sharrard WJW, Drennan JC: Osteotomy: Excision of the spine for lumbar kyphosis in older children with myelomeningocele. J Bone Joint Surg Br 1972;54B:50–60.

This review paper describes the progressive development of deformity in congenital kyphosis in myelomeningocele in the newborn, as well as satisfactory methods for the management of associated conditions.

Sponseller PD, Young AT, Sarwark JF, Lim R: Anterior only fusion for scoliosis in patients with myelomeningocele. Clin Orthop Relat Res 1999;364:117–124.

This study includes a series of patients with single major scoliosis curvatures attributable to spina bifida who were treated by anterior-only spinal fusion. The patients were followed for 2 years to determine whether the infection rate could be decreased, adequate correction and pelvic balance could be provided, and posterior surgery could be avoided.

CHAPTER 19

Spinal Cord Injury

M. Darryl Antonacci

PEDIATRIC SPINAL POSTTRAUMATIC DEFORMITY

The majority of skeletally immature individuals will develop a spinal deformity after trauma to the spinal cord. For that reason, age at the time of a spinal cord injury (SCI) in children is the most important factor in determining the type of spinal deformity that may arise. If there is injury to the vertebral growth plates, asymmetric growth arrest is possible. Those with preexisting idiopathic scoliosis or kyphosis may undergo curve progression with the loss of normal muscle tone. Vertebral column deformity resulting from chronic instability of the initial injury and abnormalities that occur after surgical intervention can also contribute to the development of deformity. The individual and combinatorial consequences of poor truncal balance, muscle asymmetry, and spasticity over time in the growing child are the dominant, dynamic factors that are involved in the development of the various types of spinal deformities to which these children are susceptible and must be thoroughly appreciated.

Spinal deformity can lead to numerous and ongoing difficulties for those who are afflicted. Chronic pain (reported to be as high as 65% in the pediatric SCI population), pelvic obliquity, pressure ulcers, and systemic autonomic dysfunction are all possible sequelae of the alteration to normal neurologic function and spinal contours. These patients often become overly reliant on their upper extremities secondary to difficulty in sitting and an inability to depend on their lower extremities for many daily activities. Pressure ulcers typically form at the apex of the curve in those who develop kyphotic deformity and on the area of convexity in those with scoliosis; pressure ulcers can occur anywhere there is insensate skin.

Epidemiology

It is difficult to know the exact number of pediatric spinal cord injuries that occur annually, because it is presumed that many injuries go unreported or are not recognized because of undetected birth-related injuries, on-scene acci-

dent fatalities, and injuries associated with intentional trauma. With these gaps in incidence acknowledged, studies have reported the total SCI estimate to be as high as 20% within the pediatric population. No gender-specific differences have been observed in younger children; however, boys in the 10- to 16-year age group have been shown to be more susceptible to SCI, and violence has become the leading cause of SCI among African American and Hispanic teenage males. Cervical spine injuries account for one third of new SCI cases in those between 0 and 12 years of age and half of the cases reported in older age groups. SCI has also been reported to be neurologically complete in 69% of those 0 to 5 years and 51% in those older than 16 years. The primary mechanisms for injury in children younger than 10 years of age are falls and motor vehicle accidents. For those older than 10 years, motor vehicle accidents and sports-related injuries are the most common causes. Additional causes of pediatric SCI include birth injury, child abuse, cervical injuries attributed to skeletal dysplasias, juvenile rheumatoid arthritis, and Down syndrome.

Spinal cord injury without radiographic abnormality (SCIWORA) is a syndrome that is primarily isolated to children and is thought to occur because of the inherent elasticity of the ligamentous spine structures in children. Dislocation with spontaneous reduction of spinal osseous structures also can occur in the pediatric population and leave no evidence of injury on plain radiographs. SCIWORA has been found to occur in roughly 10% to 30% of pediatric SCIs. With advances in magnetic resonance imaging (MRI), however, SCIWORA is perhaps no longer as widely observed. Many spinal cord injuries that might have been classified as SCIWORA in the past are now demonstrable; even ligamentous injury can often be identified.

Natural History

The relationship between age at time of spinal cord injury and spinal deformity development and/or curve progression is well supported by investigative study. Lancourt and colleagues demonstrated the incidence of scoliosis to be 100% in children with injury before the age of 10 years, 18% in those between 10 and 16 years of age, and 12% in individuals with injury occurring at the age of 17 years. Additional studies have found a 97% occurrence of scoliosis in children who were injured prior to their adolescent growth spurt, a 91% incidence of deformity in preadolescent children with SCI, and a lower rate of 52% in those who were injured after the adolescent growth spurt. In addition, individuals with paraplegia and complete SCI have been shown to develop scoliosis more frequently and to a greater degree than those with tetraplegia and incomplete lesions, respectively, in the pediatric population.

Imaging

Imaging of a posttraumatic deformity begins with full-length anterior-posterior and lateral views of the spine to comprehensively evaluate the spinal balance of the patient. Ideally, these views should be obtained with the patient standing or sitting. Bending views in the coronal and sagittal planes are helpful to discern the flexibility of the deformity and to aid in planning the surgical approach. Films should be monitored over time for curve presence, magnitude, and progression compared to previous radiographs. Radiographs should be obtained every 3 months in preadolescents with curves greater than 20 degrees and every 6 months for curves less than 20 degrees. For mature patients with curves greater than 20 degrees, radiographs can be taken every 6 months, and for curves under 20 degrees, they can be taken once a year.

MRI also has a potential role in evaluating curve enlargement. If rapid curve progression is noted, an MRI should be obtained to assess possible intrathecal pathology such as tethered cord or the presence of a syrinx.

Nonoperative Management

Children with SCI should be monitored closely for the onset of spinal deformity, as it has been demonstrated that as many as 50% of preadolescent SCI patients require later spinal fusion. Prophylactic bracing for prevention of deformity in a child has a questionable history in terms of efficacy in avoiding curve progression. Traditionally, it has been espoused that at best, prophylactic bracing might delay curve progression and perhaps afford the child several more years of growth before fusion surgery is performed.

In a recent study, Mehta and colleagues found that prophylactic bracing of curves of less than 20 degrees significantly decreased the need for surgery. In their study, 46% of patients who were initially treated with bracing required surgery compared to 80% of those who were not braced. Time to surgical correction for those with a brace was also delayed in comparison to the nonbraced group. Similar to other studies, no benefit was demonstrated in terms of delaying or surgical spinal stabilization by bracing

patients with curves greater than 41 degrees. Interestingly, however, the authors also found no impact of bracing on delaying surgery in patients who ultimately required surgery for curves between 20 and 40 degrees. This is in contrast to traditional recommendations for delaying the bracing of scoliotic curves until the patient has developed a deformity of at least 20 degrees but less than 40 degrees. The aforementioned study is important because it shows the potential for early bracing to decrease the need for surgical intervention. If fusion procedures can be avoided, more spinal flexibility can be maintained. Maintenance of spinal flexibility and motion is vitally important in patients with paralytic scoliosis, regardless of etiology. Spinal motion is required for adequate function in many activities of daily living, including driving, feeding, bladder and bowel care, and pressure relief. Spinal fusion can also compromise the ability to correct sitting posture or compensate for a loss of balance and/or spasticity.

Operative Management

As many as 60% of patients with SCI will require stabilizing surgery if injury occurs more than 1 year before skeletal maturity, whereas there is less than a 5% chance that they will develop a scoliotic curve that requires surgery once they have reached skeletal maturity. The goals of surgery are to halt progression of deformity, correct sagittal and coronal contours, level pelvic obliquity, and achieve a solid arthrodesis. Surgery is recommended for patients who are older than 10 years of age with curves greater than 40 degrees. Prior to this age, attempts at bracing to delay surgical intervention should be aggressively pursued to prevent early cessation of trunk growth. Additional indications include curve progression, pain, interference with function, and ulcer development secondary to the deformity.

Because preservation of spine flexibility is of paramount importance, as short a segment as possible should be chosen for fusion while still allowing the goals of surgery to be achieved, regardless of surgical access approach employed. It has been suggested that fusion does not have to include fixation to the pelvis as long as pelvic obliquity is corrected to 5 to 10 degrees during correction of the spinal curve. Other clinicians have found that residual pelvic obliquity in patients fused at L4 or L5 is not a clinical problem. Preservation of the lumbosacral motion segment is desirable, particularly in patients who are able to walk. However, posterior instrumentation should include fixation to the pelvis when this is the only technique for adequate correction of the spinal curve and pelvic obliquity. Some authors advocate fixation to the pelvis using the Galveston technique with pedicle screws. Pedicle screws in the sacrum of some patients with long constructs cannot accept the forces to which they are subject and have been a source of instrument failure with loss of correction.

Anterior-posterior fusion is recommended for curves that are flexible to less than 60 degrees on bending films owing to the high incidence of the development of pseudarthrosis in these patients. In addition, children younger than 10 years of age with progressive curves of greater than 60 degrees are candidates for combined anterior-posterior fusions rather than posterior-alone surgery because of concerns about pseudarthrosis and for prevention of the crankshaft phenomenon.

Postoperative complications in SCI patients are markedly higher than those in patients with idiopathic scoliosis. Patients with SCI are often nutritionally and metabolically compromised, are often osteopenic, and have poor muscle and vasomotor tone as well as respiratory insufficiency and chronic urinary tract infections. As a result, these patients are at increased risk for infection, pseudarthrosis, delayed wound healing, hardware failure, and progression of their scoliosis above and below the fusion levels. It has been suggested that these complications can be minimized by the use of combined anterior-posterior approaches utilizing rigid segmental fixation systems with adequate bone graft to reduce pseudarthrosis rates, custom-made orthotics for equalized support and skin sparing, and preoperative treatment of urinary tract infections.

ADULT SPINAL POSTTRAUMATIC DEFORMITY

Kyphotic deformity of the spine is the most common imbalance to develop following the occurrence of burst fracture. To appreciate the clinical and radiographic consequences of this outcome, it is necessary to understand what is considered normal from the perspective of the sagittal plane. In a study of 100 asymptomatic individuals more than 40 years of age, the mean thoracic kyphosis was 34 degrees (T5-12) and the lumbar lordosis was −64 degrees (bottom of T12 to top of the sacrum). When segmental sagittal plane alterations occur, regardless of cause, adjacent vertebral levels adjust to these changes with potentially disadvantaged compensatory angulation. As a result, a kyphotic deformity will cause hyperextension of adjacent segments and predispose the spine to altered facet joint kinematics, spinous process abutment, and heightened intervertebral shear with listhesis. The recruitment of adjacent segments therefore accelerates the degenerative process.

The majority of spinal fractures occur between the levels of T11 and L4. Approximately 14% to 17% of these fractures are classified as burst fractures. This region of the spine is particularly vulnerable to injury because of several factors. Beginning at the level of T11, the support that is provided by the ribs and musculature of the upper thoracic spine is no longer present. In addition, the contour of the spine transitions from the kyphotic curvature of the thoracic spine to a lordotic curvature in the lumbar spine, and facet orientation changes from coronal in the thoracic spine to sagittal in the lumbar spine. These anatomic changes increase spinal mobility in the thoracolumbar spine, exposing this area to large amounts of stress.

The treatment of burst fractures has been controversial, with proponents of both operative and nonoperative management. Generally accepted indications for surgical stabilization include new onset or progression of neurologic deficit, localized kyphotic deformity of greater than 30 degrees, canal compromise of more than 50%, and progression of deformity over time. Fortunately, only a small percentage of burst fracture patients meet these criteria, and it is the remaining majority of cases in which management debate continues.

Investigations that support operative management of burst fractures include a retrospective study by Denis and colleagues that contrasted nonoperative with operative treatment of 104 patients with burst fractures. This study found that all patients who were treated operatively experienced no neurologic sequelae, while 17% of those who were treated nonoperatively suffered neurologic deterioration. The authors concluded that stabilization and fusion of acute burst fractures without neurologic deficit had a significant advantage over conservative management. Other studies also have recommended operative treatment in most burst fracture patterns for the prevention of neurologic compromise, posttraumatic kyphosis, mechanical back pain, and the initiation of earlier ambulation.

In support of nonoperative management, Krompinger and coworkers performed a study in which patients were managed nonoperatively if they were found to have "stable" burst fractures. In this study, a stable burst fracture was defined as a two-column injury with a canal compromise of less than 50% and a kyphosis of less than 30% in neurologically intact patients. As a result, none of the patients who were managed nonoperatively showed neurologic deterioration, and only 10% were not able to return to work because of pain. Additional studies comparing nonoperative and operative management of burst fractures have found no significant difference in outcome in ability to return to work, activity level, pain level, or quality of life. In the only prospective, randomized study comparing nonoperative to operative treatment of thoracolumbar burst fractures without neurologic deficit, Wood and coworkers found that there was no significant difference in return to work or pain scores, regardless of management. This study concluded that there was no long-term advantage of operative over nonoperative treatment.

Although rare, posttraumatic deformity following burst fracture is a difficult problem. The occurrence of deformity can be attributed to unrecognized instability in the spinal column. As a result, fractures that might appear stable gradually progress to deformity after continued exposure to physiologic stresses. Furthermore, incompetency of the posterior ligamentous complex might not be appreciated when a three-column injury is present. These are instances in which nonoperative treatment can lead to a posttraumatic kyphotic deformity; however, deformity can also occur after surgery in the setting of nonunion, implant failure, or technical error.

Epidemiology

The Scoliosis Research Society Multi-Center Spine Fracture Study, published in 1991, studied 1019 spinal fractures. This study attributed 51% of fractures to motor vehicle accidents, 34% to falls, 5% to work-related events, 2% to incidents at home, and 8% to other causes. Roughly 90% of all spinal fractures occur between the levels of T11 and L4, 14% to 17% of these being burst fractures.

Imaging

Full-length anteroposterior and lateral radiographs are obtained to fully assess the spinal balance of adult SCI patients. Bending views are particularly helpful in the coronal and sagittal planes to evaluate spinal flexibility relative to the extant deformity and to facilitate surgical approach planning.

Computed tomography (CT) is an excellent method for visualizing the bony elements of the spine. In burst fractures, it is important to evaluate the condition of the posterior vertebral body. Often, the damage to this area is difficult to quantify on plain radiographs, and the integrity of this structure as well as the degree of canal compromise can be more reliably evaluated by CT.

MRI plays a very important role in the evaluation of these fractures as well. The excellent soft-tissue definition that is available with MRI makes this imaging mode essential to perform in burst fracture patients, particularly if the status of the posterior ligamentous structures is in question. Identifying this soft-tissue component of the injury is especially important in deciding on the treatment for this fracture. In addition, as with all spinal neurologic pathologies, MRI is helpful in detecting intrathecal lesions and in understanding the potential consequences of neural compression if spinal column manipulation is undertaken to correct a deformity.

Nonoperative Treatment

Nonoperative management has the advantage of avoiding the morbidity associated with a surgical procedure. Although there is no uniformly agreed-on approach to nonoperative management, kinetic bed therapy, body casting, and thoracolumbar orthoses are popular methods that are typically preceded by several days of bed rest.

One advantage of a body cast is the potential to reduce kyphosis by applying an anterior force while the patient is in a supine position on a Risser cast table. Also, cast treatment increases compliance, leading to more predictable results. The benefit of an orthosis is that it can be removed for hygiene maintenance, although compliance with 24-hour wear is an issue. Wood and coworkers followed a protocol that incorporated patient immobilization in a cast for 4 to 8 weeks during early fracture consolidation, followed by conversion to a removable brace when radiographic and clinical symptoms allow.

Operative Treatment

When operative management of posttraumatic deformity is indicated, a number of procedures have been advocated, including stand-alone posterior instrumented fusion, stand-alone anterior fusion with or without decompression, transforaminal interbody fusion with posterolateral fusion, pedicle-subtraction osteotomy, and combinations of differing anterior-posterior procedures.

Indications for surgical treatment of a kyphotic spinal deformity include localized kyphotic deformity of 30 degrees or greater, new onset or progression of neurologic deficit, or progressive worsening of kyphosis over time. Operative complications of posttraumatic deformity include risk of neurologic injury as a result of the overlay of the neural elements on the anterior vertebral bony processes and of scarring with spinal cord tethering.

Relying on posterior fusion alone in a kyphotic deformity is a risky endeavor, as it might not allow for ideal correction and stabilization of late posttraumatic thoracolumbar kyphotic deformity. This approach places large tension forces on the instrumentation, because the bending moments oppose the corrective forces that are needed to obtain spinal alignment. Similarly, for fixed kyphotic deformity, an anterior-only approach leads to a less reliable and, perhaps, inadequate correction. Often, a combination of anterior release and anterior column reconstruction with posterior instrumentation and fusion is necessary to obtain complete and lasting deformity correction.

A bilateral transforaminal approach has the advantage of an indirect circumferential fusion. In this procedure, far-lateral access portals are used to place structural interbody grafts. These grafts provide an anterior pivot point around which compressive posterior instrumentation can provide an opposing lordotic effect to the kyphotic deformity. The all-posterior approach is appealing for patients who have contraindications to anterior surgery. However, because the posterior approach does not allow for the release of contracted anterior structures, it might not be ideal for fixed deformities.

Pedicle subtraction osteotomy is an option that allows for a localized and large-degree correction of a kyphotic deformity through a posterior approach alone. Lehmer and colleagues performed 45 transvertebral osteotomies, 21 of which were done for thoracolumbar kyphosis resulting from old fractures. An average of 35 degrees of correction was obtained at each level. The authors contend that their approach allows for greater correction for a more localized deformity because the fulcrum is more anterior than the middle column fulcrum that is used in the Smith-Peterson osteotomy. The results of the pedicle-subtraction osteotomy are large, local, single-level corrections, thereby making the technique useful in acute angle kyphotic deformities. In addition, a single-staged posterior approach may result in lower morbidity for the patient. However, the procedure is technically difficult, and there is potential for significant blood loss. Furthermore, the single-segment restoration of sagittal balance is nonphysiologic, and there are limited spinal sites for safe application.

The back-front-back procedure provides the best option for complete correction of a high-magnitude kyphotic deformity. In this procedure, facetectomies and/or osteotomies are performed first via a posterior approach to remove anything that could block the eventual correction. Next, anterior release and correction of the kyphotic deformity are performed, followed by posterior instrumentation and fusion for the restoration of the posterior tension band. Steps and timing of the procedure are surgeon-dependent although the initial posterior and anterior surgeries are often performed in the same day. The obvious disadvantages to this procedure include prolonged anesthesia and the potential for large amounts of blood loss.

- Age at the time of SCI in children is the most important factor determining the onset of posttraumatic deformity. Sixty percent of patients with SCI will require surgical stabilization if injury occurs more than one year before skeletal maturity.
- SCIWORA is a result of the inherent elasticity of the ligamentous spine structures in children. This diagnosis must be considered in all pediatric trauma patients.
- Recent work has shown that bracing curves of less than 20 degrees in pediatric SCI patients decreases the need for subsequent surgery.
- Kyphotic deformity of the spine is the most common imbalance following a burst fracture.
- The majority of all spinal fractures occur between T11 and L4. This is a result of increased spinal mobility due to anatomic changes along the transition from the thoracic to the lumbar spine.

Illustrative Case Presentations

CASE 1. A Child with a Spinal Cord Injury Who Developed Posttraumatic Scoliosis

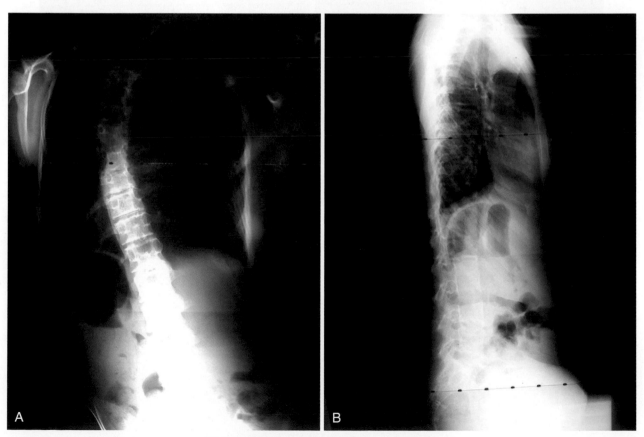

Figure 19-1. A and **B,** Preoperative radiographs.

Continued

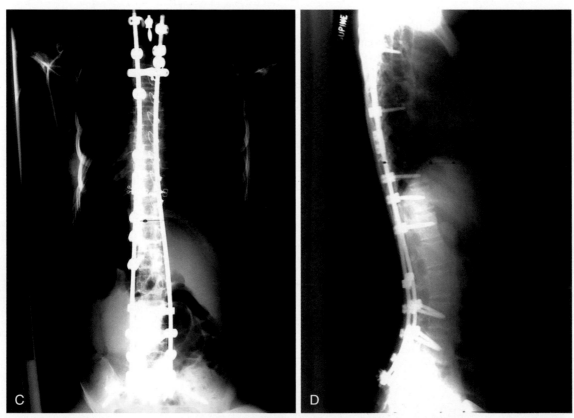

Figure 19-1, cont'd. Postoperative AP (**C**) and lateral (**D**) views. Posterior instrumentation and fusion to the pelvis were performed. Lumbar lordosis should be kept at a minimum to assist sitting posture and wheelchair use.

CASE 2. A 70-Year-Old Obese Female

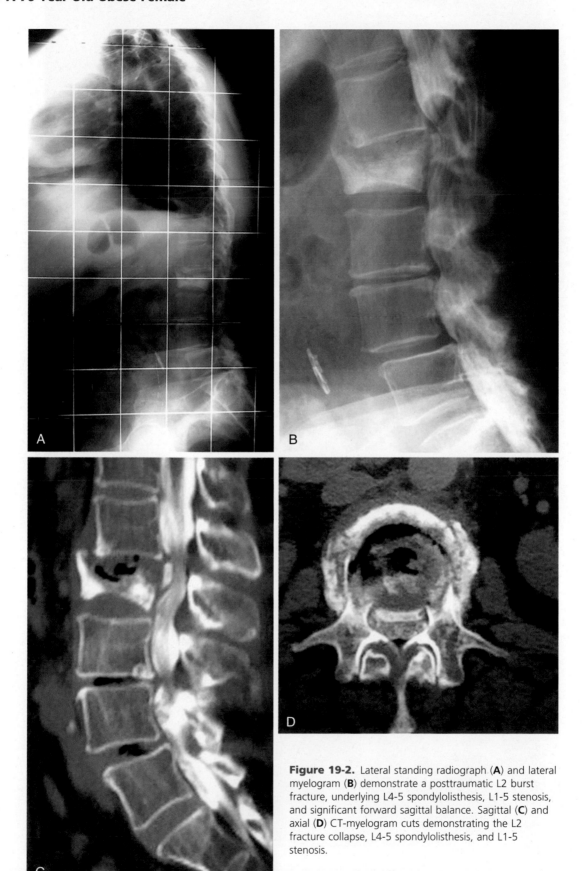

Figure 19-2. Lateral standing radiograph (**A**) and lateral myelogram (**B**) demonstrate a posttraumatic L2 burst fracture, underlying L4-5 spondylolisthesis, L1-5 stenosis, and significant forward sagittal balance. Sagittal (**C**) and axial (**D**) CT-myelogram cuts demonstrating the L2 fracture collapse, L4-5 spondylolisthesis, and L1-5 stenosis.

Continued

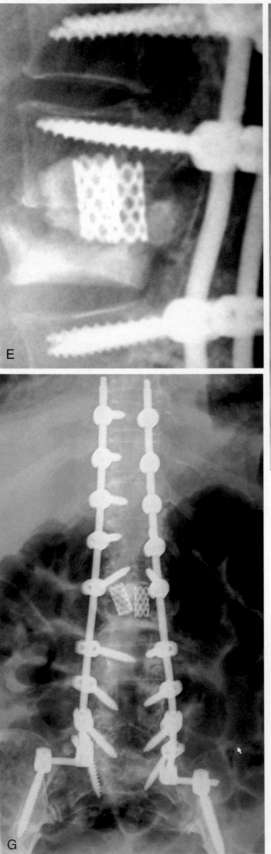

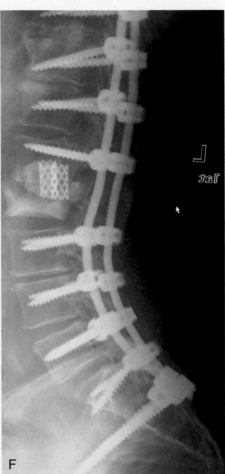

Figure 19-2, cont'd. Postoperative lateral (**E** and **F**) and AP (**G**) radiographs demonstrating partial L2 corpectomy and interbody Harms cages filled with bone cement on one side and autograft on the other via a posterior-only approach. Note lumbar central and lateral recess decompression at L1-5. Posterior spinal instrumentation and fusion from T9 to the pelvis with restoration of sagittal balance. The patient was informed but did not require possible anterior interbody support at L4-5, L5-S1.

REFERENCES

Angtuaco EC, Binet EF: Radiology of thoracic and lumbar fractures. Clin Orthop Relat Res 1984;189:43 57.

Campbell J, Bonnet C: Spinal cord injury in children. Clin Orthop 1975;112:114–123.

Denis F: The three column spine and its significance in the classification of acute thoracolumbar spinal injuries. Spine 1983;8:817–831.

Gertzbein SD: Scoliosis Research Society: Multicenter spine fracture study. Spine 1992;17:528–540.

Jacobs RR, Casey MP: Surgical management of thoracolumbar spinal injuries: General principles and controversial considerations. Clin Orthop Relat Res 1984;189:22–35

Kilfoyle RM, Foley JJ, Norton PL: Spine and pelvic deformity in childhood and adolescent paraplegia: A study of 104 cases. J Bone Joint Surg 1965;47A:659–682.

Kriss VM, Kriss TC: SCIWORA (spinal cord injury without radiographic abnormality) in infants and children. Clin Pediatr 1996;35: 119–124.

Lubicky JP, Betz RR: Spinal deformity in children and adolescents after spinal cord injury. In Betz RR, Mulcahey MJ (eds): The Child with a Spinal Cord Injury. Rosemont, IL: AAOS, 1996, pp 363–370.

Pang D, Wilberger JE Jr: Spinal cord injury without radiographic abnormalities in children. J Neurosurg 1982;57:114–129.

Polly DW, Klemme WR, Shawen S: Management options for the treatment of posttraumatic thoracolumbar kyphosis. Sem Spine Surg 2000;12:110–116.

Renshaw TS: Paralysis in the child: Orthopaedic management. In Bradford DS, Hensinger RM (eds): The Pediatric Spine. New York: Thieme, pp 118–128.

Roberson JR, Whitesides TE: Surgical reconstruction of late posttraumatic thoracolumbar kyphosis. Spine 1985;10:307–312.

Vaccaro AR, Silber JS: Post-traumatic spinal deformity. Spine 2001;26: S111–S118.

White AA, Panjabi MM: The basic kinematics of the human spine: A review of past and current knowledge. Spine 1978;3:12–20.

SUGGESTED READINGS

Bergstrom EK, Short DJ, Frankel HL, et al: The effect of childhood spinal cord injury on skeletal development: A retrospective study. Spinal Cord 1999;37:838–846.

A cross-sectional clinical review of 80 patients with acute onset of SCI before 6 years of age was performed. Scoliosis was found to occur more frequently and be more severe in those who were injured at a younger age, in paraplegics compared to tetraplegics, and in those with complete lesions compared to those with incomplete lesions.

Dearolf WW 3rd, Betz RR, Vogel LC, et al: Scoliosis in pediatric spinal cord-injured patients. J Pediatr Orthop 1990;10:214–218.

One hundred thirty children with SCI between birth and 21 years of age were reviewed to determine the progression rate of paralytic scoliosis and the effects of bracing surgery. Scoliosis develop in 97% of those who were injured prior to the adolescent growth spurt and in 52% of those who were injured after the growth spurt. Bracing was found to be effective in delaying progression in the preadolescent group.

Denis F, Armstrong GW, Searls K, Matta L: Acute thoracolumbar burst fractures in the absence of neurologic deficit: A comparison between operative and nonoperative treatment. Clin Orthop Relat Res 1984;189:142–149.

This study compared nonoperative with operative treatment of 104 patients with burst fractures. None of the patients who were treated operatively experienced neurologic sequelae, while 17% of those who were treated nonoperatively suffered neurologic deterioration. The authors concluded that stabilization and fusion of acute burst fractures without neurologic deficit had significant advantages over conservative management.

DeVivo MJ, Vogel LC: Epidemiology of spinal cord injury in children and adolescents. J Spinal Cord Med 2004;27(suppl 1):S4–S10.

The authors analyzing SCI patients from the Shriners Hospitals for Children SCI database or the National SCI Statistical Center database over a 30-year period. They found that one third of new cases of SCI, from age 0 to 12 years, were due to cervical injuries, compared to one half in those greater than 13 years of age. They also found that SCI was more likely to be complete in younger patients.

Dickman CA, Zabramski JM, Hadley MN, et al: Pediatric spinal cord injury without radiographic abnormalities: Report of 26 cases and review of the literature. J Spinal Disord 1991;4:296–305.

One hundred fifty-nine pediatric patients with acute SCI were studied. Sixteen percent of these patients sustained a SCIWORA. Thirty-two percent of these patients were younger, and 70% of these sustained complete injury. SCIWORA accounted for only 12% of injuries in the older children and was rarely associated with a complete injury.

Finch GD, Barnes MJ: Major cervical spine injuries in children and adolescents. J Pediatr Orthop 1998;18:811–814.

A population-based study of pediatric cervical spine trauma studied 32 patients younger than 15 years of age at the time of injury. Children younger than 10 years of age were found to sustain injury most commonly as a result of motor vehicle accidents, while sports or recreational activities were the main cause in those older than 10 years of age.

Gelb DE, Lenke LG, Brdwell KH, et al: An analysis of sagittal spinal alignment in 100 asymptomatic middle and older aged volunteers. Spine 1995;20:1351–1358.

One hundred adults older than age 40 years without spinal abnormality were radiographically evaluated to determine indices of sagittal spinal alignment. The authors found that total lumbar lordosis (T12–S1) averaged −64 ± 10 degrees. Lordosis increased with distal progression through the lumbar spine. Increasing age correlated to a more forward sagittal vertical axis.

Hamilton MG, Myles ST: Pediatric spinal injury: Review of 174 hospital admissions. J Neurosurg 1992;77:700–704.

A review of 174 pediatric patients with injury to the spinal column and spinal cord. SCI was found to be present in 45% of patients. Younger patients were found to be less likely to have spinal injury but had a higher incidence of neurologic injury. Anatomic and biomechanical factors are discussed as reasons for these outcomes.

Jan FK, Wilson PE: A survey of chronic pain in the pediatric spinal cord injury population. J Spinal Cord Med 2004;27(suppl 1): S50–S53.

Utilizing the Adolescent Pediatric Pain Tool and Lansky Play Performance Scale, 31 patients from age 5 months to 18 years were studied. Sixty-five percent reported chronic pain. Pain reports were classified as 48% nociceptive and 19% neuropathic. Interference with activities of daily living and play was present in only one patient. The incidence of pain in this population was found to correlate with pain in adult-onset SCI.

Knight RQ, Stornelli DP, Chan DP, et al: Comparison of operative versus nonoperative treatment of lumbar burst fractures. Clin Orthop Relat Res 1993;293:112–121.

This retrospective study looked at 22 patients with lumbar burst fractures who were treated operatively versus nonoperatively. This study found no significant difference in outcome in ability to return to work, activity level, pain level, or quality of life.

Kraemer WJ, Schemitsch EH: Functional outcome of thoracolumbar burst fractures without neurological deficit. J Orthop Trauma 1996; 10:541–544.

This study evaluated the functional outcome of 24 patients with thoracolumbar burst fractures without a neurologic deficit using the SF-36 survey and the Roland scale with a minimum 2-year follow-up. This study found no significant difference in the functional outcome of patients who were treated operatively versus nonoperatively.

Krompinger WJ, Fredrickson BE, Mino DE, Yuan HA: Conservative treatment of fractures of the thoracic and lumbar spine. Orthop Clin North Am 1986;17:161–170.

In this study, patients were managed nonoperatively if they were found to have a stable burst fracture, which the authors define as a two-column injury with canal compromise less than 50% and kyphosis less than 30% in a patient who was neurologically intact. None of the patients who were managed nonoperatively showed neurologic deterioration, and only 10% were unable to return to work because of pain.

Lancourt JE, Dickson JH, Carter RE: Paralytic spinal deformity following traumatic spinal-cord injury in children and adolescents. J Bone Joint Surg 1981;63A:47–53.

Fifty children with spinal cord injury occurring from the time of birth until the age of 17 years were evaluated for the effect of loss of muscular support on the spinal column. Age at injury was the most important risk factor for the development of scoliosis, with spasticity also significant. Forty children with SCI between the ages of birth and 18 years were reviewed.

Lehmer SM, Keppler L, Biscup RS, et al: Posterior transvertebral osteotomy for adult thoracolumbar kyphosis. Spine 1994;19:2060–2067.

This retrospective case study examined the single-stage posterior transvertebral closing-wedge osteotomy for adult thoracolumbar kyphosis on 38 patients who were available for follow-up. All patients achieved union. Ninety-three percent maintained correction averaging 35 degrees, with three patients requiring revision. Of the total, 19.5% had new neurologic deficits. Seventy-six percent of patients stated that they would repeat the surgery, and 90% said that they would recommend it to another.

Malcolm BW, Bradford DS, Winter RB, Chou SN: Post-traumatic kyphosis: A review of forty-eight surgically treated patients. J Bone Joint Surg Am 1981;63:891–899.

Forty-eight patients who were treated surgically for symptomatic posttraumatic kyphosis of the thoracic or lumbar spine 6 months or longer after the initial injury were reviewed. Presenting signs and symptoms include pain in 94%, kyphosis progression in 46%, instability in 36%, and increasing neural deficit in 27%. Posterior fusion and combined anterior and posterior fusion resulted in primary fusion in all patients. Anterior fusion alone failed in 50%. Average final deformity correction was 26%. Pain was significantly reduced in 31% and completely relieved in 67%.

Mayfield JK, Erkkila JC, Winter RB: Spine deformity subsequent to acquired childhood spinal cord injury. J Bone Joint Surg 1981;63A:1401–1411.

The cases of 40 children who had incurred a spinal cord injury between birth and the age of 18 years were reviewed for subsequent deformity at an average of 10 years after injury. All children who were injured before the adolescent growth spurt developed paralytic deformity. Scoliosis developed in 64%, lumbar lordosis developed in 20%, and 68% required spine fusion.

McAfee PC, Yuan HA, Lasda NA: The unstable burst fracture. Spine 1982;7:365–373.

With the goal of providing an optimal environment for neurologic recovery, 16 patients with unstable burst fractures of the thoracolumbar junction were treated with a modified posterolateral decompression and Harrington rod instrumentation. All 12 patients with neurologic deficits in this study improved postoperatively, including 5 of 8 with conus medullaris lesions who had a full recovery. The authors conclude that one-stage decompression and stabilization reduces the incidence of progressive kyphosis, neurologic deterioration, and mechanical back pain common in both conservative treatment and with wide laminectomy.

Mehta S, Betz RR, Mulcahey MJ, et al: Effect of bracing on paralytic scoliosis secondary to spinal cord injury. J Spinal Cord Med 2004; 27(suppl 1):S88–S92.

One hundred and twenty-three patients with cervical or thoracic SCI prior to skeletal maturity were reviewed to examine the effect of early bracing in preventing or delaying surgical fusion. The authors found that bracing of curves less than 20 degrees delayed the time to surgical correction of the deformity and that bracing of curves less than 10 degrees could prevent the need for surgery at all. Bracing for curves greater than 20 degrees did not seem to prevent surgery or delay time to surgical correction.

Wood K, Buttermann G, Mehbod A, et al: Operative compared with nonoperative treatment of a thoracolumbar burst fracture without neurological deficit. J Bone Joint Surg Am 2003;85A:773–781.

This prospective, randomized study compared operative versus nonoperative treatment of 47 consecutive patients with a stable thoracolumbar burst fracture in the absence of neurologic deficits. The average follow-up was 44 months. In the operative group, the average fracture kyphosis was 10.1 degrees at the time of admission and 13 degrees at the final follow-up. Canal compromise was 39% at admission and improved to 22% at the final follow-up. In the nonoperative group, the average kyphosis was 11.3 degrees at admission and 13.8 degrees at final follow-up. The average canal compromise was 34% at the time of admission and 19% at final follow-up. No significant difference was found in return-to-work time or pain scores. Patients who were treated nonoperatively reported less disability. The authors concluded that there was no long-term advantage of operative over nonoperative treatment.

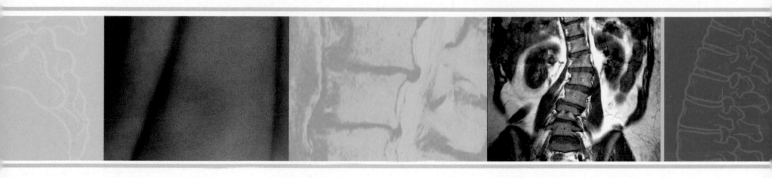

Adult Deformity

CHAPTER 20

Adult Idiopathic Scoliosis and Degenerative Scoliosis

JOHN P. KOSTUIK *and* THOMAS J. ERRICO

ADULT IDIOPATHIC SCOLIOSIS

Overview

Adult scoliosis is generally defined as a scoliotic deformity that is present after skeletal maturity, regardless of etiology or age at development (birth through adolescence or de novo after skeletal maturity). Adult spinal deformity can be subclassified into three further subsets: (1) curves that develop prior to skeletal maturity, which are usually idiopathic but may be due to congenital or neuromuscular causes; (2) curves that develop after skeletal maturity, which are typically secondary to degeneration, osteoporosis, or osteomalacia or follow extensive surgical decompression, usually for spinal stenosis; and (3) curves that develop in adults who underwent surgical treatment for scoliosis, in either the pediatric or adult age group, who present later in life with complications of spinal fusion. In this last group, the most common problems are iatrogenic flat back and accelerated degeneration of mobile adjacent vertebral segments.

Forty-five years ago, most experts believed that surgical treatment of scoliosis for adults was not indicated, with the notable exception of a patient with a progressive thoracic curve in the third decade of life, usually of idiopathic origin. Numerous clinical investigators showed that idiopathic curves could progress in the adult and might become the source of adverse clinical symptoms. Despite this, persistent conservative care was advocated by many experts who were concerned about the risks for scoliosis surgery in adults. For complicated adult curves, risks have been estimated to be 5% for death, 6% for neurologic damage, 20% for significant loss of correction, 10% for deep infection, and 40% for general postoperative medical problems.

A more aggressive and more effective surgical approach to these adult deformities ultimately became possible, first with the advent of Harrington rods, followed by the many subsequent later improvements in spinal instrumentation, such as the devices designed by Dwyer, Luque, Zielke, and Cotrel-Dubousset (Fig. 20-1). These fixation devices have overcome numerous prior technical obstacles to successful surgical treatment. At the same time, perioperative-related improvements in preoperative assessment, anesthetic techniques and intraoperative management, and spinal cord monitoring, combined with a better understanding of postoperative care, also have markedly improved our ability to deal with the complex problems of adult spinal deformities. As experience accumulated with adult patients, surgical correction was able to be offered beyond the more common idiopathic curves to include congenital curves that are usually associated with marked rigidity and kyphosis, as well as more complex neuromuscular disorders. Today, this capability is recognized not only by orthopedists but also by family physicians, internists, and, most important, patients. The field of treatment for adult scoliosis has a modern, sophisticated armamentarium and an improved success and safety record. The education of patients and physicians remains important to adequate surveillance and treatment of this condition and its contemporary issues.

Magnitude of the Current Problem

The harmful impact of progressive curvature and disability should not be underestimated in the adult patient population. Patients come to the treating physician with significant concerns of increasing pain, disturbed activities of daily living, progressing deformity, and rational and sometimes irrational concerns about the future. Patients might have recollections of a relative with a severe deformity and have fear that they are developing a similar problem. They sometimes have visions of severe debilitation, including becoming wheelchair dependent or even paraplegic. Their awareness of their loss of height and a visible cosmetic deformity is a major factor for both female and male patients. Before we discuss surgical treatments of this dis-

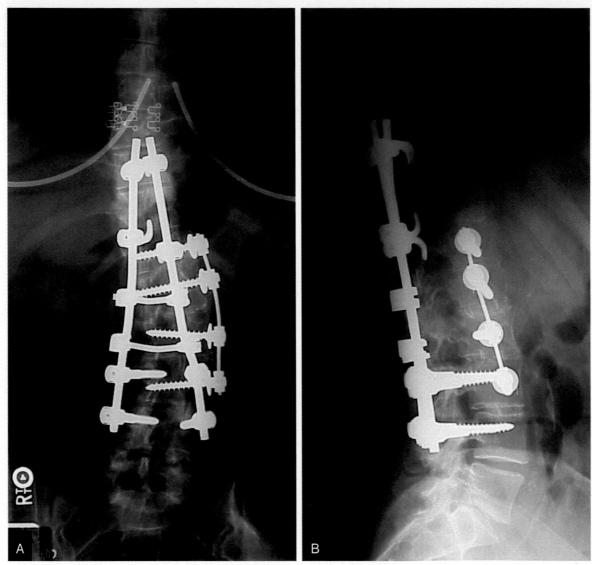

Figure 20-1. Anteroposterior (**A**) and lateral (**B**) radiographs of an anterior Zielke rod construct supplemented with a posterior Cotrel-Dubousset instrumentation and fusion.

order, it is important to understand the nature and validity of these and other patient concerns.

Incidence and Prevalence

It is generally accepted that the prevalence of curves involving the adult thoracic, thoracolumbar, and lumbar spines ranges from 1.9% to 15%. Controversy has existed as to whether a scoliotic deformity can arise de novo in later adult life. There are certainly patients whose previous radiographs show a straight lumbar spine that subsequently developed a scoliosis. It is generally thought that the majority of adult-onset lumbar scoliosis patients had a pre-existing minor lumbar curve. The prevalence of lumbar curves changes with age, starting with 2% before age 45 years and increasing to 15% after age 60. Not only does the prevalence change with age, but so does the severity of the curve(s), which shows a correlation between the Cobb angle and progression of age. The most severe curves demonstrate a predilection for females over males, but the reason is unknown. Not only do female patients have larger curves, but they more frequently complain of radicular symptoms than their male counterparts do.

Curve Progression

Despite the increased knowledge about risk factors for progression in adolescent idiopathic scoliosis that theoretically might reduce progression in some number of adults, it is not uncommon for the spinal surgeon to be presented with an adult patient with progressive scoliosis, increasing pain, loss of lumbar lordosis, or truncal imbalance. The adolescent patient with the worst prognosis for later difficulty as an adult is the one who presents with an imbalanced lumbar or thoracolumbar curve, an L5 vertebra that is not parallel to the sacrum, and a curve emanating from the lumbosacral junction. This last curve pattern presents the greatest technical difficulty for correction in the older adult and is therefore best treated surgically during adolescence rather than deferring treatment to adulthood.

Risk factors that are responsible for continued curve progression in adult life have also been determined. Thoracic curves between 50 and 75 degrees at skeletal maturity have been found to increase an average of 30 degrees over a lengthy follow-up interval. Thoracolumbar curves, 50 to 75 degrees at skeletal maturity, have also been observed to increase 22.3 degrees over the next 40 years. Lumbar curves progress the most, especially when the fifth lumbar vertebra is not well seated and the apical rotation is greater than 33%. As a general rule, it is reasonable to assume that most curves over 45 to 50 degrees at skeletal maturity will progress, on average (Fig. 20-2). Knowledge of these presentations and other factors can be used to address management of pain and disability more cogently.

Spine-Related Pain

A variety of factors have been analyzed to determine which might be important in pain complaints. Age is relevant, as in all spinal disorders. Pain also appears to reach its maximum intensity between the ages of 40 and 60 years; approximately 50% to 60% of these patients experience a level of substantial pain at one point in their lives. When the curves are greater than 45 degrees, the prevalence and severity of pain complaints increase significantly.

A comparison of patients with idiopathic scoliosis who were followed into adulthood with patients who do not have scoliosis shows a higher incidence of back pain in scoliotics. The intensity of pain is greater in the scoliosis subjects, is more continuous and generalized, and tends to have more of a neurogenic component. Radicular symptoms are more common in unstable deformities and often emanate from the L3-4 level. Particularly problematic for the treating physician is the patient who also exhibits a

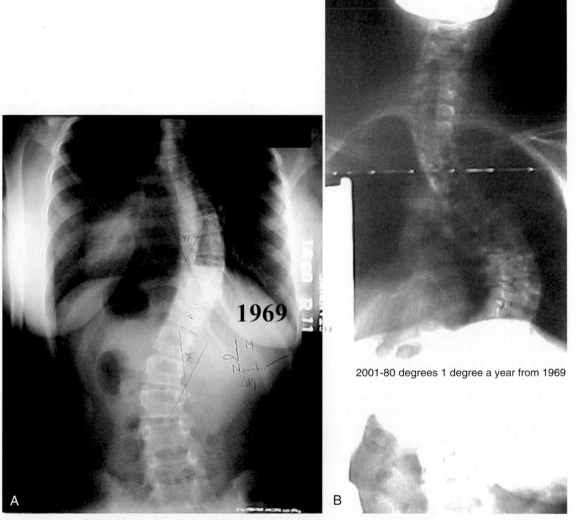

2001-80 degrees 1 degree a year from 1969

Figure 20-2. A, Right thoracic curve of 48 degrees at skeletal maturity in 1969 and age 15. **B,** Thirty-two years later, at age 47, the curve has progressed precisely 1 degree per year to 80 degrees.

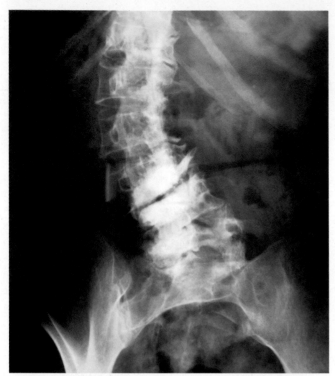

Figure 20-3. Note the degenerative changes at the apex of the curve as well as the lateral listhesis of L3 on L4 and the obliquity of the L3-4 and L4-5 end plates.

significant component of axial back pain. These pain complaints are more prevalent in lumbar curves, in which pain complaints occur in 60% of patients. Factors related to increased pain in lumbar curves are radiographic evidence of degeneration at the apex; lateral vertebral listhesis; very oblique L3 and L4 end plates; increased stiffening of the main curvature, especially in the lumbosacral area; thoracolumbar kyphosis; and loss of lumbar lordosis (Fig. 20-3). The loss of sagittal balance from a lack of lumbar lordosis is important beyond that of pain having been determined by SF 36 testing in terms of a negative significant correlation in social function, role emotion, and overall general health. The pain problems of lumbar curves are in contrast to those of thoracic curves, in which all studies agree that severe progressive pain is rarely a problem.

Comorbidities

Overall, it is thought that idiopathic scoliotic patients do suffer from more health problems than is expected in the general population. Comorbidities that may cause lumbar pain are also problematic in this population. In the older adult patient, the comorbidities of spinal stenosis and osteoporosis are common. Comorbidities associated with adult scoliosis include a higher prevalence of arthritis, heart disease, and respiratory symptoms. Nonpainful thoracic curves, especially in hyperlordosis, may cause significant pulmonary dysfunction. Scoliotic subjects, particularly women, can have a problem with self-image. Furthermore, female scoliotic patients may have lower marriage rates, difficulty becoming pregnant, and a higher incidence of

miscarriages, stillbirths, and premature births. Knowledge of these phenomena and events will affect a full evaluation of the patient.

Patient Evaluation

History

Along with the importance of obtaining a complete personal history, a family history of progressive deformity can provide an indication as to a patient's prognosis. The date of onset of the deformity should be elicited but usually is not, in itself, important. However, the history of curve progression is particularly important. Some measure of progression can be surmised from changes in how clothes fit, an observed increase in rib hump, loss of height, or an altered waistline. Ideally, a more precise definition of curve progression can be obtained from serial radiographs; unfortunately, these often have been lost or were never taken.

It is also important to discuss and understand how the deformity affects the patient's life. Many adults are reluctant to discuss the aesthetic consequences of their curve unless asked directly. Many have learned to cope with the deformity, but for others, it is a source of major concern and fear for the future. As was mentioned previously, this population may also have suffered psychologically with issues of self-image and adverse pregnancy and birth-related events.

A careful pain history should also be elicited; it can be aided by the use of pain drawings. Pain at the apex of the curve should be carefully differentiated from pain emanating from other areas, especially pain at the lumbosacral junction. Important information is pain duration and how it affects activities of daily living, occupation, social function, recreation, and sexual activities. Often, a radicular or referred component of the axial pain will be present. Sometimes this is related to the apex of the curve. A thoracic or thoracolumbar curve may present with intercostal neuralgia. This should not be confused with rib pain caused by the lower rib cage pressing on the top of the pelvis in severe curves. Leg symptoms may relate to the primary or compensatory curve and either be scleratomal in nature or have the characteristics of frank sciatica. Leg pain secondary to trochanteric bursitis should be noted and should not be confused with sciatica. Any associated bladder or bowel dysfunction is an important diagnostic and prognostic observation. Incontinence, particularly in the elderly female, should not be assumed to be secondary to myogenic causes until proven otherwise. Often, spinal stenoses can be causative of a true neurogenic bladder and not related to pelvic floor dysfunction.

Respiratory malfunction can be a presenting symptom with adult scoliosis but is far more common in paralytic or severe congenital curves and relatively rare in older idiopathic curves. Large thoracic curves give concern for the possibility of impaired pulmonary function. There is some evidence that function may start to be impaired by curves reaching 60 degrees. Exceptions are patients with idiopathic scoliosis associated with marked thoracic lordosis in whom vital capacity may be reduced significantly, even with curves of lower magnitude. Impairment of exercise performance found in adults with moderate scoliosis cannot be attributed to any important ventilatory limitation, abnormality in lung function, or impaired chemoreceptor sensitivity. The reduction likely has arisen from deconditioning and a lack of aerobic exercise. This justifies a concerted effort for the patient to participate in an aerobic conditioning program if the patient has moderate or severe curves with respiratory complaints. Death from cor pulmonale is the major concern and can occur in curves greater than 100 degrees in patients who are 45 years of age or older (Fig. 20-4). Fortunately, functionally impor-

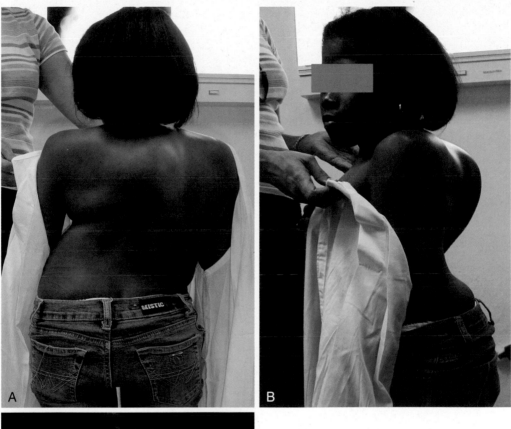

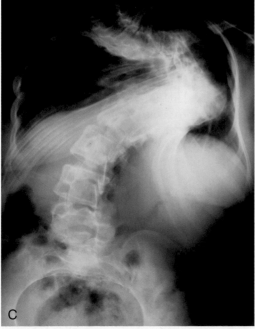

Figure 20-4. Severe 144-degree curve in a 22-year-old woman from the Dominican Republic who was experiencing mild respiratory difficulties.

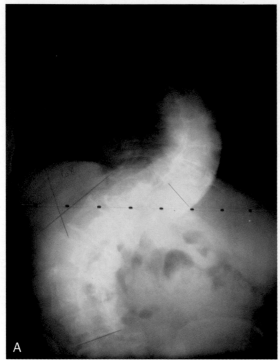

Figure 20-5. **A,** Radiograph of scoliotic deformity of a 63-year-old man. **B,** Clinical view of the patient showing rib hump, decompensation to the right, and trunk asymmetry. However, the patient had very few clinical symptoms from this deformity and required no treatment.

tant respiratory dysfunction is rarely observed, even in curves of 100 degrees or more. Vital capacity is the strongest predictor of the development of respiratory failure, followed by the scoliotic angle.

Physical Examination

As with a patient history, a complete physical examination is essential to the evaluation of all spinal disorders. Curve assessment includes evaluation of three-dimensional characteristics, including kyphosis and lordosis; the rib hump; the degree of decompensation; flexibility; pelvic obliquity; hip mobility; and deformity (Fig. 20-5). It is very important to examine the adult scoliotic thoroughly and not overlook subtle neurologic changes or mistakenly attribute them to degenerative changes and miss an underlying

neurologic cause. Therefore, the neurologic examination should be complete, and subtle neurologic findings should be assessed in both the upper and lower extremities. Special attention to neurologic findings, including spinal cord imaging studies, is warranted in left thoracic idiopathic curves. Mild clawing of the toes can indicate a tethered cord. Pediatric scoliosis and adult scoliosis are frequently present in syringomyelia associated with Chiari malformation. Physical findings might or might not be able to be correlated with image findings, but their presence and the possibility should be kept in mind.

Imaging Studies

The initial radiographic analysis includes three views: foot, standing posteroanterior, and lateral films. Focal, coned-down views can be useful in patients with pain to evaluate facets, congenital anomalies, and disc narrowing. Oblique radiographs may be taken by using Stagnara views to assess rotational deformity, particularly when a kyphosis is present. Lateral side-bending radiographs will indicate a curve's flexibility but do not predict, positively or negatively, the degree of surgical correction that might be obtained. Extension views might have greater value in determining whether an associated kyphosis is flexible, while flexion views can give similar information about lordotic deformities. Occasionally, traction films can be of value in determining whether distraction will overcome trunk decompensation. Once the routine radiographs have been obtained, a variety of ancillary imaging studies may be considered. Bone scans can be helpful in two circumstances: in the younger adult with pain who has a minor curve, to detect a possible osteoid osteoma, and in the adult with curves after laminectomy in an attempt to identify a late fracture of the remaining rim of lamina.

The presence of large curves diminishes the normal efficacy of magnetic resonance imaging (MRI) for the detection of neural compression. It has been said that in a straight spine, MRI plus computed tomography (CT) equals CT myelography. The major exception to this rule is in attempting to identify neural compression in association with significant scoliosis. If there are neurologic findings that are unexplained by plain radiographs and surgical correction is contemplated, CT myelography may be the imaging modality of choice. Its particular importance is to determine any areas of actual or potential compression, which would become important when corrective forces are applied. CT scans have little use, except when combined with myelographic enhancement. In the adult, MRI can be helpful in assessing the degree of degeneration of the lower lumbar disc levels (L4-5, L5-S1) below a curve. However, MRI is not as specific as discography is.

Other Ancillary Tests, Discography, and Facet Blocks

One of the major objectives in the evaluation of the adult with scoliosis and pain is to determine all of the sources of symptoms. When there is doubt that all sources have been identified by basic imaging and examination, special tests can provide additional, more specific information. This is of major importance when surgery is contemplated so that the surgeon can accurately assess what spinal levels to include in the fusion. It is not useful to straighten a patient's curve but unknowingly end the fusion at symptomatic levels of disc and/or facet degeneration, with resultant persistent or increased lumbar pain. Discography can be specifically helpful at the L3-4, L4-5, and L5-S1 levels and perhaps, rarely, at the apex of the curve. This is done if these levels are suspected of being a present or future

source of pain. Although the ideal approach is posterolateral, the rotational deformity might rarely necessitate a transdural approach (Fig. 20-6).

Facet blocks can also be employed in the lower lumbar spine. If discography produces pain and facet blocks provide relief, it is reasonable that fusion should incorporate that level. Conversely, should a discogram not reproduce the patient's pain and a facet block not achieve relief, then a particular level is not incorporated.

In summary, a thorough evaluation should provide the surgeon with ample knowledge of the patient's curve progression; the patient's pain history; the psychological, physical, and neurologic impact; respiratory function; and accurate imaging of the severity, location, and type of deformity. Armed with this information, a treatment plan and, if indicated, an operative plan can be outlined and discussed with the patient.

Nonoperative Care

The basic approach to nonoperative care is similar to the treatment for all chronic, painful spinal disorders and includes exercise, education, and nonsteroidal, anti-inflammatory drugs (NSAIDs). It is important to stress that modalities and exercise will not prevent curve progression but can serve to maintain flexibility and minimize symptomatology. Low-thrust aerobics, cycling, and swimming are useful adjuncts and are particularly important in preventing osteoporosis. Medical management of underlying osteoporosis is an important aspect of nonoperative care and will be especially important if the patient ever requires surgical intervention. The role of orthotics is unknown, and there is no evidence to suggest that they will prevent curve progression in the adult. However, orthotics might have some role if they are intermittently used for symptom reduction in elderly patients, but they must be rigid and fitted carefully to the patient's deformity. Frequently, however, orthotics are poorly tolerated and, once fabricated, rarely used. A patient must be equally committed to an exercise program. Owing to the relative risks of scoliotic surgery, nonoperative care is considered important to patient management; physicians should consistently and positively support appropriate levels of exercise, referring patients to therapists using well-designed programs. Follow-up of patients can reveal the emergence of surgical indications not observed previously.

Surgical Indications

The indications for surgery in an adult with an idiopathic curve are to (1) obtain pain relief, (2) improve existing deformity and prevent further progression, (3) treat current significant neurologic dysfunction (pain and/or true neurologic deficit), and (4) improve cosmetic appearance.

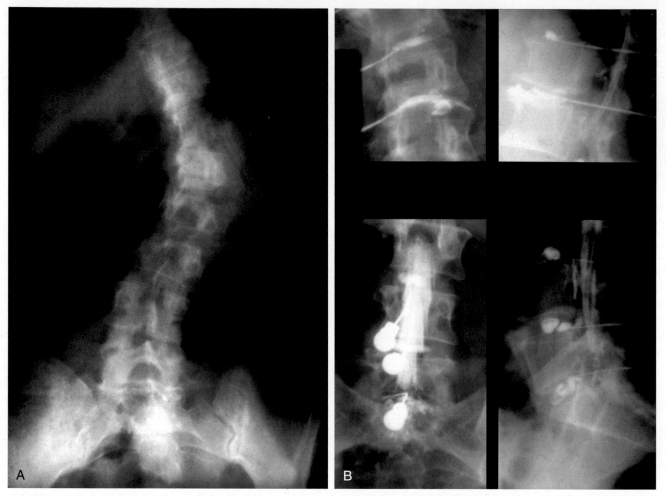

Figure 20-6. A, Radiograph of a 38-year-old woman who presented with increasing low back pain and deformity. **B,** Discography was performed to accurately localize her source of pain. Discography revealed normal L5-S1, L4-5, and L3-4 discs. No pain was reproduced. Abnormal morphology together with reproducible pain was found at the L2-3, L1-2, and T12-L1 discs.

Pain

Pain is the most common surgical indication and accounts for about 85% of surgical cases. Determining the sources of pain and predicting its surgical relief present a great challenge. The prevalence of pain and the use of a variety of investigative testing techniques have been discussed. As in any spinal disorder, the more certain the causation of pain, the more likely is a successful outcome (Fig. 20-7).

Progressive Deformity

Most patients who come to surgery for adult scoliosis have more than one indication for surgery. When unremitting pain is the major problem, it is easy to decide on a surgical solution. A dilemma exists in regard to certain patients in whom the only presenting indication is significant curve progression. Should the problem be observed or operated on at that time? There are several unknown factors to

consider. How fast is it estimated that the progression will proceed? If surgery is deferred and observation is chosen, will the patient's general health remain good or will it deteriorate, making future surgery more difficult to tolerate? Will new and better techniques become available in the future? Will fusion performed at a younger age lead to accelerated adjacent degenerative changes that will require further surgery when a delayed approach might last a lifetime? Any and all of these questions face both the patient and the surgeon.

There are two groups in whom an earlier surgery seems most prudent. The first group consists of patients with a progressive deformity who are under the age of 35 and who particularly present with lumbar or thoracolumbar curves of 45 degrees or greater. Inevitably, these curves seem to progress and develop an accelerated painful degeneration within and below the curvature. Especially in the female patient, the secondary degenerative changes can convert a lordotic scoliosis into a kyphoscoliotic deformity. If this later deformity becomes rigid, it might require a two-stage surgical correction or a kyphectomy (posterior subtraction

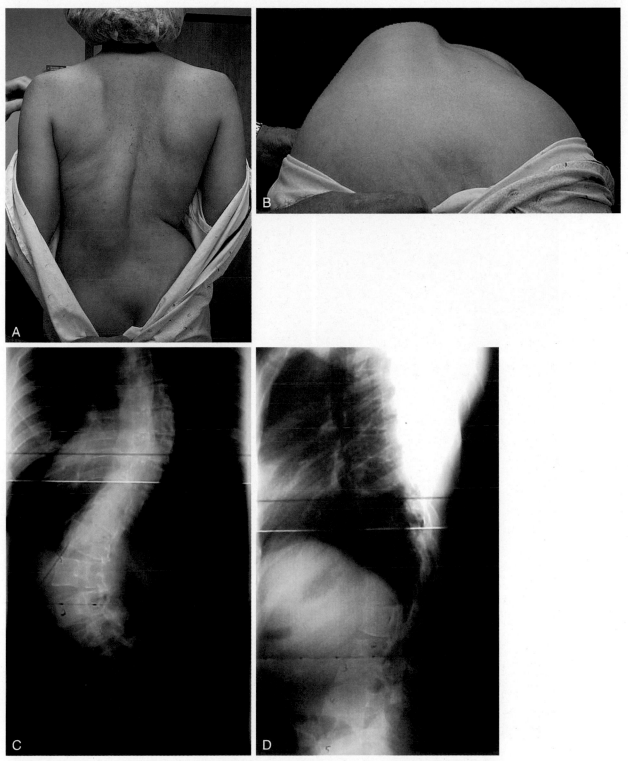

Figure 20-7. A, Clinical view of the spine of a 36-year-old female with progressive idiopathic scoliosis and well-preserved lumbosacral discs with pain over the lumbar prominence. **B,** View of the lumbar prominence demonstrated by the forward bend test. **C,** Preoperative anteroposterior radiograph. **D,** Preoperative lateral radiograph. Note the kyphosis over the curve.

Continued

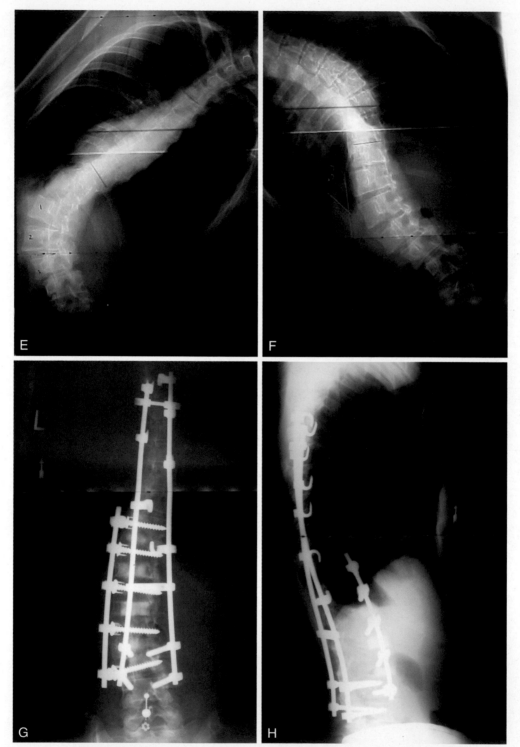

Figure 20-7, cont'd. E, Side-bending radiograph to right. **F,** Side-bending radiograph to left. Anteroposterior (**G**) and lateral (**H**) postoperative radiographs 5 years after anterior instrumentation and fusion with same-day posterior instrumentation and fusion.

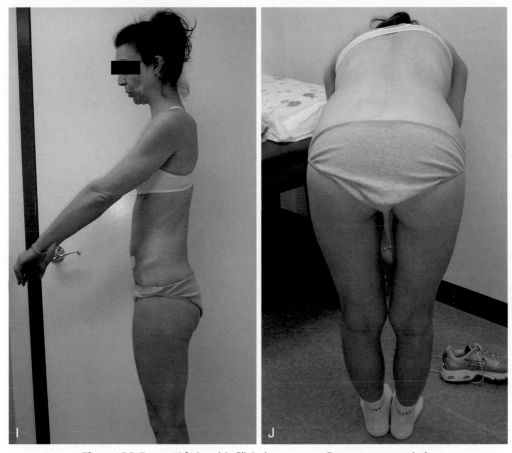

Figure 20-7, cont'd. I and **J,** Clinical appearance 5 years postoperatively.

osteotomy). In comparison, the younger adult can be treated by a one-stage anterior or posterior correction.

The second group is younger patients with a truncal imbalance of 4 cm or more whose major 40-degree or more curve extends to L3 or L4, accompanied by a compensatory curve at L4, L5, or the sacrum. The primary curve in this instance may be reduced significantly by rebalancing only the lower compensatory curve. This approach should be employed if testing has proven the lower curve to be painful. The patient should be aware that extension of the fusion could be required at a later date. By fixing the lower curve, the average degree of correction of the upper curve can be more than 40%.

Neurologic Deficit

Neurologic deficits related to associated spinal stenosis are only occasionally the prime indication for surgical intervention in adult scoliosis. With an increasingly older population, it is possible that a greater number of patients will be seen presenting with neurologically related symptoms. More commonly presented than true neurologic deficits are radicular pain complaints stemming from static or dynamic nerve compression, either within the curvature (often in the apex of the concavity) or, in some circumstances, below the curvature. Investigation of a suspected

neurologic deficit usually requires CT myelography, especially if the compression is located within the curvature. Occasionally, compression above or below the curve in a straighter area of the spine can be adequately diagnosed with MRI alone. Direct decompression of neural elements by laminectomy is usually required. Indirect decompression through curve correction or by disc height restoration, as with anterior discectomy and structural grafting, might suffice but usually only for intermittent radicular pain and not persistent nerve dysfunction. Furthermore, the adequacy of the decompression might remain in question if not directly visualized at surgery. This also applies to indirect decompression performed below the area of a fusion and achieved by spontaneous correction of a compensatory curve below the structural curve.

Cosmesis

Cosmesis is generally thought to be an uncommon indication for surgery in the adult scoliotic, with the exception of the young adult who has an unbalanced curve. However, this might be an underestimation. Body image and cosmesis probably play a greater role in the patient's decision to entertain surgery than has previously been thought. Any loss of height is a major disappointment to both male and female scoliotic patients. Their gauge of height loss is often their height relative to that of a spouse or friend. Sometimes patients are unaware of the exact amount of height loss and are shocked to discover the discrepancy between the height listed on their driver's license and their height as measured in the physician's office. Progressive rib hump and waist asymmetry are cosmetic deformities that, when associated with even moderate pain, become magnified in the patient's personal assessment of body image, self-assuredness, and overall quality of life. The thought that these conditions will worsen, that they will be more difficult to correct, and that the patient's ability to endure a major surgical procedure in the future could be lessened by time and aging are prime motivators for many patients to consider surgery at this juncture of their lives. Even if a patient's goal is predominantly cosmetic, surgical intervention might be warranted after repeated discussions with the patient and his or her close relatives to clearly define expectations. With sufficient curve flexibility, posterior segmental instrumentation is particularly useful for this purpose to obtain curve correction and overall balance and to help restore waist symmetry.

If the patient is hypokyphotic in the thoracic spine, an excellent cosmetic correction can be obtained to restore a more normal chest wall symmetry. The use of thoracoplasty (partial rib excision over four to six levels) can be used as an additional means to improve cosmetic outcome. Thoracoplasty has gained increased popularity in recent years. The reduction of rib hump is quite dramatic when done properly. The resected ribs aid in supplementing bone graft. The morbidity can be minimal. Rib excision should extend to the posterior axillary line and allow for a symmetrical junction to the adjacent remaining ribs if possible. Although there might be some loss of vital capacity in the properly selected patient, this loss will not be clinically significant.

Neuromuscular Indications

Neuromuscular curves do not follow the rules of benign curve progression as it occurs in idiopathic scoliosis. Static or progressive imbalance in the neuromuscular patient is associated with spastic, paralytic, and other muscular disorders, all of which can cause curve progression throughout the patient's lifetime. As a result of increasing world immigration, untreated adults with childhood disorders such as poliomyelitis, cerebral palsy, and other neuromuscular conditions may present in later stages without previous intervention. This is a problem that is seen more frequently now than it was 15 years ago in North America. Adult-onset disorders, such as Parkinson's disease, may present with deformities of kyphosis and kyphoscoliosis. Other indications include posttraumatic deformities following traumatic paraplegia or quadriplegia, although, again, kyphosis is more likely to ensue than scoliosis. All of these indications suggest that a focused surgical intervention is worthy of consideration.

While pain is by far the most common surgical indication and, logically, one might want to include curve progression, the latter presentation alone is a qualified indication, depending on the size, impact, and location of the curves. Cosmesis should not be undervalued or overvalued. The patient should be supported to reveal his or her feelings and should be helped to objectively evaluate the cosmetic need versus the surgical risk. Furthermore, surgeons must objectively evaluate their skills and experience with curve correction, which will significantly affect the cosmetic result.

Surgical Techniques

All noteworthy adult surgical interventions for scoliosis commenced with the use of Harrington instrumentation. It subsequently has been replaced by more modern instrumentation techniques. The ability of the surgeon to reliably and predictably stabilize and improve adult deformities effectively was significantly advanced by the advent of segmental instrumentation and the use of pedicle screw systems. This major technological and implant innovation has allowed for greater control, correction, maintenance of correction, prevention of pseudarthrosis and ease in post-operative management. Increasing familiarity with anterior surgical techniques of release, fusion, and newer instrumentation systems have made possible correction of the stiffer adult curves and restoration of sagittal balance unachievable in the Harrington era.

Overview of Spine Deformity Techniques to Correct Spinal Deformity

Spine deformity surgery in its simplest forms allows for correction of a spinal deformity either through the curve's inherent flexibility or through release of the bony and soft-tissue restraints to mobility, instrumentation to achieve and maintain correction until fusion is achieved, and finally, decompression of neural elements when necessary. Correction of the spinal deformity can be done by using posterior, anterior, or a combination of anterior and posterior surgical approaches and techniques. Techniques to create more flexibility in a stiff curve entail (1) soft-tissue release, (2) facetectomy, (3) posterior osteotomies, (4) anterior release by discectomy, and, in rare cases, (5) complete vertebrectomy. Posterior segmental instrumentation requires fixation of rods to the posterior elements by hooks, sublaminar wires or cables, and/or pedicle screws, both thoracic and lumbar. The rods are connected to each other by cross-links to further enhance stability. Anterior release and fusion may be accompanied by anterior single- or double-rod constructs fixed to the spine with vertebral body screws.

With any instrumentation technique, it is the fusion that provides the long-term success of the construct. As in all fusions in adult deformity, the use of autologous iliac crest graft is preferable and is the gold standard. Since adequate amounts for long adult fusions are sometimes difficult to harvest, supplementation is common, utilizing bone graft extenders such as cancellous allograft and demineralized bone matrix products. Anterior disc spaces may be filled with morselized bone graft or structural allograft may be utilized. The use of products such as platelet-derived factor has not been adequately proven to be of value to date. The use of specific bone morphogenic proteins such as BMP 2 and BMP 7 is supported by evidence for use in one-level fusions, but their role in long fusions associated with adult deformity surgery has yet to be defined. Techniques such as these are differentially applied, depending on specific methods employed by the surgeon in corrective surgery.

Thoracic Deformities

Treatment of thoracic deformities is usually done to manage progression of deformity and/or cosmesis and sometimes pain. The techniques that are employed are similar to those used for adolescent scoliosis. In adults, however, thoracic curves are particularly stiff related to degenerative changes, not only in the discs but also in the facet joints. The effects of progressive fibrotic changes in chronically shortened muscles in the concavity of long-standing curvatures is unknown. Overcoming forces that are resistant to correction and then maintaining the correction to the point of successful fusion is the primary challenge to the adult deformity surgeon. Because of the inherent stiffness of the curves and the difficulty in obtaining and holding powerful corrections, the use of thoracoplasty to improve the cosmetic result for the patient is not uncommon. Stiff curves with significant hypokyphosis may benefit from an anterior release if pulmonary function is adequate; otherwise, the use of wide facetectomies and rod contouring to improve thoracic kyphosis is the technique preferred.

Multiple strategies currently exist for the specific application of hooks, sublaminar wires, or pedicle screws. In the older adult, the use of pedicle screws sometimes supplemented with a sublaminar wire or cable has diminished the problem of hook pullout or fracture of laminae in the upper thoracic spine. It is important, in an effort to prevent kyphosis proximal to the instrumentation, to generally carry the proximal instrumentation to T2. One of the complications in the upper thoracic spine of the older adult is the development of junctional kyphosis due to loss of the posterior tension band immediately proximal to the instrumentation (Fig. 20-8). The use of pedicle screws at the upper level has one further theoretical advantage that might help to prevent this complication. For pedicle screw insertion in the upper spine, there is no need to destroy the superiormost ligamentum flavum or the interspinous ligaments, which is often necessary with hooks, particu-

larly when downward-going hooks are used at the top of a construct.

Rigid, severely rotated spines of 70 or more degrees, which are able to be corrected only minimally on side bending and which have been progressive, might require anterior releases prior to posterior segmental instrumentation. More recently, the use of multiple osteotomies in conjunction with thoracic screw fixation has decreased the need for anterior-posterior techniques.

Posterior Segmental Instrumentation

Overview. Although first used to describe the original Luque rod technique with sublaminar wires, the term *posterior segmental instrumentation* now describes, generically, the use of dual rods fixed to the spine by either hooks, sublaminar wires or cables, pedicle screws, or hybrid combinations. An evolution from the original Cotrel-Dubousset instrumentation to more modern systems utilizing all pedicle screws has occurred. An ongoing debate exists relative to the cost-benefit analysis between all hook, hybrid, or screw techniques. However, pedicle screw fixation from the top of the construct to the bottom of the construct has increased in popularity.

Technical Aspects of Posterior Technique. As with all deformity surgery, attention to detail in the placement of fixation points along the spine remains critical. In contrast to the situation in pediatric age groups, the presence of increased stiffness and poorer bone quality challenge the surgeon to achieve good results for the patient. Soft or osteopenic laminae are potential hazards to achieving resistance to long-term hook pullout or wire or cable pull-through. Severely rotated, stiff segments make the insertion of pedicle screws more technically difficult, especially in the apical concavities. The osteopenic bone allows bone/screw interface problems, creating either toggling of the screws, with windshield-wiper effect, or frank screw pullout.

There are many other possible curve patterns beyond those mentioned that can be explored in the literature. We shall, however, attempt to point out some of the pearls and pitfalls to achieving success. Adequate posterior release of bony and soft-tissue structures is critical for regaining flexibility within the adult deformity. While simple exposure of the posterior elements is, in and of itself, a soft-tissue release, special attention should be paid to the fibrotic scarred muscle that is often found laterally in the concavities of curvatures. Facet release, including capsules and facetectomies, not only is performed for release but also is a critical step in preparing the spine bed for instrumentation and fusion. Chevron-type osteotomies, extending from the interlaminar space laterally, resect the pars between the pedicle above and the pedicle below, greatly enhancing the ability to correct a stiff curve. The bilateral pars defects, created for improving curve flexibility, represent potential new high-risk areas for pseudarthrosis, espe-

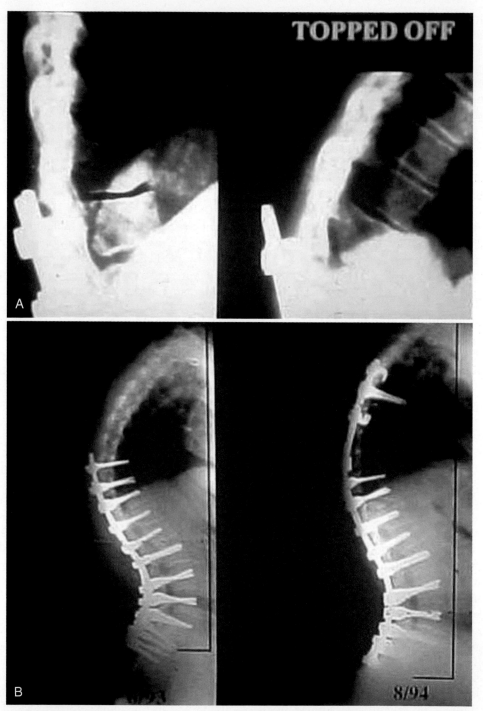

Figure 20-8. A, Topping-off (adding-on) syndrome. In addition to stopping the fusion in the area of kyphosis, the patient had osteoporosis. A fusion should never be stopped at the apex of a kyphosis. **B,** The fusion required extension proximally to T3. Screws are preferred to hooks in the upper thoracic spine, especially in the presence of osteoporosis.

cially when not located within an area of an anterior release and fusion. In contrast, pedicle subtraction osteotomy performed in areas of sharp kyphotic deformities does create an area for anterior healing to occur.

Instrumentation Planning. Generally speaking, there are geographic areas in the spine that are more difficult to expose for fusion than other areas. Any transition zone from stiffness to flexibility creates natural impediments to stable fusion within instrumentation constructs. We recognize this potentiality when we attempt to fuse the flexible lumbar spine to the sacrum. The thoracolumbar junction is similarly recognized as a region where it is difficult to obtain a successful fusion, as the relatively stiff thoracic spine, stabilized by the rib cage, meets the more flexible upper lumbar spine. These examples are naturally occurring "stiff to flexible transition zones" that are particularly prone to pseudarthrosis when included in long constructs but might not be easily recognized as transitional regions that require attention with exacting technique. Even less well recognized are iatrogenic stiff to flexible transition zones, created by the surgeon in their selection of specific techniques and instrumentation. The best example is a transition zone where an anterior fusion construct meets a posterior-only construct. Consider an anterior T10-L3 instrumentation and fusion as part of an overall posterior T4-L4 posterior instrumentation and fusion. The new iatrogenic stiff to flexible transition zones have been created at T9-10 and at L3-4. In pediatric deformity cases, in which the patient has a robust fusion response, these zones are relatively unimportant. In adults, however, with less robust fusion responses, these potential barriers or danger zones to fusion become more important potential areas of pseudarthrosis. Another iatrogenic stiff to flexible transition zone is created within a posterior construct at the juncture where bilateral pedicle screws abruptly stop and are adjacent to less secure forms of fixation, such as hooks or wires (Fig. 20-9). Similarly, as was previously mentioned, chevron osteotomies create a very definite stiff to flexible transition zone, which might be necessary for curve correction but represents a possible challenge to solid fusion. Surgeons

have often observed that pseudarthroses in long constructs often occur at the location of cross-links. This has been thought to represent a mechanical barrier to fusion by bulky cross-link to a "north-south" fusion process. It is possible, however, that a localized stiff to flexible transition zone is created by the biomechanical effect of the cross-link or perhaps a combination of the two, thereby contributing to this predilection to pseudarthrosis. In summary, a macroinstrumentation technique is a composite of microconstructs and transition zones of stiffness, and this must be recognized and considered in planning.

Tips and Hints. How do we turn the above-mentioned theoretical concepts into clinically relevant application? First, we do this by recognizing naturally occurring stiff to flexible transition zones such as the thoracolumbar junction and the lumbosacral junction. Second, we do this by recognizing whether a surgical construct plan has created iatrogenic stiff to flexible transition zones and modify the plan accordingly. Bilateral pedicle screws should be placed above and below chevron osteotomies. Surgical transitions from pedicle screws to less secure forms of fixation should be performed away from danger zones, or perhaps only pedicle screws should be utilized in that region. Cross-links at iatrogenic or natural stiff to flexible transition

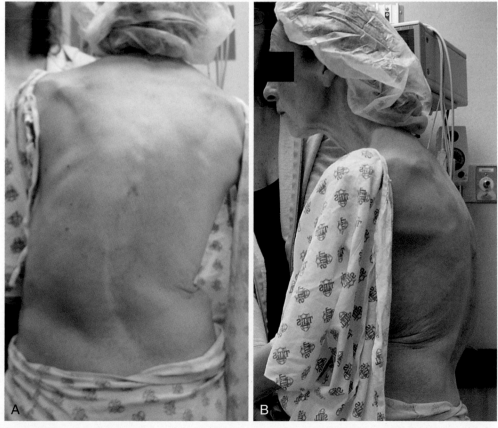

Figure 20-9. A 66-year-old woman with progressive kyphoscoliosis in adulthood. Back (**A**) and side (**B**) views.

Continued

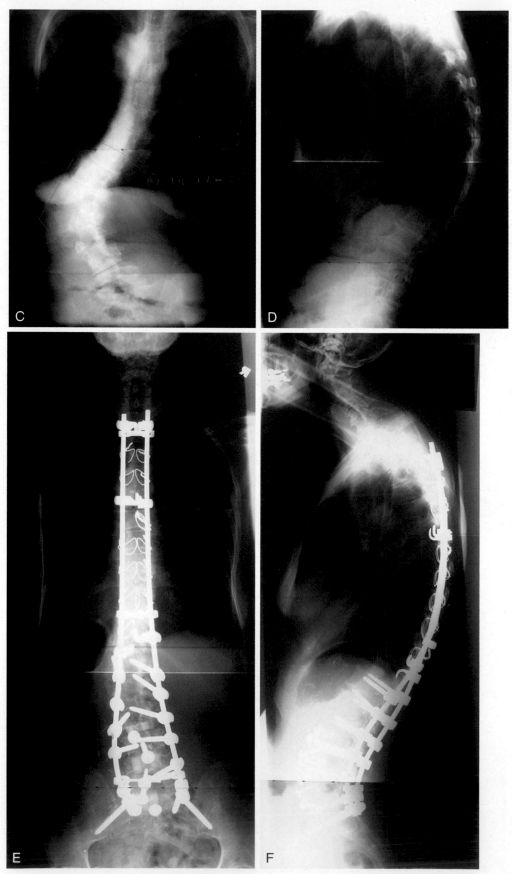

Figure 20-9, cont'd. Anteroposterior (**C**) and lateral (**D**) radiographs showing 65-degree lumbar curve. **E,** Anteroposterior radiograph 1 year postoperatively. **F,** Lateral radiograph 1 year postoperative.

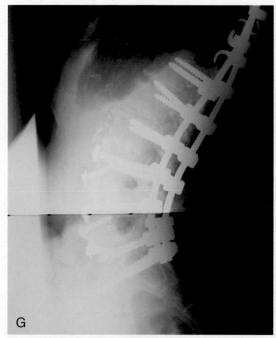

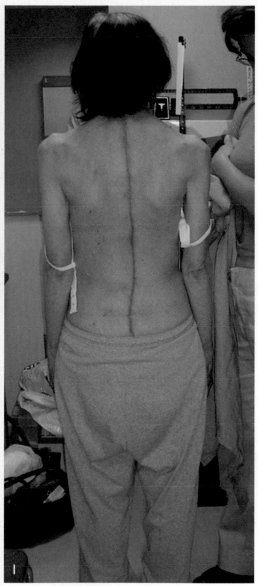

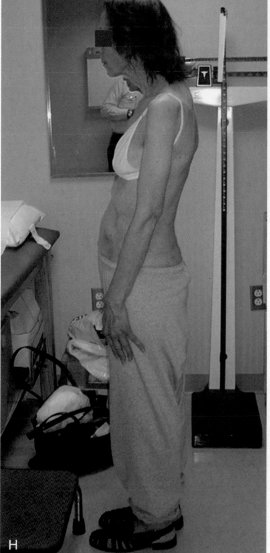

Figure 20-9, cont'd. G, Lateral radiograph showing pedicle screw fixation to L1 and transition to hook and wire fixation at the thoracolumbar junction. Also note the excellent lumbar lordosis from the anterior interbody femoral rings from L3 to S1. **H,** Lateral clinical view postoperatively. **I,** Clinical view of the back postoperatively.

Continued

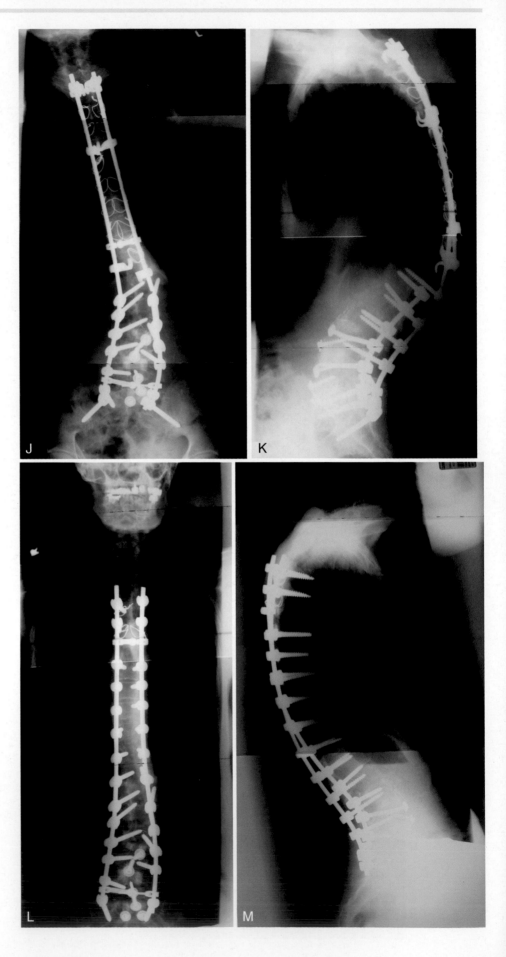

Figure 20-9, cont'd. Anteroposterior (**J**) and lateral (**K**) radiographs; 2 years postoperatively, the patient presents with pain and hardware at the transition zone of stiffness, created by the combination of the thoracolumbar junction and the zone of transition from pedicular fixation to hooks and wires. Anteroposterior (**L**) and lateral (**M**) radiographs showing revision surgery with thoracic pedicle screws and autograft and BMP (OP-1).

zones should not be utilized. Thorough decortication must be performed, and graft material must be placed carefully underneath bulky cross-links. Less bulky cross-link designs also can be chosen to lessen a risk of any impact of bulkiness on the construct. Another consideration would be to ration the use of pure cancellous iliac crest graft to danger zones to minimize the risk of pseudarthrosis.

Thoracolumbar and Lumbar Curves

The treatment of thoracolumbar and lumbar curve deformities depends to a large degree on two factors: the degree of lordosis and the source of pain. Maintaining or restoring lumbar lordosis is the single most important consideration in surgical correction to obtain a lasting, satisfactory result for the patient. Focusing on coronal plane deformity without providing adequate sagittal balance is winning a battle while losing the war. We have classified thoracolumbar and lumbar curves into four groups: (1) flexible curves that do not require fusion to the sacrum, (2) rigid deformity with kyphosis that does not require fusion of the sacrum, (3) flexible deformity with preservation of lordosis requiring fusion of the sacrum, and (4) rigid, kyphotic deformity requiring fusion to the sacrum. The latter group is becoming much more common as the age of our population increases and the ability to deal with the older adult with comorbidities has improved. Pain relief and restoration of balance should result from successful fusion and restoration of lumbar lordosis.

Group 1: Flexible Lumbar/Thoracolumbar Deformity with Preservation of Lumbar Lordosis Not Requiring Fusion to the Sacrum. These can be treated either through an anterior technique in isolation or through posterior segmental instrumentation. Generally, in the younger adult, morbidity may be less from the anterior approach. Additionally, incisional complications, the risk of incisional hernia, abdominal bulge, weakness, and umbilical shift in the younger age group (ages 20 to 40 years) are significantly less than in older age groups. As one approaches being over age 50, however, the abdominal problems related to the anterior approach increase, and the quality of the bone diminishes. Dual-rod fixation has shown lesser screw pullout and rod breakage than has use of a single rod or semiflexible rods, hence lessening the incidence of pseudarthrosis.

If the posterior approach is utilized, the use of segmental pedicle screws allows for excellent derotation and fixation. One should recognize that the pedicles at T12, L1, and L2 are frequently smaller than adjacent levels and present a problem, particularly at the concavity for the placement of pedicle screws. Over the last number of years, a posterior approach has been our preferred technique rather than an anterior approach. The latter, by necessity, can require taking down the diaphragm, which in and of itself can add to postoperative morbidity. Furthermore, anterior surgery was thought to minimize total fusion levels, especially distally, compared to posterior procedures. However, today's pedicle screw constructs might have eliminated this advantage.

Solo Anterior Instrumentation and Fusion

Overview. As was previously mentioned, the ideal candidate for anterior-only surgery is the younger adult who has a flexible thoracolumbar or lumbar curve with preserved lordosis and without indication to extend fusion to the sacrum. To achieve good results, it is critical that specific surgical techniques be employed. While the flexible Zielke threaded rod was the first system widely used in adults, the systems that are most commonly used today are solid single-rod and dual-rod instrumentation systems (Fig. 20-10).

Technical Aspects of the Anterior Technique. Once the levels to be fused have been exposed, the disc spaces are cleared, including the cartilaginous end plates, back to the posterior longitudinal ligament (Fig. 20-11). The most common mistake of the surgeon who is inexperienced in the anterior approach is performing an inadequate discectomy and end plate preparation, which limits the correction and increases the rates of both instrumentation failure and pseudarthrosis. Adequate exposure is essential so that an accurate angle of insertion can be obtained for the screws. If at all possible, the screws should be angled toward the contralateral junction of the pedicle with the vertebral body. To ensure that the opposite cortex is penetrated, a depth gauge is placed on the exposed disc space to determine the pathway and length of the screw. It is better to have 2 mm of additional length to help ensure bicortical purchase. If there is significant osteoporosis, methylmethacrylate can be used. In these instances, the screw hole is enlarged with a curette to retain the cement and enhance screw fixation. The use of low-viscosity or cooled cement will increase the working time. This technique is particularly useful in the most proximal screw to prevent pullout. The use of a derotation maneuver is now almost routine, because it has the capability to reproduce lordosis in the lumbar spine or reduce kyphosis in the thoracolumbar spine.

Autogenous bone graft is used, usually consisting of excised rib cut up into very small fragments. The autologous bone can be supplemented with morselized allograft and/or demineralized bone matrix. To increase and maintain lordosis, structural allografts can be selectively placed anteriorly in the disc space.

Limitations of the Anterior Technique. The anterior technique is possible from L5 to T9 or T10. Further extension above that level is rarely of value, since the disc spaces are so narrow that little correction can be obtained in the adult, though its efficacy has been shown in the thoracic spine of adolescents. All patients with anterior instrumentation of thoracolumbar and lumbar spine

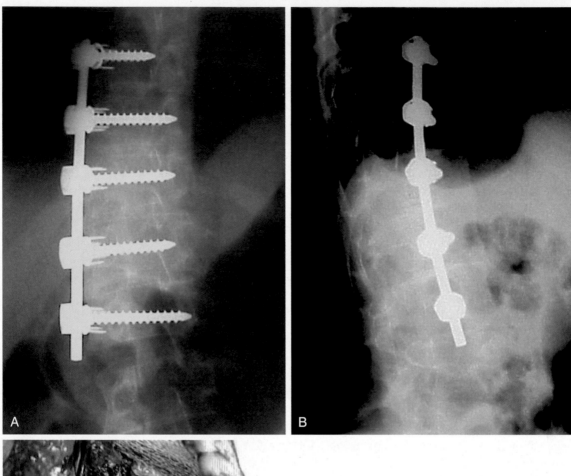

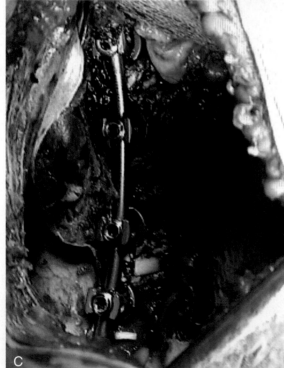

Figure 20-10. Anteroposterior (**A**) and lateral (**B**) radiographs of adult thoracolumbar curve with a solid rod. Note that lordosis has not been maintained across the instrumented segment because of the lack of structural graft in the anterior portion of the disc space. **C,** In this intraoperative photograph, structural cortical grafts have been inserted in the lowest disc space to maintain lordosis in conjunction with proper rod contouring.

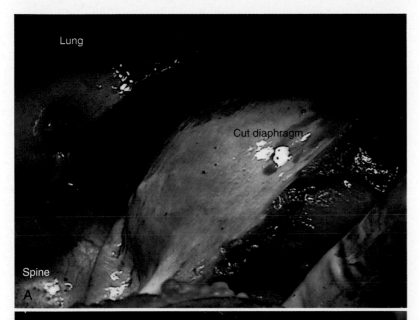

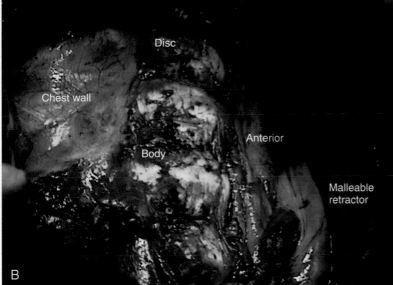

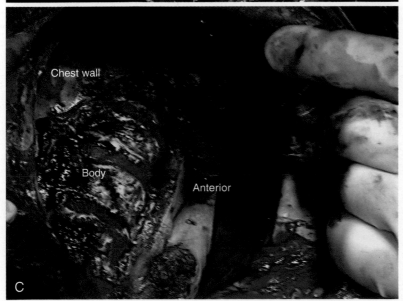

Figure 20-11. A, Anterior thoracoabdominal approaches allow for wide exposure. **B,** Anterior thoracoabdominal approach. Segmentals removed from the "valleys" of the vertebral bodies and the "hills" of the disc spaces that are exposed. **C,** Anterior thoracoabdominal approach. Multiple disc spaces are excised, with end plates removed, and are packed with Gelfoam to minimize bleeding until packed with bone.

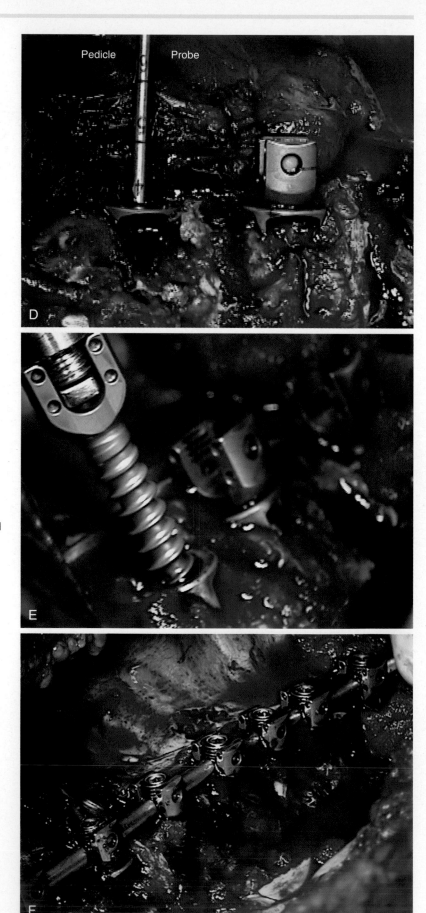

Figure 20-11, cont'd. D, Anterior thoracoabdominal approaches. Anterior vertebral body screws are placed anterolaterally. Bicortical purchase of the vertebral screws is desirable and can be achieved by pushing a pedicle probe across the vertebral body until the far cortex is felt. By carefully advancing the probe across the far cortex and measuring, the proper-sized screw can be utilized. Radiographs should verify the proper length. **E,** Anterior thoracoabdominal approaches. The screws are often inserted through staples that are thought to improve stability. **F,** Anterior thoracoabdominal approaches. A solid rod connects the individual vertebral body screws, and bone graft is carefully inserted into the disc spaces to ensure fusion.

require a total-contact custom-molded orthosis, which should be worn for 10 to 12 weeks when standing.

Surgical Results. For adult deformity, the first anterior instrumentation system that yielded good results as a stand-alone system was the Zielke instrumentation system. The Zielke device is a flexible threaded rod with nuts on either or both sides of the vertebral screws that allows for derotation and compression on the convexity of the curve. The results that can be obtained with the Zielke instrumentation have markedly improved on the results that were obtained with the original Dwyer instrumentation. The use of the derotation device further improved curve correction in the sagittal and coronal planes. Rotational deformity improved by one grade, based on the Nash-Moe method. Correction in the frontal plane for patients under 50 years of age can be 70% or more, and that for patients over 50 years of age is 60%. The noninstrumented proximal thoracic curves improve up to 30%; late loss of correction, provided that fusion is obtained, can be minimal. As was previously mentioned, with exquisite attention to surgical technique, the fusion rate can be very high. However, the Zielke system as a compression system was associated with significant loss of correction over the instrumented segment. Attention to proper derotation and the use of structural allograft anterior in the disc space can help to minimize this tendency. The use of newer solid single- and dual-rod techniques with the combined capabilities of rod rotation, compression, and distraction have helped to eliminate this problem. The use of structural anterior column support (horizontal cages and or femoral ring allograft) has also been useful.

Complications of Anterior Stand-Alone Instrumentation and Fusion. General complications include postthoracotomy syndromes, atelectasis, pleural effusion, and injury to the thoracic duct. Spine-specific complications can include instrumentation failure (either rod breakage or bone-screw interface failure), which is often associated with arthrosis and might require posterior revision instrumentation and fusion. In general, the older the patient and the stiffer the curve, the higher is the risk of postoperative complications when the anterior stand-alone technique is used.

Group 2: Rigid Kyphoscoliosis Deformity Not Requiring Fusion to the Sacrum. In these patients, anterior release is necessary, followed by posterior segmentation and fusion. Whether this is done on the same operative day or later depends on associated comorbidities, age, and blood loss, which will be discussed subsequently (Fig. 20-12). More recently, kyphectomy (posterior subtraction osteotomy) and vertebral body resection have been used, obviating the need for an anterior approach and allowing for posterior-only correction, instrumentation, and fusion.

Group 3: Flexible Deformity with Preservation of Lordosis Requiring Fusion to the Sacrum. The indications for fusion to the sacrum will be discussed in greater detail later in the chapter. Basically, if pain emanates from the lumbosacral junction in the presence of a painful, proximal deformity and/or progressive deformity, then fusion to the sacrum will be necessary. Because of the high risk of pseudarthrosis from either an anterior-alone or a posterior-alone approach, both anterior and posterior surgery are necessary. When the major lumbar curve is flexible, the anterior surgery can be performed through a minilaparotomy with a muscle-sparing midline approach. If performed prior to the posterior approach, the anterior discectomy with structural allograft for anterior column support provides the maximal amount of disc height restoration, and lumbosacral lordosis can be achieved. Conversely, this deformity can be approached by first-stage posterior segmental instrumentation with adequate sacral fixation and generally followed the same day with an anterior interbody fusion using structural allograft combined with anterior instrumentation at L4-5 and L5-Sl.

Group 4: Rigid Deformities with Associated Kyphosis Requiring Fusion to the Sacrum. As was previously mentioned, this is an increasing group, primarily owing to the current increased aging population. These patients typically require staged surgeries 3 to 7 days apart. This is because of a higher blood loss in each stage and the presence of increased comorbidities for older patients. The first stage of surgery consists of a flank incision carried distal to expose the lumbosacral junction. An anterior release of the main lumbar curve is performed with fusion, using morselized interbody grafting to either the L3-4 disc or possibly the L4-5 disc. Through the same incision, the remaining disc or discs are removed and replaced with structural femoral ring allograft together with an anterior buttress screw fixation. This is followed by a second stage of posterior release, instrumentation, and fusion, utilizing segmental pedicle screw fixation to derotate the spine and restore lumbar lordosis (Fig. 20-13).

With the increasing use of posterior subtraction osteotomy through rigid apical kyphotic segments, the need for extensive anterior release and fusion proximal to L4 can be avoided. However, anterior interbody fusion from L4 to S1 with structural allograft is still necessary to ensure a successful fusion to the sacrum.

The small direct anterior muscle-sparing incision that is employed risks significantly less morbidity in this older age group than does the flank incision. In an effort to avoid the anterior approach altogether, some surgeons perform posterior interbody fusion techniques such as transforaminal lumbar interbody fusion, but this sacrifices the ability to obtain maximal disc height restoration and lordosis from L4 to S1 in comparison to a separate anterior approach.

The problem of proximal junctional kyphosis is a significant one, particularly as one deals with an aging population. As a general principle, it is inadvisable to stop proximal instrumentation in the area of the thoracolumbar junction. If a patient has a physiologically normal thoracic kyphosis and is 50 years old or younger, often one can stop at approximately the T10 spinal region. The T10 vertebra is usually located below the apex of a thoracic kyphosis.

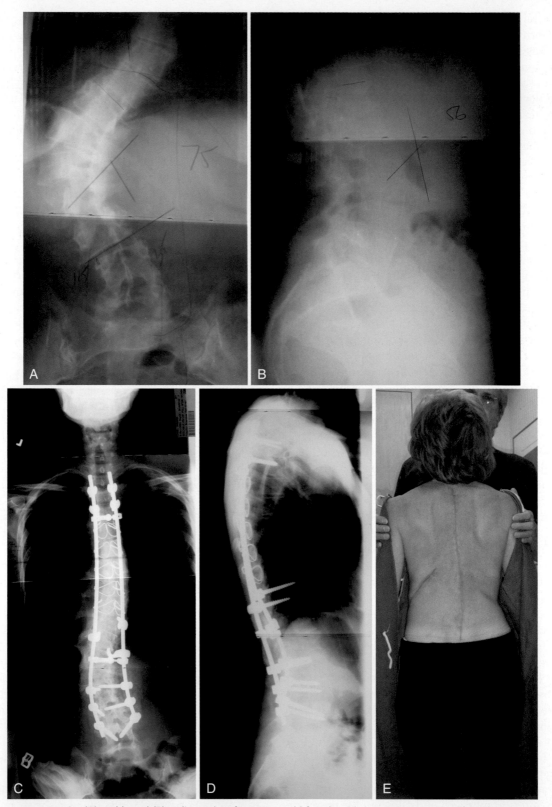

Figure 20-12. Anteroposterior (**A**) and lateral (**B**) radiographs of a 56-year-old female with a progressive curve of 75 degrees and pain located over the lumbar prominence. There was no significant lumbosacral pain, and the lumbar discs were well preserved. Postoperative anteroposterior (**C**), lateral (**D**), and clinical (**E**) appearance.

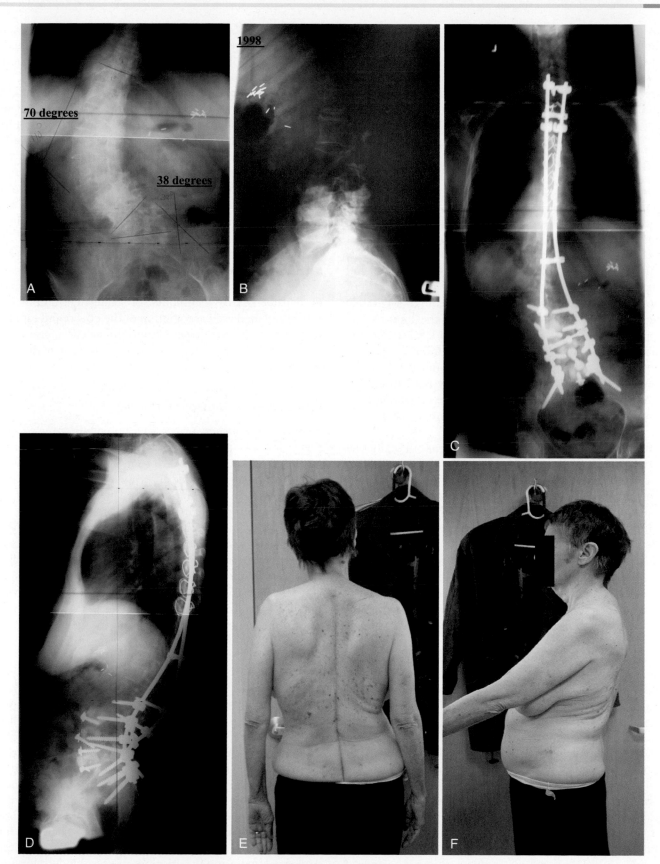

Figure 20-13. **A,** Anteroposterior radiograph. **B,** Lateral radiograph. **C,** Anteroposterior radiograph 4 years postoperatively. **D,** Lateral radiograph 4 years postoperatively. **E,** Clinical postoperative back view. **F,** Clinical postoperative side view.

Proximal instrumentation should never stop at the apex of a thoracic kyphosis. It is preferable to carry instrumentation to the high thoracic spine, with the proviso that there is less risk of a junctional kyphosis; but it can occur even there. Therefore, the proximal level of the fusion is frequently T10 if the curves allow, or instrumentation is carried up to T2 but less frequently in between.

Decision Making in Fusions to the Sacrum

By history, physical examination, radiographic evaluation, and diagnostic testing, it is relatively easy to decide which patients need fusion to the sacrum. Significant pain at the lumbosacral junction, curves emanating out of the sacrum, significant facet and disc degeneration of L4-5 and L5-S1, painful discography at L5-S1, and lumbosacral sagittal and coronal translation are all indications for the extension of fusion to the sacrum. It is more problematic to accurately determine who will be better served in the long run by stopping short of the sacrum, especially at L5, leaving only one mobile disc below a long fusion. The following conundrum exists: While it is technically demanding to achieve a long fusion to the sacrum, it is equally hard to predict the future integrity and functioning of the remaining discs below a long fusion, especially when only the L5-S1 disc remains.

Historical Perspective. Prior to the advent of segmental instrumentation during the Harrington rod era, it was very difficult to maintain lumbar lordosis when extending a fusion into the lower lumbar region, not to mention the sacrum. It was recognized in the late 1970s that, despite the best attempts at rod contouring and specialized hooks, a distraction rod inherently "corrected" lumbar lordosis while correcting coronal deformity with resultant flat-back syndrome. Furthermore, attempts to include the sacrum into long fusion constructs increased the pseudarthrosis rate dramatically. Approximately 50% of patients appeared to acquire flat back with an overall 40% pseudarthrosis rate.

The advent of segmental instrumentation, in particular Luque L-rods, as refined by the Galveston technique, improved the maintenance of lordosis and enhanced rates of fusions in the lumbosacral junction. The development of improved segmental instrumentation, particularly by that of Cotrel-Dubousset, also improved the incidence of pseudarthrosis and maintenance of sagittal balance. Further improvements resulted from better distal sacral fixation techniques, such as the use of four sacral screws, the Jackson intrasacral technique, sacral bars, or iliac screws. The additional recognition of the need for interbody fusion at L4-5 and L5-S1 for attempts at long fusion to the sacrum finally brought pseudarthrosis rates down into the low single-digit range. Initially, this was achieved with structural grafting of the distal lumbosacral junction (L4-S1), although newer posterior interbody fusion techniques seem to have the same positive results. Concerns

have been expressed that fusing the sacrum could result in subsequent degeneration of the sacroiliac joints. This is not a major problem; very few patients afterward require a sacroiliac fusion.

Stopping Short of the Sacrum. The daunting task of achieving fusion to the sacrum has often led to the seemingly attractive solution of stopping the fusion short of the sacrum. This choice brings a separate set of problems. Studies have shown that fusions that stop at L5 do not necessarily have predictable long-term adequate results. Patients who are fused short of the sacrum can develop accelerated distal disc degeneration, leading to pain and significant loss of sagittal balance. It was previously thought that the deeply seated L5 segment might protect the L5-S1 disc and allow for stopping the fusion at L5-S1. Unfortunately, this did not prove to be true. The pros and cons of saving the L5-S1 motion segment continue to be a topic of debate. Better techniques of achieving lumbosacral fusion and increased recognition of the effects and rapidity with which L5-S1 degeneration can occur increasingly may lead the surgeon to include the sacrum within the fusion.

Intraoperative Neuromonitoring

Normally, somatosensory evoked potentials are used routinely for all spinal deformity surgery. More recently, motor evoked potentials have been employed either using cranial stimulation or by applying epidural leads proximally to the instrumentation. We generally do not do Stagnara interoperative wake-up tests unless there are aberrations in spinal cord monitoring. For replacement of pedicle screws in the lumbar spine, free-running electromyograms to test the hole made for the screw as well as the screw following insertion may be employed. Despite surgical expertise in the placement of pedicle screws, rotational deformities sometimes make accurate placement of screws problematic. However, monitoring can decrease the possibility of nerve root injury.

Intraoperative Fluid Management

Patients under the age of 60 generally are allowed to predonate autologous blood. We do not currently allow patients over the age of 60 to predonate their own blood; we believe that this increases the length of stay and complications as well as postoperative efforts at rehabilitation. The use of cell-saver for intraoperative blood replacement is routine. It is important that a clear understanding between the operating surgeon and the anesthesiologist is maintained on blood replacement needs. There is a fine balance to achieve in intraoperative fluid replacement. Abnormal hydration is critical to observe: Underhydration can lead to renal problems and hemodynamic instability, and overhydration can present fluid overload for older patients. Total crystalloid administration during spine

---

BOX 20-1 ASA Physical Status Classification System

P1: A normal healthy patient
P2: A patient with mild systemic disease
P3: A patient with severe systemic disease
P4: A patient with severe systemic disease that is a constant threat to life
P5: A moribund patient who is not expected to survive without the operation
P6: A patient who has been declared brain-dead whose organs are being removed for donor purposes

The American Society of Anesthesiologists does not currently provide additional information to further define the above categories. Excerpted with permission from the 2008 annual edition of ASA Relative Value Guide of the American Society of Anesthesiologists. A copy of the full text can be obtained from ASA, 520 N. Northwest Highway, Park Ridge, Illinois 60068-2573.

---

surgery is known to predict increased lengths of stay in the intensive care unit. Other factors that can contribute to a more extensive intensive care unit stay are age, ASA (American Society of Anesthesiologists) physical status grade (Box 20-1), and additional pertinent aspects of the patient's physical condition. Blood in the form of packed red cells is administered, preferably early during the operative procedure. Certainly, by 1000 mL of blood loss, replacement hemoglobin or cell-saver hemoglobin should have been administered. Dilutional factors, including the loss of clotting factors, after 2000 mL of blood loss are to be anticipated, and clotting factors recovered through fresh frozen plasma and/or platelets might be necessary.

Postoperative Care

On awakening postoperatively, patients should be immediately assessed for neurologic functioning. Depending on the length of the surgery and the volume of blood loss, patients may be admitted into the intensive care unit for observation. Patients are generally allowed to rest for 48 hours, after which they are mobilized gradually. Fluids are permitted as soon as there are abdominal bowel sounds. Until that time, patients are allowed to take only ice chips to moisten their mouths. This significantly decreases the risk of postoperative abdominal ileus. Urinary catheters are removed only when the patients are sufficiently mobilized to allow the free use of a bedside commode or able to self-ambulate to the bathroom. There should be strict instruction to avoid the use of a bedpan with posterior incisions, since wound contamination occurs frequently in this setting, and this practice will increase the risk of wound infection. Discharge times depend on age, comorbidities, and complications. Younger adults are generally discharged within 5 to 7 days, and older adults are discharged within 10 to 12 days, depending on whether staged surgery was necessary. Abdominal binders are used solely for the comfort of the patient with an anterior abdominal incision. Bracing postoperatively depends on the quality of fixation obtained and the quality of the bone that was appreciated intraoperatively. Bracing may also be offered for a period

of 8 to 12 weeks to allow patients greater confidence in early mobilization and provide a sense of security. Patients are allowed to drive once they have decreased their narcotic intake. Return to work de-pends on the patient and his or her work environment and can vary from 6 weeks to 1 year. Generally, the average for patients over age 40 to 45 is between 3 and 4 months following surgery. Full activities, including athletic endeavors, are generally allowed at 6 months postoperatively. Patients are assessed at 6 weeks, 3 months, 6 months, 9 months, 12 months, 18 months, and 2 years postoperatively. They are then advised to return to be checked every 1 to 2 years.

Results of Idiopathic Adult Scoliosis Surgery

As was previously mentioned, pain and progressive curvature are the most important factors in considering deformity surgery for an adult. It is reasonable, given modern techniques of deformity surgery, that long-term improvement will occur in 40% to 60% of the preoperative coronal curve measurements. Regrettably, the spine literature is severely wanting in studies of assessment of pain relief, even for basic procedures such as discectomy and laminectomy. Inconsistent preoperative documentation and a variety of postoperative measurements make definitive statements difficult. Given the state of the literature, it would be reasonable to assume that approximately 70% of patients can achieve excellent relief of pain, while 15% will have partial relief, and the remaining 15% can be considered failures. Within this latter group, however, will be those who will ultimately prove to have a pseudarthrosis. If the surgeon achieves a balanced spine in both the coronal plane and the all-important sagittal plane with a solid fusion, the patient can be expected to have a highly satisfactory result.

DEGENERATIVE ADULT SCOLIOSIS

The second major category of adult scoliosis is deformity that presents de novo in the adult. This has been referred to as *collapsing scoliosis* or *senescent lumbar scoliosis*. The prevalence of de novo curves is unknown. The only certain proof that a patient has a new curve, rather than a progression from a previously unrecognized curve, is documentation of a prior normal spinal radiograph. Most surgeons would agree, however, that scoliosis arising de novo in the adult is probably degenerative in etiology and can be the source of severe symptoms. Attempts have been made to differentiate the adults with preexistent and progressing scoliosis from cases with a new curve. Significant differences and similarities have been identified. The mean age in idiopathic scoliotic patients presenting with symptoms is usually around 40 years of age, whereas the degenerative patient with a new curve usually presents around 60 years of age. The location of the low back pain is similar in both groups: radiating pain from the back into the buttocks and upper thighs. In the degenerative group, approximately 90% of patients will have leg symptoms indicative of spinal stenosis, compared to fewer than one third of the idiopathic patients. The major trigger for the stenotic pain is aggravation by spinal extension. Unlike typical degenerative stenosis, patients often are not relieved by sitting down but have to support their body weight with their arms or lie down to have pain relief.

Radiologic findings can be somewhat distinguishing but not definitive. The idiopathic patient will usually have a curve of around 50 to 60 degrees, whereas the pure degenerative patient will have a curve of 25 to 30 degrees. The idiopathic group frequently will have more of a rotational component to their curvatures as well. The degenerative group will usually demonstrate more consistent lateral translation.

Nonoperative Management

The management for adult degenerative scoliotic patients is similar to nonoperative measures described for adults who have idiopathic curves and consists of nonsteroidal anti-inflammatory medications, exercise (usually with avoidance of extension), and general aerobic conditioning. Braces and corsets can offer temporary relief, but there are no studies to prove their efficacy over time. Treatment of existent osteoporosis and prevention of further bone loss are encouraged, particularly in the female patient.

Operative Indications

The most common indication for surgery in degenerative scoliosis is nerve root symptoms and spinal stenosis. Back pain is frequently a concurrent finding. The debate about who can be treated by decompression alone and who requires decompression with fusion is unresolved. Curves under 15 degrees with unilateral single nerve root compression can benefit from a simple laminotomy if great care is taken to preserve the facets and pars interarticularis. If greater decompression is necessary or facets are sacrificed, the operation should include a fusion in situ or correction of the deformity plus fusion but only if lordosis has been preserved, which is unusual. If the patient is kyphotic, then lordosis must be restored. A patient who is fused in kyphosis is an unhappy patient who is prone to progression and increasing pain in the future.

Preoperative Evaluation

All of the preoperative tests that are recommended for the idiopathic group might also be necessary for the degenerative scoliotic. However, pulmonary dysfunction is rarely an issue unless the patient has other coexistent disease(s). If fusion is to be performed, the first question is how many vertebrae to include in the fusion. Criteria that are used to decide the extent of fusion in the adolescent are similarly applicable in the scoliotic adult and include the stable zone, the central sacral line, neutrally rotated vertebra, levels of

degenerative arthritis, displaced wedging, rotatory subluxation, and hemisacralization. It is important to understand that multiple factors must be considered in selecting the extent of fusion in adults. The most important factors in adults often turn out to be the presence and magnitude of degeneration in the lower lumbar levels. Vertebral levels with rotatory subluxation, disc space narrowing, and wedging are also important, since fusion should not be stopped above these levels. All of these findings are common and can be seen in at least 50% of adult patients. An oblique L5 takeoff and hemisacralization are seen in 25% of patients; their presence is relevant to the decision to include the lumbosacral joint. When all criteria are applied to decisions regarding the final extent of individual fusions, significant pain improvement can be achieved in 9 out of 10 patients. An important principle is to identify and incorporate all painful areas into the fusion to the best of our diagnostic abilities. If necessary, preoperative discography and facet blocks should be applied to determine the pain-associated segments.

Surgical Approaches

The first important decision is whether decompression is necessary, as assessed by preoperative findings and imaging studies. Unfortunately, there is no one criterion by which to easily establish that adequate decompression has been accomplished. Intraoperatively, the restoration of a pulsatile dura and the patency of the foramina are critical to appreciate. Postoperatively, a CT myelogram, CT scan, or MRI might prove useful to establish that an adequate decompression has been achieved.

If fusion is selected, many of the same basic strategies apply as were described previously in this chapter. Fusion in situ may be considered, although a lower rate of arthrosis will likely result with pedicle screw instrumentation. Even in this older age group, there remains a role for a combined anterior and posterior approach, particularly at unstable levels and particularly at the lumbosacral junction and to restore lumbar lordosis. As in the case of idiopathic curves, however, a posterior-only approach utilizing kyphectomy (posterior substraction osteotomy) may be used to restore lordosis. In addition, the use of posterior lumbar interbody or translumbar interforaminal fusions performed at the levels of decompression could preclude the use of anterior lumbar interbody fusions. No data exist as to which is better in achieving fusion, although there is a reasonable assumption that anterior fusion yields a lower pseudarthrosis rate with better correction of lordosis.

Surgical Results

Simmons and Capicotto reported on spinal stenosis associated with scoliosis. In a review of 40 patients (with an average age of 61.5 years) who were treated by posterior decompression and pedicle screw fixation, 93% showed marked improvement in pain. The average degree of deformity preoperatively was 37 degrees, and the average degree of deformity postoperatively was 19 degrees. There were no associated deaths, instrumentation failures, or pseudarthroses. Others have also reported on the use of pedicle fixation in the treatment of degenerative adult lumbar scoliosis. The average correction was just over 50%. Satisfactory results were obtained in approximately 85% of cases, and pseudarthrosis occurred in about 5%. The mean age was 60 years. We would agree, on the basis of our experience, that the age of patients with degenerative scoliosis was not a contraindication to surgery. Restoration of lumbar lordosis is paramount to achieving a good outcome, and use of pedicle fixation in the case of osteoporotic bone will allow this to be done.

COMPLICATIONS IN ADULT IDIOPATHIC SCOLIOSIS AND DEGENERATIVE SCOLIOSIS

Complications in the surgical treatment of adult scoliosis are common and based on numerous factors, including age, ASA status, number of stages, estimated blood loss, and spinal location of the surgery. From 40% to 100% of patients experience at least one complication, according to the literature. Differentiation is often made between minor and major complications, although there is no standard definition of either to distinguish between the two. One common distinction has been to define life-threatening complications as major and all others as minor. In considering all possible complications, it would be reasonable to assume that one third are major and two thirds are minor. Major complications would include pulmonary emboli, coagulopathy, lower-extremity paralysis, cauda equina syndrome, epidural hematoma, major vessel injury, bowel necrosis or perforation, hyponatremia syndrome of inappropriate antidiuretic hormone secretion, adult respiratory distress syndromes, myocardial infarction, generalized sepsis, deep wound infections, deep vein thromboses, genitourinary injuries, and death. Obviously, this is a sobering list of complications. Complication rates are higher for an ASA status of 2 or greater, staged procedures, increasing age, decreased pulmonary function, degree of deformity, and excessive blood loss. With careful preoperative assessment of the patient and understanding the specific risk factors for each patient, the incidence of major complications as well as the severity of each complication can optimistically be kept to a reasonable level. Despite the potential for complications, patient satisfaction rate and the percentage of patients who would undergo the same surgery under similar circumstances have been reported in the 80% to 90% range.

Infection

Infection in scoliosis surgery overall lies between 1% and 2%, based on repeated reports of the Scoliosis Research Society Morbidity Committee. This incidence is somewhat higher in the adult scoliosis population, with a rate of approximately 3% to 4%. Infection events are fewer across single-stage combined procedures than in staged or combined procedures.

Blood Loss

As with any surgical procedure, excessive blood loss is to be avoided, along with other complications such as coagulopathy or pulmonary capillary damage leading to adult respiratory distress syndrome. The average blood loss will vary in adult scoliosis surgery depending on the number of approaches and the number of levels involved in the fusion. On average, it can be assumed that approximately 5 mL per minute of surgical time (300 mL/hour) will be lost.

Pseudarthrosis

Pseudarthrosis rates will vary in adult scoliosis, depending on the length of the fusion and whether or not the fusion is extended to the sacrum. In series reported from experienced centers, pseudarthrosis rates as low as 3% to 4% have been achieved. Because of the rigid segmental instrumentation that is currently used, pseudarthrosis can be difficult to diagnose. Failure of instrumentation occurs in only a minority of pseudarthrosis patients. Pseudarthrosis might not even be diagnosed until 2 to 3 years postoperatively. In the majority of cases (two thirds), the defect can be appreciated on radiograph; in the remainder, exploration of the fusion mass might be necessary for diagnosis. One large series on pseudarthrosis noted that curvature increased an average of 7 degrees in the anterior/posterior view and kyphosis increased by a mean of 10 degrees from the time of the original arthrodesis to the time of pseudarthrosis repair. Loss of correction might be easier to document in Harrington instrumentation than in the newer forms of segmental fixation.

Staging of Surgery

Controversy exists as to the staging of surgery with patients who require anterior and posterior procedures. When combined single-stage procedures are compared to staged procedures 7 to 10 days later, morbidity from infection is less and hospital costs are 30% less in patients who underwent single-stage combined procedures. Protein and calorie malnutrition in patients increases the risk of postoperative morbidity for staged procedures. Parenteral hyperalimentation has been suggested between stages to minimize this problem. Procedures that last longer than 10 to 12 hours also have high morbidity rates. In experienced hands, regardless of the number of stages, if the anesthetic event can be limited to less than 12 hours, then finishing the entire procedure is reasonable to consider (Fig. 20-14). Decisions on staging are therefore multifactorial and based on the speed of the surgeon; the complexity of the surgery to be performed; the patient's overall medical status; and unfortunate, sometimes unpredictable, intraoperative events.

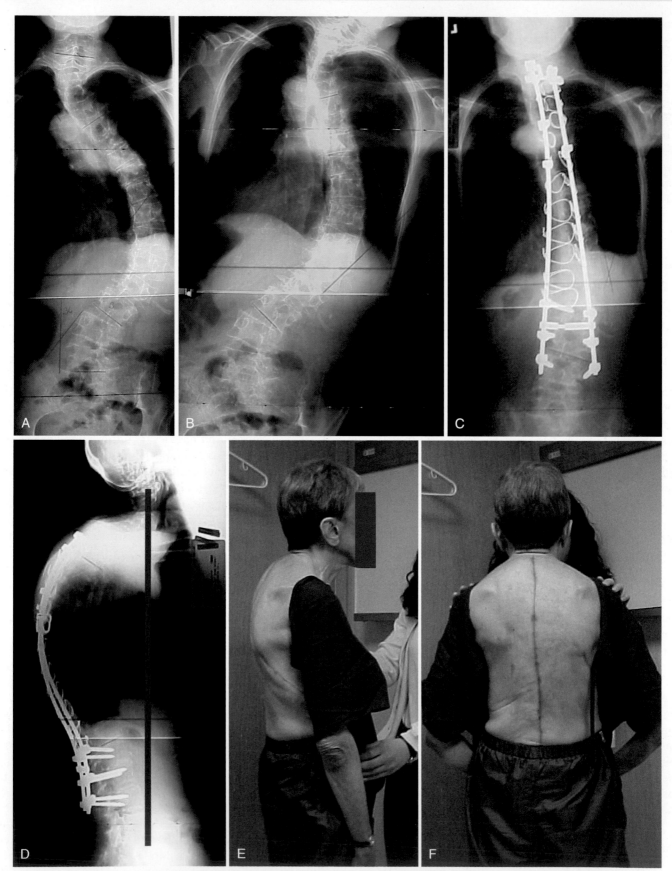

Figure 20-14. A, A 72-year-old patient with painful progression of an 80-degree thoracic curve. **B,** Right-bending films show little or no correction. **C,** Anteroposterior postoperative radiograph. Despite her age, her general medical condition was excellent. Same-day anterior release and fusion were safely performed with MOTTA mini open thoracotomy, thoracoscopically assisted, followed by posterior instrumentation and fusion surgery. **D,** Lateral postoperative radiograph. **E** and **F,** Clinical appearance of the patient postoperatively with preserved sagittal balance.

SUMMARY

Adult scoliosis comprises a diverse group of patients, whose commonality is their presentation in adulthood. Regardless of etiology or whether the condition began before or after skeletal maturity, the important clinical issues are back pain and neurologic symptoms, which are more common in patients with degenerative curves. These two types of symptoms serve as the most common indications for surgery, although curve progression and occasionally cosmesis can be important issues. In the lumbar spine, the most critical factor for success is the restoration or maintenance of lumbar lordosis. The surgical management of an iatrogenic flat back is a major undertaking, and avoidance of this problem is critical. Fusion often might have to extend into the lumbosacral junction. It is important to assess that need not only from the history, physical examination, plain radiographs, and other imaging studies but also by discography. In general, in extending a fusion to the sacrum, a combined anterior-posterior approach will minimize the possibility of instrumentation failure and pseudarthrosis. Modern internal fixation devices add to the predictability of fusion, and properly selected devices and techniques allow for the maintenance of lumbar lordosis. A realistic assessment of the patient's individualized risks of complications in the surgical treatment of adult scoliosis must be discussed in detail with the patient.

It is the advances in technology that have broadened so considerably our treatment for the different types of presenting curve pathology and ultimate patterns of kyphotic, lordotic, and scoliotic deformity. The surgeon's challenge is to diagnose the patient's individual pathology intelligently and apply the optimal surgical technology with meticulous surgical technique. Creation of surgical constructs should take into consideration transition zones and the inherent deforming forces that resist correction until fusion occurs. Using the techniques and principles outlined in this chapter will allow for a high rate of symptomatic relief and successful fusion. With continued refinements in technology and technique, the rate of success and the reduction of complications will improve further.

PEARLS & PITFALLS

PEARLS

- For pedicle screw insertion in the upper spine, there is no need to destroy the superiormost ligamentum flavum or the interspinous ligaments, which is often necessary with hooks, particularly when downward-going hooks are used at the top of a construct.
- The bilateral pars defects, created for improving curve flexibility, represent potential new high-risk areas for pseudarthrosis, especially when not located within an area of an anterior release and fusion. In contrast, pedicle subtraction osteotomy performed in areas of sharp kyphotic deformities do create an area for anterior healing to occur.
- Recognizing naturally occurring stiff to flexible transition zones, such as the thoracolumbar junction and the lumbosacral junction, recognizing whether a surgical construct plan has created iatrogenic stiff to flexible transition zones, modifying the plan accordingly can potentially minimize the risk of pseudarthrosis.
- The use of a derotation maneuver is now almost routine, because it has the capability to reproduce lordosis in the lumbar spine or reduce kyphosis in the thoracolumbar spine.
- As a general principle, it is inadvisable to stop proximal instrumentation in the area of the thoracolumbar junction. In a patient who has a physiologically normal thoracic kyphosis and is 50 years old or younger, often one can stop at approximately the T10 spinal region.

PITFALLS

- The most common mistake of an inexperienced surgeon in the anterior approach is performing an inadequate discectomy and end plate preparation, which limits the correction and increases the rates of both instrumentation failure and pseudarthrosis.
- Proximal instrumentation should never stop at the apex of a thoracic kyphosis. It is preferable to carry instrumentation to the high thoracic spine with the proviso that there is less risk of a junctional kyphosis, but even there, it may occur.
- Decisions on staging are multifactorial and are based on the speed of the surgeon; the complexity of the surgery to be performed; the patient's overall medical status; and, unfortunately, sometimes unpredictable intraoperative events.
- Further extension of an anterior technique above the T9 level is rarely of value, since the disc spaces are so narrow that little correction can be obtained in the adult, although its efficacy has been shown in the thoracic spine of adolescents.
- In general, older patients with stiffer curves are at a higher risk of postoperative complications.

Illustrative Case Presentations

CASE 1. A 58-Year-Old Female with a History of Scoliosis Since Adolescence Who Now Has Complaints of Pain in the Left Lumbar Area

Pain is worsened with standing and walking. Scoliosis radiographs demonstrate the following curves: 27 degrees right thoracic (T2-9), 72 degrees left thoracolumbar (T9-L3), and 38 degrees right lumbar (Figs. 20-15 and 20-16). Bending films demonstrate minimal flexibility of the thoracolumbar curve (65 degrees). MRI of the lumbar spine demonstrates good preservation of the L4-5 and L5-S1 discs. The patient underwent an anterior release and fusion from T10 to L3 and posterior fusion and instrumentation from T4 to L4. The postoperative thoracic and thoracolumbar curves measure 14 and 12 degrees, respectively (Figs. 20-17 and 20-18).

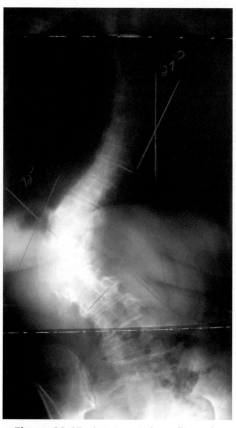

Figure 20-15. Anteroposterior radiograph.

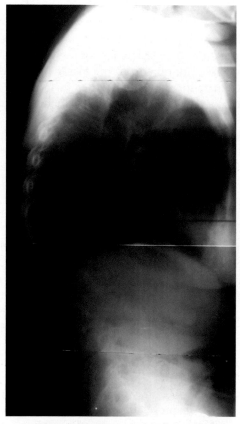

Figure 20-16. Lateral radiograph.

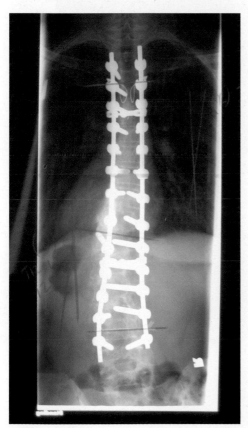

Figure 20-17. Postoperative anteroposterior view.

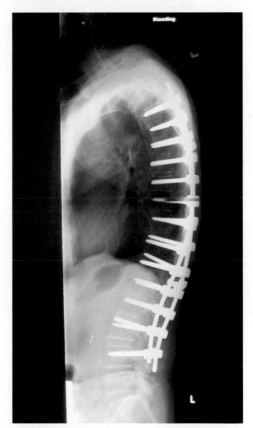

Figure 20-18. Postoperative lateral view.

CASE 2. A 36-Year-Old Female with Worsening Scoliosis Since Her Teenage Years

The patient denies pain and has had no previous treatments. Physical examination demonstrates right thoracic and left lumbar prominence. She is neurologically intact (Figs. 20-19 to 20-21).

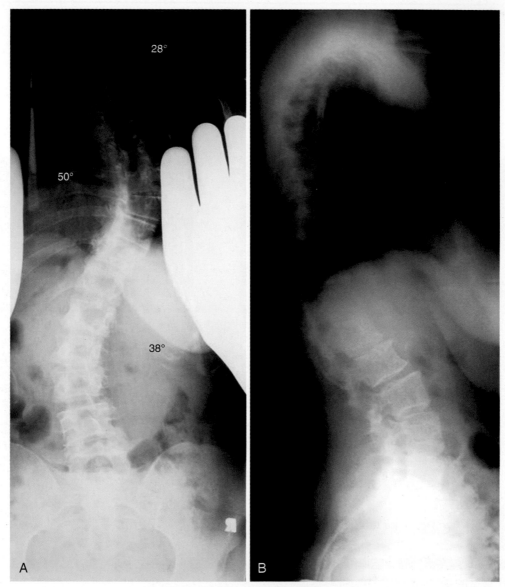

Figure 20-19. Preoperative roentgenograms.

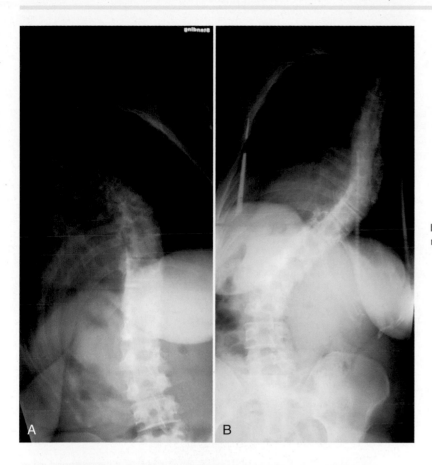

Figure 20-20. Preoperative side-bending roentgenograms.

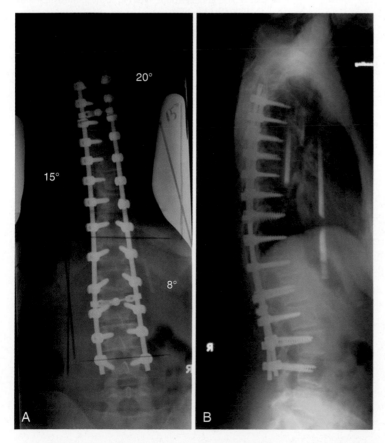

Figure 20-21. Postoperative roentgenograms showing correction at 24 months.

SUGGESTED READINGS

Bridwell HK, Edwards CC, Lenke LG: The pros and cons to saving the L5-S1 motion segment in a long scoliosis fusion construct. Spine 2003;28:S234–S242.

A clear discussion of decision making in fusing to the sacrum.

Byrd JA III, Scoles PV, Winter RB, et al: Adult idiopathic scoliosis treated by anterior and posterior spinal fusion. J Bone Joint Surg Am 1987; 9:843–850.

Minneapolis experience in anterior posterior fusion for adult scoliosis.

Cotrel Y, Dubousset J, Guillaumat M: New universal instrumentation in spinal surgery. Clin Orthop 1988;227:10–22.

One of the original descriptions of the first dual hook-rod-screw segmental instrumentation systems.

Devlin VJ, Boachie-Adjei O, Bradford DS, et al: Treatment of adult spinal deformity with fusion to the sacrum using CD instrumentation. J Spinal Disord 1991;4:1–14.

Article discussing the difficulties involved in obtaining a successful long fusion to the sacrum.

Dick J, Boachie-Adjei O, Wilson M: One stage versus two stage anterior and posterior spinal reconstruction in adults: Comparison of outcomes including nutritional status, complication rates, hospital costs and factors. Spine 1992;17:S310–S216.

An in-depth discussion of the pros and cons of deciding on staging anterior/posterior surgeries in the adult scoliosis population.

Jackson RP, Simmons EH, Stripinis D: Incidence and severity of back pain in adult idiopathic scoliosis. Spine 1983;8:749–756.

One of the early articles discussing the magnitude of the pain problem in adult idiopathic scoliosis.

Kostuik JP: Adult scoliosis. In Frymoyer J (ed): The Adult Spine: Principles and Practice. New York: Raven Press, 1991.

A textbook chapter with exhaustive detail of the experience to date with adult scoliosis.

Kostuik JP: Decision making in adult scoliosis. Spine 1979;4:521–525.

A classic early article describing how to approach surgery in adult scoliosis given the instrumentation systems that were available at the time.

Kostuik JP, Carl A, Ferron S: Anterior Zielke instrumentation for spinal deformity in adults. J Bone Joint Surg Am 1989;72:898–912.

A large series of anterior spinal instrumentations used in the adult population.

Kostuik JP, Israel J, Hall JE: Scoliosis surgery in adults. Clin Orthop 1973;93:225–234.

One of the earliest descriptions of entertaining scoliosis surgery in the adult population from the early Toronto experience.

Lauerman WC, Bradford DS, Ogilvie JW, Transfeldt EE: Results of lumbar pseudarthrosis repair. J Spin Disord 1992;5:149–157.

An excellent review of the diagnosis and treatment of pseudarthosis in the lumbar spine.

Luque ER: Segmental spinal instrumentation for correction of scoliosis. Clin Orthop 1982;163:192–198.

One of the original classic articles on Luque instrumentation by E.R. Luque, the master, himself.

Ponder RC, Dickson JH, Harrington PR, Erwin WD: Results of Harrington instrumentation and fusion in the adult idiopathic scoliosis patient. J Bone Joint Surg Am 1975;57:797–801.

A classic article outlining the use of Harrington instrumentation in the adult population.

Schwab FJ, Dubey A, Pagala M, et al: Adult scoliosis: A health assessment analysis by SF-36. Spine 2003;28:602–606.

A sophisticated outcomes assessment of adult scoliosis utilizing modern outcome measures.

Simmons EH, Capicotto WN: Posterior transpedicular Zielke instrumentation of the lumbar spine. Clin Orthop 1989;236:180–191.

One of the original articles discussing the experience with pedicle screws in degenerative conditions of the lumbar spine.

Winter RB, Lonstein JE, Denis F: Pain patterns in adult scoliosis. Orthop Clin North Am 1988;19:339–345.

An in-depth look at adult scoliosis with attention to the issue of pain and disability.

CHAPTER 21

Degenerative Spondylolisthesis

Thomas J. Errico *and* Martin Quirno

OVERVIEW

Degenerative spondylolisthesis is described as the anterior translation of one vertebral body over another adjacent vertebra in the absence of a defect of the pars interarticularis. This pathology was first described by Junghanns in 1930 as a pseudospondylolisthesis (cited in Herkowitz and Kurz and Kornblum and colleagues). The term *degenerative spondylolisthesis* was first described by Newman in 1955, based on the discovery of an intact neural arch and a slippage of the vertebrae due to degenerative arthritis of the facet joints.

The prevalence of degenerative spondylolisthesis is approximately 8.7% in the general population, with 66% of cases involving only one level and 34% involving two or more levels. Seventy percent present as anterolisthesis, and the remaining 30% present as retrolisthesis. Previous studies demonstrate a higher incidence in patients older than 50 years, especially women. The most commonly affected level is the L4-5.

Degenerative spondylolisthesis is a multifactorial disease. Disc degeneration, pregnancy, generalized joint laxity, and oophorectomy are currently believed to be the main predisposing factors. Other possible predisposing factors include sagittal orientation of the facet joints and increased pedicle facet angle, although these are currently controversial.

The slippage is believed to be secondary to the buckling of the ligamentum flavum. This process is due to the combination of one of the previously mentioned risk factors and the narrowing of the disc space due to disc degeneration. This listhesis may cause lower back pain, radicular pain, and/or symptoms of neurogenic claudication.

EVALUATION

General and surgical history should be collected to assess possible patient risk factors as well as specific symptoms. Because degenerative spondylolisthesis and lumbar stenosis commonly have similar symptomatology, the differentiating of these conditions becomes the first step toward optimal management. Patients with both lumbar stenosis and degenerative spondylolisthesis complain of back and leg pain as well as neurologic symptoms such as numbness, tingling, dysesthesia, and subjective weakness that are often exacerbated by either prolonged standing or walking. Fixed neurologic deficits may be absent or subtle in the form of reflex changes and/or mild bowel or bladder difficulties. Significant fixed motor paralysis and/or significant bowel or bladder symptoms are less common and may be seen in neglected cases or, even less commonly, in acute presentations. However, patient symptomatology does not definitively differentiate pure lumbar stenosis from degenerative spondylolisthesis.

RADIOLOGIC IMAGING

The differentiation of pure lumbar stenosis from degenerative spondylolisthesis begins with plain radiographs and dynamic lateral flexion and extension radiographs. The patient's symptoms should correlate with the pathologic anatomy that was noted on all preoperative imaging studies. More than 4 mm of anterior translation of the superior vertebral body on the inferior body constitutes degenerative spondylolisthesis. Standing lateral flexion and extension radiographs may provide additional evidence of dynamic instability to supine lateral flexion and extension views.

Magnetic resonance imaging (MRI) is gradually becoming the preferred method of documenting neural compression. Increased sophistication in the technology and interpretation of MRI scans, with or without supplemental computed tomography (CT) images, has decreased the "mandatory" usage of CT myelography for all surgical patients. Some radiologic facilities will supplement MRI images with select CT cuts through the spine areas where maximal compression has occurred. A CT image better defines the bony architecture of the spinal column, while an MRI scan better depicts the soft neural structures. The CT scan will also provide information on the extent of the neural compression due to bone involvement. Neural compression is usually due to a reduction of the spinal canal from posterior protrusion of the disc material, hypertrophy of both the facets and ligamentum flavum, and the listhesis.

TREATMENT OPTIONS

Common nonoperative measures to treat spondylolisthesis include active physical therapy, pharmacologic management, and injection techniques for steroid medications. Failure to see improvement after implementation of an adequate and coordinated program of conservative care is an indication for considering operative treatment. Since rapid neurologic deterioration is relatively rare, the vast majority of surgeries are elective.

First and foremost, decision making in lumbar stenosis involves differentiating between the two entities of stenosis and spondylolisthesis as the cause of the patient's symptomatology. Pure lumbar stenosis is frequently found in combination with significant osteoarthritic changes, often with large osteophyte formations. Pure degenerative spondylolisthesis is frequently manifested as a grade 1 spondylolisthesis of L4 on L5 and is more frequent in females than in males. There is an overlap of radiologic findings between these two entities that requires further categorization. Each level of the lumbar spine can be assessed preoperatively for individual stability based on disc height, angular motion of the end plates, translation as measured on plain radiographs, or fixed or mobile translation as evaluated on dynamic radiographs. Unfortunately, the preoperative assessment of stability loses significance after destabilizing decompressive procedures have been performed.

Increasingly, the lumbar spine is iatrogenically destabilized by hemilaminectomy, central laminectomy, concomitant discectomy, partial facetectomy, total facetectomy, and violation and destruction of the pars interarticularis. Guidelines based on biomechanical studies have suggested that it is safe to remove unilaterally or bilaterally up to 50% of either the medial or lateral facets without destabilizing the motion segment. This guideline might not apply in the clinical setting of a motion segment with more than 4 mm of fixed translation, even if the disc space is bone on bone with no angular or translational movement demonstrated on preoperative dynamic radiographs. Similarly, postoperative stability cannot be guaranteed in lumbar stenosis without translational instability even if, unilaterally, 100% of the medial facet is resected while 100% of the lateral facet is left intact (equal to a 50% facet joint resection). It is important to understand that the 50% rule means leaving 50% of a facet with functional medial and lateral components.

Clearly, violation of the pars interarticularis during a decompressive procedure creates an immediate prediliction for a painful postoperative instability. Iatrogenic violation of the pars not only produces increased instability but also decreases the probability of a successful fusion, even with the addition of instrumentation.

SURGICAL INDICATIONS

1. Persistent or recurrent back and/or leg pain or neurogenic claudication, with significant reduction of quality of life, despite a reasonable trial of nonoperative treatment (minimum of 3 months)
2. Progressive neurologic symptoms
3. Bladder or bowel symptoms

The main goal in treatment of spinal stenosis with degenerative spondylolisthesis is decompression of both the exiting and traversing nerve roots. The role of arthrodesis, with or without instrumentation, in the treatment of spinal stenosis with degenerative spondylolisthesis is controversial. In a retrospective review of 290 patients who underwent decompression laminectomy with 10-year follow-up, the reported outcome was excellent in 69% of patients, good in 13%, fair in 12%, and poor in 6%. The reoperation rate for pseudarthrosis was only 2.7%. A prospective randomized study conducted by Herkowitz and Kurz compared the results at 3 years' follow-up of decompression alone versus decompression and intertransverse arthrodesis in patients with one level of spinal stenosis and degenerative spondylolisthesis. Only 44% of patients with decompression without fusion reported a satisfactory outcome, compared to 96% of patients reporting the same outcome who received decompression plus fusion. Patients who underwent concomitant arthrodesis had significantly better results. Moreover, despite the pseudarthrosis rate of 36% in patients who underwent decompression and in situ fusion, all had good to excellent results. Significant progression of the slip did not occur in either group. The authors concluded that patients with degenerative spondylolisthesis and stenosis should undergo concomitant arthrodesis at the time of decompression.

Mardjetko and colleagues attempted a meta-analysis of the literature on degenerative spondylolisthesis. This meta-analysis demonstrated that patient outcome was significantly better when concomitant arthrodesis was performed ($P < 0.0001$). A satisfactory clinical result was found in 69% of the 260 patients who received decompression without spinal arthrodesis; progression of the spondylolisthesis occurred in 31% of these patients. Ninety percent of patients who had a surgical decompression with posterolateral arthrodesis achieved a satisfactory clinical outcome, with progressive listhesis in only 17%.

An instrumented arthrodesis has been shown to produce higher fusion rates; however, the clinical outcome of decompression with instrumented spinal fusion for this entity is not completely known. Fischgrund and colleagues examined 67 patients who had undergone decompression and arthrodesis with or without instrumentation. Patients who underwent the instrumented arthrodesis demonstrated an 87% fusion rate, while the patients who underwent a noninstrumented arthrodesis had a 45% fusion rate. However, the higher fusion rate of the instrumented group did not improve their clinical outcome. A landmark follow-up study of longer duration by Kornblum and colleagues reviewed 47 of the original patients who were diagnosed with single-level symptomatic spinal stenosis and spondylolisthesis and were treated with decompression and in situ arthrodesis. These patients were observed over 5 to 14 years, with an average follow-up of 7 years and 8 months. The researchers found that the long-term clinical outcome was excellent or good in 86% of patients who had solid arthrodesis but only 56% in the patients who developed a pseudarthrosis. Significant differences in residual back and lower-limb pain were discovered between the two groups, the solid fusion group performing significantly better in the symptom, severity, and physical function categories on self-administered questionnaires. Patients who achieved a solid fusion had improved clinical results, which demonstrated the benefit of a successful arthrodesis over pseudarthrosis with respect to back and lower-limb symptomatology compared to their prior short-term studies.

When reviewing the current literature, one might conclude that patients who at least have an arthrodesis attempted, even if this results in pseudarthrosis, will have better short-term results than will patients who have no attempt at arthrodesis. Although this "fibrous union" might benefit patients in the short term, long-term results deteriorate in patients who do not have a solid fusion. On the basis of the literature, one can conclude that patients who receive instrumentation at the same time as arthrodesis will have a higher fusion rate. A higher fusion rate when instrumentation is used, along with the desirable long-term clinical effect of achieving a solid fusion, makes the case for using instrumentation in the treatment of degenerative spondylolisthesis. Because fusion performed with instruments will improve the likelihood of a solid fusion, this would suggest that an instrumented arthrodesis in the treatment of degenerative spondylolisthesis is preferred over noninstrumented fusion.

CONCLUSIONS

Degenerative spondylolisthesis is a highly prevalent pathology that affects patients older than 50 years of age, especially women. The increasing life expectancy due to new medical and sanitary technological outbursts will increase the incidence of this disease in the future. The proper long-term quantification of diagnostic and treatment methods will allow larger patient pools to be assessed in a more cost-effective manner.

Decision making in lumbar degenerative spondylolisthesis involves differentiating between the two entities of stenosis and spondylolisthesis as the cause of the patient's symptomatology. This is properly obtained through correlation of symptoms and radiographic evaluation. There must be a consideration of the extent of disease, adequacy of decompression, and instability that may be surgically produced.

The latest surgical evidence proves that instrumentation is associated with better fusion percentages and fewer long-term complications when compared to noninstru-

mentation. New long-term studies will prove whether instrumentation also leads to significantly better clinical outcomes.

There is still a paucity of evidence focusing on the effectiveness of bone morphogenetic protein and dynamic stabilization devices on degenerative spondylolisthesis and how they influence the patient's outcome. Future studies could show a promising replacement for current therapies.

PEARLS & PITFALLS

- Differentiation between degenerative spondylolisthesis and spinal stenosis is the first step toward optimal management. Identifying the etiology of symptoms is of primary importance.
- Three major types of pain patterns can present in these patients. It is important to understand the patterns' different mechanisms to identify where symptoms come from.
- Neurogenic claudication can be caused either by pure spinal stenosis (hypertrophy of ligamentum flavum or encroaching facet osteophytes) or by spinal stenosis secondary to degenerative spondylolisthesis. This symptom is presented by pain along the buttock and both legs brought on by walking or standing. It is often associated with tingling, numbness, and weakness in the legs and is relieved by flexing the spine. It is thought to result from oxygen deprivation of the cauda equina in cases of severe lumbar stenosis. This symptom does not usually present in pure degenerative low-grade spondylolisthesis.
- Radicular pain is associated with numbness, paresthesias, and sensory or motor deficit in the specific motor root distribution. It is due to compression of the nerve root in the lateral recess or in the foramen. The pain is secondary to mechanical compression as well as a local inflammatory reaction. This pattern is usually present in patients with some level of spondylolisthesis, although it can appear in pure forms of stenosis, secondary to facet hypertrophy, intervertebral disc herniation, or osteophytes from the posterolateral corner of the vertebral end plate.
- Mechanical low back is the third and last kind of pain. It is referred as pain related to the posture and activities of daily life. It is thought to be due to abnormal distribution of load across the vertebral end plate following disc degeneration. This pattern produces a characteristic "pain catch" in the lower back when the patient rises from a forward bent posture, followed by pain climbing up the body. It is secondary to instability and abnormal increase in vertebral translation. The presence of this pain does not help to differentiate which process is behind it, although it usually is more associated with a slippage instability.
- Patient symptomatology does not definitively differentiate pure lumbar stenosis from degenerative spondylolisthesis. Therefore, the next step begins with analyzing plain radiographs and dynamic lateral flexion and exten-

sion radiographs. More than 4 mm of anterior translation of the superior vertebral body on the inferior body constitutes degenerative spondylolisthesis. Standing lateral flexion and extension radiographs can provide additional evidence of dynamic instability to supine lateral flexion and extension views. This is a controversial issue because there actually is no evidence that the range of motion is increased or unchanged in flexion-extension lateral radiographs when degenerative spondylolisthesis patients are compared to normal patients.

■ When considering surgical treatment, the orthopedic surgeon has to take into consideration that for the primary condition of degenerative spondylolisthesis not associated with spinal stenosis, the choice of fusion is unambiguous, instrumentation being weighed in the balance. Most recently, research appears to indicate that an instrumented arthrodesis, as opposed to a noninstrumented procedure, could provide the patient's best opportunity for long-term clinical benefit, owing to a substantially lower incidence of pseudarthrosis. However, there is also evidence that instrumentation has a higher complication rate and shows no significant difference in comparison with noninstrumentation in patients' health quality of life in the short term. It is generally accepted that instrumentation has to be indicated whenever there is evidence of higher grades of listhesis (2 or higher) and clinical or radiologic signs of instability. Its use in lower grades should also be considered according to the latest evidence.

Illustrative Case Presentations

CASE 1. A 73-Year-Old Female Who Presented with Back Pain, Pain Down the Posterior Aspect of Both Legs, and Bilateral Lower-Limb Numbness (Fig. 21-1)

The patient had a history of atrial fibrillation and pacemaker implantation. Physical examination revealed power 5/5, reduced sensation in left leg L3 to S1, and absent knee and ankle reflexes. There was no improvement following epidural steroid injection (Fig. 21-1E). Treatment was with bilateral laminotomy at L4-5 and insertion of a Coflex interspinous implant (Fig. 21-1F and G).

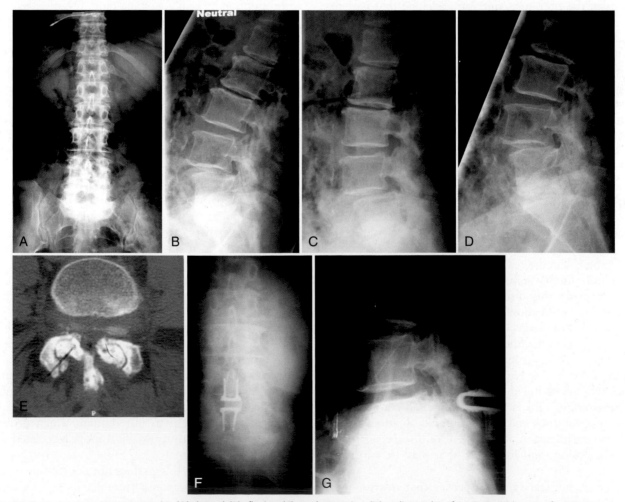

Figure 21-1. Preoperative anteroposterior (**A**), lateral (**B**), flexion (**C**), and extension (**D**) radiographs of L4-5. **E,** CT image of L4-5. Postoperative anteroposterior (**F**) and lateral (**G**) radiographs.

CASE 2. A 63-Year-Old Male Who Complained of Progressive Low Back Pain of 6 Years' Duration (7 out of 10 in Intensity, Worst While Standing) That Radiates to the Right Buttock and Calf (Fig. 21-2)

The patient also referred to tingling and muscle weakness in his lower right leg. He denied bowel or bladder disturbances. The patient tried physical therapy and epidural injections, although neither helped. He had no prior significant medical or surgical history. Physical examination revealed no pain on palpation; spine range of motion was within normal limits; he exhibited negative bilateral straight leg raising; and muscle strength was 5/5 in all quadrants. Preoperative diagnoses included spinal stenosis from L3 to L5 and degenerative spondylolisthesis at L4-5. L3-5 laminectomy was performed with segmental pedicle screw fixation and iliac crest bone grafting.

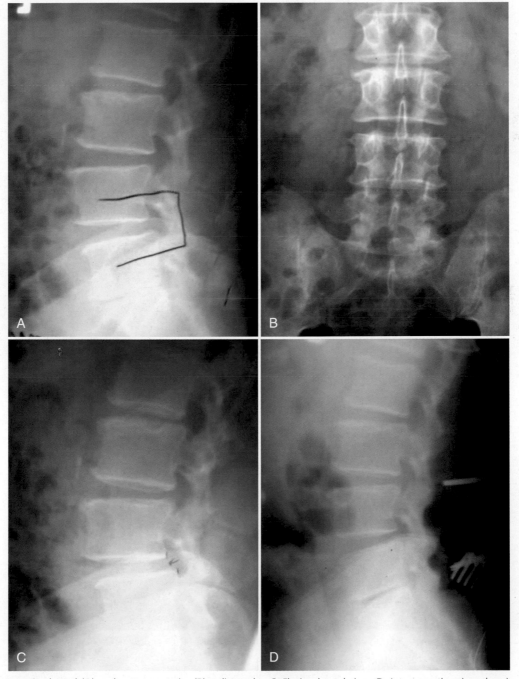

Figure 21-2. Preoperative lateral (**A**) and anteroposterior (**B**) radiographs. **C,** Flexion lateral view. **D,** Intraoperative view showing reduction of mild spondylolisthesis.

Continued

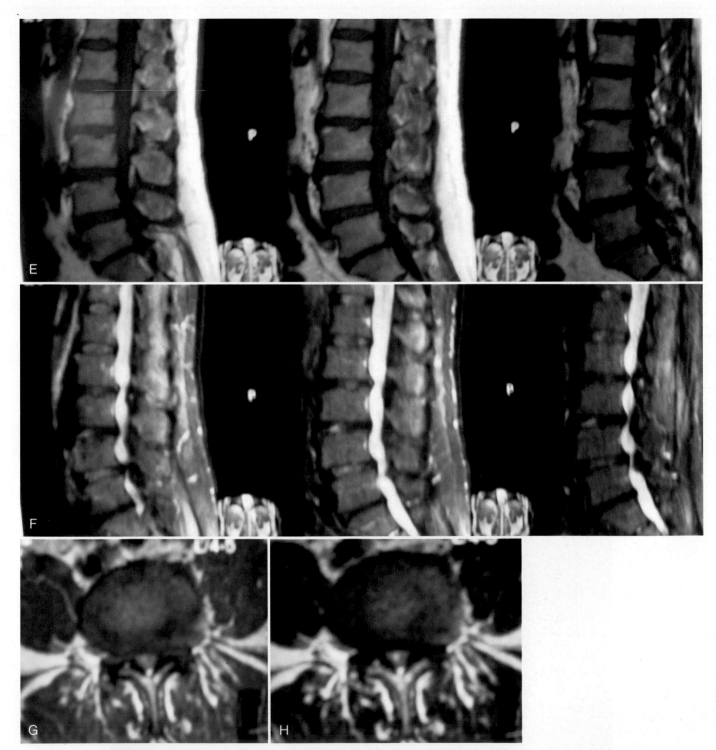

Figure 21-2, cont'd. T1 (**E**) and T2 (**F**) lumbar MRI, lateral views. T1 (**G**) and T2 (**H**) MRI at the L4-5 level.

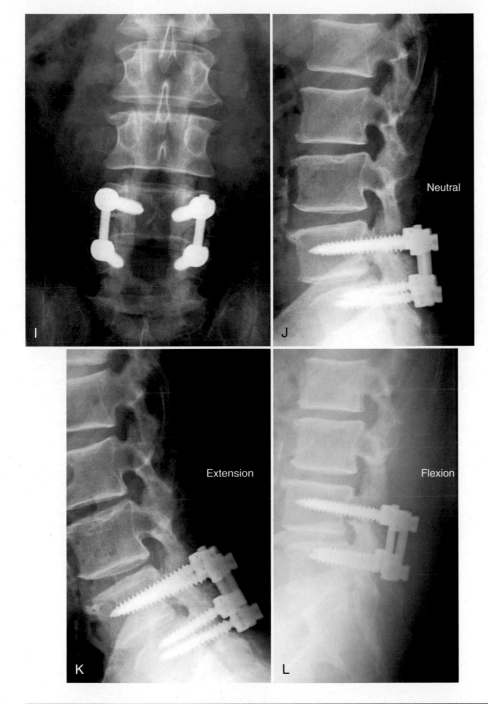

Figure 21-2, cont'd. Postoperative anteroposterior (**I**) and lateral neutral (**J**) views. **K,** Flexion. **L,** Extension.

SUGGESTED READINGS

Epstein NE: Decompression in the surgical management of degenerative spondylolisthesis: Advantages of a conservative approach in 290 patients. J Spinal Disord 1998;11:116–122.

This retrospective study reviews 290 patients with degenerative spondylolisthesis who were treated with 249 laminectomies and 41 fenestration procedures over an average of 3.2 levels. The authors conclude that decompression alone successfully managed degenerative spondylolisthesis because only 8 patients (2.7%) required secondary fusion.

Fischgrund JS, Mackay M, Herkowitz HN, et al: 1997 Volvo Award winner in clinical studies: Degenerative lumbar spondylolisthesis with spinal stenosis: A prospective randomized study comparing decompressive laminectomy and arthrodesis with and without spinal instrumentation. Spine 1997;22:2807–2812.

This prospective study analyzed the influence of transpedicular instrumentation on the operative treatment of 76 patients with degenerative spondylolisthesis and spinal stenosis.

Gibson JN, Grant IC, Waddell G: The Cochrane review of surgery for lumbar disc prolapse and degenerative lumbar spondylosis. Spine 1999;24:1820–1832.

This is a Cochrane review of randomized controlled trials that intends to collate the scientific evidence on surgical management for lumbar disc prolapse and degenerative lumbar spondylosis.

Herkowitz HN: Spine update: Degenerative lumbar spondylolisthesis. Spine 1995;20:1084–1090.

This review article presents a detailed description of the pathophysiology, clinical presentation, and nonoperative and operative intervention of degenerative lumbar spondylolisthesis.

Herkowitz HN, Kurz LT: Degenerative lumbar spondylolisthesis with spinal stenosis. A prospective study comparing decompression with decompression and intertransverse process arthrodesis. J Bone Joint Surg Am 1991;73:802–808.

This is a prospective study of 50 patients that were being treated for spinal stenosis and degenerative spondylolisthesis. Patients were sequentially, alternatively treated with either laminectomy or laminectomy and bilateral lateral intertransverse process fusion. Three-year follow-up results demonstrated that patients that had laminectomy and fusion had better radiographic and clinical outcomes.

Iguchi T, Wakami T, Kurihara A, et al: Lumbar multilevel degenerative spondylolisthesis: Radiographical evaluation and factors related to anterolisthesis and retrolisthesis. J Spinal Disord Tech 2002;15:93–99.

The authors of this review examined the radiographs of 3259 outpatients with low back disorders for age, gender, level, direction, degree of slip, lumbar lordosis, pedicle facet angle, facet shape, and disc height.

Kornblum MB, Fischgrund JS, Herkowitz HN, et al: Degenerative lumbar spondylolisthesis with spinal stenosis: A prospective long-term study comparing fusion and pseudoarthrosis. Spine 2004;29:726–734.

This is a prospective study of 47 patients with single-level symptomatic spinal stenosis and spondylolisthesis. Patients were treated with posterior decompression and bilateral posterolateral fusion with autogenous bone graft. Eight-year follow-up results demonstrated that patients with a solid fusion had better clinical outcomes than patients with pseudoarthrosis.

Love TW, Fagan AB, Fraser RD: Degenerative spondylolisthesis: Developmental or acquired? J Bone Joint Surg Br 1999;81:670–674.

This study compares the radiographs and CT scans of 118 patients over the age of 55 years to those of a control group under the age of 46 years. The authors conclude that the increased angle of the facet joint is the result of arthritic remodeling and not the primary cause of degenerative spondylolisthesis, contradicting previous evidence.

Mardjetko SM, Connolly PJ, Shott S: Degenerative lumbar spondylolisthesis: A meta-analysis of literature 1970–1993. Spine 1994;19:2257S–2265S.

This is an extensive meta-analysis that focuses on etiology and statistics, as well as the specific recommended treatments, up to 1993.

Matsunaga S, Sakou T, Morizono Y, et al: Natural history of degenerative spondylolisthesis: Pathogenesis and natural course of the slippage. Spine 1990;15:1204–1210.

This retrospective study intends to clarify the specific mechanism and progression of disc slippage based on the clinical and radiographical analysis of 40 patients.

Newman PH: Spondylolisthesis: Its cause and effect. Ann R Coll Surg Engl 1955;16:305–323.

This was the first article to introduce the term degenerative spondylolisthesis. It also focuses on the causes and consequences of degenerative spondylolisthesis on the basis of the author's experience.

Rosenberg NJ: Degenerative spondylolisthesis: Predisposing factors. J Bone Joint Surg Am 1975:57:467–474.

This retrospective study analyzed 20 skeletons and 200 patients with degenerative spondylolisthesis and established that this disease occurred four times more frequently in females, six to nine times more frequently at the interspace between the fourth and fifth lumbar vertebrae than at adjoining levels, three times more frequently in blacks than in whites, and four times more frequently if the fifth lumbar vertebra was sacralized.

Sengupta DK, Herkowitz HN: Degenerative spondylolisthesis: Review of current trends and controversies. Spine 2005;30(6 suppl):S71–S81.

This is a complete and extensive review of the management and controversies involved in degenerative spondylolisthesis. The authors also present their recommendations.

Thomsen K, Christensen FB, Eiskjaer SP, et al: 1997 Volvo Award winner in clinical studies: The effect of pedicle screw instrumentation on functional outcome and fusion rates in posterolateral lumbar spinal fusion: A prospective, randomized clinical study. Spine 1997;22:2813–2822.

This is a prospective randomized clinical study that intends to evaluate supplementary pedicle screw fixation (Cotrel-Dubousset) in posterolateral lumbar spinal fusion.

CHAPTER 22

Osteoporosis

EERIC TRUUMEES

INTRODUCTION AND EPIDEMIOLOGY

Osteoporosis, the most common metabolic bone disorder, is becoming more pervasive with the aging of populations worldwide. Initially, as with hypertension or hypercholesterolemia, this bone loss is clinically silent. Later, patients might notice progressive kyphosis or sustain a low-energy fracture. Although hip fractures have garnered a great deal of attention, osteoporotic spinal compression fractures were thought to be benign, self-limited entities. More recent studies are ascribing an ever-increasing list of sequelae to spinal fractures. Population-wide studies have found that vertebral compression fractures (VCFs) increased mortality rates even in patients who never presented to their physician for evaluation.

There are 35 million people at risk for osteoporosis in North America alone (Box 22-1). This number is expected to triple over the next three decades with the aging of the population. Until a universally employed method of early osteoporosis detection and aggressive treatment has been instituted, the health care delivery system will experience a deluge of osteoporosis-related problems. VCF is the most common manifestation of spinal osteoporosis and is estimated to affect one third of all North Americans at some point during their lifetime. Outnumbering hip and wrist fractures combined, there are 700,000 cases of VCF per year in the United States. In a population-based European study, a 12% prevalence was recorded in men and women aged 50 to 79 years. The direct medical costs associated with these fractures have been estimated at $13.8 billion annually in the United States alone. Annual direct costs are projected to exceed $60 billion, or $164 million per day, by 2030. The indirect costs in lost productivity and human pain and suffering are incalculable.

Osteoporosis will affect the practice of spinal deformity surgeons in a number of ways. Often, osteoporosis is the root cause of the deformity and pain. Patients might present with acute onset of pain with or without noticeable deformity. Alternatively, patients might report a gradual loss of height with increasing upper thoracic kyphosis. This deformity could be associated with muscular pain,

pain from the ribs rubbing on the ilium, or chronic midline pain from deficiency of the anterior column. The fractures themselves can be classified in a number of ways. Morphologically, three general fracture configurations are common: VCFs, osteoporotic burst fractures, and sacral insufficiency fractures.

Even for deformity surgeons who do not see patients with acute compression fractures, osteoporosis can complicate the treatment plan of other spine interventions. For example, the surgical strategy for instrumented stabilization of a degenerative scoliosis must consider the patient's bone stock and the reliability of fixation in an osteoporotic patient. Thus, while fractures are the main manifestation of spinal osteoporosis, the clinician must have a solid understanding of the biology and biomechanics of osteoporosis in treating any spinal condition in an osteoporotic patient population.

PATHOPHYSIOLOGY AND PATHOMECHANICS

In osteoporosis, both the crystalline (inorganic) and collagenous (organic) phases of bone are lost. Normal bone is a composite of mineral, protein, water, and cells, the exact composition of which varies by anatomic site, age, diet, and disease. Up to 70% of bone's dry weight is in the mineral phase. The largest component of bone's mineral phase is hydroxyapatite $[Ca_{10}(PO_4)_6(OH)_2]$, the loss of which weakens resistance to compressive loading. The remaining 30% is organic matrix, of which 90% is collagen. Collagen, an extremely low solubility protein, is composed of three polypeptide chains of 1000 amino acids. Loss of the organic matrix of bone makes it more brittle.

Bone is an extremely dynamic and well-organized tissue. The apatite crystal arrangement is modulated at the molecular level, and the strain patterns of the trabecular network are modulated at the organ level. The synergy of the molecular, cellular, and tissue components of bone yield a relatively lightweight tissue with a tensile strength nearly that of cast iron. At the microscopic level, bone

---

BOX 22-1 Risk Factors for Osteoporosis

- Advanced age
- Endocrine abnormalities
  - Hypercortisolism
  - Hyperthyroidism
  - Hyperparathyroidism
  - Hypogonadism
- Other diseases
  - Tumors
  - Chronic disease
  - Expression of abnormal collagen or bone matrix genes
- Inactivity or immobilization
- Dietary issues
  - Calcium-deficient diet
  - Alcoholism
  - Body mass index < 22 kg/m^2
- Smoking

---

consists of two forms: woven (or primitive) and lamellar bone. Lamellar bone begins to form 1 month after birth, and by age 4 years, most normal bone is lamellar. Lamellar bone is characterized by highly organized, stress-oriented collagen, which gives it anisotropic properties. That is, the mechanics of loading lamellar bone depend on the direction of force application. Typically, bone is strongest parallel to the long axis of the collagen molecules.

In the mature skeleton, lamellar bone is found in two forms: trabecular (spongy or cancellous) and cortical (dense or compact). Trabecular bone exhibits much greater metabolic activity with eight times greater turnover. This trabecular bone represents 20% of the total bone mass and is found in the metaphyses and epiphyses of long bones as well as in the cuboid bones (including the vertebrae). In trabecular bone, internal beams or spicules form a three-dimensional branching lattice that is aligned along areas of mechanical stress. Cortical bone, on the other hand, has four times the mass of trabecular bone. While trabecular bone varies widely according to the stress applied to it, cortical bone has a fairly uniform density and makes up 80% of total bone mass. Cortical bone forms the "envelope" of cuboid bones and the diaphysis of long bones.

Bone contains three main cell types: osteoblasts, osteocytes, and osteoclasts. Osteoblasts and osteocytes arise from the same lineage but differ in both location and function. Throughout life, the body constantly remodels bone by removing old bone and creating new bone.

Pathophysiology of Bone Loss

Osteoporosis stems from changes in the normal balance between bone formation and bone resorption. In osteoporosis, there is a decrease in the rate of bone formation relative to the rate of destruction. In contradistinction, osteomalacia represents a difficulty in bone mineralization in the context of normal osteoid production. Given the lower rates of formation in osteoporosis, overall bone mineral density decreases. Moreover, unbalanced osteoclast activity disrupts the normal connectivity of boney trabeculae. Therefore, the bone is weakened both in a material and an architectural sense. While there are a number of environmental, genetic, and pharmacologic factors that affect the development of osteoporosis, the root etiology of this disregulation is not yet understood and is probably multifactorial.

Osteoporosis is a disease state that is characterized by a decrease in both the organic and inorganic phases of bone. With age, everyone loses bone mass at approximately 0.5% per year, but not everyone develops osteoporosis. The two most important determinants for the development of osteoporosis are the peak bone mass and the rate of bone loss.

Peak bone mass is achieved in the early part of the fourth decade. The single most effective way to prevent the devastating complications of VCF is to increase peak bone mass in pubertal patients. Eating disorders such as anorexia and exercise-induced amenorrhea lead to profound osteoporosis. Several studies have documented increasing rates of osteoporosis among young women. Lack of weight-bearing exercise and changes in dietary habits have been implicated. These disorders are especially worrisome because they affect women at a relatively early age, when their bone mass should be reaching its peak.

After peak bone mass is achieved, bone is gradually lost with age. The rate of loss is accelerated through decreased exposure to gonadal hormones (i.e., menopause) as well as genetic, environmental, and nutritional conditions and chronic disease states. Estrogen deficiency is directly implicated in accelerated bone osteoporosis at up to 2% to 3% per year for 10 years. The mechanism of bone loss resulting from normal aging is poorly understood, but its rate is equivalent in women and men. Other risk factors associated with osteoporosis are listed in Box 22-1.

Pathomechanics of Osteoporosis

Osteoporosis has a number of critical mechanical effects. For our purposes, three effects are most important. First, osteoporotic bone is at risk for fracture. Second, operative management of spinal disorders in patients with osteoporosis has increased risk for instrumentation failure. Third, osteoporosis has a number of implications for the development and progression of spinal deformity, including spondylolisthesis, scoliosis, and, of course, hyperkyphosis.

Osteoporosis and a high rate of falls contribute to a higher incidence of spine fractures in the elderly than in other age groups. These injuries can occur with very little energy delivered to the spine and can affect any level from the atlantoaxial complex to the sacrum. Multilevel fractures are also frequently encountered. This distribution of injuries reflects the influence of both mechanical and physiologic factors. There is likely a complex interplay between arthrosis, ligament elasticity, muscular changes, and the underlying bone weakness. Spondyloarthrosis and ligament ossification exert a relative stiffening effect on the midcervical spine (C4-7). The upper cervical spine, particularly the atlantoaxial complex, maintains mobility.

In the cervical spine, hyperextension is the most common injury vector in the elderly. Large retrospective studies have documented the predominance of upper cervical injuries in this group. Lomoschitz and colleagues reviewed 225 cervical spine injuries in patients age 65 and older to define the association between age, fracture pattern, and causative mechanism. The authors subdivided these patients into young elderly (65 to 75 years) and old elderly (75 years and older). Admission radiographs, injury mechanism, clinical status, and neurologic status were reviewed. In the young elderly, motor vehicle accidents were the main mechanism of injury. In the old elderly, a fall from seated or standing height predominated. In patients over age 75, multilevel injuries and fractures that were at risk for neurologic deterioration were common (greater than 50%).

Dens fractures are archetypical for osteoporotic fractures of the cervical spine. These fractures represent 10% of all cervical spine injuries and are the most common spinal column fracture in the elderly. The critical role of the dens in atlantoaxial stability ensures its relevance as a significant cause of morbidity at any age.

In the thoracolumbar spine, for example, decreased bone mineral content increases the vulnerability to vertebral fracture with axial load. VCFs are the archetypical thoracolumbar injury. These injuries are discussed in detail subsequently.

Aside from the sudden displacement or collapse associated with an osteoporotic fracture, osteoporosis also increases the risk for the more gradual loss of alignment and balance associated with spinal deformity and degeneration. For example, loss of bone strength increases the risk of progression of virtually all types of spondylolisthesis: degenerative, isthmic, and iatrogenic. Case reports also describe pars elongation in patients with osteoporotic bone leading to spondylolisthesis. Interestingly, the focal bone density at the level of slip is typically somewhat higher than that for nonlisthetic controls. This likely represents the sclerotic interface between the moving bones.

Similarly, the presence of osteoporosis is associated with increased risk of deformity progression with either idiopathic or degenerative scoliosis. Given the persistence of osteopenia after treatment for idiopathic scoliosis, even in teenage girls, the question of its role in scoliosis pathophysiology remains. Some studies suggest that decreased bone mass on the convexity will foster curve propagation.

Beyond spondylolisthesis and scoliosis, however, hyperkyphosis is the key feature of osteoporotic patients. An upper thoracic hyperkyphosis, the so-called dowager's hump, can be seen with fracture or in the absence of frac-

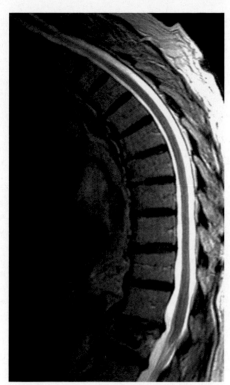

Figure 22-1. This sagittal T2-weighted MRI demonstrates a patient with a healed thoracolumbar compression fracture. While she has some focal, residual kyphosis from the fracture, the larger part of her deformity lies in the upper thoracic spine, where the end plates appear to be intact.

ture (Fig. 22-1). Thoracolumbar junction fractures tend to accelerate the progression of this hyperkyphosis, and this type of fracture is usually the injury that leads to loss of sagittal balance. Currently, a debate is raging as to whether cementation of the spine increases the risk for additional fracture by increasing stiffness or whether decreasing the deformity can actually normalize the weight-bearing axis and protect adjacent segments.

Finally, ligamentous and muscular factors are underestimated as a cause of deformity. Several studies have shown progressive kyphosis in osteoporotic patients without significant fracture or bone irregularity. Disc degeneration and spondylotic factors as well as muscular factors have been implicated.

CLINICAL PRESENTATION AND EVALUATION

Symptoms of osteoporosis are not usually evident until low-energy or fragility fractures occur. The most common sites for these fractures are the spine, ribs, hips, and wrists. The patient will then report localized pain in these areas. Diffuse bone pain is a feature of osteomalacia and is not seen with osteoporosis.

Prior to fracture, osteoporosis is identified on the basis of screening studies in at-risk populations. The potential

TABLE 22-1. Comparison of Osteoporosis and Osteomalacia

	Osteoporosis	Osteomalacia
Definition	Bone mass decreased	Bone mass variable
Mineralization	Normal	Decreased
Age of onset	Generally elderly	Any age
Etiology	Endocrine abnormality	Vitamin D deficiency
	Age	Abnormality of vitamin D pathway
		Idiopathic
		Hypophosphatemic
		Renal tubular acidosis
		Hypophosphatasia
Symptoms	Pain referable to fracture	Generalized bone pain
Signs	Tenderness at fracture	Generalized tenderness
Laboratory Findings		
Serum Ca^{2+}	Normal	↓ or normal (↑ hypophosphatasia)
Serum P	Normal	↓ or normal (↑ renal osteodystrophy)
Alkaline phosphatase	Normal	↑ (not hypophosphatasia)
Urinary Ca^{2+}	High or normal	Normal or ↓ (↑ in hypophosphatasia)
Bone biopsy	Normal	Abnormal

for osteoporosis or other abnormal bone states should be considered in any patient encounter. If a patient presents with pain, exclude fracture. If a fracture is present without an appropriate high-energy mechanism, an evaluation for bone loss is undertaken.

Similarly, in any patient who has a progressive spinal deformity, underlying bone weakness should be considered among the potential etiologies. In an at-risk patient who is due to undergo surgery, with or without instrumentation, the impact of bone mineral loss on the potential for postoperative fracture, spondylolisthesis, or instrumentation failure should impel the surgeon to consider an osteoporosis workup.

The goals of evaluation in osteoporosis are as follows: First, identify decreased bone mineral density; second, exclude the osteopenia of malignancy, osteomalacia, or secondary osteoporosis; third, assess the bone turnover state (Table 22-1).

Osteoporosis Etiologies and Assessment

Every physician, including orthopedic and spine surgeons, must ensure that their at-risk patients have been screened and, if necessary, treated for osteoporosis. Patient outcomes after primary prevention greatly exceed those of fracture stabilization. Risk factors for osteoporosis were discussed earlier in the chapter. World Health Organization criteria for screening tests are listed in Box 22-2.

The osteoporotic patient population is divided into three etiologic categories: type I (postmenopausal), type II (senile), and type III (secondary). Type I osteoporosis affects women more often than men (although hypogonadic men will get this form of osteoporosis as well). Most patients with type I osteoporosis show signs or symptoms in their 50s and 60s with fractures of trabecular bone (such

---

BOX 22-2 World Health Organization's DEXA Screening Criteria

All Patients
- Who have sustained a low-energy fracture
- Who have osteopenia on plain radiographs
- With diseases that place them at risk for osteoporosis
- Who are taking medications that place them at risk for osteoporosis

Women
- Postmenopausal
- Older than 65 years
- Younger than 65 with one or more risk factors
- Who have been on hormone replacement therapy for prolonged periods
- Who are considering hormone replacement therapy, if bone mineral density will affect decision

DEXA, dual-energy X-ray absorptiometry.

---

as the wrist and spine) predominating. Type II osteoporosis affects men and women equally, arises in the 70s and 80s, and increasingly affects cortical bone.

Various medications and disease states may precipitate secondary or type III osteoporosis. Elevated endogenous or exogenous cortisol levels are among the most common offenders and are deleterious to bone mass, owing to decreased calcium absorption across the intestinal lumen, increased calcium loss from the kidney, and direct inhibition of bone matrix formation. Alternate-day dosing of corticosteroids decreases bone damage. Calcium, vitamin D, and antiosteoporotic medications can counter some of the deleterious effects.

Plain radiographs are the least accurate and least precise method of assessing bone density. A decrease in bone mass of at least 30% is necessary to detect osteopenia on plain films. A more accurate measurement of bone mass is critical in the diagnosis of osteoporosis both as a means of diagnosis and to gauge response to treatment. Bone density is a major determinant of fracture threshold in osteoporotic patients, along with other factors, including cardiovascular status, medications, neuromuscular disorders, body habitus, and falls.

Evaluation algorithms begin with a screening dual-energy X-ray absorptiometry (DEXA) scan. Severity of bone loss is classified by the T-score, which represents the number of standard deviations a patient's bone mineral density is above or below normal young adult bone. Bone mineral density more than 1 standard deviation less than the mean young adult value is defined as osteopenia. Below 2.5 standard deviations from the mean, patients are defined as having osteoporosis. The patient with bone mineral density below 2.5 standard deviations with prevalent fragility fractures has severe osteoporosis. For each standard deviation below the norm, fracture risk increases 1.5-fold to 3-fold. A T-score of −1 implies a 30% chance of fracture. The Z-score is also occasionally used. This value compares the patient's bone with age-matched controls. Patients more than 2 standard deviations away from age-normal should be investigated for neoplasia or osteomalacia.

Laboratory evaluation in osteoporosis is used mainly to exclude other causes of osteopenia, such as osteomalacia. Laboratory studies may be abnormal in osteomalacia, which should be suspected when the product of the serum calcium level multiplied by the serum phosphate level remains chronically below 25 mg/dL. Serum alkaline phosphatase levels are elevated, and 24-hour urinary calcium excretion may be less than 50 mg. Occasionally, serum blood tests alone are insufficient to exclude the diagnosis of osteomalacia, at which time a transiliac bone biopsy might be indicated. For younger patients and women with a questionable menstrual history, a hormonal profile, including sex hormones, thyroid-stimulating hormone, thyroxine, and parathyroid hormone (PTH), should be ordered.

In patients with unusual fracture patterns or histories that are suggestive of malignancy or infection, laboratory evaluation may include erythrocyte sedimentation rate, white blood cell count with differential, C-reactive protein, serum protein electrophoresis, urine protein electrophoresis, and prostate antigens.

If no clearly identifiable cause of osteopenia is encountered, iliac crest bone biopsy and marrow aspirations might be indicated. Most typically, these procedures are performed in patients under age 50 with idiopathic osteopenia, when osteomalacia is highly suspected, or in chronic renal failure patients with skeletal symptoms. Two weeks before the biopsy, tetracycline is administered twice each day for 3 days. This dose is repeated in the 3 days immediately prior to biopsy. This tetracycline binds to newly mineralized osteoid and permits the determination of mineralization rates. In osteoporosis, a normal mineralization pattern should be encountered. Here, two distinct bands of fluorescence, representing the tetracycline labels, are noted. With impaired mineralization, on the other hand, the examiner records a single band of fluorescence.

In a patient with known osteoporosis, bone biomarker assays are being increasingly requested to provide information complementary to that of densitometry. These biomarkers include markers of bone formation, such as bone-specific alkaline phosphatase (an osteoblast enzyme) and osteocalcin (a bone matrix protein), and markers of bone resorption, such as collagen degradation products in the urine (cross-linked telopeptides and pyridinolines). These markers offer improved prediction of future fracture risk and a sensitive means to monitor therapy effectiveness.

Many spine surgeons refer their patients to an endocrinologist for this workup, but it is incumbent on the surgeon to ensure that an appropriate workup has been undertaken.

Assessment of Osteoporotic Compression Fractures

When a patient has sustained a fracture related to osteoporosis, the workup begins with a careful history. The fracture occurs in the context of minimal to no trauma and leads to focal, intense, deep midline spine pain. Fracture pain must be differentiated from muscular pain, which is more typically diffuse or paravertebral pain. These systems should be primarily mechanical in that the pain varies in intensity. Usually, fracture pain is worse with loading and relieved with recumbency. Ask about associated neck pain and thoracic or lumbar radicular complaints.

Understand the time course of the patient's symptoms as well as the course of any previous fractures. Patients with night pain, fevers, chills, unusual weight loss, or bowel or bladder changes require more intense investigation. Medical history is investigated to ascertain appropriate treatment of underlying osteoporosis, including a history of cancer, tuberculosis, systemic infection, or other fractures. In the setting of concomitant head injury or dementia, a clear history and precise symptom localization might be impossible.

Unfortunately, multiple underlying comorbidities, decreased mental status, and degenerative changes in anatomy can compromise the history and physical examination. Therefore, heightened suspicion and meticulous examination are critical in elderly patients.

Assess the patient's general condition and sagittal spinal balance. Body shape, difficulty breathing, and obesity can all affect the likelihood of effective bracing. Elderly patients with odontoid fractures might be asymptomatic or experience only mild suboccipital tenderness. Restricted cervical range of motion and tenderness prompt immediate immobilization and thorough evaluation.

In patients with thoracolumbar injuries, look for associated rib tenderness; coexisting and iatrogenic rib fractures are common in osteoporotic patients. Acute VCF and burst fractures are typically point tender over the spinous process. Undertake a complete neurologic examination. Although major neurologic deficits are rare (0.05%), many of these patients have significant stenosis or neuropathic causes of neurologic decline. Sacral insufficiency fractures can cause pain in the tailbone or sacroiliac joint regions. Often, this pain will be felt in a bandlike distribution across the low back. Maneuvers that stress the sacroiliac joint will cause severe pain in these patients.

When osteoporotic or low-energy fractures occur, they are classified morphologically. They are described first on the basis of spinal level and then on the basis of fracture pattern. By far the most common pattern is the thoracolumbar VCF; cervical fractures are not rare, even with minimal trauma.

VCFs are subdivided into fractures of the superior end plate, the inferior end plate, and both end plates. The fractures can lead to a crushing pattern (vertebra plana), a biconcave pattern, or a wedge deformity. Further, lateral compression deformities can worsen preexisting coronal plane deformities. In the lumbar spine, these fractures may include collapse of the central portion of both the superior and inferior end plates; this has been termed a *biconcave* or *codfish vertebra*. In the thoracic spine, the anterior portion of the superior end plate is most typically involved and leads to a wedge compression fracture.

Not all osteoporotic thoracolumbar fractures are compression fractures. The senile burst fracture represents increased axial loading and failure of the middle column with retropulsion of bone into the spinal canal. Somewhat less common, but by no means rare, are extension injuries that occur when the patient falls backward onto the apex of kyphosis. It is critical to distinguish burst and extension injuries from compression fractures, as these injuries are typically not suited to percutaneous stabilization (Fig. 22-2). Sacral insufficiency fractures can occur in the context of insufficiency fractures of the pelvis with concomitant pubic ramus fractures or as isolated injuries.

With cervical spine injuries, neurologic involvement ranging from greater occipital nerve palsy to quadriparesis is not uncommon. Spinal cord injury, radiculopathy, and a worsening of preexisting neurogenic claudicatory symptoms are occasionally seen with thoracolumbar fractures, typically those with a bursting pattern.

In patients with known fractures, the goals of imaging are to determine the extent of vertebral collapse, the location and extent of any lytic process, the visibility and degree of pedicular involvement, the presence of cortical destruction, the presence of epidural or foraminal stenosis, and the age or acuity of the fracture.

Several of these goals are achieved through plain radiography. With standing radiographs, overall sagittal and coronal spinal balance is apparent. Thoracolumbar fractures are readily discovered, but sacral and odontoid fractures can be difficult to see. Determination of the age or acuity of the fracture is more difficult. Comparison films,

including old chest radiographs, can be helpful, but apparent sclerosis can represent healing or merely compressed bone. Spot films, particularly at the thoracolumbar junction, aid in visualization. During early patient management for acute fracture, plain radiographs should be followed serially over the short term to assess for further collapse.

Scrutinize plain radiographs for signs of posterior cortical compromise such as widened pedicles and more than 50% height loss. Look for end plate erosion that is suggestive of infection or pedicular destruction (winking owl sign), as seen in malignancy. Fractures above T6 are more likely to represent neoplasm.

Yet interpretation of plain radiographs is limited by degenerative changes that obscure radiographic landmarks. Mild spondylolisthesis, segmental ossification of the annulus fibrosis, and osteophytes at the facet joints represent overlapping radiologic findings of both spondylosis and trauma. Canal involvement and fracture acuity are more readily determined with magnetic resonance imaging (MRI). The edema that is seen in acute fractures is reflected by increased signal on T2 or short T1 inversion recovery sequences. Acutely, fractures demonstrate decreased T1 signal, and both T1 and T2 marrow signal changes normalize over time. MRI can reveal several key features that differentiate malignant from osteoporotic compression fractures, including pedicular and soft-tissue extension.

Avascular necrosis of the vertebral bone (Kummel's disease) is an increasingly recognized cause of chronic, unhealing compression fractures. Such continuing collapse of the vertebra after minor trauma is particularly common in patients with known risk factors for avascular necrosis, such as previous radiation therapy or chronic corticosteroid use. On MRI, these fractures demonstrate the "double-line sign" of discrete fluid collections within a vacuum cleft with areas of diminished T2 signal surrounding the cleft.

In patients who are unable to undergo MRI, a computed tomography (CT) scan offers high bone and soft-tissue contrast and clearly delineates posterior cortical compromise. Fracture acuity can then be determined by bone scan. Both MRI and CT demonstrate sacral insufficiency fractures. On bone scan, these lesions may have the classic "H" configuration or may appear as a linear band of increased uptake in the region of the sacral ala (Fig. 22-3).

NONOPERATIVE CARE

Nonoperative care of the osteoporosis patient with spinal deformity requires treatment of both the osteoporosis and the deformity. Each aspect of the patient's disease state affects the management options for the other.

Osteoporosis Management

Treatments for osteoporosis have had variable success because of delayed and inaccurate diagnosis, insufficient understanding of the disease process, and inadequate

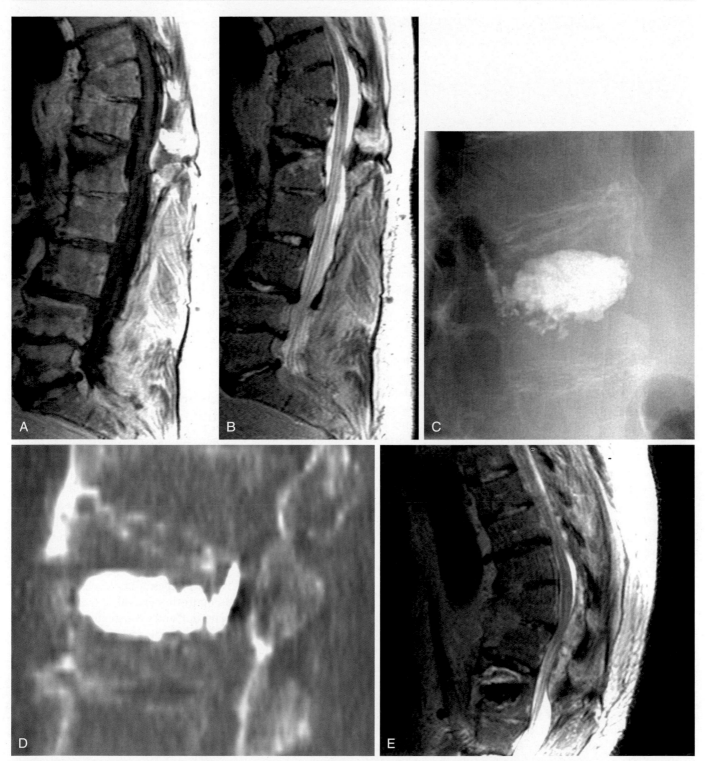

Figure 22-2. This patient sustained a three-column extension injury after a fall onto his back. This injury was misidentified as a compression fracture. The trabeculae are not compressed together but rather have been distracted (**A** and **B**). Despite this unstable injury mechanism, the patient underwent a vertebroplasty (**C**), which was complicated by leakage of polymethyl methacrylate (PMMA) (**D**). Later, an epidural hematoma developed, and the patient lost motor function in his lower extremities (**E**).

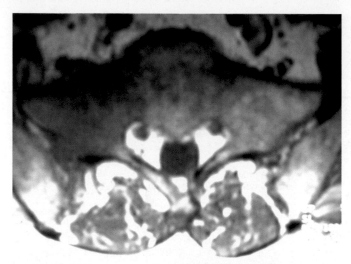

Figure 22-3. This axial T1 MRI demonstrates a sacral ala fracture with diminished T1 signal intensity. Note how the fracture extends anteriorly to contact the descending L5 nerve.

follow-up. Appropriate treatment begins before the first fracture, with calcium, physiologic vitamin D, and mild weight-bearing exercise. Tai chi has been favored because it also improves the patient's balance. These measures are intended to decrease bone resorption and to mineralize osteoid, but they do not increase total bone mass. Studies show that individuals who take calcium have a quarter of the hip fractures of individuals with low calcium intake. However, excess calcium can be harmful.

In menopausal women, estrogen supplementation might be appropriate. Estrogen receptors have been identified in bone-forming cells. Estrogen acts to block the action of PTH on osteoblasts and marrow stromal cells, and estrogen supplementation decreases bone loss by acting to counter the effect of unopposed PTH activity. Without estrogen, osteoblasts and marrow stromal cells secrete increased levels of interleukin (IL-6), which stimulates the osteoclasts to resorb bone. Estrogen does not appreciably alter bone formation rates; therefore, the primary effect of estrogen therapy lies in the maintenance of bone mass, but women who take estrogen have fewer fractures. Recent studies appear to show increased rates of coronary artery disease, stroke, pulmonary embolus, and cancer in women who are on hormone replacement therapy. The potential of untoward side effects of estrogen has increased interest in the selective estrogen receptor modulators such as raloxifene (Evista). These agents appear to have bone-preserving effects similar to those of estrogen without the cancer and coronary complications.

More aggressive pharmacologic management is indicated in patients with fractures or with femoral T-scores less than −2.5. Calcitonin, administered via either subcutaneous injection or nasal spray, decreases osteoclastic bone resorption. Over the short term, calcitonin enhances bone formation, leading to a slight net bone accretion.

Over the long term, however, osteoblastic activity slows, and bone mass stabilizes.

The bisphosphonates have dramatic effects in suppressing bone resorption and in preventing fractures of the hip and vertebral bodies. These agents act in two ways to inhibit bone resorption. First, they directly stabilize the bone crystal, making it more resistant to osteoclastic bone resorption. Second, they directly inhibit the activity of the osteoclast. Thus, bisphosphonates may help to preserve bone architecture as well as overall density. Weekly forms of these agents are now available with better compliance and no increase in toxicity.

Currently, PTH is undergoing clinical trials in the treatment of osteoporosis. Intermittent administration of PTH is anabolic and leads to early dramatic increases in bone mass, especially in areas of trabecular bone. The long-term safety and efficacy of these protocols have not yet been established. Ultimately, for patients with severe osteoporosis, combination therapies linking an anabolic agent with an antiresorptive agent along with calcium and vitamin D supplementation could prove to be the most rational treatment.

Nonoperative Management of Osteoporotic Spine Fractures

The goals of management for osteoporotic fractures of the spine include decreased pain, early mobilization, preservation of sagittal and coronal spinal stability, and prevention of late neurologic compromise. During the initial, painful interval, patients who present to their physicians are typically offered pain medications and braces. Limited activity and often bed rest are advised or self-imposed. In the osteoporotic population, bed rest is associated with an additional 4% loss of bone mineral density and should be discouraged for all fracture types.

The group of osteoporotic cervical spine fractures is quite variable in presentation and management. Those that place the spinal cord in jeopardy are most likely treated operatively, but most low-energy fracture patterns can be immobilized in a collar. Dens fractures are particularly problematic and have a 6% to 64% collective nonunion rate. This risk is increased in fractures through the waist of the dens.

For thoracolumbar and sacral fractures, the period of acute pain usually lasts 4 to 6 weeks, but in some circumstances, the pain persists beyond 3 months. Narcotic pain medications may be continued until the patient can bear weight comfortably. In the elderly patient population, use of narcotics may be associated with as many functional problems as the underlying fracture. Nasal calcitonin and bisphosphonates, while useful in the treatment of osteoporosis, may also be effective in decreasing fracture-related pain.

For many osteoporotic fractures from the atlas to L5, braces have been recommended to maintain alignment and

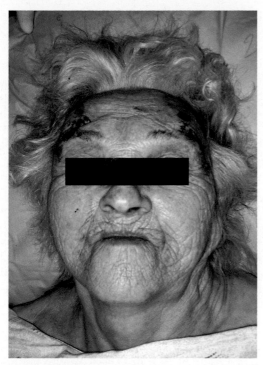

Figure 22-4. This elderly female with a displaced type II dens fracture was placed in a halo three times at two institutions before being transferred to our center. Each time, the halo pins loosened, and the device was displaced. Only the standard four-pin arrangement was employed. Typically, in patients with poor bone, six- or eight-pin fixation would be sought. In this case, the patient underwent successful operative stabilization.

decrease fracture pain. These patients' borderline pulmonary function limits tolerance of full-contact braces and halos. Halo complications, including pin loosening, are more common in these patients (Fig. 22-4). More rigid braces might even accelerate bone loss. Limited contact orthoses, such as a tri-pad Jewett extension or Cash braces, are deemed easy to fit and wear, but variable rates of compliance have been cited. Elderly patients often have a body habitus that is not particularly braceable (short, obese trunk). Further, patients with shoulder problems will have difficulty donning and doffing the brace. Unfortunately, there is no satisfactory method for bracing sacral fractures.

Physical therapy might aid the patient's recovery to mobility. Therapy efforts should be directed toward proprioception training and extensor muscle strengthening, which have clearly been shown to improve function and decrease the risk of an additional fracture.

Previously, these VCFs were thought to be benign, self-limited injuries with few, if any, significant long-term sequelae. This conception arose from the group of nearly two thirds of VCFs that were never reported by patients to their physicians. Further, in many of the cases that are brought to medical attention, symptoms respond rapidly to simple nonoperative treatment. On the basis of recent population-wide studies, it is becoming increasingly evident that any VCF can have significant functional and physiologic effects, such as acute and chronic pain, recurrent fracture, kyphotic deformity, gastrointestinal dysfunction, pulmonary dysfunction, functional decline, increased hospitalization rates, and, ultimately, increased mortality.

Acute VCFs are variably painful. While some patients note only mild and transient symptoms, others require hospitalization. Further, while most patients report significant symptomatic improvement in the first 4 weeks, the period of acute pain can persist for months. Once the period of acute pain subsides, chronic pain disorders can develop. Many of these appear to arise from the change in the sagittal balance of the spine. The risk of developing chronic pain increases with the number of vertebral fractures.

This pain is intensified from many typical daily activities such as standing, sitting, or bending. In many of these patients, standing tolerance decreases to only a few minutes. Pain is relieved on lying down, but the increase in bed rest, just as in patients with acute fractures, only serves to accelerate bone loss.

Also, increased kyphosis and VCFs are associated with decreased truncal strength and with greater back-related disability, annual number of bed-days, and annual number of limited-activity days. The loss of strength and decrease in activity level increase the risk of additional fractures. Various studies have cited increased risks of additional spinal fractures from 5 to 25 times baseline. Similarly, the risk of hip fracture rises five times in patients who sustain a VCF. In one study of physical function, common tasks such as walking, bending, dressing, carrying bags, climbing stairs, rising from a supine position, and rising from a seated position were assessed. Only 13% of VCF patients were able to accomplish these activities without difficulty, 40% had difficulty, and 47% required assistance.

The deformity that is associated with each of these fracture types can have multiple physiologic implications. Taken together, the osteoporotic body habitus is characterized by loss of height and thoracic hyperkyphosis (the dowager's hump). Abdominal protuberance and loss of lumbar lordosis might also be noted. Many otherwise active elderly patients complain bitterly about the cosmetic effects of these changes. Beyond the cosmetic effects, compression on the abdominal viscera by the rib cage or by loss of height through the lumbar spine leads to decreased appetite, early satiety, and weight loss. One recent paper found that women with hyperkyphosis secondary to osteoporosis were at risk for refractory reflux esophagitis, which unfortunately also limits treatment with oral bisphosphonates. Similarly, thoracic hyperkyphosis leads to compression of the lungs and, subsequently, decreased pulmonary function with an increased risk of pulmonary death. Lung function, as measured by forced vital capacity and forced expiratory volume, is significantly reduced in patients with thoracic or lumbar fractures.

BOX 22-3 Consequences of Vertebral Compression Fractures

- Intractable pain
- Physiological impact
- Increased mortality
- Recurrent fracture
- Kyphotic deformity
- Gastrointestinal dysfunction
- Pulmonary dysfunction
- Functional decline
- Increased hospitalization

The precise risk of neurologic deficit after VCF is not known; it is probably uncommon but not as rare as was first thought. Interestingly, a tardy neurologic decline may occur up to 18 months from the initial injury. These late neurologic changes are thought to represent dysfunction of the spinal cord as it drapes over the apex of the kyphosis. Women who sustain osteoporotic VCFs report a number of debilitating psychological effects, including crippled body image and self-esteem, depression, and anxiety (Box 22-3).

The 5-year survival rate after osteoporotic spine fracture is significantly worse than that for age-matched peers (61% versus 76%) and is comparable to survival rates after hip fracture. Excess mortality increases with the number of fractures.

Management of Other Spinal Deformity in Osteoporosis Patients

With the addition of antiosteoporotic medications, the nonoperative management of spinal deformity in the osteoporosis patient population comprises the typical elements common to deformity management elsewhere. These relatively fragile patients require much closer follow-up and are more technically difficult to manage, however.

The same combination of spinal deformity and axial height loss leads to relatively unique pain syndromes such as rib cage on ilium pain. Here, the combination of thoracolumbar kyphosis and height loss drops the lower ribs onto the ilium with consequent painful rubbing. Physical therapy often helps the patient regain enough extensor strength to decrease pain, but some patients require regular rib blocks.

SURGICAL MANAGEMENT IN OSTEOPOROTIC PATIENTS

Surgical management of osteoporosis patients is divided into two types: surgical treatment for complications of osteoporosis, such as VCFs, and management of other spinal conditions.

At least 150,000 compression fractures per year are refractory to nonoperative measures and require hospitalization, with protracted periods of bed rest and intravenous narcotics. Fractures that are less likely to improve with standard medical management include those of the thoracolumbar junction (T11-L2), those with bursting patterns, wedge compression fractures with more than 30 degrees of sagittal angulation, those with vacuum shadow in fractured body (ischemic necrosis of bone), and those with progressive collapse in office follow-up (Box 22-4).

For patients with intractable pain that limits ambulation, early consideration of percutaneous polymethyl methacrylate (PMMA) vertebral body augmentation (VBA) through either vertebroplasty or kyphoplasty is warranted. In ambulatory patients, such VBA procedures are reserved for patients who demonstrate continued collapse on follow-up radiographs or those who fail to improve clinically after a reasonable nonoperative window (Boxes 22-5 and 22-6).

BOX 22-4 Fractures That Are Less Likely to Improve with Standard Medical Management

- Thoracolumbar junction (T11-L2)
- Bursting patterns
- Wedge compression fractures with greater than 30 degrees of sagittal angulation
- Vacuum shadow in fractured body (ischemic necrosis of bone)
- Progressive collapse in office follow-up

BOX 22-5 Indications for VBA

- Primary osteoporosis
- Secondary osteoporosis
- Multiple myeloma
- Osteolytic metastasis

BOX 22-6 Relative Contraindications to Percutaneous VBA

- Neurologic symptoms
- Young patients
- Pregnancy
- High-velocity fractures
  - Fractured pedicles or facets
  - Burst fracture with retropulsed bone
- Medical issues
  - Allergy to devices
  - Allergy to contrast medium
  - Bleeding disorders
  - Severe cardiopulmonary difficulties
  - Technically not feasible
  - Vertebra plana
  - Multiple painful vertebral bodies
- Active infection

Of course, there are a number of other osteoporotic fractures of the spine. Some unstable cervical spine fractures may require operative management. There have been trends away from the use of halo braces in these frail patients. A more comprehensive review of these injuries is beyond the scope of this chapter.

Vertebral Body Augmentation

Vertebral body augmentation (VBA) procedures are another means of treating patients with continuing vertebral collapse or intractable pain after VCF. Vertebral augmentation with PMMA variably restores strength and stiffness to a fractured body. Strength reflects the ability of the vertebral body to bear load and can protect against future fracture of the treated segment. Stiffness limits micromotion within the compromised vertebral body. The clinical importance of this distinction is not certain, but limitation of micromotion is ostensibly the source of symptom relief. See Boxes 22-5 and 22-6 for indications and contraindications to VBA.

Both kyphoplasty and vertebroplasty strive to gain access to the vertebral body through a small, 1-cm incision. Then, 8- to 11-gauge instruments are placed into the body. With vertebroplasty, the vertebra is filled with liquid PMMA through an 11-gauge needle. With kyphoplasty, a balloon tamp is used to first create a void in the bone and to attempt fracture reduction. This instrumentation also allows placement of more viscous cement through an 8-gauge delivery system. The more viscous cement, placed in a known void, may lower rates of cement extravasation.

These procedures may be performed under general anesthesia or with local anesthesia and intravenous sedation. The patient is turned prone on a radiolucent table or frame and bolstered to allow partial postural reduction of the fracture. The critical first step in either procedure is to obtain true anteroposterior (AP) and lateral images with fluoroscopy. Most typically, a transpedicular route to the vertebra is selected. In some thoracic cases, the narrow and straight pedicle precludes appropriate medialization, and an extrapedicular approach is required. Kyphoplasty is performed through bilateral approaches; vertebroplasty may be performed unilaterally or bilaterally.

Beginning with AP fluoroscopy, an 11-gauge Jamshidi needle is positioned at 10 o'clock or 2 o'clock on the pedicular ring. Unlike the situation with pedicle screws, the goal is not to proceed "straight down the barrel" but rather to medialize through the cylinder of the pedicle. Therefore, start at the lateral border and aim medially. Once in bone, verify the trajectory on the lateral image. If the AP and lateral images do not demonstrate a clearly intrapedicular position, an en face or oblique view is useful.

Under lateral fluoroscopy, advance the Jamshidi needle to the midway point of the pedicle. Return to the AP view and verify the tip position. Until the Jamshidi needle has passed through the posterior cortical margin of the vertebral body, it must be lateral to the medial pedicle wall on the AP image. If the needle has been medialized appropriately, return to the lateral image and advance to 1 to 2 mm past the posterior vertebral body margin. Now the needle should be just barely across the medial pedicle border on the AP view.

While several different systems and needles are employed for vertebroplasty, most require advancement of the cannulas into the central portion of the vertebral body. Then PMMA is mixed and delivered under live fluoroscopy. In kyphoplasty, additional instruments are employed. Remove the Jamshidi stylet and place a guide pin through it to the midway point in the body. Then, remove the Jamshidi needle. The osteointroducer instruments are passed over the guide pin. The blunt dissector of the osteointroducer and the guide pin are removed, leaving the working cannula in place just anterior to the posterior cortical margin of the vertebral body. In soft bone, a bone void filler is passed through the cannula to the midway point in the body. Again, check the AP view for appropriate medialization. If the void filler is past the outer third, advance to within 2 mm of the anterior cortex. The void filler should be halfway between the medial pedicle outline and the spinous process. Better medialization allows for more aggressive anterior placement. For harder bone, use the provided drill to prepare the path for the bone void filler. Live fluoroscopy is recommended in approaching the anterior cortex. The guide pin can be used to palpate the anterior cortex. Switch to the AP view to verify final drill placement. The drill should appear to touch the spinous process.

Insert the inflatable bone tamp (IBT) to within 4 mm of the anterior cortex. Inflate the balloon to 50 psi to maintain its position and tamponade the bone. Place instruments through the opposite pedicle in a similar fashion. Once the contralateral balloon has been placed, inflate both IBTs in 0.5-mL increments. Monitor AP, lateral, and oblique images for IBT position in relation to the cortices. Sequentially inflate the IBTs until an inflation end point has been reached:

- Realignment of vertebral end plates
- Maximum balloon pressure (>220 psi) without decay
- Maximum balloon volume: 4 mL for 15/3, 6 mL for 20/3
- Cortical wall contact

The void created by the IBT is typically filled with PMMA, much as occurs with vertebroplasty. Newer calcium phosphate and hydroxyapatite cements are also being tested. Extra sterile barium is added to the powder to increase its radiopacity. For vertebroplasty, the PMMA is injected into the body in a fairly liquid state to allow it to interdigitate between the crushed trabeculae of the fracture. For kyphoplasty, the PMMA is placed into bone filler devices. The surgeon should wait until it reaches a toothpaste consistency. Remove the balloons and apply the PMMA under continuous fluoroscopy. Inject slightly more bone void filler than the final IBT inflation volume. The wound may be closed with a suture or Steri-Strip. No braces or particular postoperative precautions are needed.

There are few appealing treatment options for sacral insufficiency fractures. If there is a concomitant pubic ramus fracture, limited weight bearing on the affected side and walker ambulation are recommended. For bilateral fractures, a walker helps the patient to decrease weight bearing through the fracture to a degree. Unfortunately, there is no effective bracing for these injuries. Similarly, the early experience of VBA procedures for these injuries is limited. For fractures with significant displacement or neurologic compromise, operative reduction and stabilization are occasionally required.

Osteoporotic burst fractures (senile burst fractures) are more common than was previously thought. Any fracture with more than 50% height loss will have associated posterior cortical compromise. In many cases, this compromise takes the form of buckling of the cortex, and if the canal occlusion is less than 33%, VBA procedures may be considered in selected cases. On the other hand, if significant comminution exists, VBA should not be undertaken because of the increased risk of cement extravasation. In patients with neurologic injury, open surgery might be required.

Open surgery is indicated in osteoporotic patients only in the context of significant or progressive neurologic deficit or deformity. Unfortunately, operative intervention is associated with high morbidity and mortality in this frail patient population. Similarly, spinal instrumentation systems often fail in osteoporotic bone. Often, anterior-posterior surgeries are required to achieve adequate fixation, and screws are augmented with PMMA to increase their pullout strength. Alternatively, a hybrid approach that utilizes PMMA for anterior column reconstruction and short-segment transpedicular instrumentation may be appropriate in some cases (Fig. 22-5).

One of the goals of VBA procedures is to interrupt the cycle of decline that is seen in patients with VCFs. Unfortunately, there have been no randomized trials yet comparing nonoperative management with VBA. However, a number of case series have demonstrated that vertebroplasty and kyphoplasty procedures tend to be well tolerated and associated with 70% to 95% rates of pain relief.

In 2000, Grados and colleagues reported the first long-term outcomes of osteoporotic vertebral body compression fractures treated by percutaneous vertebroplasty. Pain significantly decreased from a mean of 80 mm before the

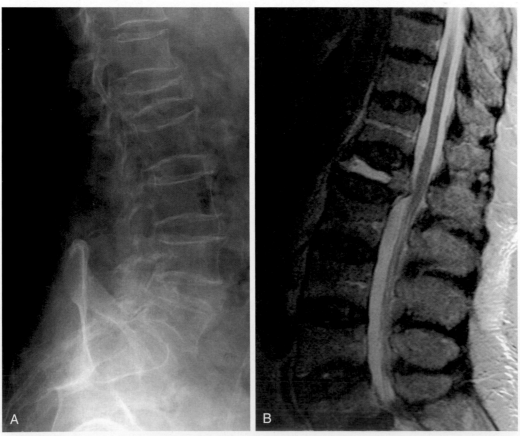

Figure 22-5. This patient sustained a burst fracture with a clinically worsening conus injury (**A** and **B**).

procedure to 37 mm after 1 month. Results were stable over time at 34 mm at final follow-up. There were no severe treatment-related complications. The vertebral deformity did not progress in any of the injected vertebrae. A slight but significant increase in adjacent segment fracture risk was reported. Kaufmann and colleagues performed a retrospective review of 80 treatment sessions in 75 patients with painful osteoporotic VCFs. Garfin and colleagues note that 95% of patients treated with either kyphoplasty or vertebroplasty can expect significant improvement in pain and functional status. Kyphoplasty conferred the additional advantage of 50% increase in vertebral height. Lieberman and colleagues reported a phase I efficacy study of the kyphoplasty IBT in the treatment of symptomatic VCF. Seventy consecutive procedures were performed in 30 patients. There were no major technique-related complications. A mean 47% height restoration was encountered in 70% of the fractures. Bodily Pain and Physical Function scores demonstrated significant improvement.

Vertebroplasty and kyphoplasty are associated with the same types of complications. That is, no particular complications have been reported from use of the balloon tamp or from attempted reduction. Complications can be categorized as medical, anesthetic, instrument placement, or PMMA problems. More common than any of these groups, though, are additional fractures and failure to improve. In most cases, failure to improve is due to inappropriate patient selection. Like any spine procedure, there must be close agreement between the history, physical examination, and

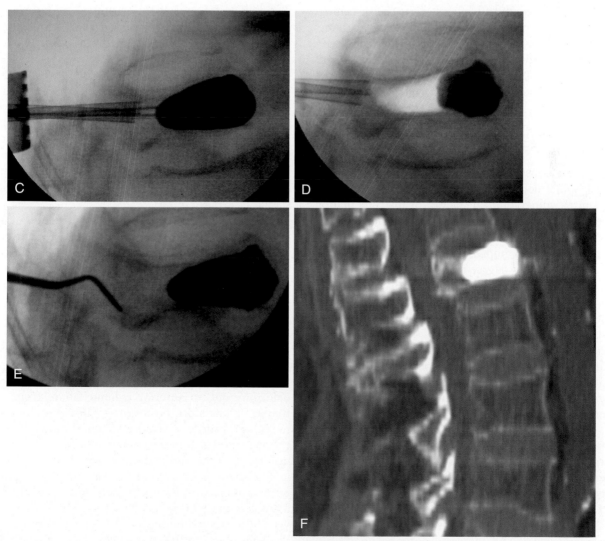

Figure 22-5, cont'd. She was not thought to be an acceptable candidate medically for an anterior corpectomy. Instead, she underwent mini-open posterior decompression and PMMA stabilization after reduction of the fracture with both a balloon tamp (**C** and **D**) and direct compression with a woodson (**E**). Postoperative sagittal CT reconstructions (**F**) demonstrate reasonable reduction and excellent height restoration. The patient noted gradual improvement in her bowel and bladder function over the next 6 months.

imaging findings. The more diffuse the patient's pain, the less likely the patient is to benefit from VBA. The natural history of spinal osteoporosis includes a significant jump of at least five times the risk of additional fractures after the first fracture has occurred. Placement of PMMA into the spine can increase the risk of adjacent segment fracture. The correction of proper weight-bearing axis with kyphoplasty can decrease the risk of additional fracture.

Medical and anesthesia issues are not unusual in this elderly patient population. On the other hand, VBA procedures are not significantly physiologically taxing. More likely are technical errors related to misplacement of the vertebroplasty needles or kyphoplasty instrumentation. High-quality imaging and meticulous surgical technique with frequent evaluation of both AP and lateral fluoroscopy should decrease this risk. The most devastating complications of VBA procedures have come from extravasation of PMMA. In vertebroplasty, up to a 6% leak risk per level has been identified. Many of these leaks are asymptomatic, but one potential benefit of kyphoplasty is the placement of more viscous cement into a cavity of known volume. High-quality, live image intensification during placement, additional radiopacifying agent, avoidance of high-risk fracture patients, and placement of the most viscous PMMA possible can decrease this risk.

Operative Fixation in the Osteoporotic Spine

In planning a reconstruction or stabilization procedure in the at-risk spinal deformity patient, recognize the osteoporotic spine's vulnerability to failure of instrumentation and hence loss of correction. Because trabecular bone exhibits eight times greater metabolic activity than cortical bone, the mechanical impact of osteoporosis affects it earlier and to a greater degree than cortical bone.

Bone mineral density is linearly related to screw insertion torque and pullout strength. Thus, the surgeon's tactile sense of purchase when placing the screw does relate to construct strength. Bone mineral density is the single stronger predictor of pullout strength of pedicle screws, sublaminar wires, hooks, and other spinal implants. Normalization of bone mineral density improves construct stability more than bicortical purchase does.

When spine surgery is contemplated in the at-risk patient, careful assessment of bone quality is critical. Once the degree of bone loss has been established, relevant surgical strategy decisions can be made. Changes may include the following:

1. A decision to cancel the surgery: Any operative intervention is planned on the basis of a careful risk/benefit assessment. Because osteoporosis decreases the chance of surgical success and increases potential morbidity, the surgeon might counsel the patient to avoid operative intervention altogether.

2. A decision to delay the surgery: In the era of improving antiosteoporotic medications, it might be prudent to delay an elective procedure to allow for maximal management of the osteoporosis. Pulsed PTH therapy (Forteo) reaches peak effectiveness between 1 year and 18 months. During this time, a sustained rehabilitation effort might also allow improved extensor muscle strength, which, in turn, improves the patient's capacity for postoperative mobilization and recovery.

3. A decision to decrease the scope of the surgery: In some frail osteoporotic patients, major corrective procedures might be averted in favor of surgery with more modest goals, such as in situ stabilization.

4. A decision to increase the scope of the surgery: In other patients with poor bone stock, larger surgeries are necessary to achieve the same stability that a smaller procedure might have achieved in patients with better bone. Examples of increased surgical size include the addition of anterior procedures, additional levels fused (to allow for more fixation points), addition of osteotomy procedures, and more aggressive forms of instrumentation (combined sacral and pelvic fixation, for example).

Often, successful fixation in osteoporotic patients simply requires that best practice principles be used in all cases.

In other cases, surgical strategy is revised to account for the deficient bone stock. For example, one recent paper found that the threshold bone mineral density, as measured by quantitative CT, for successful ventral spinal instrumentation was 0.22 g/cm. Clearly, for patients with lower bone density, adjunctive posterior stabilization should be considered.

Other specific changes to operative technique are recommended to improve fixation strength. Most frequently, changes consist of additional fixation points, whether this means adding levels to a posterior construct or adding a posterior stabilization after an anterior procedure. For example, in a patient with normal bone, the corrective power of transpedicular instrumentation might obviate anterior release and fusion. In osteoporotic patients, on the other hand, the surgeon must be careful not to excessively preload the screws. In these patients, an anterior approach might be necessary. Similarly, for patients with kyphotic deformity due to anterior column failure from fracture, tumor, or infection, posterior stabilization alone is likely to fail, as cantilever forces lead to cut through of the screws through the surrounding bone and often into the cranial disk space of the end vertebra (Fig. 22-6).

For osteoporotic patients who are undergoing long posterior stabilization for spinal deformity, caudal fixation is a problem as well (Fig. 22-7). The osteoporotic sacrum has very little screw-holding power. At the very least, large-diameter, bicortical screws should be placed. Anterior column support should be considered as well. Unlike patients with good-quality bone in whom posterior inter-

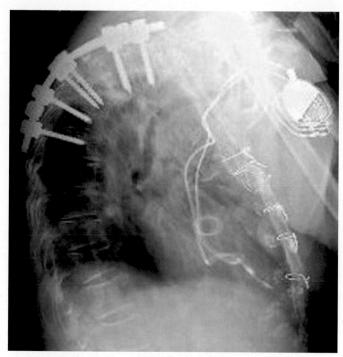

Figure 22-6. This is an example of a man who had had a relatively short posterior upper thoracic fusion performed for complaints of progressive kyphosis. After the surgery, he continued to drift further into kyphosis. This lateral radiograph demonstrates kyphosis above and below thoracic instrumentation.

body access, such as a transforaminal lumbar interbody fusion, can give suitable anterior column support, these cages with small footprints are likely to subside into their

bone. In these patients, a formal anterior lumbar interbody fusion should be considered. At the very least, use bilateral cage placement or placement of larger footprint cages.

Along the same lines, whereas anterior correction and fixation of spinal deformity are often adequate in patients with good bone quality, fixation in osteoporotic patients is marginal, and supplementary posterior fixation is often recommended.

Other means to improve holding power include PMMA screw tract augmentation, use of laminar hooks and other neutralization implants to "protect" the screws, unique screw designs, optimized screw trajectories, increased use of transverse connectors, and bicortical purchase.

Adding PMMA to the screw tract significantly increases pullout strength. A number of techniques have been described, but placement of a Jamshidi needle or Kyph-X bone void fillers (Kyphon, Sunnyvale, CA) into the vertebral body allows 1.5 mL of PMMA to be placed under image guidance without disrupting the tapped threads. Most authors recommend cementing the vertebral body only and not the pedicles (Fig. 22-8). Hydroxyapatite and calcium phosphate cements have been employed for this purpose as well, but they have more difficulty handling characteristics of the elderly osteoporotic patient group and have dubious benefits for this group.

PMMA may be added to the vertebral body for other reasons as well, typically to improve the axial stiffness of the body in cases of anterior column deficiency (tumor and

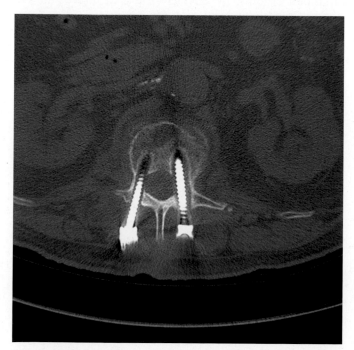

Figure 22-7. This axial CT scan demonstrates pedicle screw pullout in an osteoporotic patient.

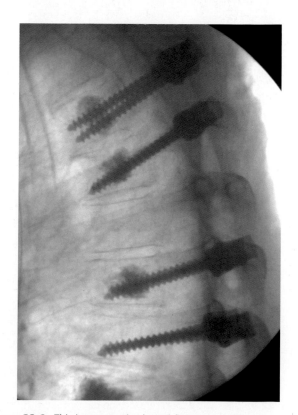

Figure 22-8. This intraoperative lateral fluoroscopic image demonstrates PMMA supplementing pedicle screw fixation.

fracture predominantly). Here, PMMA injection functions in lieu of strut graft anterior column reconstruction or transpedicular bone grafting. One advantage lies in the immediate restoration of strength and stiffness. Some surgeons recommend percutaneous PMMA injection (vertebroplasty and kyphoplasty) at the cranial level of the construct and the levels above and below to decrease the risk of fracture at those levels (Fig. 22-9).

Bicortical purchase certainly improves pullout strength and fatigue life of both anterior and posterior constructs. Unfortunately, bicortical placement adds surgical risk. The benefits of bicortical placement outweigh the risks for sacral screws, which are below the bifurcation of the great vessels, and for anterior constructs.

In most posterior situations, unicortical screws are most common. The strength of these consults can be improved by optimization of the screw's trajectory. Triangulated screw placement significantly improves pullout strength. Bilateral screws placed in a triangulated pattern with a transverse connector allow the screws to hold all the bone between the screws rather than merely the bone within the threads of each screw individually.

Pedicle screws and, where possible, anterior vertebral body screws should be aimed toward the stronger bone of the subchondral plate. In the sacrum, both techniques are advised. Aim bicortical screws upward through the disc space or through the sacral promontory. When sacral fixation is in doubt, augmented instrumentation such as alar screws, S2 pedicle screws, and intrasacral rods have been recommended, and all yield similar improvements in construct stability. For larger constructs in markedly osteoporotic patients, however, fixation to the pelvis is much more reliable.

In osteoporotic patients and all others, maximizing pedicle screw diameter will improve pullout strength and decrease the risk of fatigue failure of the screw. Screw length is linearly related to pullout strength, but little difference is seen with self-drilling or self-tapping designs. If formal tapping is undertaken, undertapping by 1 mm leads to greater pullout strength than does undertapping by 0.5 mm.

Expanding screws, designed to work like drywall screws, have been designed and are in testing. More typically, neutralization implants are added. For fusions that end above the sacrum, some authors recommend placing an infralaminar hook under the caudalmost pedicle screw to neutralize pullout forces. Similarly, translaminar facet screws and sublaminar and spinous process wiring have been used to augment transpedicular constructs when formal decompressive procedures are not required (Box 22-7).

Other aspects of deformity surgery that place additional stress on the bone-implant interface must also be altered in patients with osteoporosis. Do not distract or compress against the implants themselves. Rather, use lamina spreaders or other devices on the cortical posterior elements. For interbody fusions, use distractors placed directly in the interspace. Compressing or distracting against the screws tends to loosen the screws, as even optimally placed and sized screws will not completely fill the pedicle. Early toggling from distractors will increase the likelihood of windshield-wipering of the implants in the postoperative period. Similarly, in situ bending maneuvers should be done with extreme caution if at all. While modern implant systems such as polyaxial screw designs do have some "give," and various insertion instruments such as "towers" and "persuaders" can force an imperfectly contoured rod into the screw assembly, these maneuvers risk ultimate construct failure.

Soft-tissue and skeletal mechanical principles concerning end levels for fusions are even more important in osteoporotic patients. While ending a fusion at the apex of kyphosis is problematic in any patient, the risk is higher in osteoporotic patients. Here, rapid and dramatic sagittal imbalance can be seen either with or without compression fracture. Even ending a construct at a high-stress transition zone should be avoided. Many surgeons recommend avoiding L1 as a cranial termination point, citing kyphotic collapse at the thoracolumbar junction. Depending on the local facet morphology and the number of transitional

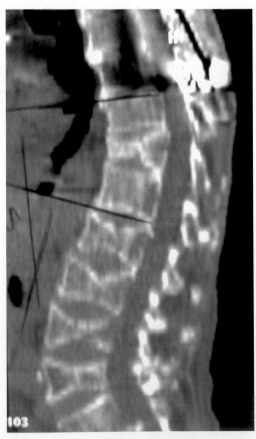

Figure 22-9. This sagittal CT reconstruction demonstrates osteoporotic and kyphotic collapse at the thoracolumbar junction in a patient who had recently undergone thoracic spine surgery.

BOX 22-7 Methods to Improve Fixation in Osteoporotic Patients

Approach Changes

- Liberally add anterior column support
  - Anterior lumbar interbody fusion to long posterior procedures to reduce axial pistoning through open disc spaces
  - Cement augmentation
  - Corpectomy with strut graft reconstruction to minimize cantilever forces on screws and prevent kyphotic collapse; PMMA can be used in vertebral bodies above and below construct as well
- Liberally add posterior fixation to anterior procedures
- Add more levels and fixation points (at least bilateral screws in each fused level)
- Avoid termination at transition zones or apex of kyphosis

Instrumentation Changes

- Use longer, larger-diameter screws when possible
- Add cross-links
- Augment screws with PMMA if necessary
- Use additional neutralization implants, such as translaminar facet screws, hooks, and wires, if possible
- In the future, expanding screws or coated screws could prove useful

Trajectory Changes

- In the sacrum, seek bicortical purchase
- Medialize
- Aim toward denser bone below the vertebral end plate

Decompression—Limit Iatrogenic Destabilization

- Minimize facet resection
- Preserve midline elements where possible

Fusion Technique—Bias Race from Loosening to Solid Fusion

- Optimize graft material
  - Use of bone morphogenetic proteins might lead to accelerated healing, thereby decreasing risk of failure of the screw-bone interface
- Optimal fusion technique, including full exposure of posterolateral elements, especially lateral pars
  - Careful resection of facet capsules, insert bone shim into facet

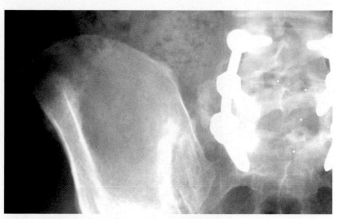

Figure 22-10. The fluffy periosteal reaction on this AP radiograph demonstrates a stress fracture through the ilium in this osteoporotic patient after an aggressive iliac crest bone harvest.

sagittal balance and appropriate skeletal loading. Compromised extensor musculature allows the spine to collapse into kyphosis above or below the instrumentation. Similarly, careful preservation of the regional blood supply supports rapid graft incorporation and biases the race toward fusion and against construct failure.

PEARLS & PITFALLS

PEARLS

- VCFs are the most common manifestation of spinal osteoporosis and are estimated to affect one third of all North Americans at some point during their lifetime.
- In osteoporosis, there is a decrease in the rate of bone formation relative to the rate of destruction. With age, everyone loses bone mass at approximately 0.5% per year, but not everyone develops osteoporosis.
- Osteoporosis has the following mechanical effects: (1) It increases the risk of bone fracture; (2) it increases instrumentation failure in the operative management of spinal disorders; (3) it increases the development and progression of spinal deformity, including spondylolisthesis, scoliosis, and hyperkyphosis.
- Evaluation algorithms for osteoporosis begin with a screening DEXA scan.
- The two most important determinants for the development of osteoporosis are peak bone mass and rate of bone loss. The most effective way to prevent complications of VCF is to increase peak bone mass in pubertal patients.
- Begin preemptive medical treatment with calcium, physiologic vitamin D, and mild weight-bearing exercise. More aggressive pharmacologic management consisting of calcitonin or bisphosphonates is indicated in

levels and floating ribs, it might be more appropriate to end those constructs at T10. Similarly, posterior cervical constructs ending at C7 have been seen to fall into kyphosis, and some surgeons recommend extension of the fixation into the upper thoracic spine (to T3, for example).

Osteoporotic patients are subjected to other increased risks after surgery as well. If a bone graft is harvested, they have an increased rate of ilium stress fractures (Fig. 22-10). Similarly, more of the facet and lateral pars must be preserved during decompression procedures to avoid iatrogenic instability (Fig. 22-11).

The importance of soft-tissue and muscular tension has been grossly underappreciated in thoracolumbar reconstruction. Recent studies have documented a linear relationship between the degeneration and loss of mechanical strength of a patient's bone, ligament, and muscle. Meticulous handling of the extensor muscles followed by a tight fascial closure improves the muscle's ability to promote

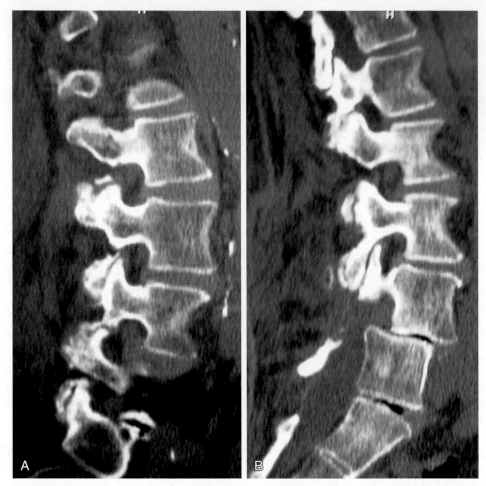

Figure 22-11. This patient had undergone a relatively wide lumbar laminectomy and complained of persistent low back pain thereafter. A CT scan was ordered, and the sagittal reconstruction demonstrates a stress fracture through the pars (**A**). The patient did well in a brace for 18 months. Subsequently, he returned with more back pain. The new CT scan demonstrates progression to spondylolisthesis (**B**).

patients with fractures or with DEXA femoral T-scores less than −2.5.

- Patients with VCF usually present with an acute onset of pain with or without noticeable deformity.

- For patients with intractable pain, percutaneous PMMA vertebral body augmentation (VBA) through either vertebroplasty or kyphoplasty is possible. Open surgery is indicated in progressive neurologic deficit or deformity.

PITFALLS

- The clinician must have a solid understanding of the biology and biomechanics of osteoporosis in treating any spinal condition in an osteoporotic patient popula-

tion. Many spine surgeons will refer their patients to an endocrinologist for this workup, but it is incumbent on the surgeon to ensure that an appropriate workup has been undertaken.

- Fractures that are less likely to improve with standard medical management include those of the thoracolumbar junction (T11-L2), those with bursting patterns, wedge compression fractures with more than 30 degrees of sagittal angulation, those with vacuum shadow in the fractured body (ischemic necrosis of bone), and those with progressive collapse in office follow-up.

- High-quality imaging and meticulous surgical technique should decrease the risks of VBA. The most devastating complications of VBA procedures have come from extravasation of PMMA.

Illustrative Case Presentation

CASE 1. A 76-Year-Old Male Presented with a Long History of Low Back Pain That Was Ostensibly Related to Scoliosis

The patient was a heavy smoker with chronic obstructive pulmonary disease, diabetes, and previous myocardial infarction. He weighed more than 240 pounds, had been on steroids for at least 10 years, and was known to have developed osteoporosis. AP radiographs demonstrated worsening of his previous deformity with a lateral compression fracture (note the vacuum cleft within the bone). On the basis of the patient's intractable pain, a kyphoplasty procedure was offered (Fig. 22-12A). Gradual restoration of some of the lost height is being achieved with the balloons (Fig. 22-12B). The postoperative film demonstrates a reasonable, partial reduction (Fig. 22-12C). The patient's pain improved immediately.

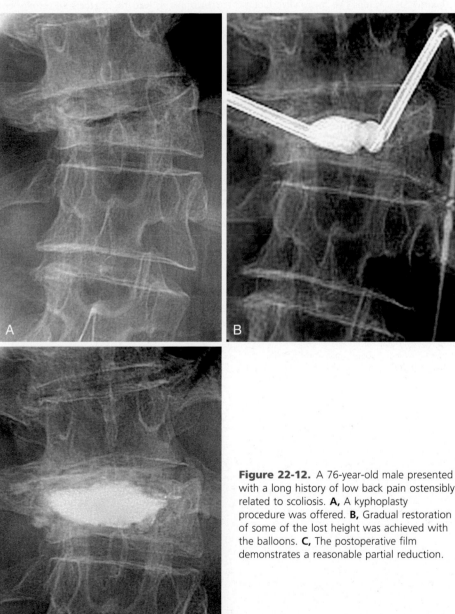

Figure 22-12. A 76-year-old male presented with a long history of low back pain ostensibly related to scoliosis. **A,** A kyphoplasty procedure was offered. **B,** Gradual restoration of some of the lost height was achieved with the balloons. **C,** The postoperative film demonstrates a reasonable partial reduction.

REFERENCES

Adachi JD, Loannidis G, Berger C, et al: The influence of osteoporotic fractures on health-related quality of life in community-dwelling men and women across Canada. Osteoporos Int 2001;12:903–908.

Aerssens J, Boonen S, Joly S, Degueker J: Variations in trabecular bone composition with anatomical site and age: Potential implications for bone quality assessment. J Endocrinol 1997;155:411–421.

Babayev M, Lachmann E, Nagler W: The controversy surrounding sacral insufficiency fractures: To ambulate or not to ambulate? Am J Phys Med Rehabil 2000;79:404–409.

Bauer DC, Sklarin PM, Stone KL: Biochemical markers of bone turnover and prediction of hip bone loss in older women: The study of osteoporotic fractures. J Bone Miner Res 1999;14:1404–1410.

Becker C: Clinical evaluation for osteoporosis. Clin Geriatr Med 2003;19: 299–320.

Belkoff SM, Maroney M, Fenton DC, Mathis JM: An in vitro biomechanical evaluation of bone cements used in percutaneous vertebroplasty. Bone 1999;25(2, suppl):23S–26S.

Benoist M: Natural history of the aging spine. Eur Spine J 2003;12(suppl 2):S86–S89.

Benzel EC, Larson SJ: Postoperative stabilization of the posttraumatic thoracic and lumbar spine: A review of concepts and orthotic techniques. J Spinal Disord 1989;2:47–51.

Berlemann U, Schwarzenbach O: Dens fractures in the elderly: Results of anterior screw fixation in 19 elderly patients. Acta Orthop Scand 1997;68:319–324.

Bostrom MP, Lane JM: Future directions: Augmentation of osteoporotic vertebral bodies. Spine 1997:22(24, suppl):38S–42S.

Buckwalter J, Einhorn T, Simon S: Orthopaedic Basic Science: Biology and Biomechanics of the Musculoskeletal System, 2nd ed. Rosemont, IL: American Academy of Orthopaedic Surgeons, 2000.

Cheng JC, Guo X, Sher AH: Persistent osteopenia in adolescent idiopathic scoliosis: A longitudinal follow up study. Spine 1999;4: 1218–1222.

Chung SK, Lee SH, Kim DY, Lee HY: Treatment of lower lumbar radiculopathy caused by osteoporotic compression fracture: The role of vertebroplasty. J Spinal Disord Tech 2002;15:461–468.

Coen G, Ballanti P, Fischer MS, et al: Serum leptin in dialysis renal osteodystrophy. Am J Kidney Dis 2003;42:1036–1042.

Cortet B, Houvenagel E, Puisieux F, et al: Spinal curvatures and quality of life in women with vertebral fractures secondary to osteoporosis. Spine 1999;24:1921–1925.

Cranney A, Adachi JD: Corticosteroid-induced osteoporosis: A guide to optimum management. Treat Endocrinol 2002;1:271–279.

Dennison E, Cole Z, Cooper C: Diagnosis and epidemiology of osteoporosis. Curr Opin Rheumatol 2005;17:456–461.

Eleraky MA, Masferrer R, Sonntag VK: Posterior atlantoaxial facet screw fixation in rheumatoid arthritis. J Neurosurg 1998;89:8–12.

Faciszewski T, McKiernan F: Calling all vertebral fractures classification of vertebral compression fractures: A consensus for comparison of treatment and outcome. J Bone Miner Res 2002;17:185–191.

Fritton JC, Myers ER, Wright TM, van der Meulen MC: Loading induces site-specific increases in mineral content assessed by microcomputed tomography of the mouse tibia. Bone 2005;36: 1030–1038.

Garfin SR, Reilly MA: Minimally invasive treatment of osteoporotic vertebral body compression fractures. Spine J 2002;2:76–80.

Garfin SR, Yuan HA, Reiley MA: New technologies in spine: Kyphoplasty and vertebroplasty for the treatment of painful osteoporotic compression fractures. Spine 2001;26:1511–1515.

Gasser JA, Ingold P, Grosios K, et al: Noninvasive monitoring of changes in structural cancellous bone parameters with a novel prototype micro-CT. J Bone Miner Metab 2005;23(suppl):90–96.

Gold DT: The nonskeletal consequences of osteoporotic fractures: Psychologic and social outcomes. Rheum Dis Clin North Am 2001;27: 255–262.

Grados F, Depriester C, Cayrolle G, et al: Long-term observations of osteoporotic fractures treated by percutaneous vertebroplasty. Rheumatology (Oxford) 2000;39:1410–1414.

Hadjipavlou AG, Nicodemus CL, al-Hamdon FA, et al: Correlation of bone equivalent mineral density to pull-out resistance of triangulated pedicle screw construct. J Spinal Disord 1997;10:12–19.

Hans D, Biot B, Schott AM, Meunier PJ: No diffuse osteoporosis in lumbar scoliosis but lower femoral bone density on the convexity. Bone 1996;18:15–17.

Hasserius R, Karlsson MK, Jonsson B, et al: Long-term morbidity and mortality after a clinically diagnosed vertebral fracture in the elderly: A 12- and 22-year follow-up of 257 patients. Calcif Tissue Int 2005;76:235–242.

Hitchon PW, Brenton MD, Black AG, et al: In vitro biomechanical comparison of pedicle screws, sublaminar hooks, and sublaminar cables. J Neurosurg 2003;99(1, suppl):104–109.

Hitchon PW, Brenton MD, Coppes JK, et al: Factors affecting the pullout strength of self-drilling and self-tapping anterior cervical screws. Spine 2003;28:9–13.

Iida T, Abumi K, Kotani Y, Kaneda K: Effects of aging and spinal degeneration on mechanical properties of lumbar supraspinous and interspinous ligaments. Spine J 2002;2:95–100.

Jaovisidha S, Kim JK, Sartoris DJ, et al: Scoliosis in elderly and age-related bone loss: A population-based study. J Clin Densitom 1998; 1:227–233.

Kayanja MM, Togawa D, Lieberman IH: Biomechanical changes after the augmentation of experimental osteoporotic vertebral compression fractures in the cadaveric thoracic spine. Spine J 2005;5: 55–63.

King GJ, Kostuik JP, McBroom RJ, Richardson W: Surgical management of metastatic renal carcinoma of the spine. Spine 1991;16: 265–271.

Knoller SM, Meyer G, Eckhardt C, et al: Range of motion in reconstruction situations following corpectomy in the lumbar spine: A question of bone mineral density? Spine 2005;30:E229–E235.

Korovessis P, Konstantinou D, Piperos G, et al: Spinal bone mineral density changes following halo vest immoilization for cervical trauma. Eur Spine J 1994;3:206–208.

Kuklo TR, Lehman RA Jr: Effect of various tapping diameters on insertion of thoracic pedicle screws: A biomechanical analysis. Spine 2003;28:2066–2071.

Lehman RA Jr, Kuklo TR, Belmont PJ Jr, et al: Advantage of pedicle screw fixation directed into the apex of the sacral promontory over bicortical fixation: A biomechanical analysis. Spine 2002;27: 806–811.

Lieberman I, Reinhardt MK: Vertebroplasty and kyphoplasty for osteolytic vertebral collapse. Clin Orthop Relat Res 2003;415(suppl): S176–S186.

Lombardi I Jr, Oliveira LM, Mayer AF, et al: Evaluation of pulmonary function and quality of life in women with osteoporosis. Osteoporos Int 2005;16:1247–1253.

Lomoschitz FM, Blackmore CC, Mirza SK, Mann FA: Cervical spine injuries in patients 65 years old and older: Epidemiologic analysis regarding the effects of age and injury mechanism on distribution, type, and stability of injuries. AJR Am J Roentgenol 2002;178: 573–577.

Lotz JC, Hu SS, Chiu DF, et al: Carbonated apatite cement augmentation of pedicle screw fixation in the lumbar spine. Spine 1997;22: 2716–2723.

Lu WW, Zhu Q, Holmes AD, et al: Loosening of sacral screw fixation under in vitro fatigue loading. J Orthop Res 2000;18:808–814.

Mathis JM: Percutaneous vertebroplasty: Complication avoidance and technique optimization. AJNR Am J Neuroradiol 2003;24: 1697–1706.

McKiernan F, Faciszewski T: Intravertebral clefts in osteoporotic vertebral compression fractures. Arthritis Rheum 2003;48:1414–1419.

Moore DC, Maitra RS, Farjo LA, et al: Restoration of pedicle screw fixation with an in situ setting calcium phosphate cement. Spine 1997; 22:1696–1705.

Myer BS, Belmont PJ Jr, Richardson WJ, et al: The role of imaging and in situ biomechanical testing in assessing pedicle screw pull-out strength. Spine 1996;21:1962–1968.

Neumann P, Ekstrom LA, Keller TS, et al: Aging, vertebral density, and disc degeneration alter the tensile stress-strain characteristics of the human anterior longitudinal ligament. J Orthop Res 1994;12: 103–112.

Noorda RJ, Wuisman PI, Fidler MW, et al: Severe progressive osteoporotic spine deformity with cardiopulmonary impairment in a young patient: A case report. Spine 1999;24:489–492.

Oleksik A, Lips P, Dawson A, et al: Health-related quality of life in postmenopausal women with low BMD with or without prevalent vertebral fractures. J Bone Miner Res 2000;15:1384–1392.

Pitzen T, Franta F, Barbier D, Steudel WI: Insertion torque and pullout force of rescue screws for anterior cervical plate fixation in a fatigued initial pilot hole. J Neurosurg Spine 2004;1:198–201.

Riggs BL, Melton LJ 3rd: The worldwide problem of osteoporosis: Insights afforded by epidemiology. Bone 1995;17(5, suppl): 505S–511S.

Robertson PA, Plank LD: Pedicle screw placement at the sacrum: Anatomical characterization and limitations at S1. J Spinal Disord 1999;12:227–233.

Ruland CM, McAfee DC, Warden KF, Cunningham BW: Triangulation of pedicular instrumentation: A biomechanical analysis. Spine 1991; 16(6, suppl):S270–S276.

Ryken TC, Clausen JD, Traynelis VC, Goel VK: Biomechanical analysis of bone mineral density, insertion technique, screw torque, and holding strength of anterior cervical plate screws. J Neurosurg 1995;83:325–329.

Sarikaya S, Ozdolap S, Acikgoz G, Erdem CZ: Pregnancy-associated osteoporosis with vertebral fractures and scoliosis. Joint Bone Spine 2004;1:84–85.

Schneider DL, von Muhlen D, Barrett-Connor E, Sartoris DJ: Kyphosis does not equal vertebral fractures: The Rancho Bernardo study. J Rheumatol 2004;31:747–752.

Shea JE, Miller SC: Skeletal function and structure: Implications for tissue-targeted therapeutics. Adv Drug Deliv Rev 2005;57: 945–957.

Shipp KM, Purse JL, Gold DT, et al: Timed loaded standing: A measure of combined trunk and arm endurance suitable for people with vertebral osteoporosis. Osteoporos Int 2000;11:914–922.

Silverman SL: Quality-of-life issues in osteoporosis. Curr Rheumatol Rep 2005;7:39–45.

Silverman SL, Azria M: The analgesic role of calcitonin following osteoporotic fracture. Osteoporos Int 2002;13:858–867.

Sinaki M: Critical appraisal of physical rehabilitation measures after osteoporotic vertebral fracture. Osteoporos Int 2003;14:773–779.

Sinaki M, Brey RH, Hughes CA, et al: Balance disorder and increased risk of falls in osteoporosis and kyphosis: Significance of kyphotic posture and muscle strength. Osteoporos Int 2005;16:1004–1010.

Tabrizi P, Bouchard JA: Osteoporotic spondylolisthesis: A case report. Spine 2001;26:1482–1485.

Thomas E, Richardson JC, Irvine A, et al: Osteoporosis: What are the implications of DEXA scanning 'high risk' women in primary care? Fam Pract 2003;20:289–293.

Tosteson AN, Gabriel SE, Grove MR, et al: Impact of hip and vertebral fractures on quality-adjusted life years. Osteoporos Int 2001;12: 1042–1049.

Truumees E, Lieberman I: Minimally invasive spinal decompression and stabilization techniques. In Benzel E (ed): Spine Surgery: Techniques, Complications, Avoidance, and Management. Philadelphia: Elsevier, 2005, pp 1274–1308.

Vogt MT, Gabriel SE, Grove MR, et al: Degenerative lumbar listhesis and bone mineral density in elderly women: The study of osteoporotic fractures. Spine 1999;24:2536–2541.

Yamaguchi T, Sugimoto T, Yamauchi M, et al: Multiple vertebral fractures are associated with refractory reflux esophagitis in postmenopausal women. J Bone Miner Metab 2005;23:36–40.

Zhilkin BA, Doktorov AA, Denisov-Nikol'skii YI: Structure of human vertebral lamellar bone in age-associated involution and osteoporosis. Bull Exp Biol Med 2003;135:405–408.

Zmuda JM, Sheu YT, Moffett SP: Genetic epidemiology of osteoporosis: Past, present, and future. Curr Osteoporos Rep 2005;3:111–115.

SUGGESTED READINGS

Bai B, Kummer FJ, Spivak J: Augmentation of anterior vertebral body screw fixation by an injectable, biodegradable calcium phosphate bone substitute. Spine 2001;26:2679–2683.

A biomechanical study that compared vertebral body screw fixation strength in normal spines and spines that were augmented with biodegradable calcium phosphate. Results demonstrated that the spines that were augmented with calcium phosphate were significantly stronger than were the spines in the control group. The study concluded that calcium phosphate is a safer alternative to PMMA while providing the same benefits.

Barr JD, Barr MS, Lemley TJ, McCann RM: Percutaneous vertebroplasty for pain relief and spinal stabilization. Spine 2000;25:923–928.

A retrospective study of patients treated for vertebral compression fractures and spine neoplasms with percutaneous vertebroplasty. Results demonstrated that patients with vertebral compression fractures had a significant amount of relief of pain due to vertebroplasty, while those with neoplasms obtained stabilization but did not consistently have pain relief.

Baur A, Stäbler A, Brüning R, et al: Diffusion-weighted MR imaging of bone marrow: Differentiation of benign versus pathologic compression fractures. Radiology 1998;207:349–356.

A prospective evaluation of patients with acute or malignant causes of vertebral compression fractures that were evaluated with the use of MR imaging. Using T1-weighted images, this study demonstrated that benign causes of vertebral fractures were hypointense or isointense compared to normal marrow space while malignant causes were hyperintense compared to normal marrow.

Brown JP, Josse RG: 2002 clinical practice guidelines for the diagnosis and management of osteoporosis in Canada. CMAJ 2002;167(10, suppl):S1–S34.

The recommendations of the Scientific Advisory Council of the Osteoporosis Society of Canada concerning the diagnosis and management of osteoporosis. Four key factors were identified: low bone mineral density, prior fragility fracture, age, and family history of osteoporosis. Various treatments were also suggested and thoroughly discussed.

Cook SD, Barberá J, Rubi M, et al: Lumbosacral fixation using expandable pedicle screws: An alternative in reoperation and osteoporosis. Spine J 2001;1:109–114.

A retrospective clinical and radiographic review of patients who were treated with an expandable pedicle screw for the following reasons: osteoporosis, previous pedicle instrumentation, intraoperative screw relocation, construct reinforcement, and sacral anchoring. Results demonstrated a high rate of fusion and a low rate of screw breakage. This study determines that expandable screws are a viable option for spinal instrumentation.

Kaufmann TJ, Jensen ME, Schweickert PA, et al: Age of fracture and clinical outcomes of percutaneous vertebroplasty. AJNR Am J Neuroradiol 2001;22:1860–1863.

A retrospective study of patients with different ages of vertebral compression fractures that had undergone percutaneous vertebroplasty. The results demonstrated that percutaneous vertebroplasty was efficious regardless of the age of the vertebral compression fracture.

Kayanja MM, Ferrara LA, Lieberman IH: Distribution of anterior cortical shear strain after a thoracic wedge compression fracture. Spine J 2004;4:76–87.

A biomechanical study of the effect of anterior cortical strain at the level above and below a thoracic vertebral fracture. The results demonstrated that anterior cortical strain was concentrated at the apex of the thoracic curve. Also, the vertebra one segment above the compression fracture had the most increased anterior cortical strain and therefore the most risk for secondary fracture.

Lieberman I, Dudeney S, Reinhardt M-K, Bell G: Initial outcome and efficacy of "Kyphoplasty" in the treatment of painful osteoporotic vertebral compression fractures. Spine 2001;26:1631–1638.

An efficacy study of an inflatable bone tamp usage in the treatment of symptomatic osteoporotic compression fractures. The indications for treatment included painful primary or secondary osteoporotic vertebral compression fractures. The treatment levels treated ranged from T6 to L5, but the majority were performed at the thoracolumbar junction. Results demonstrated early improvement of pain and mobility as well as restoration of vertebral body height.

Lowe T, O'Brien M, Smith D, et al: Central and juxta-endplate vertebral body screw placement: A biomechanical analysis in a human cadaveric model. Spine 2002;27:369–373.

A biomechanical study of the thoracic and lumbar spine. This study demonstrated that bicortical placement of screws into the body of a vertebra is stronger than unicortical placement. Also, placement of a screw close to the end plate with a staple produced the highest yield strength.

Mika A, Unnithan VB, Mika P: Differences in thoracic kyphosis and in back muscle strength in women with bone loss due to osteoporosis. Spine 2005;30:241–246.

A prospective study of female patients who were followed to access the association of thoracic kyphosis, bone mineral density, and back extensor strength. The results demonstrated that there was no significant correlation between bone mineral density and thoracic kyphosis.

Nguyen HV, Ludwig S, Gelb D: Osteoporotic vertebral burst fractures with neurologic compromise. J Spinal Disord Tech 2003;16:10–19.

A retrospective study of patients with osteoporotic burst fractures with neurologic compromise that had operative decompression and stabilization treatment. All the patients had thoracolumbar fractures. Operative stabilization allowed for significant neurologic recovery, but patients remained disabled secondary to pain.

Sinaki M, Wollan PC, Scott RW, Gelczer RK: Can strong back extensors prevent vertebral fractures in women with osteoporosis? Mayo Clin Proc 1996;71:951–956.

A cross-sectional study of female patients with osteoporosis who were assessed for bone mineral density, muscle strength, level of physical activity, and radiographic findings in the spine. The results demonstrated that there was a negative correlation between back extensor strength and the number of vertebral compression fractures as well as bone mineral density and the number of vertebral compression fractures. The authors concluded that increased back strength can be an effective treatment of an osteoporotic spine.

Suk SI, Kim JH, Lee SM, et al: Anterior-posterior surgery versus posterior closing wedge osteotomy in posttraumatic kyphosis with neurologic compromised osteoporotic fracture. Spine 2003;28:2170–2175.

A retrospective study comparing the surgical results between combined anterior-posterior procedures and posterior closing wedge osteotomy procedures in patients with posttraumatic kyphosis and neurologic compromise secondary to osteoporotic fractures. The results demonstrated that the posterior closing wedge osteotomy procedure led to a better surgical result with significantly less operative time and blood loss.

Tracy JK, Meyer WA, Flores RH, et al: Racial differences in rate of decline in bone mass in older men: The Baltimore men's osteoporosis study. J Bone Miner Res 2005;20:1228–1234.

A prospective evaluation of older black and older white men in the Baltimore Men's Osteoporosis Study. The study found that older black men had a higher adjusted bone mineral density than did older white men and that the decline in bone mass was greater in older white men than in older black men.

Truumees E, Hilibrand A, Vaccaro AR: Percutaneous vertebral augmentation. Spine J 2004;4:218–229.

A literature review of the pathophysiology, evaluation, treatment, and complications of vertebral compression fractures.

CHAPTER 23

Adult Neoplasia

CARLOS A. BAGLEY *and* ZIYA L. GOKASLAN

OVERVIEW

Cancer affects approximately 1.4 million Americans every year. Despite recent advances and improvements in the care of these patients, approximately half will eventually succumb to their disease, a rate that has remained relatively unchanged over the last half century. In 2001, cancer ranked second only to heart disease in terms of mortality in the United States, accounting for approximately 23% of all deaths. The most common causes of death in oncology patients are complications related to metastasis of their primary disease. The skeletal system is the third most common site for metastases, behind the lungs and liver. Within the skeletal system, the spinal column is the most commonly affected site. In fact, metastases are the most common type of neoplastic lesion found in the spinal column, comprising up to 90% of all spinal tumors in some series. Autopsy studies also demonstrate that upward of 90% of cancer patients will have spinal metastatic deposits at the time of death. Of patients with spinal metastases, up to 50% will require some form of treatment for their spinal metastasis, and 5% to 10% will require surgery.

CLASSIFICATION

The lungs are the most common source of neoplasia in men and women, accounting for 32% and 25% of all cases, respectively, followed by breast/prostate cancer (10%/15%) and colorectal cancer (10%). A 30-year review of the literature published in 1988 by Brihaye and colleagues found that in nearly 1500 patients with symptomatic metastatic disease to the spine, 16.5% of the metastases arose from breast cancer, 15.6% from lung cancer, 9.2% from prostate cancer, and 6.5% from kidney cancer. Overall, these four tumor types accounted for over 50% of all spinal metastases. Furthermore, 10% to 20% of metastases to the spine have no known primary.

Breast cancer is by far the most common source of metastatic tumor deposits to the spine. In fact, as many as 85% of women with breast cancer will develop skeletal metastases during the course of their disease. The clinical course of these metastatic deposits can vary greatly between patients. Lesions may behave rather indolently in some, whereas the behavior may be much more aggressive in others. Breast cancer cells typically spread to the spine via the azygous venous system, most commonly to the thoracic region. Although solitary lesions do occur, multiple, often noncontiguous levels are most often involved.

As was mentioned above, lung cancer is the second most common source of metastatic disease to the spine and the most common type of cancer in adults. Spinal lesions are often multiple and usually present late in the overall disease course. Of the different lung cancer subtypes, the adenocarcinomas are the most common type to present with symptomatic spinal metastases that warrant therapeutic intervention. Other subtypes, such as squamous cell, are far more aggressive and often have massive lung and liver involvement by the time symptomatic spinal metastasis develops. Lung cancer cells may enter the pulmonary venous system, subsequently reaching the heart, after which they may spread to the entire skeletal system. In addition, spinal involvement can result from direct tumor invasion of the anterior elements.

Prostate cancer is generally considered a disease of the elderly, many cases being diagnosed after the age of 70 years. Prostate cancer can spread to the lumbosacral spine by entering the pelvic venous system. Although spinal metastases can occur at any point during the disease process, it is uncommon for these to become symptomatic until very late.

Renal cell carcinoma represents a significant portion of the spinal metastases that come to clinical attention. As was mentioned above, it is the fourth most common source of spinal metastases. In addition, renal cell carcinoma will often present initially with spinal metastases. These lesions, unlike breast or lung carcinomas, will most often have a single level of spinal involvement in addition to the renal mass. This fact has tremendous implications in the development of the surgical treatment plan for these patients (see the section entitled "Surgery").

Most patients with spinal metastases will be found to have multilevel disease. In most cases, however, only one level is symptomatic at the time of clinical presentation. The thoracolumbar spine is the most common region of the spine to be affected by both primary and metastatic disease. In fact, between 70% and 80% of symptomatic primary and metastatic tumors occur in this region. This may be due in part to the small size of the vertebral body and the small size of the spinal canal in the thoracic region, in addition to the typical routes by which the most common metastatic tumors spread, as discussed above.

No single staging system exists for metastatic spinal tumors. These lesions are staged independently on the basis of the primary tumor type and the extent to which it has spread. The TNM classification takes into account the size and extent of the primary tumor (T), regional lymph node involvement (N), and distant metastases (M). The clinical stage for the tumor is determined by the physical findings as well as the results of radiographic and laboratory testing. The pathologic stage of the tumor is determined by histologic examination of the tumor specimens that are obtained at the time of biopsy or surgery. In most cases, the pathologic stage most accurately predicts the prognosis.

TREATMENT OPTIONS

Surgery

In the setting of metastases, the goals of surgery are the preservation of neurologic function, pain control, and immediate stabilization of the spine. In addition, for a minority of patients with a single, intraosseous metastasis, the potential to cure or significantly alter the overall prognosis exists. The generally agreed-on indications for surgical intervention for osseous vertebral neoplasms are (1) radioresistant tumor, (2) severe neurologic compromise, (3) evidence of spinal instability or bony compression, and (4) tumor recurrence despite maximum previous radiation treatment.

In considering surgical interventions, a number of patient factors must be taken into account. The first is the patient's expected survival. No consensus exists in the literature regarding the expected length of survival of patients who could benefit from surgical intervention. In addition, survival is something that is extremely difficult to predict for the individual patient, despite our best attempts. Some authors have proposed requirements of 3- to 6-month expected survival; however, this is not universally agreed upon. Therefore, each patient's prognosis must be assessed individually.

Defining spinal instability in the setting of neoplasia remains somewhat controversial in the literature. For the occipitocervical junction, ligamentous structures and bony articulations are critical for stability of this region. The

cruciate ligament, along with the apical and alar ligaments, provides the bulk of the stability at C1 and C2. In the thoracic and lumbar spinal regions, the biomechanics of stability are quite different. A significant body of literature has been devoted to this issue in the setting of trauma, whereas very little exists solely in the face of neoplasia. Denis's three-column model for spinal instability is widely accepted as a biomechanical model for thoracolumbar trauma and has applications to neoplastic processes that involve this region of the spine. This model divides the spinal column into three columns. The anterior column consists of the ventral half of the vertebral body, the ventral annulus fibrosus, and the anterior longitudinal ligament; the middle column consists of the dorsal half of the vertebral body, the dorsal annulus fibrosus, and the posterior longitudinal ligament; the posterior column consists of the pedicles, laminae, ligamentum flavum, and interspinous and supraspinous ligaments.

Based on Denis's model, the criteria for defining spinal instability in the setting of trauma are (1) two or more column injury, (2) more than 50% loss of vertebral body height, (3) more than 20 to 30 degrees of kyphotic angulation, or (4) involvement of the same level in two or more adjacent levels. In addition to these factors, the quality of the surrounding bone must be taken into consideration in patients with neoplastic disease of the thoracic and lumbar spines. Furthermore, the cervicothoracic and thoracolumbar regions are very high-stress regions of the spine. This is due in part to the rather abrupt transition from the mobile cervical spine to the rigid thoracic spine to the mobile lumbar spine. This abrupt transition increases the risk of developing fractures and instability in these regions, especially in the setting of neoplastic invasion. These factors must be taken into account in considering surgical intervention on the spine.

The overall surgical goal varies depending on the histology and stage of the tumor. Patients with a solitary spinal metastasis might have the potential for long-term survival; therefore, one can justify surgery that offers en bloc tumor removal with negative margins. For some extremely aggressive tumors, such as sarcomas, a wide, compartmental resection is required to remove more remote microscopic deposits. For patients with widely metastatic disease and a symptomatic metastasis, the goal should be to restore spinal stability and relieve neurologic compression. In these patients with widespread disease, cure is not possible, so the goal of surgery is palliative, and an intralesional resection is a more reasonable option.

Numerous surgical approaches have been described to deal with neoplastic processes of the vertebral column. Metastatic lesions may less commonly involve solely the posterior elements. These lesions are therefore best approached dorsally via a limited laminectomy and resection. In addition, anterior laterally placed lesions may be approached through dorsolateral approaches in the thoracic and lumbar spines. These include both costotransversectomies and transpedicular approaches. Although this provides a less direct route to the pathologic area, certain situations might call for such an approach. These situations include patients that medically are unable to tolerate a more ventral approach and cases in which anatomic structures can provide a formidable obstacle, as in the case of the innominate vessels and the aortic arch at the second and third thoracic vertebral levels.

The bulk of spinal metastases involve the vertebral body; therefore, anterior approaches provide the most direct route to these lesions. Because the posterior elements are the only remaining intact anatomic structure, their removal by laminectomy can actually make the patient worse by leading to progressive kyphosis. Numerous ventral approaches to the spine have been described. In the occipitocervical junction, options include transoral, extended "open door" maxillotomy, and transmandibular circumglossal approaches. Each affords its own unique view of the clivus and C1-2 region anteriorly. Owing to the intricate anatomy of these transoral and transfacial approaches, an access surgeon should likely be involved in these cases. In addition, issues such as the need for a tracheostomy and gastrostomy tube postoperatively for a period of time should be discussed with the patient during preoperative counseling. The middle and lower cervical regions may be approached via a standard anterior lateral approach. Care must be taken during this approach to avoid injury to the trachea and esophagus as well as the recurrent laryngeal nerve.

Several ventral approaches to the cervicothoracic, thoracic, and thoracolumbar regions have been described in the literature. High cervical vertebrectomies may be approached through a median sternotomy. The trapdoor exposure, described by Nazzaro, Arbit, and Burt, is a ventral method for exposing high thoracic region lesions that involve T3 and T4 levels. This exposure combines a standard ventral approach to the cervical spine with both a partial median sternotomy and a ventrolateral thoracotomy. Lower-level thoracic lesions may be effectively approached through a dorsolateral thoracotomy, whereas a thoracoabdominal approach provides exposure for decompression and stabilization of the thoracolumbar spine.

The lumbosacral spine may likewise be exposed via a myriad of ventral and dorsal approaches. Retroperitoneal and transperitoneal approaches may be used for direct ventral exposure of the spine at this level. Dorsolaterally, the transpedicular route allows for both dorsal and ventral decompression. Large sacral lesions may require a more extensive approach in which both ventral and dorsal exposure and decompression are required. This might require a multidisciplinary team approach to expose the ventral spine, protect the abdominal viscera, and close the large defect left from the tumor resection. In addition, because of the biomechanics of the lumbosacral region, additional fixation involving the pelvis might be required.

The type of anterior column reconstruction that is performed after a vertebrectomy depends on the anticipated survival of the patient. When a reasonable survival is expected (typically longer than 6 months), reconstruction with a biologic material is preferred. Graft options include autologous and cadaveric strut grafts (usually fibula or rib) as well as metallic cage implants that are packed with either autologous harvested bone or cancellous allograft bone chips. The use of bone graft for anterior reconstruction requires that postoperative radiation be delayed to prevent fusion failure (see "Radiotherapy").

Patients who have a relatively limited life expectancy might be more suitable candidates for anterior column reconstruction with polymethyl methacrylate (PMMA). The advantage of this technique is that it provides immediate stability of the spinal column. In addition, there is no convincing evidence in the literature that the presence of PMMA interferes with local radiation therapy or that radiation affects the compressibility, shear strength, or durability of methyl methacrylate. Therefore, it is the authors' view that radiation therapy may be delivered without delay when PMMA is used for anterior reconstruction.

Various methods have been proposed to anchor the PMMA to the rostral and caudal vertebral bodies of the vertebrectomy defect. These include chest tube techniques, Steinmann pins, and fixation screws. It is the authors' preference to use the chest tube technique described by Errico and Cooper, owing to its excellent stability and because Steinmann pins or screws are not required, as they can cause significant artifact on postoperative magnetic resonance imaging (MRI) scans.

In addition to the reconstruction of the anterior column, posterior instrumentation is often required to supplement the anterior construct. This can be done in a single session through a single or double approach, as well as in a staged fashion. Cases involving reconstruction of the cervicothoracic and thoracolumbar regions are under particularly high stress, as was discussed above. Furthermore, severe kyphotic deformity from anterior column failure can be indicative of posterior column incompetence. This often necessitates both ventral and dorsal rigid internal fixation to provide durable stability. Options of dorsal fixation include hooks, rods, wires, cables, or plates with lateral mass and or pedicle screws. In the occipitocervical region, combinations of occipital screws and wires along with cervical lateral mass and pedicle screws have been demonstrated to provide adequate stability in the face of neoplastic processes. In addition, pedicle screw fixation has been shown to provide excellent results in terms of pain relief and restoration or preservation of mobility in patients with neoplastic spinal lesions.

Radiotherapy

Radiation therapy has long been the treatment of choice for spinal metastases and for certain primary lesions.

In fact, numerous studies from the 1960s and 1970s demonstrated no difference in outcome between patients who were treated with radiation therapy alone and those who were treated with laminectomy with or without radiation treatment. The major criticism of these studies, however, was that, given that spinal metastases are usually ventral, laminectomy alone was an inappropriate surgical choice as the sole operative procedure in the majority of these cases. Nonetheless, radiation therapy has been shown to improve pain control in 50% to 90% of patients and to improve neurologic function in approximately 40% of patients with metastatic cord compression. The patients in whom the neoplastic process was diagnosed earlier fared the best. In fact, in patients who were treated early, the tumor histology had very little influence on the treatment outcome, whereas it had a much more profound effect when patients were treated late in their course. Metastatic tumors such as breast, prostate, and small cell ("oat cell") lung cancer, along with primary tumors such as plasmacytomas and hemangiomas, are very sensitive to radiation and therefore are excellent candidates for this treatment option. Radiation-resistant tumors such as renal cell carcinoma and sarcomas respond relatively poorly to radiation treatment alone and are best treated with a combination of surgical resection and radiation.

In evaluating patients with possible neoplastic cord compression for radiation therapy, it is important to determine whether the source of compression is from the tumor mass or from bony fragments. Patients with significant neoplastic bony destruction will often have concomitant pathologic vertebral fractures. In a significant proportion of these cases, there will be retropulsion of vertebral body fragments into the spinal canal that might impinge on the spinal cord. Radiation therapy has no chance of relieving the compression in these cases. In addition, the bony destruction might result in destabilization of the spinal column, which could predispose the patient to future neurologic injury. These patients are best managed with surgical decompression and stabilization (if needed) if their overall medical condition permits.

The standard radiation treatment protocol for palliation of spinal metastases is 300 cGy daily fractions to a total dose of 3000 cGy. A single posterior field or opposed fields are used to encompass the involved segments plus one to two spinal levels above and below. The tolerance of the spinal cord and cauda equina to radiation therapy is the major limiting factor in treating with higher doses of radiation. Higher doses increase the risk of developing radiation-induced myelopathy with resultant loss of spinal cord function. A recent review of the Mayo Clinic's experience with patients who required reirradiation for recurrence of malignant spinal lesions found that at a median follow-up period of 4.2 months, nearly 70% of the patients remained ambulatory. The median total radiation dose in the reirradiated segment was 5425 cGy. This study demonstrates that in select patients with limited life expectancy, reirradiation can still have a role.

After the decision to proceed with radiation therapy has been made, the timing must still be carefully considered. Several studies have shown that radiation therapy has deleterious effects on wound healing as well as bone healing and graft incorporation. The negative effects that radiation has on skin healing have been well documented. The operative incision must be taken into account in developing a radiation treatment plan to prevent potentially disastrous wound dehiscence and infection. In addition, a great deal of literature from animal models points to preoperative and immediate postoperative radiation as having the most significant negative effects on bony fusions. Delayed radiation therapy (more than 21 days), however, has not been shown to have this same negative effect. The negative effects of radiation also appear to be more profound with posterior than anterior graft fusions. This is presumably due to the increased blood supply of the anterior column and the reliance of posterior grafts on adjacent tissues (which are also negatively affected by the radiation treatment) for fusion. The authors advocate a 3- to 4-week delay following surgical intervention before initiating radiation therapy when a bone graft has been placed.

Chemotherapy

Chemotherapeutic options can be divided into antitumoral drugs and drugs that prevent or ameliorate the effects of the tumor. Antitumor chemotherapy has a relatively limited role in the treatment of spine metastases. Germ cell tumors are particularly chemosensitive; therefore, these agents have a role in the treatment of patients who harbor these lesions. Systemic chemotherapy is often the first line of treatment for these patients, even in the face of epidural spinal cord compression.

A small number of metastatic tumors, namely breast and prostate cancer, have variable numbers of surface hormone receptors. This makes these lesions susceptible to chemotherapeutic agents that act to block these receptors. Agents such as tamoxifen have been used systemically with fair clinical results. Spinal metastatic lesions from these tumors might or might not possess the same concentration of hormone receptors. Therefore, primary lesions in the breast or prostate might respond, whereas the metastatic lesion might not respond to the same degree.

Dexamethasone has been shown to reduce the spinal cord edema and pain associated with some spinal column tumors. Dosage schemes range from low dose (16 mg per day in divided doses) to very high dose (96 mg per day in divided doses). The optimal dose that is necessary to treat patients with acute spinal cord compression is somewhat controversial. In addition, it is unclear whether high doses are associated with improved neurologic outcomes when compared to low to moderate doses. High-dose steroids are associated with significantly higher rates of complications such as hyperglycemia, gastrointestinal ulceration and perforation, and avascular necrosis of the hip. In addition, steroids can affect the yield of biopsy specimens of undiagnosed spinal masses. Lymphoma and thymomas are particularly sensitive to this oncolytic steroid effect, and this can prevent or delay their diagnosis.

Bisphosphonates are a class of drugs that inhibit osteoclast activity and therefore suppress bone resorption. They have been shown to be quite effective in treating malignancy-associated hypercalcemia. Pamidromate, the most commonly used drug in this class, has been shown to reduce or delay the onset of pathologic fracture in cancer patients when used in combination with systemic antitumoral therapy. This has been shown to be effective for breast cancer, multiple myeloma, and osteolytic metastases.

Other Treatment Options

Vertebroplasty is a relatively new technique that has been added to the armamentarium of treatment options for cancer patients with vertebral body lesions. This technique, which was developed in France in the late 1980s, involves the percutaneous injection of PMMA into a fractured vertebral body. This reinforces the vertebral body and therefore alleviates the pain associated with these destructive processes. Percutaneous balloon kyphoplasty is a recent modification of this technique that involves inflation of a balloon within a collapsed vertebral body to restore vertebral body height and reduce the degree of kyphotic deformity prior to the injection of the PMMA. These techniques have been used extensively in recent years for the treatment of painful primary and metastatic, osteolytic vertebral processes. Fourney and colleagues reported on a series of 56 consecutive cancer patients who underwent vertebroplasty and kyphoplasty at the M.D. Anderson Cancer Center over a 2-year period. The authors noted improvement or complete relief of pain in 84% of the patients within 72 hours of the procedure. They found that this pain relief was quite durable and maintained statistical significance through the follow-up period of 1 year. They did not report any deaths or complications associated with these procedures during the study period. Although vertebroplasty and kyphoplasty are not direct treatments for the tumor, these results demonstrate a clear palliative role for both these procedures in the treatment of cancer patients.

PEARLS & PITFALLS

PEARLS

- Excisional surgery is recommended for Tokuhashi prognostic score greater than 9.
- Tokuhashi scoring system's surgical recommendations:
  - Score 2–3: Wide surgical excision reduces incidence of local recurrence
  - Score 4–5: Marginal intralesional resection
  - Score 8–10: Nonoperative
- Optimize nutritional status preoperatively.
- Consider parental feeding and plastic surgery consult.

PITFALLS

- Anticipate large blood volume loss.
- Optimize hemodynamic status with blood transfusions.
- Monitor volume status intraoperatively and postoperatively to reduce cardiac risk.

Illustrative Case Presentation

CASE 1. A 39-Year-Old Female with A History of Breast Carcinoma Presented with Acute-Onset Low Back Pain, Bilateral Lower-Extremity Weakness, and Bowel and Bladder Dysfunction.

Plain radiographs (Fig. 23-1A) showed complete collapse of the L2 vertebra, and MRI (Fig. 23-1B) revealed severe compression of the cauda equina. The patient underwent a two-stage procedure: Stage 1 consisted of a retroperitoneal approach, L2 corpectomy, reconstruction with a distractable cage, correction of the kyphotic deformity, fixation with plate/screws, and fusion; and stage 2 consisted of posterior thoracolumbar pedicle screw fixation and fusion. One year later, following additional radiation therapy locally, the patient was neurologically intact and pain free (Fig. 23-1C).

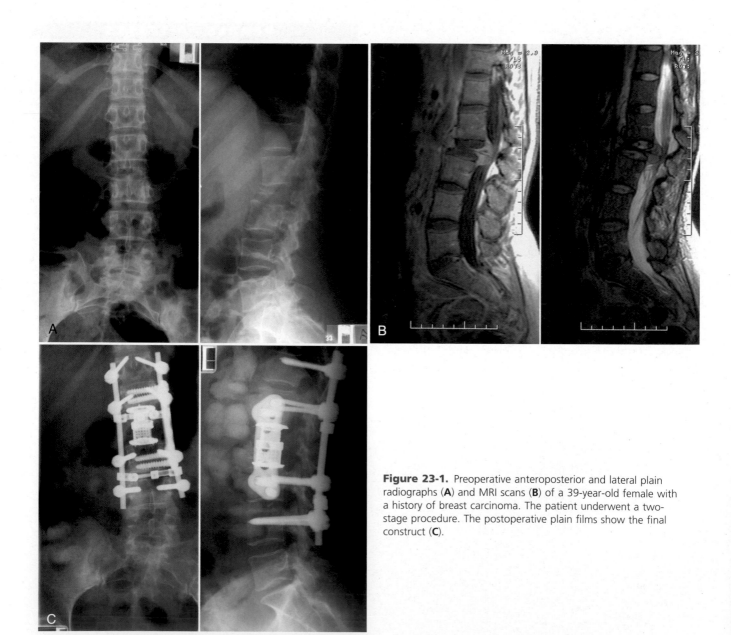

Figure 23-1. Preoperative anteroposterior and lateral plain radiographs (**A**) and MRI scans (**B**) of a 39-year-old female with a history of breast carcinoma. The patient underwent a two-stage procedure. The postoperative plain films show the final construct (**C**).

REFERENCES

Berenson JR, Lichtenstein A, Porter L, et al: Efficacy of pamidronate in reducing skeletal events in patients with advanced multiple myeloma: Myeloma Aredia Study Group. N Engl J Med 1996;334:488–493.

Black P: Spinal metastasis: Current status and recommended guidelines for management. Neurosurgery 1979;5:726–746.

Bouchard JA, Koka A, Bensusan JS, et al: Effects of irradiation on posterior spinal fusions: A rabbit model. Spine 1994;19:1836–1841.

Brihaye J, Ectors P, Lemort M, Van Houtte P: The management of spinal epidural metastases. Adv Tech Stand Neurosurg 1988;16:121–176.

Denis F: The three column spine and its significance in the classification of acute thoracolumbar spinal injuries. Spine 1983;8:817–831.

Emery SE, Brazinski MS, Koka A, et al: The biological and biomechanical effects of irradiation on anterior spinal bone grafts in a canine model. J Bone Joint Surg Am 1994;76540–76548.

Errico TJ, Cooper PR: A new method of thoracic and lumbar body replacement for spinal tumors: Technical note. Neurosurgery 1993;32:678–680.

Gokaslan ZL, Romsdahl MM, Kroll SS, et al: Total sacrectomy and Galveston L-rod reconstruction for malignant neoplasms: Technical note. J Neurosurg 1997;87:781–787.

Jackson RJ, Gokaslan ZL: Occipitocervicothoracic fixation for spinal instability in patients with neoplastic processes. J Neurosurg Spine 1999;91:81–89.

Schiff D, Shaw EG, Cascino TL: Outcome after spinal reirradiation for malignant epidural spinal cord compression. Ann Neurol 1995;37:583–589.

Seol HJ, Chung CK, Kim HJ: Surgical approach to anterior compression in the upper thoracic spine. J Neurosurg Spine 2002;97:337–342.

Sundaresan N, Galicich JH, Lane JM, et al: Treatment of neoplastic epidural cord compression by vertebral body resection and stabilization. J Neurosurg 1985;3:676–684.

Tomita K, Kawahara N, Kobayashi T, et al: Surgical strategy for spinal metastases. Spine 2001;26:298–306.

Walsh GL, Gokaslan ZL, McCutcheon IE, et al: Anterior approaches to the thoracic spine in patients with cancer: Indications and results. Ann Thorac Surg 1997;64:1611–1618.

York JE, Wildrick DM, Gokaslan ZL: Metastatic tumors. In Benzel EC, Stillerman BC (eds): The Thoracic Spine. St. Louis: Quality Medical Publishing, 1999, pp 392–411.

SUGGESTED READINGS

Abdu WA, Provencher M: Primary bone and metastatic tumors of the cervical spine. Spine 1998;23:2767–2777.

This is a detailed review of the clinical manifestations, evaluation, diagnostic images, treatments, and tumor staging according to the Weinstein, Boriani, Biagini system of primary bone and metastatic tumors of the cervical spine.

Bell GR: Surgical treatment of spinal tumors. Clin Orthop Relat Res 1997;335:54–63.

This study describes the different surgical techniques that can be used to treat spinal tumors. It focuses on the fact that selection of technique is based largely on the location of the tumor within the spine.

Bilsky MH, Lis E, Raizer J, et al: The diagnosis and treatment of metastatic spinal tumor. Oncologist 1999;4:459–469.

This review addresses tumor metastases to the spine. It concludes that radiation therapy remains the primary treatment for metastatic spinal tumor but that advances in radiation therapy, chemotherapy, and surgery have changed the roles of each and lead to improved patient outcomes.

Cahill DW: Surgical management of malignant tumors of the adult bony spine. South Med J 1996;89;653–665.

This article addresses the diagnosis and therapy of malignant tumors of the bony spine, emphasizing the common primary tumors of the spine and even more common metastatic lesions. Specific tumor types and therapeutic approaches at different levels of the spine are addressed, and newer techniques available to the treating clinician are reviewed.

Fourney DR, Abi-Said D, Lang FF, et al: Use of pedicle screw fixation in the management of malignant spinal disease: Experience in 100 consecutive procedures. J Neurosurg Spine 2001;94:25–37.

This study focuses on the use of pedicle screw fixation in the management of malignant spinal column tumors. It concludes that for selected patients with malignant spinal tumors, pedicle screw fixation after tumor resection can provide considerable pain relief and restore or preserve ambulation with acceptable rates of morbidity and mortality.

Fourney DR, Abi-Said D, Rhines LD, et al: Simultaneous anterior-posterior approach to the thoracic and lumbar spine for the radical resection of tumors followed by reconstruction and stabilization. J Neurosurg Spine 2001;94:232–244.

This study reviews the results of treating patients with anterior and posterior tumors in whom surgery was performed via a simultaneous anterior-posterior approach. It concludes that the procedure is a safe and feasible alternative for the exposure of tumors of the thoracic and lumbar spine that involve both the anterior and posterior columns.

Fourney DR, Schomer DF, Nader R, et al: Percutaneous vertebroplasty and kyphoplasty for painful vertebral body fractures in cancer patients. J Neurosurg Spine 2003;98:21–30.

This study aims to assess the safety and efficacy of minimally invasive vertebroplasty and kyphoplasty for painful vertebral body fractures in cancer patients. It concludes that the procedures provided significant pain relief in a high percentage of patients and that this appeared to be durable over time.

Fourney DR, York JE, Cohen ZR, et al: Management of atlantoaxial metastases with posterior occipitocervical stabilization. J Neurosurg Spine 2003;98:165–170.

The authors of this study review their experience with a surgical strategy that emphasizes posterior stabilization of the spine and avoidance of poorly tolerated external orthoses such as the rigid cervical collar or halo vest for the treatment of atlantoaxial spinal metastases. The authors reviewed 19 consecutively treated patients with C1 or C2 metastases.

Gokaslan ZL, York JE, Walsh GL, et al: Transthoracic vertebrectomy for metastatic spinal tumors. J Neurosurg 1998;89:599–609.

This study provides a clear perspective of results that can be expected in patients who undergo anterior vertebral body resection, reconstruction, and stabilization for spinal metastases that are limited to the thoracic region. A total of 72 patients were evaluated in a retrospective fashion.

Jackson RJ, Gokaslan ZL: Spinal-pelvic fixation in patients with lumbosacral neoplasms. J Neurosurg Spine 2000;92:61–70.

The authors describe their experience with a modification of the Galveston technique, originally described by Allen and Ferguson in the treatment of scoliosis, to achieve rigid spinal-pelvic fixation in patients with lumbosacral neoplasms. A total of 13 patients received this procedure with seemingly good outcomes.

Jackson RJ, Loh SC, Gokaslan ZL: Metastatic renal cell carcinoma of the spine: Surgical treatment and results. J Neurosurg Spine 2001;94:18–24.

This retrospective article addresses the role and benefits of the surgical treatment for metastatic renal cell carcinoma of the spine in 79 patients. It concludes that in selected patients with metastatic RCC of the spine, resection followed by stabilization can provide pain relief and neurologic preservation or improvement.

Nazzaro JM, Arbit E, Burt M: "Trap door" exposure of the cervicothoracic junction: Technical note. J Neurosurg 1994;80:338–341.

This report describes a trapdoor exposure of the cervicothoracic junction. This method provides full bilateral anterior exposure from the C4 through at least the T3 vertebral levels, as well as unilateral anterolateral access to the upper thoracic spine.

Panjabi MM, Oxland TR, Kifune M, et al: Validity of the three-column theory of thoracolumbar fractures: A biomechanic investigation. Spine 1995;20:1122–1127.

This study validated the three-column theory of fractures by correlating the multidirectional instabilities and the vertebral injuries to each of the three columns, using a biomechanic trauma model.

Patchell RA, Tibbs PA, Regine WF, et al: Direct decompressive surgical resection in the treatment of spinal cord compression caused by metastatic cancer: A randomised trial. Lancet 2005;366(9486):643–648.

This randomized multicenter study addresses the efficacy of direct decompressive surgery in treatment for spinal cord compression caused by metastatic cancer. It concludes that direct decompressive surgery plus postoperative radiotherapy is superior to treatment with radiotherapy alone for patients with spinal cord compression caused by metastatic cancer.

Tokuhashi Y, Matsuzaki H, Toriyama S, et al: Scoring system for the preoperative evaluation of metastatic spine tumor prognosis. Spine 1990;15:1110–1113.

This assessment system for the prognosis of metastatic spine tumors was evaluated for 64 patients who had undergone surgery. The total score obtained for each patient can be correlated with the prognosis while being valuable in predicting it. However, the prognosis could not be predicted from a single parameter.

CHAPTER 24

Inflammatory Arthropathies

Joseph M. Zavatsky, Christopher Zarro, Baron S. Lonner, *and* Jeffrey M. Spivak

There are many inflammatory diseases that can affect the musculoskeletal system, including the spine. Spondyloarthropathies are a group of related inflammatory joint diseases that can affect the spine and are associated with the major histocompatibility complex (MHC) class I molecule HLA-B27. The term *seronegative spondyloarthropathy* refers to conditions in which serologic tests are typically negative for rheumatoid factor, a nonspecific indicator of other rheumatologic disease. These conditions include ankylosing spondylitis, Reiter's syndrome, psoriatic arthritis, and inflammatory bowel disease. Rheumatoid arthritis is another inflammatory disease that is usually serologically positive for rheumatoid factor and can also affect the spine. Of the inflammatory conditions mentioned, the two most prevalent and potentially devastating conditions that affect the spine are ankylosing spondylitis (negative for rheumatoid factor) and rheumatoid arthritis (positive for rheumatoid factor), which will be the focus of this chapter.

ANKYLOSING SPONDYLITIS

Ankylosing spondylitis (AS) is the third most common form of chronic arthritis in the United States. The incidence of AS is 1 to 3 per 1000 of the general population. Males are more commonly affected than females, with a ratio of about 4:1. AS is a seronegative inflammatory disease that affects the hips, sacroiliac joints, and spine. There is an association between HLA-B27 and AS. An antecedent bacterial infection with *Klebsiella pneumoniae* has been proposed to cause an autoimmune disorder due to molecular mimicry between HLA-B27 and *Klebsiella* antigens.

In AS, the site of inflammation is at the junction of fibrous tissue and bone, such as the insertions of tendons and ligaments. This process leads to erosion of bone and ossification of the tendons and ligaments. In the spine, this occurs at the insertion of the annulus fibrosus on the vertebral body as well as the paravertebral zygapophyseal joints. Erosion here leads to squaring of the vertebrae, and ossification leads to syndesmophytes (nonmarginal) flush with the lateral borders of the vertebrae and the classic "bamboo spine" caused by calcification of the facet joints

and longitudinal ligaments (Fig. 24-1). The progression of ankylosis often causes patients to assume a kyphotic posture, ultimately leading to fixed deformities of the cervicothoracic, thoracic, and lumbar spines. These deformities result in difficulty with horizontal gaze, ambulation, and activities of daily living. The autofusion of the spinal column and subsequent decrease in movement and elasticity result in altered biomechanics of the spine, rendering it susceptible to a variety of disorders, including fracture, dislocation, progressive spinal deformity, atlanto-occipital or atlantoaxial subluxation, and spinal stenosis. The rigidity and immobility of the AS spine give it a propensity to develop osteoporosis, further increasing the risk of fracture.

Clinical Presentation and Examination

Patients typically present during the second through fourth decades of life with low back pain, morning stiffness, chest wall pain, and difficulties with activities of daily life. Additional orthopedic manifestations include enthesopathy and pain in the Achilles tendon and plantar fascia. Nonorthopedic manifestations include anterior uveitis and ileitis or colitis, which may be present in up to 25% of patients. Cardiopulmonary manifestations include aortic and mitral regurgitation, aortic stenosis, aortitis, and restrictive pulmonary disease resulting from decreased chest wall expansion.

Physical examination requires a systematic examination of the entire patient. Early in the disease, evaluation of the sacroiliac joints often reveals tenderness to palpation and reproduction of symptoms with flexion, abduction, and external rotation. Hip pathology may be evident with performance of a Thomas test to assess for hip flexion contractures. Diminished spinal mobility will also be present and can be assessed with the Schober test: Points 10 cm above and 5 cm below the posterior superior iliac spine are marked in the midline with the patient fully erect. The patient then fully flexes, and there should be at least 5 cm of excursion between these points. In AS, the excursion is less than 5 cm. Once autofusion of the costovertebral joints occurs, chest expansion measured at the fourth intercostal

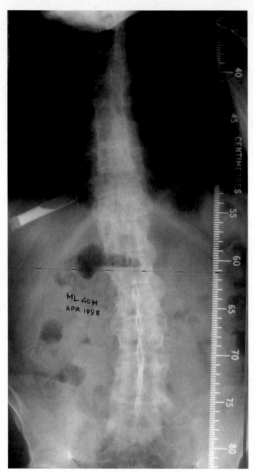

Figure 24-1. Advanced changes in ankylosing spondylitis with appearance of bamboo spine and obliteration of the sacroiliac joint. *(From Benzel EC [ed]: Spine Surgery: Techniques, Complication Avoidance, and Management, 2nd ed. Philadelphia: Elsevier, 2004.)*

space is limited to less than 2.5 cm as determined by a tape measure around the chest with the differential between full inspiration and expiration. Additionally, the clinical assessment of deformity can be performed by measuring the chin-brow angle, occiput-to-wall distance, and gaze angle. The chin-brow angle is formed by the vertical line drawn from the chin to the brow with the patient's hips and knees fully extended. The occiput-to-wall distance is the horizontal distance from the occiput to the wall with the hips and knees extended and the patient's buttocks and heels against the wall. It is a measure of sagittal balance.

Radiographic evaluation of the spine must include assessment of the sacroiliac joints, as they are often the first involved; a Ferguson view of the pelvis, an anteroposterior view with tube directed 30 degrees cephalad, is necessary to determine the degree of sacroiliitis: Grade 0 is normal-appearing joints, grade 1 is suspicious for pathology, grade 2 is minimal sacroiliitis, grade 3 is moderate, and grade 4 is ankylosis. As the disease progresses, osseous changes in the cervical, thoracic, and lumbar spines lead to the characteristic bamboo spine.

According to the modified New York criteria, AS is diagnosed by back pain in a patient younger than 40 years

that persists for at least 3 months, is associated with morning stiffness, and improves with exercise. There are limitation of movement of the lumbar spine in the sagittal and coronal planes and decreased chest expansion compared to the normal for age and sex. On plane films of the spine, there will be unilateral or bilateral sacroiliitis. Tissue typing is not included in any set of diagnostic criteria, although there is a high degree of association between HLA-B27 positivity and AS. Approximately 90% of AS patients are positive for the HLA-B27 antigen, but fewer than 10% of patients who are HLA-B27-positive manifest the signs and symptoms of AS.

Perioperative Considerations

The indications for surgical management of AS are to lessen pain, improve function, correct deformity, and treat fractures. Prior to surgical intervention, AS patients should have preoperative pulmonary evaluations, which include a careful history and physical examination, a chest radiograph, pulmonary function tests, and evaluation by the anesthesiologist. Fibrotic upper lung fields, ankylosed ribs, and exaggerated thoracic kyphosis restrict chest wall and diaphragmatic expansion. This places the pulmonary system at great risk for complications such as difficulties with postoperative extubation, atelectasis, and pneumonia. Additionally, preoperative echocardiogram and evaluation by a cardiologist should be considered to assess for aortic stenosis and aortic or mitral regurgitation.

Owing to the fragility of the spinal column, in patients with spinal fractures all prestabilization transfers should be supervised by a spine care physician. Preoperative anesthesia consultation should be sought owing to the difficulty with intubation as a result of the kyphotic deformity and inability to extend the neck. Fiber-optic intubation should be employed by the anesthesiologist to avoid any translational movement of the cervical spine, which can result in neurologic impairment. Owing to the deformity of the spine, surgical positioning on a standard operating room table might not be possible. Modifications using bolsters, rolls, and pillows might be required.

Spinal Fractures

Diffuse spinal ossification and inflammatory osteitis create a fused, brittle spine that is susceptible to fracture even by minor trauma. The fused or bamboo spine becomes osteopenic following long-term immobility making the spine vulnerable. Three recognized patterns of vertebral fractures exist. These include simple vertebral compression fractures, transversely oriented shear fractures, and stress fractures associated with pseudarthrosis. Simple vertebral compression fractures are injuries that occur early in the course of disease and are related to osteoporosis. They typically result in stable kyphosis. Transversely oriented shear fractures are acute fractures that disrupt the ossified supporting ligaments and usually traverse the disc space. Stress fractures associated with pseudarthrosis are subacute injuries that tend to occur in the thoracolumbar region.

Fractures in AS patients can occur at all levels of the spine. The magnitude of the forces necessary to fracture the spine of an AS patient is much less than that in a patient with a normal spine. Normally, preload is absorbed by spinal ligaments, discs, and facet joints. In patients with AS, ossification of the soft-tissue structures, along with exaggerated spinal kyphosis and decreased lumbar lordosis, creates a rigid, brittle spine that is prone to fracture. Impaired mobility leading to increased vulnerability to falls also occurs.

In the AS patient, calcification of the annulus fibrosus reduces the movement and elasticity of the intervertebral disc, making it the point of least resistance when the spine is involved in trauma. It is important to note the difficulty in making the initial diagnosis of spinal fractures in this patient population. This is due to several factors, such as increased density of ossified ligaments, distortion of the normal anatomy due to kyphosis, and increased osteopenia. Also, often a low-energy trauma results in the injury with little or no displacement of the fracture occurring.

Many patients with AS do not realize their injuries, owing to their baseline pain. Therefore, when an injury of the spine is suspected in these patients, imaging should include the entire spine and not just the symptomatic region. One must have a high index of suspicion and a realization of the drastic consequences that can occur. The physician should use advanced imaging techniques to make the diagnosis. Magnetic resonance imaging (MRI) allows visualization of intramedullary edema, disc space injury, spinal cord injury, and epidural hematoma. Bone scans can be used, but it is difficult to differentiate degenerative changes from acute trauma. Thin-cut computed tomography (CT) scans with coronal and sagittal reformats can allow visualization of the fracture. Once diagnosed, vertebral fractures should be managed with three basic principles in mind: reduction of fracture, early stabilization, and minimization of patient transfers.

Cervical fractures are a serious and possibly life-threatening complication of AS. It has been reported that 60% to 70% of cases result in neurologic deficits. There is a 35% mortality rate, which is nearly double that of normal fractured spines. It is important to evaluate any change in neck pain and head position in these patients because there might be minimal trauma or a remote history of trauma. The minor nature of the trauma and frequency of baseline pain in these patients result in delays in the recognition and management of cervical fractures. Cervical injuries account for up to 75% of all spine fractures in AS patients. Fractures at all cervical levels have been reported, but the lower cervical segments (the fifth through seventh cervical spine segments) are the most common. The mechanism of spinal cord injury in AS patients is often from hyperextension of the neck. The kyphotic deformity results in a forwardly flexed neck, at risk with falling both forward and backward. It is important to note the frequency and ease of hyperextension injuries in these patients in performing endotracheal intubation. In this situation, the anesthesiologist will often place the normal patient in the neutral to hyperextended neck position. This poses a problem to the AS patient with a rigid cervical spine. Awake nasotracheal fiber-optic intubation is helpful to avoid neurologic injury. Another area of concern is with emergency medical personnel and the application of cervical collars in the acute setting. These collars keep the normal neck in neutral position, which for the AS patient is a position of dangerous hyperextension. This hyperextension can result in an iatrogenically induced fracture through the ossified intervertebral discs. Owing to the instability of these fractures, collars, orthoses, and neutral axial halo vest traction are not adequate for immobilization. These conventional mechanisms of immobilization have led to failed union, fracture displacement, and progression of neurologic deficit. Thus, in the case of a patient with AS and with a suspected cervical spine injury, the spine should be immobilized in the position in which it typically presents. Modification of standard technique, such as elevation of the head and placement of sandbags on each side, as well as halo cast immobilization with kyphotic bars will assist in safely immobilizing the patient. Fracture reduction when necessary can be applied through halo traction in line with the original deformity. The vector of traction should be superior and anterior or in line with the nonfractured position of the spine, and most cases can be reduced with less than 10 pounds of weight.

Thoracic and lumbar fractures occur less frequently than do cervical fractures, at 14% and 5%, respectively. Fractures of the thoracic and lumbar spines in AS patients can be of three types: shearing/distraction-extension injuries, wedge compression, and pseudarthrosis-associated. In general, upper thoracic fractures are relatively stable, owing to a rigid sternum and rib cage, but should be closely observed, since they can lead to a progressive kyphotic deformity. About 25% of patients present initially with neurologic deficits, but most present with increasing pain. There has been much confusion between fractures of the thoracolumbar spine and inflammatory changes in these patients. Fractures commonly occur through the intervertebral disc or vertebral body. The mechanism of injury is through a distraction-extension force. Bony deformation and stress fracture occur most commonly in the thoracolumbar and lumbosacral junctions. This occurs because of increased stress in the region resulting from a progressive loss of lumbar lordosis and subsequent flattening with an axial load to the lumbar spine. As this happens, the apex of the normal kyphosis migrates distally to the thoracolumbar junction, placing it at the center of a two-lever arm: the thoracic spine and rib cage above and the lumbar spine and sacrum below. A rare complication of thoracolumbar vertebral fractures is the occurrence of visceral complications such as a disruption of the aorta due to extension injury. This is a devastating complication with a mortality rate of 90%.

Fractures in AS lead to instability in flexion, extension, and rotation. Therefore, surgical procedures must control all directions of instability. In surgically stabilizing fractures, at least three segments above and below the lesion should be instrumented. Careful preoperative evaluation of the patient's spine in both the coronal and sagittal planes should be performed so as not to end a point of fixation at a level where a significant deformity exists. Owing to the common presence of osteoporosis, obtaining solid fixation using conventional surgical techniques can be problematic. Wiring into osteoporotic bone is not advisable, as the wires might cut through the posterior elements. Hooks, when utilized, may pull out. Therefore, the authors' standard means of fixation is via screws. However, osteoporotic bone reduces screw mechanical fixation strength and can lead to clinical failure. To enhance mechanical fixation in osteoporotic bone, various techniques can be implemented, including augmentation using polymethyl methacrylate. When used in small amounts (3 mL per screw) prior to screw insertion, polymethyl methacrylate has been shown to reinforce the screw/bone interface strength. The combination of a pedicle screw with a sublaminar hook at the caudal end of a construct leads to an increase in pullout strength compared to a pedicle screw alone in osteoporotic bone. This technique may be implemented at the terminal end of the construct. Finally, an expandable pedicle screw has been shown to increase biomechanical stability without the risk of bicortical fixation.

Anterior instrumentation is fraught with technical challenges resulting from underlying osteoporosis, which can lead to loosening. Loosening of the anterior instrumentation can lead to vascular injuries of the aorta as well as damage to the esophagus from pressure necrosis. Additionally, the anterior approach is more difficult in these patients, owing to the kyphotic angle and forward flexion of the spine. Therefore, a posterior-only approach is favored in most cases.

Deformity

In AS, chronic inflammation of the spine leads to progressive fusion in a caudal-to-cranial fashion and progressive increases in cervical and thoracic kyphosis. The sagittal imbalance and stiffness of both the spine and hips lead to a stooped posture, inability to lie flat in bed, and difficulty with horizontal gaze. The location of the deformity must be identified in order to plan surgical intervention. If the deformity corrects with sitting, the hips are the likely culprit; if the deformity remains while sitting but corrects when lying supine, the thoracolumbar spine is the primary cause; however, if it persists while lying supine, the cervicothoracic spine is to blame, the so-called chin-on-chest deformity. This latter deformity can make the patient prone to falls and to difficulty eating, and once the location of primary deformity has been identified, the surgeon can plan a corrective osteotomy.

In 1958, Urist described an extension osteotomy of the cervical spine at C7-T1 in an awake, seated patient to facilitate neurologic monitoring. Correction at the cervicothoracic junction improves a chin-on-chest deformity and oral hygiene, as well as facilitating swallowing. McMaster reported the results of 15 patients who were treated prone, under general anesthesia utilizing neuromonitoring, thereby decreasing the risk of air embolus compared to the seated position and maintaining the ability to assess function. A halo can be used intraoperatively to assist with reduction and stability. Additional benefits of the C7-T1 level include a wide spinal canal and lateral masses and usually the absence of the vertebral arteries coursing through the foramen transversarium. Magnetic resonance angiography is helpful to assess the location of the vessels intraoperatively.

Osteotomies of the lumbar spine are used to correct sagittal imbalance of the thoracolumbar spine and can be performed at levels below the cord and conus, typically the third lumbar vertebra. Various osteotomies have been described, including an opening-wedge, polysegmental closing-wedge, and monosegmental closing-wedge or pedicle subtraction osteotomy (Figs. 24-2 and 24-3). Van Royen and DeGast performed a meta-analysis of various osteotomies for fixed kyphotic deformity in 856 patients. They reported a mean correction of 40.3 degrees for opening-wedge and polysegmental osteotomies and 36.5 degrees for closing-wedge osteotomies. They concluded that, although no one technique was superior to the others, the complications associated with closing-wedge osteotomies were less severe. Opening-wedge osteotomies have been associated with aortic rupture. Pedicle subtraction osteotomy is favored.

Complications

In the general population, spinal epidural hematoma occurs rarely in comparison to intracranial epidural hematoma, but its incidence is much higher in AS. Its etiology may be traumatic or nontraumatic, resulting from coagulopathy, vascular malformation, and iatrogenic or idiopathic causes. Spinal epidural hematoma complicating AS can result from trivial neck trauma and usually presents as incomplete spinal cord injury with rapidly progressive deterioration. The speculated mechanism has been bleeding from disrupted epidural veins, diseased hypervascular epidural soft tissue, and fractured bone, leading to an expanding hematoma confined within a rigid spinal canal. Clinically, the hematoma follows a rapid course, manifesting as an incomplete cord injury with rapidly deteriorating neurologic status. Most patients experience ascending weakness and numbness within several hours after injury as a result of external compression from the enlarging hematoma. The prognosis is poor. CT with or without myelography, as well as MRI, can be used to demonstrate spinal epidural hematoma. MRI can detect ligamentous injuries, herniated discs,

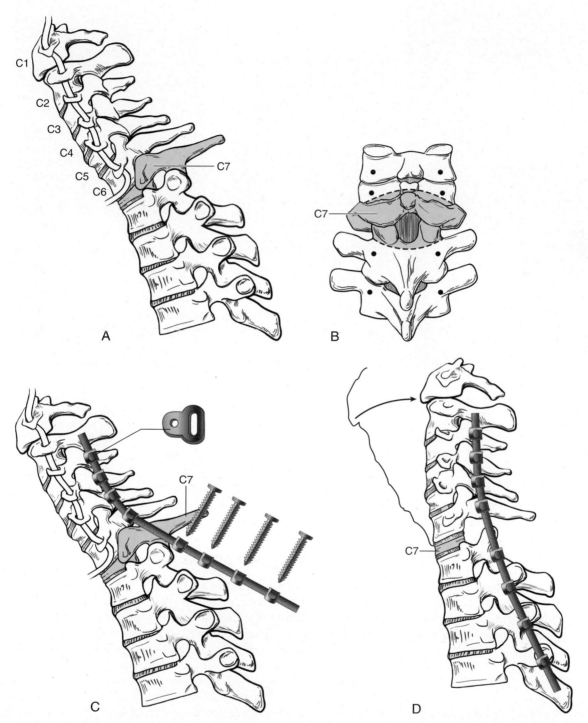

Figure 24-2. A, Cervical osteotomy to correct flexion deformity. The inset shows the area of bone to be removed from C7. The margins of the C6 and T1 laminae should be undercut to prevent impingement on closure of the osteotomy. **B,** The C8 nerve root should be thoroughly decompressed. **C,** The proximal segment of the spine is instrumented, and drills are prepared in the distal segment before completion of the osteotomy to prevent translation. **D,** As soon as the osteotomy is completed, the spine should be stabilized immediately. *(Redrawn from Webb JK, Sengupta DK: Posterior cervicothoracic osteotomy. In Vaccaro AR, Albert TJ [eds]: Tricks of the Trade of Spine Surgery. New York: Thieme, 2002.)*

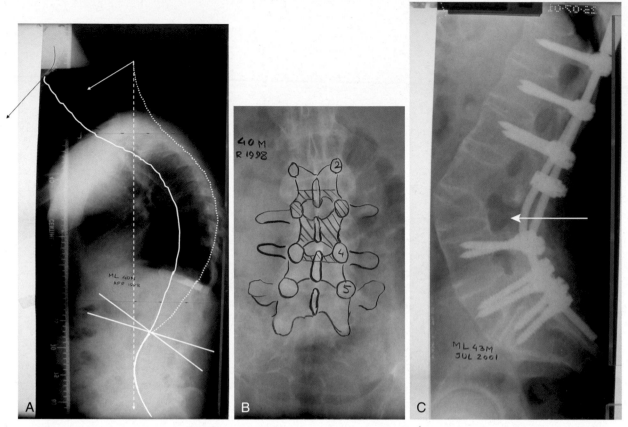

Figure 24-3. A, Preoperative planning indicated that only 30 degrees of corrective osteotomy at the L3 level would adequately restore the sagittal balance but not the gaze angle, which needed around 50 degrees of correction. **B,** A 20-degree osteotomy is therefore planned at the L3 level, and the amount of bone to be resected is marked out. Posterior closing-wedge osteotomy is performed with subtraction of the L3 pedicle. **C** and **D,** Three more polysegmental osteotomies were performed in the thoracic spine, with around 10 degrees of correction at each level, to compensate for the deliberate undercorrection at the lumbar spine. The net effect was total visual angle correction by 50 degrees and, at the same time, adequate correction of the sagittal balance.

and hemorrhage or edema within the cord, but its use might be limited by the inability to use monitoring devices or traction equipment that is typically required in these patients following injury. The treatment of a patient with a clinically significant epidural hematoma is emergent evacuation followed by stabilization of the injured segments. Clinically insignificant hematomas associated with fractures should be monitored carefully in an intensive care unit setting for any evolving neurologic deficit. Strict avoidance of anticoagulation medications should be employed.

Summary

AS is a spondyloarthropathy characterized by involvement of the sacroiliac joints and spine. The disease primarily affects the axial skeleton, leading to progressive deformity in a caudal-to-cranial direction. Surgery should be considered for those with a painful progressive deformity that causes functional disability and difficulty with horizontal gaze. Closing-wedge osteotomies have the lowest complication rates. Any patient with back or neck pain, even if after minor trauma, should be considered to have a fracture

until proven otherwise. Great care must be taken while transporting and positioning the patient to avoid extension injuries.

RHEUMATOID ARTHRITIS

Rheumatoid arthritis (RA) is a relatively common, chronic, progressive, inflammatory, autoimmune disease characterized by the destruction of synovial joints, ligaments, and bone. The prevalence of RA is 0.5% to 1.5% in the U.S. population, affecting twice as many women as men. Patients usually present between the ages of 20 and 45 years, complaining of pain, stiffness, and progressive joint swelling secondary to synovitis. Chronic synovial inflammation can also lead to destruction of the joints, ligaments, and bones in the cervical spine. The etiology of this condition is unclear, but there appears to be a genetic association. A positive rheumatoid factor is present in 85% of patients with RA and is clinically associated with an increased severity of symptoms and more aggressive disease.

The most common areas of disease involvement include the hands and feet, followed by the cervical spine. Radiographic evidence of lumbar pathology has also been docu-

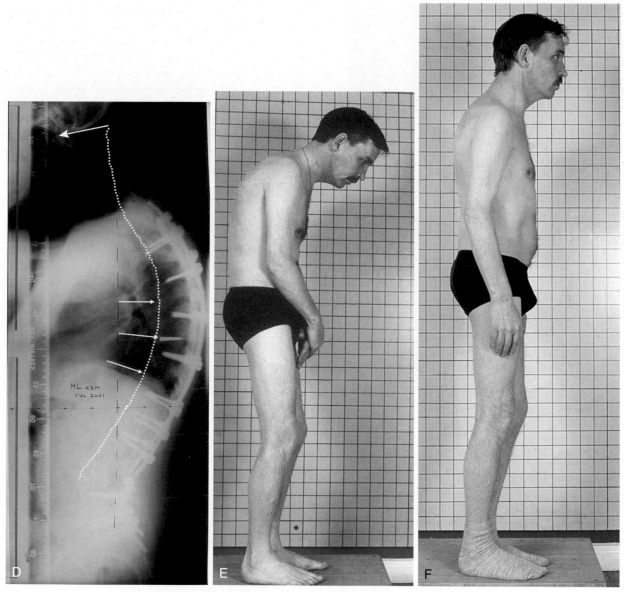

Figure 24-3, cont'd. E and **F,** Preoperative and postoperative clinical photographs show satisfactory correction of both the sagittal balance and visual angle. *(From Benzel EC [ed]: Spine Surgery: Techniques, Complication Avoidance, and Management, 2nd ed. Philadelphia: Elsevier, 2004.)*

mented in patients who have been diagnosed with RA, although clinically relevant lumbar disease is much less common than is cervical involvement. Studies suggest that the cervical spine can become involved within 2 years following diagnosis of RA. Radiographic evidence of cervical instability has been reported in 43% to 86% of RA patients. The documented prevalence of cervical subluxation in RA patients varies widely secondary to population and diagnostic criteria used.

Pathophysiology

Cervical instability is a consequence of the destruction of synovial joints, ligaments, and bone. Pannus formation, a fibrous inflammatory tissue, is characteristic of RA in the cervical spine. Synovitis and pannus formation can result in erosion of the bony surfaces and facet capsules of these joints, in addition to damaging the transverse, apical, and alar ligaments, which can cause instability (Fig. 24-4). This can result in pain, bony subluxation, and eventually spinal cord or brain stem compression. Compression of these structures can occur directly, from the synovial pannus that forms, or indirectly, from cervical subluxation. Rheumatoid patients can present with any combination of the three main types of cervical instability: atlantoaxial subluxation, cranial settling (atlantoaxial impaction), and subaxial subluxation.

The most common form of cervical instability in RA patients is atlantoaxial subluxation, which represents approximately 65% of all cervical instability (Fig. 24-5).

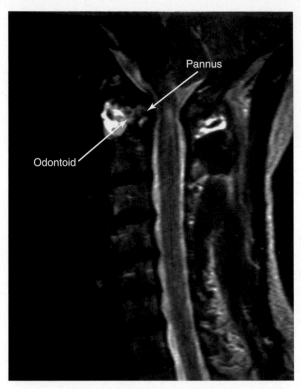

Figure 24-4. T2-weighted MRI scan demonstrating bony destruction of the tip of the odontoid and pannus formation reducing the space available for the cord.

The atlantoaxial and occipitoatlantal articulations are the only spinal segments without intervertebral disks, which could explain the preponderance of pathology in this area. Atlantoaxial subluxation can result from the destructive synovitic process that occurs at the atlanto-odontoid and atlantoaxial joints. This process can occur at the synovial

bursa that exists anteriorly at the odontoid articulation with the arch of C1 and posteriorly at the odontoid articulation with the transverse ligament. Most atlantoaxial subluxation occurs anteriorly, resulting in anterior subluxation of C1 on C2, but can also occur laterally and posteriorly. Anterior instability is commonly the result of transverse ligament weakening or rupture at the site of the synovial bursa that separates the posterior aspect of the dens from the transverse ligament. Instability in any direction can also result from bony erosion at the base of the odontoid process, resulting in fracture. As anterior subluxation progresses, the space available for the cord decreases. This can result in cord compression and possible neurologic compromise.

Cranial settling, also known as atlantoaxial impaction or pseudobasilar invagination, occurs alone or in combination with atlantoaxial instability in approximately 20% of rheumatoid patients (Fig. 24-6). Destruction of the atlanto-occipital and atlantoaxial articulations can occur with collapse of the lateral masses. This can result in atlantoaxial impaction and cranial migration of the odontoid. Cranial settling carries the worst prognosis, relative to the other forms of instability, with a greater incidence of myelopathy, brain stem injury, and sudden death secondary to compression of the respiratory center of the medulla oblongata. Additionally, compression of the anterior spinal and vertebral arteries can result in ischemic neurologic injury, transient ischemic attack, and vertebrobasilar insufficiency.

Subaxial subluxation occurs, frequently at multiple levels, producing a stepwise deformity in approximately 15% of RA patients (Fig. 24-7). Subaxial instability can occur as a result of the incompetence of the facet joints secondary to destruction of the articular cartilage and erosion of the lateral masses, weakening of the facet cap-

Figure 24-5. Lateral cervical (**A**) flexion and (**B**) extension radiographs of a 58-year-old woman with long-standing rheumatoid arthritis, neck pain, and signs of myelopathy demonstrating C1-2 instability.

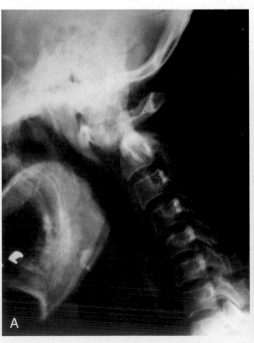

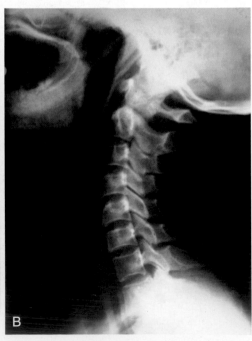

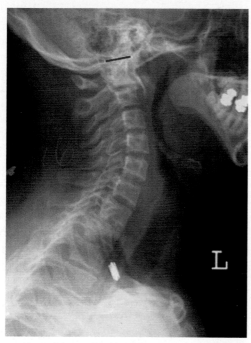

Figure 24-6. Lateral radiograph demonstrating cranial settling evidenced by protrusion of the tip of the odontoid above McRae's line.

sules and interspinous ligaments. Although radiographic changes associated with degenerative disk disease are usually present, the synovitic process associated with RA has not been observed in the disk or annular tissue. As opposed to cervical degenerative arthritis, RA usually lacks osteophyte formation and more commonly involves the C2-3 and C3-4 levels. Plain lateral radiographs with the neck in a neutral position may not reveal the instability, so it is important to obtain lateral flexion-extension views. These views can also be useful in determining whether the subaxial subluxation is fixed or mobile. Subaxial subluxation can result in painful instability as well as myelopathy due to canal stenosis and spinal cord compression.

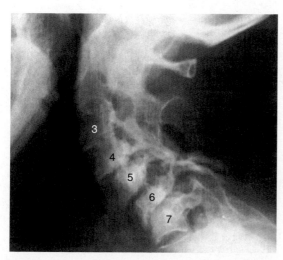

Figure 24-7. Lateral radiograph demonstrating stepwise subaxial subluxation across the C3-7 vertebrae along with erosions of the facet joints and spinous processes.

Clinical Presentation

The clinical manifestations of cervical spine involvement in rheumatologic disease can be subtle, and patients can often be asymptomatic. A detailed and careful history and physical examination are crucial in the evaluation of spinal involvement in the RA patient. The most common complaint is neck pain, which may be present in up to 80% of patients. Stiffness, crepitus, and painful range of motion are common symptoms. Patients may also complain of occipital headaches, ear pain, and facial pain secondary to compression of the greater occipital nerve, greater auricular nerve, and trigeminal nucleus, respectively. Joint crepitation and instability of the upper cervical spine can be elicited with range of motion. A positive Sharp-Purser test, which is a clunking sensation caused by the spontaneous reduction of a subluxed atlantoaxial joint with neck extension, has been described.

Cranial settling can cause vertebrobasilar insufficiency, resulting in symptoms that may include vertigo, tinnitus, and visual and equilibrium disturbances. Brain stem compression can present as vertical nystagmus and Cheyne-Stokes respirations. Cheyne-Stokes is a bizarre breathing pattern characterized by a period of apnea, followed by gradually increasing depth and frequency of respirations. Brain stem compression can also be associated with sleep apnea and sudden death.

Symptoms other than pain have been reported in 7% to 34% of rheumatoid patients. Patients may complain of hand clumsiness, difficulty handling small objects, or a change in handwriting. Objective neurologic findings can be difficult to interpret in RA patients. Motor strength testing and even signs of myelopathy can be masked by peripheral musculoskeletal manifestations of the disease, including multiple joint involvement and tendon pathology. Signs of cervical myelopathy should be ruled out and include a wide-based gait, hyperreflexia, and positive Babinski and Hoffmann signs. Lhermitte's sign suggests myelopathy, with patients complaining of electric shocks traveling down their spine or upper extremities with neck flexion. Additionally, a positive scapulohumeral reflex can suggest upper motor dysfunction above C3. A scapulohumeral reflex is elicited by tapping the spine of the scapula and acromion in a caudal direction. An abnormal response results in elevation of the scapula or abduction of the humerus, suggesting upper motor dysfunction. As the disease progresses and severe myelopathy develops, urinary retention and incontinence can occur. In contrast to the radiographic findings, which appear early, neurologic deficits, however subtle, usually manifest later in the disease process. Therefore, the physician must be diligent in examining the patient to detect these changes associated with neurologic compression in the cervical spine.

Radiographic Parameters

Plain radiographs are primarily utilized for the radiographic evaluation of the cervical spine in rheumatoid patients. Although MRI is superior for the evaluation of spinal cord compression and synovial pannus involvement, the routine use of MRI for screening rheumatoid patients or following progression of the disease is impractical. There is no standard screening protocol for radiographic evaluation of the cervical spine in RA patients, but certain patients should be given special consideration. All RA patients who require intubation for a surgical procedure should receive an initial series of radiographs, including anteroposterior, neutral lateral, and flexion-extension lateral views. Additionally, patients who have had cervical symptoms for more than 6 weeks, any neurologic signs or symptoms, evidence of rapid progressive peripheral carpal or tarsal involvement, or rapid overall functional decline should have cervical spine radiographs.

Anterior atlantoaxial subluxation can be assessed by measuring the anterior atlantodental interval (AADI) on a lateral cervical spine radiograph (Fig. 24-8). This is obtained by measuring the distance from the midposterior margin of the anterior arch of C1 to the anterior surface of the odontoid. If this interval measures more than 3 mm in an adult or 4 mm in a child, then it is considered abnormal, and the spinal cord might be at risk of injury. If the spine is anteriorly unstable, the AADI is most pronounced with cervical flexion. The dynamic interval, measured as the change in AADI with flexion and extension, can also be clinically important as a measure of relative instability.

Traditionally, the AADI has been used clinically to follow patients with RA that affects the cervical spine. However, several studies have shown that the AADI does not correlate with the risk of neurologic injury. The posterior atlantodental interval (PADI) has been shown to be a more sensitive test for detecting the risk of neurologic injury.

The PADI, also known as the space available for the cord, is measured from the posterior aspect of the odontoid to the anterior margin of the C1 lamina (see Fig. 24-8). Careful interpretation of the PADI in rheumatoid patients must be taken because this might not represent the true space available for the spinal cord. Soft-tissue compression from a periodontoid synovial pannus might not be appreciated on plain lateral radiographs but is well identified with MRI. In a long-term series, the PADI has been evaluated and compared to the AADI. A PADI less than or equal to 14 mm had a 97% sensitivity in detecting patients with paralysis. More important, the negative predictive value using the PADI was 94%; therefore, if the PADI was greater than 14 mm, there was a 94% chance that the patient would not have paralysis. The posterior atlantodental interval may also be utilized to predict postoperative neurologic recovery. Patients with a PADI less than 10 mm prior to surgery had a poor prognosis for neurologic recovery, whereas patients with a PADI of 14 mm or greater had a significant improvement of motor function after surgery. These data suggest that a PADI less than 14 mm is a relative indication for surgical stabilization.

Cranial settling of the odontoid can be measured by several different techniques. It was originally defined on plain lateral radiographs of the cervical spine as encroachment of the odontoid above the margins of the foramen magnum, or McRae's line (Fig. 24-9). McRae's line connects the midpoint of the anterior and posterior margins of the foramen magnum, or basion and opisthion, respectively. These landmarks are often difficult to delineate, so alternative methods have been described. Chamberlain's line is defined by a line drawn from the posterior margin

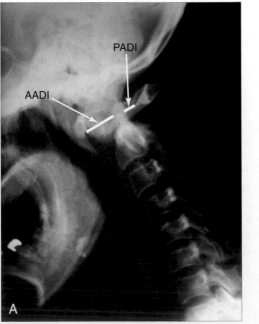

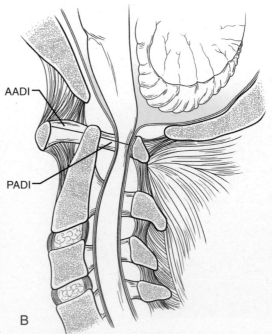

Figure 24-8. A, Lateral flexion radiograph of 58-year-old rheumatoid arthritis patient demonstrating an increased AADI and decreased PADI. **B,** Illustration of upper cervical spine depicting the AADI and PADI.

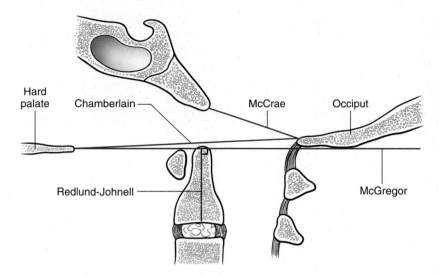

Figure 24-9. Evaluation of cranial settling. The tip of the odontoid should not protrude above McRae's line or protrude more than 4.5 mm above McGregor's line. The tip of the odontoid should not protrude more than 3 mm above Chamberlain's line; projection 6 mm above this line is considered pathologic. Redlund-Johnell values less than 34 mm in men and less than 29 mm in women are diagnostic of cranial settling.

of the hard palate to the opisthion. The odontoid should not project more than 3 mm above this line. The landmarks that define McGregor's line are often easier to see and include the posterior margin of the hard palate and the caudalmost point of the occiput. Projection of the tip of the odontoid more than 4.5 mm above this line is considered pathologic. Because the tip of the odontoid can often be difficult to define secondary to osteopenia or erosion, additional methods have been described to assess cranial settling.

The Ranawat and Redlund-Johnell methods for evaluating cranial settling do not rely on the tip of the odontoid for measurement. For the Ranawat method, on a lateral radiograph, a line is drawn transversely through the axis of the atlas. A second line is drawn vertically along the long axis of the odontoid from the center of the C2 pedicle to the line drawn traversing the atlas (Fig. 24-10). The distance from the center of C2 to the atlas is measured; values less than 15 mm for men and less than 13 mm for women define cranial settling. The Redlund-Johnell method measures the distance from McGregor's line to the midpoint of the inferior end plate of C2 (see Fig. 24-9). Values less than 34 mm in men and less than 29 mm in women are diagnostic for cranial settling.

Subaxial subluxation tends to occur at multiple levels, producing a stepwise deformity on plain lateral radiograph. As was previously stated, C2-3 and C3-4 are more commonly involved, and osteophyte formation is usually lacking in rheumatologic disease, which is in contrast to cervical degenerative disease. Subluxation may be quantified on lateral radiographs as translation, expressed in millimeters, as the distance of forward slip of the cranial vertebra relative to the caudal vertebra. Multiple definitions of pathologic subluxation exist. Abnormal subluxation has been described as greater than 4 mm or 20% of listhesis of the vertebral body diameter. Alternatively, subluxation can be measured as the minimum anteroposterior canal distance behind the slipped vertebra. This method might more accurately reflect the space available for the spinal cord. Boden and colleagues found that all patients with

subaxial subluxation and paralysis had a sagittal subaxial anteroposterior canal measurement less than or equal to 14 mm.

Although CT and CT myelography can provide useful information in RA patients with cervical disease, MRI has the capacity to directly identify spinal cord compression, particularly compression caused by soft tissue. The finding of a rheumatoid pannus or odontoid erosion on MRI is specific for RA and can aid the surgeon in diagnosis and treatment. The cervicomedullary angle can also be measured on MRI by drawing a line parallel to the long axis of both the upper cervical spine and the medulla (Fig. 24-11). The resulting angle obtained by the intersection of these lines is the cervicomedullary angle. This angle is normally between 135 and 175 degrees. With progressive disease, this angle can decrease as the brain stem drapes over the ventrally compressive odontoid. One study reported neurologic signs of C2 irritation, cervicomedullary compression, and myelopathy in 100% of patients

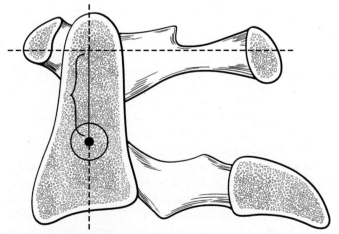

Figure 24-10. Ranawat and colleagues described a method for evaluating cranial settling. The solid red line marks the distance between a vertical line drawn from the center of the C2 pedicle to a line drawn through the transverse axis of the atlas. As this distance decreases, the severity of cranial settling increases.

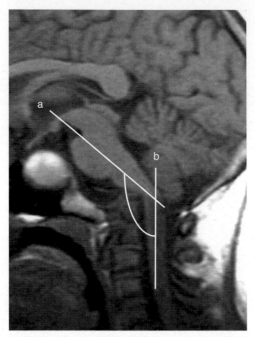

Figure 24-11. T1-weighted MRI scan of the craniocervical junction in a patient with atlantoaxial impaction. The cervicomedullary angle is defined by the angle subtended between lines drawn parallel to the long axis of the brain stem (a) and to the cervical spinal cord (b).

with a cervicomedullary angle less than 135 degrees. Dynamic flexion-extension MRI has been described as a tool that can help to identify dynamic compression before static compression is apparent. One study reported that a cervical cord diameter less than 6 mm in flexion carries a theoretical risk for neurologic injury.

Natural History

The literature is limited on reports describing the natural history of untreated rheumatic cervical spine disease. This is in large part due to the effective medical therapies that exist. Additionally, most studies are retrospective and have small sample sizes. However, these studies report that 40% to 80% of RA patients with atlantoaxial subluxation demonstrate radiographic progression over time. Seropositivity for rheumatoid factor, more extensive peripheral joint involvement, male gender, and corticosteroid use are factors that have been associated with more extensive cervical involvement. Although the prevalence of radiographic progression of cervical instability in RA patients is high, associated neurologic deficits have been variably reported in only 7% to 58% of patients. Pellicci and colleagues reported that 80% of the RA patients who had cervical involvement showed radiographic progression, but only 36% had neurologic progression. The large disparity between radiographic and neurologic progression might be explained by the variable classification systems used to assess neurologic function and the difficulty in assessing often subtle neurologic findings in patients with often severe musculoskeletal manifestations of the disease.

TABLE 24-1. Ranawat Grading for Myelopathy

Grade	Severity
I	Normal
II	Weakness, hyperreflexia, altered sensation
IIIA	Paresis and long-tract signs, ambulatory
IIIB	Quadriparesis, nonambulatory

Although rheumatoid patients are likely to have radiographic progression of their cervical disease, the likelihood of developing neurologic deterioration is lower.

Boden and associates retrospectively reported on 73 RA patients with an average follow-up of 7 years. Of the 73 patients, 42 (58%) developed paralysis. No significant neurologic deficit occurred with observation in 31 patients who were treated nonoperatively. In the 42 patients in whom paralysis developed, 7 were treated nonoperatively. Six of the 7 patients who were treated nonoperatively had progressive neurologic deterioration. All seven of these patients died within 4 years of the onset of paralysis, five from neurologic compression. Of the 35 patients who had operative intervention, 25 (71%) experienced marked neurologic improvement.

Conversely, once neurologic symptoms develop, the natural history appears to be that of progressive neurologic deterioration, which can ultimately lead to sudden death. When myelopathy is present, the mortality rate increases substantially, and most patients treated without surgery die within 1 year. Sudden death occurs in approximately 10% of rheumatoid patients with cervical involvement as a result of brain stem compression. Unfortunately, the poor correlation of radiographic instability parameters in patients with cervical RA and impending neurologic injury makes identifying surgical candidates difficult.

Several grading systems have been developed to assess disease severity and progression, as well as treatment outcomes. Ranawat and colleagues described a grading scale for myelopathy, but this system lacks the ability to differentiate mild degrees of myelopathy (Table 24-1). Zeidman and Drucker modified the Nurick classification of myelopathy to include hand function, and this might be more useful (Table 24-2). The Japanese Orthopaedic Association scoring system measures both upper- and lower-extremity motor and sensory function in addition to bladder function. This 17-point classification system is more inclusive and has been shown to have higher interobserver and intraobserver reliability in the assessment of cervical myelopathy.

Predictors of Neurologic Recovery

There are multiple risk factors that do not appear to strongly correlate with postoperative neurologic recovery. These include age, sex, preoperative duration of paralysis, AADI prior to stabilization, and the degree of preoperative subaxial subluxation measured by percentage of slip.

Several factors have been associated with the potential for postoperative neurologic recovery. Using the Ranawat

TABLE 24-2. Zeidman and Drucker's Classification of Myelopathy

Grade	Radiculopathy	Myelopathy	Gait	Hand Function
0	Present	Absent	Normal	Normal
I	Present	Present	Normal	Slight
II	Present	Present	Mildly abnormal	Functional
III	Present	Present	Severely abnormal	Unable to button
IV	Present	Present	With assistance only	Severely limited
V	Present	Present	Nonambulatory	Useless

classification, the severity of preoperative neurologic deficit appears to correlate with postoperative neurologic recovery, and patients with more severe deficits tend to have poorer neurologic recovery.

Multiple radiographic parameters have been evaluated in their correlation with postoperative neurologic improvement. Boden and colleagues found that the PADI correlates with postoperative neurologic recovery. Patients with a PADI of 14 mm or greater tended to have significant motor recovery after appropriate surgical intervention. Patients with a preoperative PADI less than 10 mm did not experience significant postoperative neurologic improvement. Patients with a postoperative subaxial sagittal canal diameter less than 14 mm and/or a postoperative pseudarthrosis might also achieve less neurologic recovery.

Nonoperative Treatment

Currently, early and aggressive medical treatment can preserve joint function and alter the natural history of the disease. Disease-modifying antirheumatic drugs, such as antimalarial drugs, methotrexate, sulfasalazine, and gold, are the mainstay of medical treatment. Newer drugs that block the effects of tumor necrosis factor–alpha (TNF-α) have also had a favorable effect on the natural course of the disease. Aggressive treatment with disease-modifying antirheumatic drugs can delay and possibly prevent the development of atlantoaxial instability.

The high prevalence and early appearance of cervical involvement in patients with rheumatoid disease warrant screening with cervical spine plain radiographs on diagnosis. Regular follow-up for patients with cervical disease includes a detailed neurologic examination and cervical radiographs to assess for disease progression.

Soft cervical collars can be utilized for symptomatic patients with minor acute pain. This treatment modality can also be used for elderly patients and those who are deemed to be poor surgical candidates. Soft collars can alleviate acute neck pain but do not adequately stabilize the cervical spine and probably do not alter the natural course of disease in the cervical spine. Physical therapy can be used to strengthen the cervical muscles and for postural training, with patients being taught to avoid cervical flexion. Pain medication can also be utilized to treat acute pain, but once chronic narcotic medication becomes necessary for pain relief, surgical intervention becomes an option.

Surgical Management

Patients with unremitting chronic pain or progressive or new-onset neurologic deficit are usually surgical candidates. The goals of surgery are to achieve stability through bony fusion and to decompress the neural elements. Additionally, because of the apparent increased morbidity in patients with more profound neurologic symptoms, even with surgical intervention, earlier operative intervention may result in better outcome. Because of the risk of cord impingement due to cervical instability that can occur with standard intubation techniques, awake, nasotracheal fiberoptic intubation should be strongly considered.

Plain lateral radiographs that demonstrate a PADI less than 14 mm warrant an MRI to evaluate the true space available for the cord and any soft-tissue compression. Any patient with neurologic deficit should have MRI evaluation. If the MRI demonstrates a cervicomedullary angle less than 135 degrees or any evidence of cord compression, then posterior atlantoaxial fusion should be considered. Posterior C1-2 fixation techniques include Brooks or Gallie wiring, Magerl transarticular screws, or Harms C1-2 lateral mass screws and rods. The latter technique is currently in favor, owing to predictable stabilization and fusion rates.

Because of the high postoperative morbidity of patients with cranial settling and their poor prognosis for neurologic recovery, any evidence of cord compression warrants a more aggressive approach. In patients with atlantoaxial subluxation and cranial settling, cervical traction may be appropriate. If normal cervical alignment is achieved, then an occipitocervical fusion can be performed. If compression of the cervical cord is not relieved with traction, C1 laminectomy and occipital decompression or odontoid resection should be considered along with occipitocervical fusion. If odontoid resection is performed to relieve cord compression, posterior C1-2 fusion can be considered rather than occiput–C2 fusion, especially if cranial settling is due to C1-2 joint disease with relative sparing of the occiput–C1 joints.

Patients with subaxial subluxation with a posterior subaxial canal diameter less than 14 mm warrant an MRI to evaluate the true space available for the cord. Operative stabilization may be considered if any cord impingement is observed or any significant degree of instability is present. In most cases, posterior cervical fusion is the procedure of choice. However, in the presence of irreducible subaxial subluxation, anterior decompression alone or in combination with posterior fusion may be considered. When atlantoaxial and subaxial subluxations occur concomitantly, all pathology should be addressed simultaneously. The fusion should extend down to the caudalmost segment involved, to avoid junctional deterioration below the long fusion mass. This can result in the fusion extending from the occiput to the thoracic spine.

Outcomes after surgical arthrodesis are good when patients have not developed severe myelopathy. As a result, surgery has been proposed when patients, even without neurologic findings, demonstrate specific radiographic criteria, including atlantoaxial instability and a PADI less than or equal to 14 mm, atlantoaxial impaction greater than or equal to 5 mm rostral to McGregor's line, or subaxial subluxation with a sagittal canal diameter less than or equal to 14 mm.

Complications

A high rate of perioperative complications has been attributed to the overall debilitation of this patient population. The most common complications of cervical spine surgery in patients with RA include infection and wound dehiscence (up to 25%), wire breakage and loss of reduction, pseudarthrosis (5% to 20%), and late subaxial subluxation below a fusion mass. Late subaxial subluxation has been shown to occur with a higher frequency following occiput–C2 fusions as compared to C1-2 fusions. The overall perioperative mortality rate has been reported to be between 5% and 10%, with higher rates in patients with concomitant cardiovascular disease or atlantoaxial impaction.

Summary

In most patients with RA, neck pain is the most common symptom, but it usually occurs without significant neurologic deficit. Early and aggressive medical treatment of RA, particularly with the newer pharmacologic therapy, can preserve joint function and alter the natural history of the disease. This may delay and possibly prevent the development of atlantoaxial instability and neurologic compromise. The primary goal in the management of patients with RA and cervical spine involvement is to prevent permanent neurologic deficit. Patients with cervical involvement should be evaluated regularly to identify any subtle changes in their neurologic examination. Measuring the PADI and measuring the subaxial sagittal canal diameter on plain lateral radiographs are reliable screening tools to identify high-risk patients who might warrant further imaging with MRI or CT myelography. If instability with neurologic deficit develops or cord compression is identified, surgical decompression and stabilization should strongly be considered. With proper decompression and solid fusion, pain relief is usually achieved, and postoperative neurologic recovery is predicated on preoperative neurologic status. Perioperative complications are not uncommon and tend to occur more frequently in patients who have developed severe myelopathy.

PEARLS & PITFALLS

PEARLS

- Ninety percent of patients with AS are positive for HLA-B27.
- AS patients are at an increased risk for fracture and neurologic deterioration.
- AS patients are often osteoporotic and therefore require additional fixation compared to standard techniques.
- Closing-wedge osteotomies have fewer complications in the management of kyphotic deformity.
- Advances in the medical treatment of RA, including newer pharmacologic agents, have altered the natural history of the disease and can delay or prevent cervical instability.
- The PADI and subaxial anteroposterior canal diameter measured on lateral cervical radiographs are reliable screening tools to identify patients who are at risk for neurologic injury.
- Patients with neurologic signs should have MRI evaluation to check for soft-tissue involvement or cord compression.
- Patients with a preoperative PADI of 14 mm or greater tend to have significant motor recovery after appropriate surgical stabilization, and patients with a PADI less than 10 mm might not experience significant postoperative neurologic improvement.
- Patients with a postoperative subaxial sagittal canal diameter less than 14 mm and/or postoperative pseudarthrosis might achieve less neurologic improvement.

PITFALLS

- Cervical spine extension during immobilization after trauma and during intubation can cause significant bony and neurologic injury.
- Fractures can be missed without the use of advanced imaging techniques in the workup of minor trauma.
- Neurologic signs and symptoms can be difficult to elicit in RA patients secondary to peripheral musculoskeletal manifestations of the disease.
- Radiographic progression of cervical involvement in RA patients does not correlate with the development of neurologic deterioration.
- The PADI on lateral cervical radiographs might not accurately evaluate the space available for the cord secondary to soft-tissue compression.
- Once neurologic signs develop in RA patients, the natural history appears to be that of progressive neurologic deterioration, which can ultimately lead to sudden death.
- Perioperative morbidity and mortality rates in RA patients are relatively high.

Illustrative Case Presentation

CASE 1. A 44-Year-Old Man with Paraparesis Who Had Been Involved in a Car Accident

He also sustained an unstable extension fracture at C6-7 necessitating anteroposterior cervical spine instrumentation (Fig. 24-12).

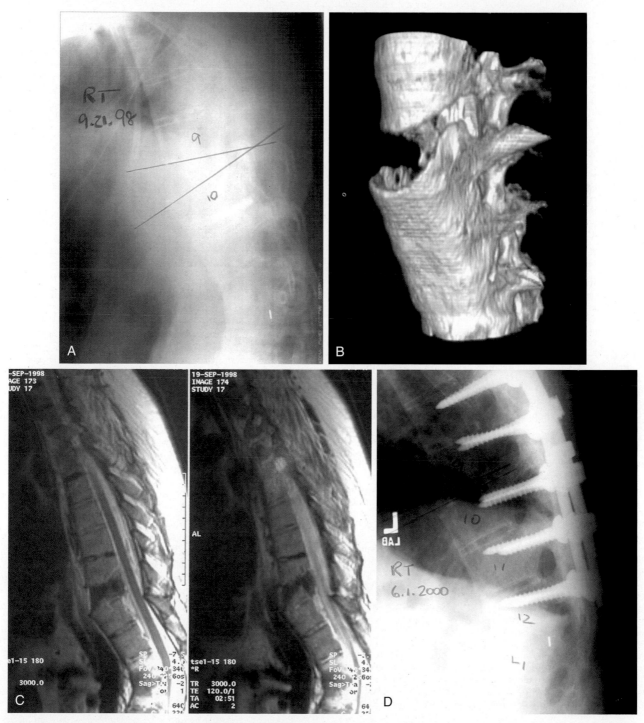

Figure 24-12. A, Lateral radiograph reveals a fracture at T9-10. He also sustained an unstable extension fracture at C6-7 that necessitated anteroposterior cervical spine instrumentation. **B,** Three-dimensional CT scan shows the three-column extension fracture across the caudal end of T9 and facets with posterior dislocation of T9 relative to T10. **C,** Sagittal T2-weighted MRI shows the posterior compression of the spinal cord by the T10 lamina. **D,** Postoperative lateral radiograph at 2 years' follow-up shows posterior fixation with pedicle screws and rods from T8 to T10. *(From Benzel EC [ed]: Spine Surgery: Techniques, Complication Avoidance, and Management, 2nd ed. Philadelphia: Elsevier, 2004.)*

REFERENCES

Boden SD, Dodge LD, Bohlman HH, et al: Rheumatoid arthritis of the cervical spine: A twenty year analysis with predictors of paralysis and recovery. J Bone Joint Surg Am 1993;75:1282–1297.

Braun J, Bollow M, Remlinger G, et al: Prevalence of spondyloarthropathies in HLA-B27 positive and negative blood donors. Arthritis Rheum 1998;41:58–67.

Bridwell K, DeWald R: The Textbook of Spinal Surgery. Philadelphia: Lippincott-Raven, 1997.

Broom M, Raycroft J: Complications of fractures of the cervical spine in ankylosing spondylitis. Spine 1988;13:763–766.

Brophy S, Pavy S, Lewis P, et al: Inflammatory eye, skin and bowel disease in spondyloarthritis: genetic, phenotypic, and environmental factors. J Rheumatol 2001;28:2667–2673.

Bundschuh C, Modic MT, Kearney F, et al: Rheumatoid arthritis of the cervical spine: Surface-coil MR imaging. AJNR Am J Neuroradiol 1988;151:181–187.

Clark C, Goetz D, McNeles A: Arthrodesis of the cervical spine in rheumatoid arthritis. J Bone Joint Surg Am 1989;71:381–392.

Cook SD, Salkeld SL, Whitecloud TS: Biomechanical evaluation and preliminary clinical experience with an expansive pedicle screw design. J Spinal Disord 2000;13:230–236.

Crockard HA: Surgical management of cervical rheumatoid problems. Spine 1995;20:2584–2590.

Crockard HA, Calder I, Ransford AO: One-stage transoral decompression and posterior fixation in rheumatoid atlanto-axial subluxation. J Bone Joint Surg Br 1990;72:682–685.

Detwiler K, Loftus C, Godersky J, et al: Management of cervical spine injuries in patients with ankylosing spondylitis. J Neurosurg 1990;72:210–215.

Dvorak J, Grob D, Baumgartner H, et al: Functional evaluation of the spinal cord by magnetic resonance imaging in patients with rheumatoid arthritis and instability of upper cervical spine. Spine 1989;14:1057–1064.

Exner G, Kluger B, Richter M, et al: Treatment of fracture and complication of cervical spine with ankylosing spondylitis. Spinal Cord 1998;36:377–379.

Fast A, Parikh S, Marin E: Spine fractures in ankylosing spondylitis. Arch Phys Med Rehab 1986;67:595–597.

Finkelstein JA, Chapman JR, Mirza S: Occult vertebal fractures in ankylosing spondylitis. Spinal Cord 1999;37:444–447.

Foo D, Rossier A: Post traumatic spinal epidural hematoma. Neurosurgery 1982;11:25–32.

Fox M, Onofrio B, Kilgore J: Neurological complications of ankylosing spondylitis. J Neurosurg 1993;78:871–878.

Gelman M, Umber J: Fractures of the thoracolumbar spine in ankylosing spondylitis. Am J Roentgenol 1978;130:485–491.

McMaster M: Osteotomy of the cervical spine in ankylosing spondylitis. J Bone Joint Surg Br 1997;79:197–203.

Murray G, Persellin R: Cervical fracture complicating ankylosing spondylitis: A report of eight cases and review of the literature. Am J Med 1981;70:1033–1041.

Neva MH, Kaarela K, Kauppi M: Prevalence of radiological changes in the cervical spine: A cross sectional study after 20 years from presentation of rheumatoid arthritis. J Rheumatol 2000;27:90–93.

Oda T, Fujiwara K, Yonenobu K, et al: Natural course of cervical spine lesions in rheumatoid arthritis. Spine 1995;20:1128–1135.

Pellicci PM, Ranawat CS, Tsairis P, et al: A prospective study of the progression of rheumatoid arthritis of the cervical spine. J Bone Joint Surg Am 1981;68:342–350.

Ranawat CS, O'Leary P, Pellicci P, et al: Cervical spine fusion in rheumatoid arthritis. J Bone Joint Surg Am 1979;61:1003–1010.

Redlund-Johnell I, Petterson H: Radiographic measurements of the cranio-vertebral region. Acta Radiol Diagn 1984;25:23–28.

Savolaine E, Ebraheim N, Stitgen S, et al: Aortic rupture complicating a fracture of an ankylosed thoracic spine. Clin Orthop Relat Res 1991;272:136–140.

Tetzlaff J, Yoon H, Bell G: Massive bleeding duing spine surgery in a patient with ankylosing spondylitis. Can J Anaest 1998;45:903–906.

Trent G, Armstrong GWD, O'Neil J: Thoracolumbar fractures in ankylosing spondylitis: High risk injuries. Clin Orthop Relat Res 1988;227:61–66.

Urist M: Osteotomy of the cervical spine: Report of a case of ankylosing rheumatoid spondylitis. J Bone Joint Surg Am 1958;40:833–843.

Van Der Linden S, Valkenburg H, Cats A: Evaluation of diagnostic criteria for ankylosing spondylitis: A proposal for modification of the New York Criteria. Arthritis Rheum 1984;27:361–368.

Van Royen B, DeGast A: Lumbar osteotomy for correction of thoracolumbar kyphotic deformity in ankylosing spondylitis: A structured review of three methods of treatment. Ann Rheum Dis 1999;58:399–406.

Wittenberg RH, Lee K, Shea M, et al: Effect of screw diameter, insertion technique, and bone cement augmentation of pedicular screw fixation strength. Clin Orthop Relat Res 1993;296:278–287.

Wu C, Lee S: Spinal epidural hematoma and ankylosing spondylitis: Case report and review of the literature. J Trauma 1998;44:558–561.

Zeidman SM, Drucker TB: Rheumatoid arthritis: Neuroanatomy, compression, and grading of deficits. Spine 1994;19:2259–2266.

Zoma A, Sturrock RD, Fisher WD, et al: Surgical stabilization of the rheumatoid cervical spine: A review of indications and results. J Bone Joint Surg Br 1987;69:8–12.

SUGGESTED READINGS

Falope ZF, Griffiths ID, Platt PN, et al: Cervical myelopathy and rheumatoid arthritis: A retrospective analysis of management. Clin Rehabil 2002;16:625–629.

A retrospective review of 40 patients with RA was performed. The 18 patients who were treated nonsurgically had a 5-year mortality rate of 73%, and no neurologic improvement was noted. Twenty-two patients were treated surgically and had a 5-year mortality rate of 27%; 30% of patients improved one Ranawat grade, and 55% of nonambulators (Ranawat grade IIIB) became ambulators.

Kawaguchi Y, Matsuno H, Kanamori M, et al: Radiologic findings of the lumbar spine in patients with rheumatoid arthritis, and a review of pathologic mechanisms. J Spinal Disord Tech 2003;16:38–43.

Lumbar radiographic findings were noted in 57% of 106 patients with RA. In descending frequency of occurrence, these included disk space narrowing, postural anomaly, olisthesis, end plate erosion, and facet erosion. End plate erosion correlated most closely with clinical symptoms.

Matsunaga S, Sakou T, Onishi T, et al: Prognosis of patients with upper cervical lesions caused by rheumatoid arthritis: Comparison of occipitocervical fusion between C1 laminectomy and nonsurgical management. Spine 2003;28:1581–1587.

Nineteen patients were treated surgically compared to 21 patients who were treated nonsurgically. Improvement was found in 68% of patients who underwent surgery. The survival rate for surgical patients was 84% at 5-year follow-up and 37% at 10-year follow-up. In the nonsurgical patients, no neurologic improvement was reported; neurologic deterioration was found in 76% of patients during the follow-up period, and no patient survived beyond the 8-year follow-up.

Nakstad P, Server A, Josefsen R: Traumatic cervical injuries in ankylosing spondylitis. Acta Radiol 2004;45:222–226.

The authors assess the usefulness of advanced imaging for the diagnosis and management of cervical spine fractures in patients with ankylosing spondylitis.

O'Dell JR: Therapeutic strategies for rheumatoid arthritis. N Engl J Med 2004;350:2591–2602.

This article is a comprehensive review of the current pharmacologic agents available, current recommendations, and future direction in the medical treatment of rheumatoid arthritis.

Omura K, Hukuda S, Katsuura A, et al: Evaluation of posterior long fusion versus conservative treatment for the progressive rheumatoid cervical spine. Spine 2002;27:1336–1345.

Seventeen seropositive patients with RA with mutilating joint involvement were assessed. Eleven patients underwent surgical treatment, and six patients underwent nonsurgical management. Patients who underwent surgical stabilization improved, or the progressive natural history of the disease was interrupted. Patients without surgical intervention went on to experience sudden death from minor trauma or became bedridden.

Riew KD, Hilibrand AS, Paulumbo MA, et al: Diagnosing basilar invagination in the rheumatoid patient: The reliability of radiographic criteria. J Bone Joint Surg Am 2001;83:194–200.

Standard screening radiographs in 131 patients with rheumatoid arthritis were not sensitive, nor did they have a negative predictive value for basilar invagination. MRI or tomography is recommended when the diagnosis of basilar invagination is suspected on plain radiographs.

Simmons E, DiStefano R, Zheng Y, et al: Thirty-six years experience of cervical extension osteotomy in ankylosing spondylitis: Techniques and outcomes. Spine 2006;31:3006–3012.

The authors report on their experience, clinical outcomes, and adverse events with cervicothoracic osteotomies for the treatment of ankylosing spondylitis.

CHAPTER 25

Revision Deformity Surgery

MATTHEW E. CUNNINGHAM, DAVID A. BOMBACK, *and* OHENEBA BOACHIE-ADJEI

OVERVIEW

This chapter focuses on the management of patients who have had previous surgery for correction of spinal deformity that requires further surgical intervention. Patients who present with failed surgical correction or with new surgical issues are typically complex and require a thorough physical examination and complete diagnostic evaluation. A combination of laboratory, radiologic, and electrodiagnostic testing often provides critical information in formulating a diagnosis and plan for revision surgery. A treatment plan can then be established, consisting of any required provocative preoperative testing followed by revision surgical management and comprehensive postoperative care.

Revision spine deformity surgery, also known as salvage reconstruction, presents several challenges to the spine surgeon. The biologic environment for fusion is often unfavorable and requires meticulous attention to both optimizing preparation of the intended fusion bed and stabilizing the reconstructed spine with implants. Additional technical considerations, including osteotomies and subtotal vertebrectomies, are also quite complex and require special training. Both the patient and surgeon need be aware that the risks and complications of revision deformity surgery are significantly greater than those of primary procedures. Nevertheless, successful outcomes can be obtained with careful preoperative, intraoperative, and postoperative decision making.

CLASSIFICATION

Clinical Presentation

Typical complaints at presentation for patients who are undergoing revision surgery are back or leg pain, increasing spine deformity, neurologic involvement, or any combination of these. Patients usually present several years after the index corrective procedure, but it is not uncommon for patients to report symptom-free intervals of 20 years or longer following their index surgeries. Symptoms may have an insidious onset and may be the result of motion segment degeneration below a long fusion or indolent infection, which can take months or years to be noticed by the patient, or they may be more precipitous in their onset because of the immediate loss of mechanical stability in the setting of instrumentation failure secondary to a pseudarthrosis. It is very important to characterize the nature, intensity, and duration of complaints to best utilize this information logically in diagnosis and ultimately treatment. Although tedious, the art of eliciting a complete and accurate historical vignette and performing a complete physical examination is what provides the practitioner with the most critical information for diagnosing the problem.

Pain that occurs in the area of previous surgery can be secondary to several pathologic processes. Pseudarthrosis is a particularly common etiology in this regard, is often overlooked as a possibility, and should be considered to be the diagnosis until proven otherwise. Posteroanterior, lateral, and oblique radiographs of the fusion mass; computed tomography (CT) scans with reconstructions; and bone scans are all instrumental for evaluating for the bony healing defect. Pathognomonic of pseudarthrosis is the presence of failed or broken implants, which are commonly associated with this process. Other etiologies to consider include indolent infection, prominent instrumentation, or crankshafting (in an adolescent population) in addition to less likely mechanisms, including acute fracture within the fusion mass or superimposed spinal stenosis. Vague pain symptoms that are difficult to localize are more consistent with indolent infection, crankshaft, or diffuse spinal stenosis, whereas point tenderness is consistent with a suppurating infection, acute fracture of the fusion mass, or prominent implants. Evaluation of these etiologies requires the imaging listed previously and might also require magnetic resonance imaging (MRI) or CT myelography in addition to blood work to evaluate markers for correlates of infection (e.g., complete blood count, erythrocyte sedimentation rate, C-reactive protein). Although implants can certainly be painful, this is a diagnosis of exclusion; all other etiologies, in particular pseudarthrosis and infec-tion, need to be formally eliminated as diagnoses prior to concluding that the symptoms are due to symptomatic implants.

The pain generator might not be based within the fusion mass proper but rather could be at a level adjacent to it proximally or distally. It is important to elicit the specific character of the pain, its chronicity, and any diurnal variability. An inflammatory process would classically be expected to generate complaints of morning stiffness that gradually gets better with activity during the day. The patient might report that the complaints are responsive to, and relatively well controlled with, over-the-counter anti-inflammatory medications. Pain symptoms that are worst at the end of the day or that are associated with activity suggest a mechanical origin of the pain such as might be seen with generalized junctional degeneration. More specifically, if mechanical symptoms are aggravated with sitting, positions of flexion, or vibratory movements, a discogenic source of the pain should be sought. Radicular symptoms should raise diagnostic suspicion of a disc herniation or spinal stenosis. Systematic and logical application of the historical vignette will guide imaging and other evaluations that might be required to confirm the diagnosis.

Increasing deformity is commonly attributable to one of three causes: pseudarthrosis, crankshaft phenomenon, or the adding-on phenomenon. The patient presents complaining of "falling forward" or "leaning to the side" or has the subjective sensation that this is happening. The patient is usually aware of the progressive nature of the deformity and might relate a history of balance difficulty with ambulation, a loss of height, waistline asymmetry, or an increase in a rotational prominence. Fixed sagittal imbalance, or flat-back syndrome, often presents with low back pain, hip flexion deformity and contracture, and quadriceps fatigue. On physical examination, coronal decompensation can be measured clinically by using a plumbline from C7 to the gluteal fold and can be monitored serially to document progression. Sagittal plane decompensation can be demonstrated by viewing the standing patient from the side and noticing the loss of natural sagittal contour or the frank forward thrust of the shoulders anterior to the hips. Sagittal and coronal imbalance can be monitored both radiographically, with full-length spine radiographs, and by using plumblines dropped from T1 to the back of the S1 vertebral body or the center sacral line, respectively.

Clinical clues to the etiology of progressive deformity can be provided by careful scrutiny of the history and physical examination, radiographs and supplementary imaging, and review of the prior operative reports. Deformity that is related to pseudarthrosis occurs due to a defect within the fusion mass itself. A failure to achieve arthrodesis at a particular level or levels can then lead to coronal imbalance,

sagittal imbalance, or both and, as was mentioned previously, is frequently accompanied by pain. Failure to use autogenous bone graft or osteogenic factors at the principal operation and poor arthrodesis technique are risk factors for pseudarthrosis. Meticulous decortication of the posterior elements and placement of either rib autograft or iliac crest autograft is crucial for a successful union. The crankshaft phenomenon is seen only in skeletally immature individuals. This occurs in patients with infantile or juvenile scoliosis who have undergone a posterior spinal fusion alone. The healthy anterior vertebral apophyses allow for continued growth and subsequently a rotational deformity. These patients present with a significant rotational deformity, frequently with excessive rib prominences. By definition, crankshafting can be diagnosed only in a growing individual. Finally, the adding-on phenomenon refers to a new deformity above or below the prior surgical site. This may also be described as junctional deformity or lengthening of the curve. It is caused by unpredictable remaining spinal growth and/or inadequate selection of fusion levels at the index procedure. Rotation is not nearly as severe as that seen in crankshaft cases. The presentation can be one of sagittal or coronal decompensation on either end or on both ends of a previous fusion. Junctional kyphosis, a specific subset of junctional deformity, commonly develops cranially to a fusion mass when fusions are terminated in the midthoracic or thoracolumbar spine.

Physical Examination

Prior to a comprehensive spine examination, a pertinent general medical examination needs to be performed. Fever might indicate an underlying infection and must be thoroughly evaluated. On pulmonary auscultation, wheezes, rales, or rhonchi might suggest underlying pulmonary or cardiac disease. Salvage surgery is frequently lengthy in duration, and it is critical that the patient be systemically healthy enough to undergo such an event. The abdomen and thorax should be inspected in anticipation of anterior surgery, and prior surgical incisions should be noted. Lower-extremity pain should mandate a hip and knee examination to rule out local pathology, and palpation of distal pulses should be performed to evaluate large-vessel peripheral vascular disease.

After completion of a relevant medical examination, the spine examination is performed to evaluate pain, document deformity, and assess neurologic status. Inspection of the prior surgical incision reveals erythema, drainage, prominent implants, and cutaneous healing potential. The entire spine, including the sacroiliac joints, is palpated both in the midline and along the paraspinal musculature. Points of maximal tenderness must be noted and correlated to the spinal levels that were previously instrumented. Standing posture is observed, and sagittal and/or coronal decompensation is noted. Subtleties of stance need to be appreciated: Are one knee and hip flexed to compensate for coronal imbalance, or are both hips and knees flexed to correct sagittal imbalance? With the patient's hips and knees extended, a plumbline should be dropped from the vertebra prominens, and the magnitude and direction of horizontal displacement from the gluteal fold should be recorded. Similarly, a visual estimation of the sacrovertebral angle allows for quantification of forward tilt. The Adams forward-bending test permits documentation of thoracic and lumbar rotational prominences. Trunk range of motion must be measured in flexion, extension, and lateral bending; this measurement also allows an estimation of curve flexibility. Gait and station are evaluated, with emphasis on global spinal balance and hip abductor/extensor weakness or contracture. A detailed neurologic examination is an essential component of the clinical examination. Thorough motor and sensory testing of upper and lower extremities must be performed and documented, with emphasis placed on unambiguously defining deficits that the patient has at presentation. Normal and pathologic reflexes, balance, and tension signs must also be included in the assessment, along with assessment of rectal tone as indicated by the clinical scenario.

Diagnostic Evaluation

A complete diagnostic workup encompasses a medical, radiologic, electrodiagnostic, and occasionally interventional evaluation. The medical assessment should fulfill two criteria: clearing the patient for surgery and addressing specific issues pertinent to each individual's circumstance. Medical clearance consists of routine blood work, a chest radiograph, electrocardiogram, and echocardiogram (in males over 40 years and females over 50 years of age). If anterior thoracic surgery is necessary, pulmonary function tests are recommended as well. Attention is then directed toward patient-specific problems, such as infection or pseudarthrosis. A preoperative complete blood count with differential, erythrocyte sedimentation rate, and C-reactive protein should be obtained for diagnostic purposes and baseline values. Finally, radionuclide bone scans (e.g., technetium, gallium, or labeled white blood cells) can help to detect the presence of a spinal infection. If a prior surgical site is draining or there is evidence of a fluid collection, aspiration and/or swabbing of this site (after meticulous sterile preparation) can be performed, although cultures from draining wounds frequently are not helpful for guiding management. Antibiotics are held until the cultures return unless there is clear evidence of infection or systemic manifestation of sepsis. Preferably, cultures can be obtained in the operating room, where biopsies of bone and soft tissue can be collected simultaneously.

Preoperative diagnostic imaging can be critical in formulating the treatment plan. The radiologic evaluation begins with full-length standing posteroanterior and lateral views of the entire spine to assess global coronal and sagittal balance. In addition, the presence of scoliosis, kyphosis,

pelvic obliquity, shoulder asymmetry, and any prior instrumentation is documented. Areas proximal or distal to a prior fusion are assessed for junctional degeneration or decompensation. The fusion mass itself is assessed for evidence of crankshafting or pseudarthrosis. Supine oblique radiographs are often helpful in establishing the latter diagnosis; 70% of pseudarthroses can be detected with the addition of oblique views. In addition, coned-down views of an area of interest (e.g., lumbosacral junction) can prove to be useful.

Three-dimensional imaging and provocative testing provide detailed and novel information to confirm clinical diagnoses. CT scans can highlight bony detail such as bridging trabecular bone if a pseudarthrosis is in question. Spinal stenosis is typically evaluated with multisequence MRI examinations, which are also used to evaluate patients for canal or neuroforaminal compromise. However, metallic instrumentation makes visualization of the spine difficult with MRI. Revision surgical candidates who are being evaluated for spinal stenosis can be assessed by a CT-myelogram, which has better ability to visualize the stenosis in this setting. However, the status of intervertebral discs distal to the instrumentation can be evaluated with MRI. MRI examination of intervertebral discs is often an important preoperative test in considering terminating a fusion in the distal lumbar spine. More commonly, patients with suspected discogenic back pain and positive MRI findings can have their diagnoses confirmed by using provocative discography. The authors recommend testing multiple disc spaces during this examination, if possible, to decrease false-positive results.

Neurodiagnostics encompasses nerve conduction studies, electromyography, somatosensory evoked potentials, and motor evoked potentials. Such electrodiagnostic testing can be extremely useful in both the preoperative and the intraoperative setting. Patients who present with radicular symptoms and/or weakness can be evaluated preoperatively with electromyography and nerve conduction studies. In addition, cases that involve significant deformity correction or shortening, placement of thoracic pedicle screws, placement of intracanicular implants (e.g., hooks, wires), or any complex cervical reconstruction should have intraoperative spinal cord monitoring with somatosensory evoked potentials, motor evoked potentials, and electromyography. If motor evoked potentials are not available, a Stagnara wake-up test must be performed after the correction and before completion of the surgery.

Physiatric and pain management consultations can also offer valuable modalities and therapies that can mitigate or control pain symptoms. Patients with symptoms of spinal stenosis might elect to undergo epidural steroid injections or selective nerve root blocks. Similarly, facet injections or instrumentation injections (injecting local anesthetic adjacent to a prominent implant) not only can temporarily reduce the pain, but also might offer a solution for permanent relief. These interventions should be seen as providing a dual service of both symptomatic treatment and aid in confirming the diagnosis. The surgeon who takes on the challenge of revision deformity surgery should be equipped with as much information as possible before proceeding to operative intervention.

TREATMENT OPTIONS

After the patient has been fully assessed and a working diagnosis has been established, the surgeon can formulate a treatment plan to best address the clinical problems. Preoperative planning involves assessing the patient's general state of health, including any particular risk factors that might have an adverse effect on surgical outcome. Patients who have overwhelming medical comorbidities or patients with insufficient physiologic reserves to tolerate the stresses of the operating room might not be suitable candidates for revision surgery. Medical clearance and risk stratification are mandatory for all patients, regardless of age, as is preoperative medical optimization from pharmacologic, physiologic, and nutritional standpoints. Planned surgical intervention is much better delayed for the patient who is at increased risk for complications secondary to medical or nutritional issues, such as uncontrolled diabetes or hypertension, anemia, physical deconditioning, or occult pulmonary or genitourinary infection. Revision spine deformity surgery demands a tremendous physiologic response from the patient, and properly preparing the patient for the procedure will increase the chances of an optimal outcome.

Modifiable risk factors, such as cigarette smoking and poor bone density, should be addressed well in advance of surgery. Patients should be counseled to quit smoking at some time prior to the surgery, owing to the known detrimental effects of nicotine on wound healing and union rates, but there is no generally agreed-on length of time for presurgical abstinence. In addition to the problems with healing, heavy smokers have poorer postoperative pulmonary recovery and may be at increased risk for longer duration of mechanical ventilation and pneumonia. Bone density can occasionally be apparent on preoperative radiographs; however, by the time mineralization differences are noted on plain radiographs, the amount of bone loss is excessive (greater than 30%). The current standard for assessing bone density is DEXA (dual-energy X-ray absorptiometry). DEXA is much more sensitive and accurate than are plain films or quantitative CT and, if positive for osteopenia or frank osteoporosis, can be used to monitor response to pharmacologic treatment. For patients with diagnosed osteopenia or osteoporosis, preoperative treatment with antiresorptive bone medications (e.g., bisphosphonates) or bone anabolic agents (e.g., PTH/Forteo) must be considered in collaboration with the medical consultant.

Each aspect of the planned surgical revision procedure needs to be carefully considered and discussed with the patient. Many of these concerns will be included in the informed consent document, including intraoperative bleeding, neurologic injury, infection, and the possibility of paralysis or death. It is important to discuss these issues with the patient preoperatively to assess the patient's agreement with the preoperative plan and to prevent potential problems postoperatively. If the patient agrees to accept blood transfusion, preoperative blood donation by the patient or a direct donor can limit the amount of indirect donor blood transfused intraoperatively or postoperatively. In addition, blood preservation techniques such as hypotensive anesthesia and intraoperative salvage with cell saver can further limit the use of communally banked blood. Intraoperative monitoring, if it is to be used, must be arranged, and the patient must be made aware that this system is not infallible or without its own risks. Finally, the actual surgical intervention itself needs to be outlined, and methods for reconstruction need to be planned on the basis of the patient's needs as developed in the preoperative evaluation. Revision deformity procedures include posterior spinal fusion (PSF), anterior spinal fusion followed by PSF (or vice versa), PSF with extension-type (Smith-Petersen) osteotomy, PSF with pedicle subtraction or decancellation osteotomy, and vertebral resection with PSF. With this array of bony procedures and the addition of spinal instrumentation and bone grafts, deformity correction and stabilization are possible for the most complex reconstruction requirements.

Before working out the details of what will be performed in the operating room, the operating surgeon must obtain a copy of the patient's prior operative reports. This simple action will provide a surprisingly large amount of useful information, including the instruments that are needed to remove existing implants (depending on the manufacturer) and any problems that were encountered in the prior procedures (e.g., anomalous vasculature or dural ectasia). Intraoperative surprises should be avoided whenever possible, particularly when this is within the control of the operating surgeon. Having the required instruments to remove the existing implants can make that portion of the operation go quite smoothly. In addition, a variety of revision implants, including large-diameter pedicle screws, dual-diameter connectors, and sacropelvic fixation instrumentation, may be required during the reinstrumentation and should be available. If both iliac crests have been harvested in the past, commercially available bone graft substitutes or biologic agents, particularly bone morphogenetic protein and demineralized bone matrix, can be planned to be used with allograft or as autograft extenders.

The final decision the surgeon must make is whether or not to stage the reconstruction. This determination can be made preoperatively or intraoperatively and is based on medical comorbidities, estimated surgical blood loss, length of surgery, hemodynamic parameters, and the surgeon's expertise in executing both procedures in a timely fashion. Preoperative factors that would necessitate staging a reconstruction include ruling out or treating an infection of the spine in the region of planned implant or graft placement or when multiple osteotomies are planned and blood loss is expected to be excessive. Intraoperative parameters that prompt surgical staging include total surgical time in excess of 12 hours, unanticipated excessive blood loss, devastating neurologic injury, and hemodynamic changes that make safe anesthesia management difficult. If surgery is to be staged, the authors recommend waiting a week to 2 weeks between procedures for improved nutrition, coagulation, hematologic, and cardiopulmonary status. For staged procedures, the authors favor interval hyperalimentation administration.

SPECIAL COMPLICATIONS: HOW TO AVOID AND TREAT

Pseudarthrosis

The most common late complication following adult spine deformity surgery is pseudarthrosis occurring in the fusion mass, with resultant pain and patient dissatisfaction. Complaints of pain associated with the pseudarthrosis are almost universal and correlate with lower SRS-24 outcomes measurements. Patients may demonstrate radiographic changes, including loss of implant fixation (>60%), deformity progression (50%), disc space collapse (19%), and motion on stress views as well as the classic intraoperative finding of gross motion (94%) at the pseudarthrosis site. Increased rates of pseudarthrosis are seen with age over 55 years, fusions spanning more than 12 vertebrae, and thoracolumbar (T10-L2) kyphosis over 20 degrees. Recent rates of pseudarthrosis from primary deformity surgeries range from 11% to 17%, and rates for revision surgery range from 0% to 15%. Pseudarthroses are often present at more than one level in the fusion mass.

Appropriate surgical intervention has the goals of limiting or eliminating pain symptoms, restoring sagittal balance and arresting progressive deformity, and protecting neurologic function. The preoperative patient workup should include determination of previous surgery (anterior or posterior only or combined procedures), as well as standard imaging and laboratory assessments. Anterior procedures are required in the setting of pseudarthrosis after failed anterior fusion attempts and where anterior column structural support must be added. Posterior revision procedures are the mainstay of treatment of pseudarthroses, either alone (in certain clinical settings) or in combination with anterior fusions. Posterior procedures involve exposure of the implants and bone in the region of the diagnosed pseudarthrosis, removal of implants, mechanical testing of the fusion mass, and then bony preparation and reinstrumentation. The standard of care has become circumferential fusions at the pseudarthrosis site, along with anterior and posterior osteotomies to allow restoration of proper sagittal balance of the spine. A recent report challenged this dictum for pseudarthroses of the thoracic spine; in a small series of patients, posterior-only procedures were shown to be uniformly successful in treating the pseudarthroses.

Studies describing surgical outcomes for dedicated revision procedures for pseudarthrosis are limited but are supportive of the role of revision reconstruction. In a 2001 study, Voos and colleagues reported on 17 patients with pseudarthroses in a population of 27 patients who were subjected to combined anterior-posterior fusions with osteotomies and had three pseudarthroses postoperatively (11%), with only one persistent pseudarthrosis present from the original population (6%). In a 1997 study, Buttermann and colleagues reported on 38 patients with pseudarthroses after lumbar fusions who underwent anterior-posterior fusions with anterior structural grafts of either tricortical autograft or femoral ring allograft. They found 4 patients in the allograft group ($N = 26$ patients, $N = 64$ levels) to have residual pseudarthroses and none in the autograft group, for a cumulative successful pseudarthrosis treatment rate of 89%. These findings suggest that appropriate surgical intervention can lead to predictable success in treatment of this difficult problem.

Fixed Sagittal Imbalance (Flat-Back Syndrome)

The loss of normal lumbar lordosis can be multifactorial, but the most common reported cause is iatrogenic, secondary to distraction (Harrington) instrumentation to the lower lumbar spine or sacrum. Other etiologies include hypolordotic lumbar fusion for spondylolisthesis, other malaligned fusions, pseudarthrosis with progression of deformity, thoracolumbar kyphosis, decompensation of inferior or superior adjacent segments secondary to inadequate scoliosis fusion length or segmental degeneration, hip flexion contractures, and hip extensor weakness. The result is positive sagittal imbalance with anterior translation of the plumbline and the body's center of gravity. Patients attempt to compensate for this imbalance by hyperextending the remaining mobile spine segments (mid/upper thoracic and cervical spine) as well as by flexing the hips and knees. These compensatory maneuvers allow the patient to stand upright and/or to achieve horizontal gaze.

The loss of lumbar lordosis directly correlates with the number of caudad levels included in the fusion: Aaro and colleagues, in a 1983 report, showed that patients treated with Harrington instrumentation stopping at T12 averaged 38 degrees of lumbar lordosis, whereas those whose fusions terminated at L4 and L5 averaged only 21 degrees and 16 degrees, respectively. Further study by this and other groups demonstrated decreased lordosis in patients who were fused to the sacrum and normal lordosis in those who were instrumented cephalad to L3.

Patients with flat-back syndrome often complain of painful fatigue in the cervical, upper thoracic, or lower lumbar region. Physical examination reveals obvious flattening of the lumbar region with an obligatory forward tilt of the trunk. A biomechanical study by Tveit and colleagues from 1984 demonstrated that increased paraspinal muscle forces are necessary to maintain erect posture in this patient population and suggested that this was a likely contributory source to the fatigue symptoms. Moreover, more than 50% of patients who are treated with Harrington rods have degenerative cervical changes on radiographs at late follow-up. Using an explanation similar to the first, this could be due to persistent attempts to achieve horizontal gaze with neck extension that result in increased stresses placed on the cervical spine.

The goal of corrective surgery in the management of flat-back syndrome is the restoration of physiologic (or supraphysiologic) lordosis and sagittal balance. Normal sagittal balance is such that the vertical axis falls within 2.5 cm of the posterior aspect of the sacral end plate. An osteotomy is typically performed as the principle corrective maneuver for loss of lordosis; the type and location depend on the site of the deformity, the magnitude of the deformity, and the presence of a solid anterior fusion. The osteotomy can be an opening-type or a closing-type (shortening-type) procedure and can be performed as a stand-alone posterior construct or combined with anterior column support.

Posterior correction alone can be achieved with a Smith-Petersen (extension-type) osteotomy or a pedicle subtraction (or decancellation) osteotomy. A Smith-Petersen osteotomy entails resection of the posterior elements with undercutting of the cephalad spinous process. The entire inferior articular facet of the cephalad vertebra and the superior articular facet of the caudad vertebra are excised; the pars interarticularis is transected. The osteotomy can be repeated at multiple levels, and sagittal correction is achieved via posterior compression with segmental instrumentation; this results in distraction anteriorly through the anterior longitudinal ligament and disc space. It is important to note that this osteotomy lengthens the anterior column and, as a result, can destabilize the spine if the instrumentation fails prior to bony fusion. Additionally, this anterior distraction can injure calcified great vessels or result in superior mesenteric artery syndrome. For these reasons, it has been recommended to add anterior releases and fusion in conjunction with the Smith-Petersen osteotomies. An average of 1 degree of correction can be expected for each millimeter of posterior bone resection, yielding 5 to 20 degrees of total segmental correction.

When a larger deformity exists or in the presence of a solid anterior fusion, it is necessary to remove bone from the anterior column in addition to the posterior elements to obtain adequate correction. The pedicle subtraction osteotomy, or transpedicular decancellation osteotomy, is a three-column posterior closing-wedge osteotomy with the anterior column acting as the hinge. An eggshell varia-

tion, or transpedicular vertebrectomy, which was popularized by Heinig, is the preferred technique of the authors if larger corrections are needed. The operation consists of removal of all posterior elements at the level of the desired correction, including the pedicles and facet joints. The cephalad disc might or might not be included. A posterior wedge of bone or a complete decancellation is then performed.

The authors prefer three levels of rigid transpedicular fixation both above and below the level of the osteotomy. The osteotomy is usually performed at L3 or L2 to protect conus medullaris and spinal cord function. For an L3 osteotomy, removal of the entire neural arch of L3 and resection of any overhanging lamina from L2 or L4 are performed. The dura and nerve roots are completely mobilized, and the transverse processes and pedicles are excised. This frees the L2 and L3 nerve roots bilaterally, as well as the central dura. Copious bleeding may occur as the resection continues laterally down the pedicles, but hemostasis can be obtained with bipolar electocautery, bone wax, and thrombin-soaked Gelfoam. Then the posterior wedge decancellation procedure is carried out by careful elevation of the dura off the posterior wall of the vertebral body. Prior to decancellation, it is important to place temporary fixation on the side away from the surgeon to prevent inadvertent collapse as the osteotomy is completed. This can be moved from side to side as the surgeon moves from one pedicle to the next. The osteotomy is closed by compression through the instrumentation and/or by gradual extension of the operating table. A single-level osteotomy delivers an average of 30 degrees of correction.

In some instances, bony apposition is insufficient at the level of the osteotomy; in this case, the authors prefer to insert an autograft-filled cage through a posterior lumbar interbody fusion approach. Anterior surgery or adjacent segment posterior lumbar interbody fusions may be added in cases of concomitant pseudarthrosis, compromised bone stock, or extension to the sacrum. Pelvic fixation should be considered for fusions that extend to or above the thoracolumbar junction. Advantages of the pedicle subtraction osteotomy include significant sagittal correction at a single level, the ability to achieve coronal correction (modifying the technique to a biplanar osteotomy), preservation of anterior column length, and promotion of rapid fusion by compressed, interdigitating cancellous bone. Drawbacks include its technically demanding nature, significant blood loss, and risk of neurologic injury.

Vertebral column resection, or vertebrectomy, is a shortening procedure that should not be utilized for isolated flat-back syndrome; it can be useful, however, in patients with fixed sagittal imbalance and concomitant degenerative or adult scoliosis with severe coronal plane deformities or hyperkyphosis. Dramatic correction can be achieved at a single level, but the procedure is extremely challenging and should be performed only by a surgeon who is experienced with this technique. Complication rates are as high as 60%.

Coronal Imbalance

Coronal plane imbalance with lateral trunk shift is usually associated with rotational deformity. Patients often complain of an inability to maintain an upright posture; in some instances, flank pain may be caused by impingement of the concave side rib cage on the iliac crest. Significant coronal decompensation with translation can lead to nerve root entrapment or traction, resulting in a radiculopathy.

Coronal imbalance can occur because of curve progression within a prior fusion site or at adjacent levels. If the etiology lies within the prior operative site, a pseudarthrosis, fracture, or crankshaft phenomenon is the likely culprit. When the imbalance occurs proximally or distally to the prior fusion, the cause may be inadequate fusion length (the adding-on phenomenon), juxtafusion disc degeneration with loss of disc height and progressive instability, severe facet degeneration, facet joint or pars interarticularis fracture, or dislodgement of a terminal implant prior to arthrodesis at that level.

Treatment of pure coronal imbalance is quite challenging, given the frequent rotation that is associated with this scenario. Therefore, the best treatment is prevention: Care should be taken in planning fusion levels. The surgeon should consider including an additional caudal level in the presence of angular instability, translational instability (anterolisthesis or retrolisthesis), laminectomy, discectomy, oblique takeoff, or disc degeneration at that level.

For severe and rigid deformities, a circumferential release with multilevel discectomies and fusion, or osteotomies through an existing fusion mass at multiple levels, provides the desired balanced correction in the coronal plane without stressing the correction at a single level with one osteotomy. In the presence of a pseudarthrosis in the thoracic spine, a vascularized rib graft with its intercostal pedicle can be considered. In the lumbar spine, iliac crest autograft or rib autograft supplemented with anterior structural grafts for distal levels should suffice. Supplementation with bone morphogenetic protein can also be contemplated. An extension to the sacropelvic region is the most sound option for patients with significant oblique takeoff of L4 or L5 or for patients with degenerative disc disease at L4-5 or L5-S1 and those that had a long fusion past the thoracolumbar junction. This entails anterior structural graft placement and unilateral or bilateral Galveston-type fixation posteriorly.

Junctional Deformity (Adding-on Phenomenon)

Progressive deformity in juxtaposition to a fusion performed for spinal deformity correction can result from the adjacent segments that were not previously included in the fusion. This complication is most frequently encountered where inappropriately short deformity fusions were performed on younger patients with significant growth remaining in an effort to preserve motion segments. Other settings in which such junctional deformities are seen include neuromuscular deformity and in proximity to large uninstrumented curves. Attempts to prevent this type of junctional deformity and to optimize postsurgical balancing of the spine have led to the routine assessment of curve flexibility in addition to standard standing AP and lateral full-length radiographs, leading to various recommendations for vertebrae to include in a particular fusion.

Surgical goals for junctional deformity are to correct or at least arrest the deformity, to restore spine balance, to relieve pain symptoms if these are present, and to preserve and protect neurologic function. Proper assessment of the patient preoperatively should include determination of the rigidity of the minor or compensatory curves and selection of appropriate extensions of the index fusion. Anterior discectomies and fusion might be required for rigid or large deformities or where anterior column structural support is needed. Osteotomies of the fusion mass might be also be required if overall sagittal and coronal balance cannot be achieved via mobilization of the junctional deformity segments. Typically, posterior-only procedures are utilized to provide direct extensions of the existing fusion mass to include the involved junctional segments.

Adjacent Segment Degeneration (Junctional Degeneration)

Deterioration of the motion segments proximal or distal to a fusion mass is referred to as *adjacent segment* or *junctional degeneration*. This deterioration may be in the form of desiccation of adjacent discs and degenerative disc disease or degeneration of facet joints and arthrosis of adjacent levels often accompanied by a new deformity such as kyphosis. The true etiology of junctional degeneration has not been established. Suggestions for causation include (1) compromised stability of adjacent levels secondary to the stripping of soft tissues and local damage incurred during the index fusion or (2) increased rate of normal wear and tear at adjacent levels incurred by the increased motion imparted by the long fusion segment. Junctional degeneration is encountered after posterior fusions for Scheuermann's disease or neuromuscular scoliosis and can be seen proximal to short thoracic fusions done for thoracolumbar scoliosis. Perhaps the best-recognized example of junctional degeneration is in the lumbar intervertebral discs below long deformity fusions; however, there is controversy over whether this degeneration is clinically relevant. The experience from patients who have undergone limited lumbar fusions for degenerative disease suggests that degenerative discs adjacent to lumbar fusion masses did not have a predictable negative impact on clinical outcomes.

Surgical goals for junctional degeneration are pain relief, correction of spinal imbalance, correction of deformity if this is present, and protection and preservation of neurologic functioning. Lesions in the thoracic spine are typically amenable to posterior-only procedures and simple extensions of the fusion mass to include the degenerative involved segment. Lumbar lesions should be worked up with appropriate three-dimensional imaging to evaluate the neural elements and rule out stenosis or impingement as well as to evaluate the status of the discs at subjacent levels of a planned fusion extension. Extensions of the fusion mass might require anterior procedures if anterior support is needed, especially as this pertains to the lumbosacral junction, but posterior-only procedures typically are sufficient.

Crankshaft Phenomenon

The term *crankshaft phenomenon* was coined by Dubousset as a progression of rotational and angular deformity within a posterior spinal fusion in young patients as a result of continued growth and not due to pseudarthrosis within the fusion mass. Crankshaft deformity has been reported in populations including those with paralytic, congenital, and idiopathic scoliosis diagnoses that have been subjected to posterior-only fusions at young ages. The Risser stage and status of the triradiate cartilage at the time of surgery do not predict the risk of crankshaft deformity, but peak height velocity and a multivariate method using chronologic/skeletal ages and rib vertebral angle difference are effective. In that residual anterior spinal growth drives the crankshaft deformation, standard care of patients of skeletal age 10 years or younger, or Risser 0 or 1, has become combined anterior and posterior fusions, which successfully prevent the deformity. However, when adolescent idiopathic patients are examined as a subpopulation, the magnitude of crankshaft deformity is typically small, and this finding has led to the recommendation that these patients do not need anterior-posterior fusions.

Surgical goals are to arrest and correct the deformity, to restore balance of the spine, to preserve and protect neurologic functioning, and to alleviate pain symptoms if these are present. In that the deforming force is the continued anterior growth of the spine, anterior or combined anterior and posterior procedures are the mainstay of treatment. Anterior procedures should include complete discectomies and fusion with anterior column support and grafting within the prior fusion mass. Posteriorly, surgical intervention includes removal of appropriate implants and mechanical testing of the fusion mass to evaluate pseudarthrosis and may include osteotomies to correct deformity and to restore proper spine balance prior to replacement of instrumentation.

Painful Instrumentation

Pain is the most common presentation in patients who require revision deformity surgery. Many patients report a history of chronic pain with continued narcotic use. Often, it is impossible to wean these patients off such medications if the source of their pain (e.g., the spine) is not addressed. Nevertheless, a preoperative and postoperative consult with a chronic pain specialist should be ordered. These specialists can also help with diagnostic injections in the preoperative period.

The pain may be coming from prominent instrumentation, pseudarthrosis, infection, fracture, degenerative disc disease, facet arthrosis, instability, spinal stenosis, or nerve root compression. The revision surgeon needs to be aware that the diagnosis of prominent or painful implants is strictly a diagnosis of exclusion. All other potential etiologies should be ruled out prior to removal of instrumentation. Symptomatic relief with peri-implant injections of local anesthetic supports this diagnosis. If no specific site is particularly painful, all of the implants are usually removed, and the entire extent of the fusion is explored. The exception is in a patient with prominent instrumentation and site-specific pain. In this case, offending implants are removed, and the fusion is explored in the area of pain for evidence of a pseudarthrosis. All fibrous tissue is removed with a rongeur or large curette to allow for careful inspection of bony union. If a nonunion is identified, it should be treated as described earlier.

If the fusion appears solid and implants are removed, postoperative bracing is often recommended. Bone removal is frequently necessary to remove screws, hooks, or rods, and the fusion might thus become biomechanically weaker. Consequent loss of coronal or sagittal plane correction may be encountered in the setting of a weakened fusion mass. External support protects the fusion and decreases fracture risk.

Infection

An infection in a postoperative spine patient falls into one of three groups: (1) early infection, prior to fusion; (2) late infection, after fusion has been achieved; (3) late infection with a pseudarthrosis. In all cases of presumed infection (concordant laboratory values and imaging studies), antibiotics should be held until operative cultures can be obtained. Multiple superficial and deep cultures should be sent to pathology as well as specimens of soft tissue and bone.

When an infection is present in the immediate or early postoperative period, the fusion has not yet taken. Here, every attempt is made to eradicate the infection while leaving the implants in place. This often involves multiple visits to the operating room with meticulous debridement and copious irrigation with antibiotic solution. All loose bone graft can be removed or irrigated and replaced, according to the surgeon's preference. The patient is started on broad-spectrum antibiotics, which are then modified according to culture results and infectious disease input. If the infection cannot be eradicated, all instrumentation is removed, and a postoperative brace is issued.

A late infection alone in the presence of a solid fusion is the easiest subset to treat. All instrumentation is removed, and all infected tissue is debrided, including removal from screw and rod tracts. A high-speed burr or small curettes can be quite helpful. After the debridement and irrigation are complete, it is wise to pack the wound open with peroxide-soaked gauze or close the incision over drains. Repeat debridements should occur every other day until the wound is clean enough to be definitely closed over drains. If the condition of the soft tissues or the shape of the wound prohibits wound closure, a vacuum-assisted wound closure system may be utilized. Antibiotics are selected on the basis of organism, and duration of treatment is usually 6 to 8 weeks.

The final scenario, a late infection with concomitant pseudarthrosis, is the most challenging to manage from both a surgical and an infectious disease standpoint. The metallic implants serve as foreign bodies where bacteria can flourish, while the instability of the nonunion often requires rigid structural support in the form of instrumentation. Treatment often requires meticulous debridement and irrigation followed by revision instrumentation. Management of the pseudarthrosis itself was covered in a previous section. Wound closure over drains and a prolonged course of intravenous antibiotics (based on culture sensitivity) are necessary. Occasionally, some patients who have had multiple infections require chronic suppressive antibiotic therapy.

Postoperative Management

In the postoperative period, the patient is cared for by a multidisciplinary team composed of the surgical team, medical consultant, nursing staff, rehabilitation staff, social worker, and appropriate ancillary consultations, including nutrition and pain management. Initial management includes maintenance of wound drains and chest tube, wound care, routine laboratory assessments, and intravenous fluid to support the patient until the return of bowel function and reinitiation of enteral nutrition. Parenteral perioperative antibiotics are given routinely for not less than 48 hours, and parenteral pain medications are provided until the patient is able to tolerate a solid diet. Orthoses (thoracolumbosacral orthosis) are routinely used in osteoporotic patients, those who have undergone osteotomies, and those for whom the surgeon wants to otherwise "protect" the internal fixation. Mobilization begins postoperative day number one and consists of "logroll" training and progression to ambulation as tolerated, as well as posture and balance training. Patients have daily dressing changes and wound checks and full bedside motor-sensory examinations. Oral nutrition is initiated with clear liquids on passage of flatus and is advanced as tolerated to full diet, complete with protein or other supplementation, as directed by the nutritionist. The patient meets with the social worker on a regular basis to determine the patient's needs, and when the multidisciplinary team thinks that the patient has made an adequate hospital convalescence, the team helps to arrange a fluid transition to home or a rehabilitation facility.

Complications

Adult deformity surgery has a late complication rate that has recently been estimated to be between 12% and 48%. Revision deformity surgeries that specifically require osteotomies have complication rates of 33% to 60%. Minor perioperative complications include deep venous thrombosis without embolus, urinary tract infection, superficial wound infection, dural tear and pneumonia without respiratory compromise, prolonged gastrointestinal dysfunction including ileus requiring nasogastric suction, and intravenous catheter infection. Major perioperative complications include deep wound infections, pneumonia, cardiovascular embarrassment, implant failure or dislodgement, pulmonary embolus, neurologic deficits, cauda equina syndrome or paralysis, and death. Late complications include deep wound infections (4%), pseudarthrosis (4% to 11%), junctional degeneration requiring revision, and instrumentation problems requiring a second procedure (12% to 15%). A comparison of complication rates between primary and revision adult deformity surgeries does not demonstrate significant differences, but revision patients did have significantly lower self–image, and patients who required revision for pseudarthrosis had lower SRS-24 total scores.

SUMMARY

Revision surgery in the adult deformity patient population is technically challenging and is associated with a high rate of complications. However, when properly performed, revision deformity surgery has a tremendous positive impact on the patient's quality of life. Surgical indications need to be clear, preoperative planning must be complete, and both patient and surgeon need to be aware of the goals of the intended surgery. Postoperative care is approached on a team basis with close coordination between orthopedic, rehabilitation, medical, social work, and other consultants.

PEARLS & PITFALLS

- Revision deformity surgery can be intellectually and technically very challenging. Use of a multidisciplinary team approach and proper education of the patient as to what to expect from the surgery are important factors to optimize success.
- Pseudarthrosis is the most common late complication of adult deformity surgery. Pseudarthroses correlate with poorer patient satisfaction, implant breakage and loosening, and perceived pain. Diagnosis can be made by static or dynamic radiographs, nuclear medicine bone scans, or three-dimensional imaging such as CT

scans, but the "gold standard" is surgical exposure and assessment. Pseudarthroses must be debrided and stabilized and might require combined anterior and posterior fusions or osteotomies to restore sagittal and coronal balance in affected patients.

■ Flat-back syndrome is often the result of distraction (Harrington) instrumentation and results in a posterior fusion with a relatively elongated posterior column. Forward trunk station, with resultant muscular back pain, and complaints of "falling forward" are very common. Surgical intervention involves shortening of the posterior column either by segmental Smith-Petersen osteotomies and compressive segmental instrumentation or by posterior closing-wedge osteotomies, including pedicle subtraction osteotomy and decancellation osteotomy. Smith-Petersen osteotomies can produce 5 to 10 degrees of correction per level, while decancellation osteotomy can produce 30 degrees of lordosis in a single level. Bleeding can be profuse in using the decancellation osteotomy, and the surgical team should be in constant coordination with their anesthesiologist to manage volume replacement intraoperatively and postoperatively.

■ Coronal imbalance is often associated with rotational deformity and clinically with trunk shift. Radiographs should be analyzed to determine whether the imbalance is secondary to an angulation within the fusion mass (possibly requiring anterior osteotomies and revision posterior fusion) or outside of the fusion mass (possibly manageable with an extension posterior fusion).

■ Junctional deformity (the adding-on phenomenon) is typically encountered when inappropriate fusion levels are chosen, and deformity occurs proximal or distal to a fusion. Typically, posterior-only fusions can be used to extend fusion from the existing fusion mass to stabilize and correct the added-on segments. Care must be taken to maintain coronal and sagittal balance.

■ Adjacent segment degeneration is thought to be secondary to increased stresses transferred below and above the fusion mass. There is preliminary evidence to suggest that MRI assessments of discs below long fusions show signs of degeneration, but strict clinical correlation and alteration in outcomes are lacking. If preoperative studies demonstrate degeneration of segments below the planned lowest vertebra of a fusion, consideration of further degeneration at that level and inclusion of it into the index fusion should be made.

■ Crankshaft deformity after posterior-only spinal fusions in young patients can be definitively avoided by performing combined anterior and PSFs. There is limited evidence to suggest that use of rigid segmental instrumentation with pedicle screws in posterior-only spine fusions could be able to overcome the crankshaft phenomenon in patients who have surgery prior to their peak growth velocity, but large studies have not yet validated this observation. Surgical goals are to arrest the deformity and to restore physiologic coronal and sagittal balance.

■ Painful instrumentation is a diagnosis of exclusion and should be applied only after infection, pseudarthrosis, ongoing degeneration or stenosis, and other pain generators have been ruled out. Peri-implant injections of local anesthetics can help to confirm the diagnosis, as can tenderness to gentle palpation over prominent implants. Definitive treatment in the setting of a solid fusion is implant removal and otherwise requires revision of instrumentation.

■ Infection must be treated aggressively in the postoperative setting. Early infections are managed with irrigation and debridement, implants being maintained if needed for stability or maintenance of deformity correction. Late infections can allow removal of implants if no pseudarthroses are present, but spinal stability must be maintained if the infection is to be definitively eradicated.

■ Complication rates for revision deformity surgery range from 33% to 60%, and patients who require these surgeries tend to have more pain, lower SRS scores, and poorer self-image. Revision surgical outcomes can be good when care is taken to achieve sagittal balance and patient goals emphasize restoring function and limiting pain symptoms.

Illustrative Case Presentations

CASE 1. Pseudarthrosis

A 53-year-old woman presented with 1 year of back and bilateral leg pain. She had previously undergone posterior lumbar decompression and fusion along with combined anterior and posterior spine instrumented fusion from T12 to S1 and from L4 to S1, respectively, for spinal stenosis and scoliosis (Fig. 25-1A). Lumbar stiffness, first noted at 1 year from surgery, ultimately was diagnosed as an L3-4 pseudarthrosis (Fig. 25-1B), and the patient was counseled that revision surgery was necessary. Medical and anesthesia consults were obtained, and a full preoperative workup was completed.

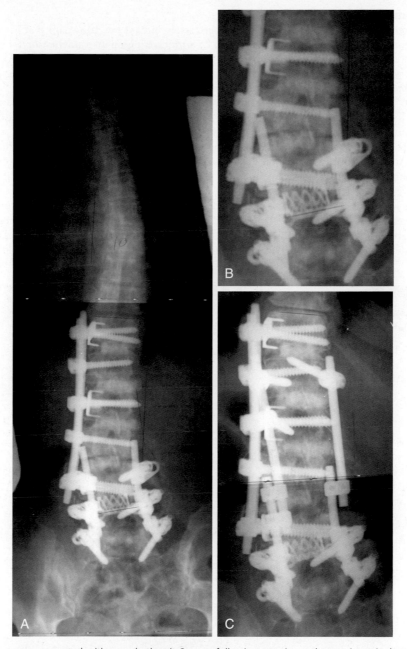

Figure 25-1. A 53-year-old woman presented with pseudarthrosis 3 years following anterior and posterior spinal arthrodesis for scoliosis. **A,** Preoperative anteroposterior full-length radiograph at presentation showing good coronal alignment. **B,** Preoperative anteroposterior close-up view at the L3-4 level illustrating transverse lucency of pseudarthrosis. **C,** Postoperative anteroposterior radiograph illustrating revision instrumentation and healing of pseudarthrosis.

At 3 years and 1 month after her index procedure, she returned to the operating room for exploration of the fusion mass and revision fusion. Because neither progressive nor significant deformity was present at the pseudarthrosis site, the decision was made that osteotomies would not be needed for the revision surgery. After removal of a portion of the instrumentation, an obvious pseudarthrosis was confirmed at L3-4. The pseudarthrosis site was debrided from the posterior exposure, and posterior elements were debrided of scar and soft tissue from L1 to S1, excluding the site of the prior decompression. A revision posterolateral spinal fusion with instrumentation was then performed from L1 to S1, with placement of pedicle screws from L1 to L4 and attachment to prior instrumentation to S1 (Fig. 25-1C). At this time, decortication of the bony fusion surfaces was completed, and these were packed with autogenous bone graft taken from the left iliac crest. To further increase the probability of fusion at the pseudarthrosis site, an EBI bone stimulator was also implanted, with electrodes applied to the posterolateral fusion graft. The patient had no adverse events postoperatively and was completely asymptomatic by 6 months postoperatively from the revision surgery. She underwent elective removal of the EBI stimulator 10 months following the revision surgery and remains symptom free 2 years after the first revision surgery.

CASE 2. Flat-Back Syndrome

A 34-year-old man presented with a 4- to 5-year history of progressively intense low back pain that interfered with his activities of daily living. He had undergone posterior spine fusion from T8 to L5 with Harrington instrumentation for scoliosis 18 years previously. Radiographs at presentation were notable for lumbar hypolordosis, measured to be 18 degrees (Fig. 25-2A). He was given the diagnosis of flat-back syndrome and was counseled that revision surgery was required to restore alignment and sagittal balance. Medical and anesthesia consults were obtained, and a full preoperative workup was completed.

Our surgical plan was to remove the Harrington instrumentation, explore the fusion mass, perform extension-producing osteotomies, and reinstrument with extension of the fusion mass to the pelvis. By utilizing the old scar and continuing distally, the spine was exposed from T8 to the sacrum posteriorly out to the transverse processes, Harrington instrumentation was identified, and the distal portion was removed. No pseudarthrosis was identified in the fusion mass. Pedicle screws were placed bilaterally at L1, L2, L4, and S1 and on the right at L5. An iliac screw was placed on the left side to augment the distal fixation. A posterior lumbar fusion was then completed at L5-S1 by using a carbon cage and local autograft bone. At this point, a posterior lumbar transpedicular decancellation closing-wedge osteotomy was performed at the L3 level, and the table was placed in extension to close the osteotomy site. The wound was irrigated, bony surfaces were prepared with a high-speed burr, and the remainder of the instrumentation was placed and tightened. A bone stimulator was placed just prior to closure, owing to the patient's preoperative history of smoking. His postoperative course was uneventful, and his lumbar spine was restored to 63 degrees of lordosis (Fig. 25-2B). He returned to the operating room 2.5 years later for removal of his bone stimulator. He remains without complaints 7.5 years after his index revision surgery.

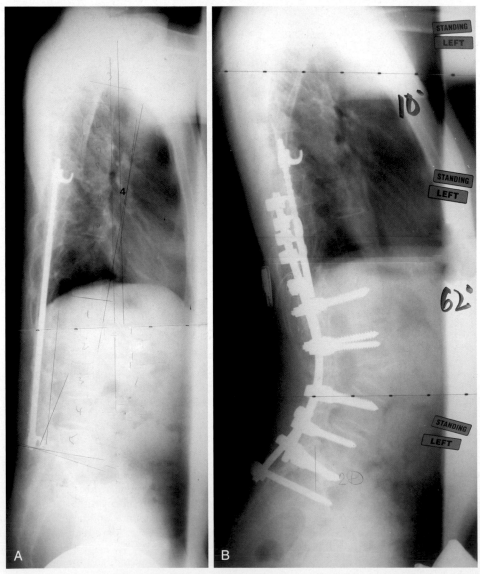

Figure 25-2. A 34-year-old man presented with painful flat-back deformity 18 years after posterior spine fusion with Harrington instrumentation. **A,** Preoperative lateral full-length radiograph demonstrating loss of lumbar lordosis (L1-S1 measured 18 degrees by Cobb method). **B,** Postoperative lateral full-length radiograph demonstrating restoration of lumbar lordosis (L1-S1 measured 63 degrees by Cobb method) and sagittal alignment.

CASE 3. Junctional Deformity

An 81-year-old woman presented with the complaint that she had pain and deformity in her upper back in the 8 months since her last surgery. She had had four spine surgeries in the past, beginning with two posterior lumbar decompression and fusion procedures. These did not control her mild scoliosis deformity (18 degrees), and lumbar deformity progressed postoperatively from the second procedure to 40 degrees. She was treated with staged posterior and anterior spinal fusions from T9 to S1 and from T12 to S1, respectively (Fig. 25-3A). Radiographs and a CT scan demonstrated T8 compression fracture and acute kyphosis proximal to the prior instrumented fusion (Fig. 25-3B). She was given the diagnosis of junctional deformity and counseled that she needed revision posterior spine fusion to extend the fusion to T2 and an extension osteotomy through the compression fracture to allow deformity correction.

She was evaluated by medical and anesthesiology consultants preoperatively, was cleared by both, and completed full preoperative surgical evaluation. Owing to the osteoporosis that was noted on her preoperative radiographs, a decision was made to use thoracic pedicle screws and to augment the fusion with OP-1 putty and other allograft extenders for the local bone graft. The spine was exposed from T2 to T11 out to the transverse processes, and prior instrumentation was visualized. Facetectomies were then performed from T2-3 down to T7-8, and pedicle screws were placed in the thoracic levels. The proximal extent of the prior instrumentation was loosened, and T9 pedicle screws were removed. T8 vertebral osteotomy was then performed. The wound was irrigated, and proximal rods were placed and connected to the distal rods by using parallel connectors (Fig. 25-3C). Bony surfaces were prepared for fusion with a high-speed burr, and a combination of OP-1 putty, local bone, and allograft was placed in the intended fusion bed. The wound was closed in layers over a drain. The patient tolerated the procedure well, had no immediate postoperative complications, and is without symptoms 3 months postoperatively.

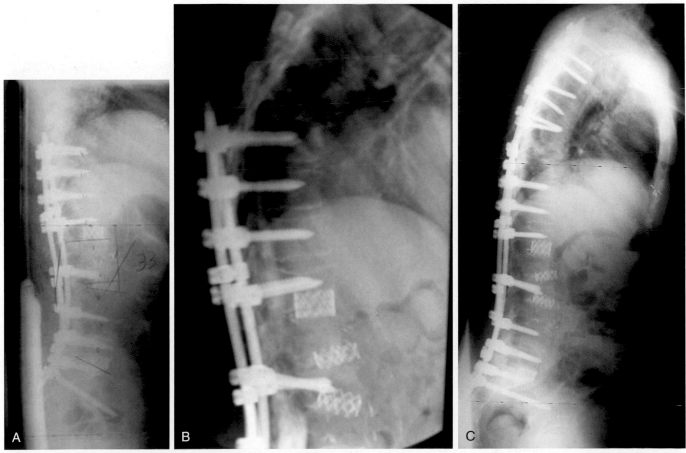

Figure 25-3. An 81-year-old woman with osteoporosis presented with compression fracture and junctional deformity 8 months following revision anterior and posterior surgery. **A,** Full-length lateral radiograph preceding compression fracture. **B,** Scout image from CT examination showing a compression fracture of T8 vertebral body. **C,** Postoperative lateral full-length radiograph illustrating deformity correction, restoration of sagittal balance, and revision instrumentation utilizing thoracic pedicle screws.

CASE 4. Adjacent Segment Degeneration (Junctional Degeneration)

A 58-year-old woman presented with complaints of pain in her back for several years and new radicular pain in her right leg. She had undergone Harrington rod instrumented posterior spinal fusion from T6 to L3 for adolescent idiopathic scoliosis 15 years prior. She had had intermittent back pain since the time of the operation that was tolerable, but with the new leg pain, she sought medical attention. Radiographs at presentation demonstrated a fusion mass down to the L4 level and lateral listhesis of L4 on L5 of approximately 1.5 cm (Fig. 25-4A). A myelogram demonstrated central, lateral, and foraminal stenosis at the L4-5 level (Fig. 25-4B). She was given the diagnosis of distal junctional degeneration and associated spinal stenosis and was counseled that she would need revision surgery.

After preoperative assessment and clearances by internal medicine and anesthesiology, the patient submitted to anterior and posterior procedures under a single anesthesia. A thoracolumbar incision and a retroperitoneal dissection technique were used to expose the lumbar spine with the patient in a left lateral decubitus position. Segmental vessels were identified, dissected free, and ligated prior to performing complete discectomies at L4-5 and L5-S1. Allograft-filled titanium mesh Harms cages were then placed at each of these levels. The spontaneous ankylosis of L3-4 was then taken down, complete discectomy was performed, and the disc space was filled with allograft. Wounds were irrigated and closed in layers, and the patient was repositioned for the second procedure. Utilizing the prior posterior scar, the spine was exposed from the thoracolumbar spine to the sacrum out to the transverse processes. The Harrington instrumentation was identified, and the distal extent of this implant was removed. Pedicle and iliac screws were placed distally, and claw hooks were placed proximally. Laminectomy of L4 and extensive decompression of L4-5 was completed. Bony surfaces for fusion were prepared with a high-speed burr; bone graft was placed; and quarter-inch ISOLA rods were placed, connected to the other implants, and tightened (Fig. 25-4C). Wounds were irrigated and closed in layers. The patient tolerated the procedures well, had no immediate postoperative complications, and remains without complaints 2.5 years postoperatively.

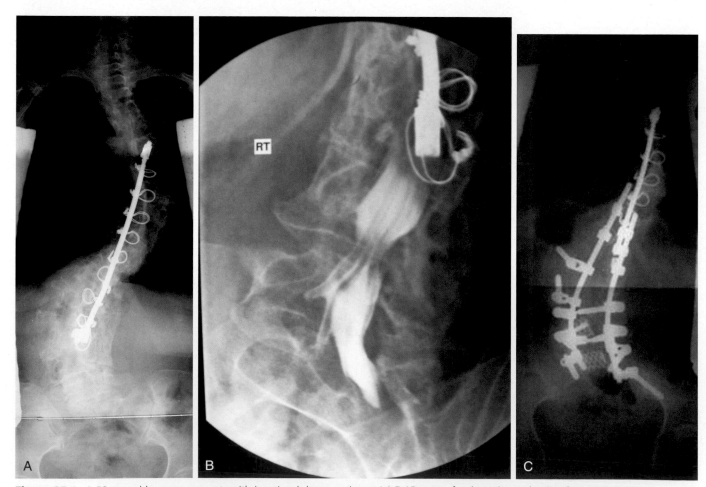

Figure 25-4. A 58-year-old woman presents with junctional degeneration at L4-5 15 years after long thoracolumbar fusion. **A,** Preoperative anteroposterior full-length radiograph at presentation showing listhesis and disc space narrowing at L4-5 and prior Harrington instrumentation. **B,** Preoperative myelogram image demonstrating central and foraminal stenosis at the L4-5 level. **C,** Postoperative anteroposterior full-length radiograph illustrating revision fusion and instrumentation connected to prior hardware and extending to pelvis. L4-5 laminectomy and bond canal decompression are not visible, owing to fusion mass and instrumentation.

CASE 5. Crankshaft Deformity

A 15-year-old boy presented with progressive spine deformity and difficulty breathing for the past few years. He was a full-term boy who was noted to have scoliosis early in life and had a poorly described muscular dystrophy diagnosed later in life. At the age of 8 years (Fig. 25-5A), he underwent posterior spine fusion for a 63-degree thoracic curve with Luque instrumentation. Five years later, he was treated for provisional diagnosis of the adding-on phenomenon (junctional deformity), and he underwent surgery for instrumentation removal and revision to control the proximal and distal deformities. At presentation, he had significant decompensation coronally, with a plumbline from the occiput 8 cm to the left of the gluteal fold, the T1 plumbline in midline, and the T8 plumbline 8 cm to the right of the gluteal fold. Radiographs that were brought with the patient demonstrated a 65-degree curve from T3 to L2 with Luque instrumentation in place (Fig. 25-5B), while current films showed this curve to be 100 degrees with an apparent solid posterior fusion (Fig. 25-5C). The clinical and radiographic findings were detailed to the patient and his parents, and the diagnosis and pathology of crankshaft deformity were explained. The opinion was given that optimal treatment would require revision surgery with osteotomies for deformity correction and fusion of the spine both anteriorly and posteriorly to prevent continued or recurrent curve progression.

The patient submitted to pediatric and anesthesia evaluations, pulmonary function testing, electrocardiography, and echocardiogram analysis. Pulmonary function tests revealed significant restrictive disease and a vital capacity of 26% of predicted. Electrocardiograms and echocardiograms demonstrated no change from prior examinations. Blood gas assessment was acceptable, with no evidence of retention of carbon dioxide. The patient and his parents were given informed consent documents with risks including but not limited to infection, pseudarthrosis, instrumentation-related problems, respiratory complications including tracheostomy, prolonged intubation and ventilator dependency, residual deformity, the possible need for multiple future surgical procedures, and death. He underwent combined anterior and posterior spinal fusion surgeries, including posterior osteotomies and posterior segmental instrumentation from T3 to L4 (Fig. 25-5D). He tolerated the procedure well and was discharged from the hospital to home on postoperative day 7. He has been followed by his local physician (the patient lives at quite a distance from our institution), has been doing well, and remains without complaints 5 years postoperatively.

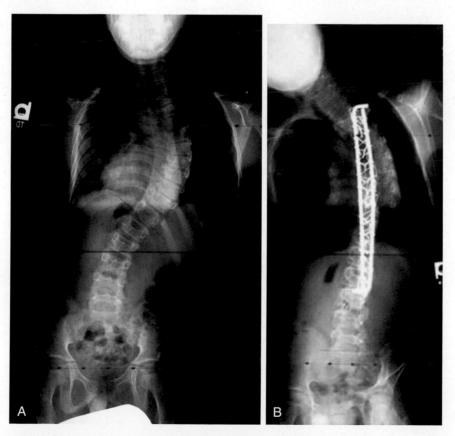

Figure 25-5. A 15-year-old boy presented with crankshaft phenomenon 7 years after index posterior spine fusion. **A,** Anteroposterior radiograph at age 8 years prior to any surgical intervention. The thoracic curve measured 63 degrees by the Cobb method. **B,** Anteroposterior radiograph at age 13 years prior to revision surgery for presumed adding-on phenomenon. With Luque instrumentation in place, the thoracic curve measured 65 degrees by the Cobb method.

Continued

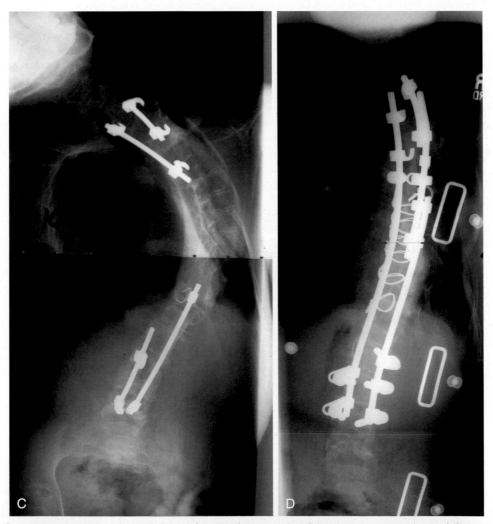

Figure 25-5, cont'd. C, Anteroposterior radiograph at presentation demonstrating discontinuous compression and distraction instrumentation. The thoracic deformity has progressed in the interval to 100 degrees by the Cobb method. **D,** Postoperative anteroposterior full-length radiograph illustrating revision segmental instrumentation and restoration of coronal balance. The thoracic curve measured 42 degrees by the Cobb method.

CASE 6. Failed Implants

A 19-year-old woman presented with the complaint of back pain that she had been experiencing since being involved in a motor vehicle accident 2 years previously. She had suffered multiple injuries, including a lumbar spine fracture that was originally missed but several months later was treated with posterior spinal fusion from T10 to L4. Pain in the vicinity of the proximal extent of the implants, in addition to motion through the intended fusion segment with flexion and extension lateral views, led to the diagnosis of painful implants and implant failure (Fig. 25-6A). She was counseled that she required revision surgery to achieve bony stability of the injured portion of her spine and that this would require anterior and posterior spinal fusion procedures.

After preoperative assessment and clearances by internal medicine and anesthesia, the patient submitted to anterior and posterior procedures under a single anesthesia. The anterior procedure was performed through a thoracoabdominal retropleural and retroperitoneal approach to expose the T11-L4 disc spaces. Complete discectomies were performed, allograft was placed within the prepared disc spaces, and femoral ring structural allograft was used at the L3-4 interspace with a blocking screw. Wounds were irrigated and closed in layers, and the patient was repositioned for the second procedure. By utilizing the prior scar and continuing proximally and distally, exposure of the spine was completed out to the transverse processes. The prior instrumentation was removed, the fusion mass was explored, and pseudarthrosis was identified. Pedicle screws were placed proximally and distally, and the pseudarthrosis sites were debrided and prepared for revision fusion with a high-speed burr. The remainder of the T10-L4 fusion bed was also prepared with a high-speed burr; bone graft was placed; and quarter-inch ISOLA instrumentation was placed, connected to the pedicle screws, and tightened (Fig. 25-6B). Two sublaminar wires were placed proximally, and the wound was irrigated and closed in layers over a drain. The patient tolerated the procedure well, had no difficulties in the immediate postoperative period, and remains without complaints 9 years postoperatively.

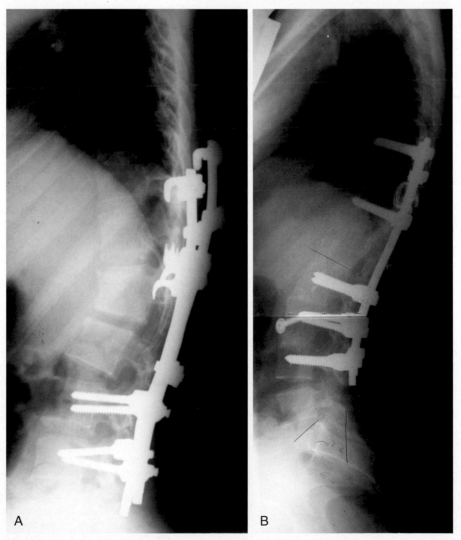

Figure 25-6. A 19-year-old woman presented 2 years after a car accident with failed instrumentation. **A,** Preoperative lateral radiograph illustrating proximal instrumentation disengagement from the posterior spinal elements. **B,** Postoperative lateral radiograph showing healed anterior and posterior fusion masses, corrected sagittal plane balance, and revision instrumentation with thoracic pedicle screws.

REFERENCES

Aaro S, Ohlen G: The effect of Harrington instrumentation on the sagittal configuration and mobility of the spine in scoliosis. Spine 1983;8:570–575.

Allen BL Jr, Ferguson RL: The Galveston technique of pelvic fixation with L-rod instrumentation of the spine. Spine 1984;9: 388–394.

Berven S, Kao H, Deviren V, et al: Treatment of thoracic pseudarthrosis in the adult: Is combined surgery necessary? Clin Orthop Relat Res 2003;411:25–31.

Boachie-Adjei O: Role and technique of and eggshell osteotomies/vertebral column resections. Instr Course Lect 2006;55:583–589.

Burton DC, Asher MA, Lai SM: Scoliosis correction maintenance in skeletally immature patients with idiopathic scoliosis: Is anterior fusion really necessary? Spine 2000;25:61–68.

Eck KR, Bridwell KH, Ungacta FF, et al: Complications and results of long adult deformity fusions down to L4, L5, and the sacrum. Spine 2001;26:E182–E192.

Hamill CL, Bridwell KH, Lenke LG, et al: Posterior arthrodesis in the skeletally immature patient: Assessing the risk for crankshaft: Is an open triradiate cartilage the answer? Spine 1997;22:1343–1351.

Heinig CF: Egshell procedure. In Luque ER (ed): Segmental Spinal Instrumentation. Thorofare, NJ: Slack, 1984, pp 221–230.

Kesling KL, Lonstein JE, Denis F, et al: The crankshaft phenomenon after posterior spinal arthrodesis for congenital scoliosis: A review of 54 patients. Spine 2003;28:267–271.

King HA, Moe JH, Bradford DS, Winter RB: The selection of fusion levels in thoracic idiopathic scoliosis. J Bone Joint Surg Am 1983; 65:1302–1313.

Lagrone MO: Loss of lumbar lordosis: A complication of spinal fusion for scoliosis. Orthop Clin North Am 1988;19:383–393.

Law WA: Osteotomy of the spine. Clin Orthop Relat Res 1969;66: 70–76.

Lee CS, Nachemson AL: The crankshaft phenomenon after posterior Harrington fusion in skeletally immature patients with thoracic or thoracolumbar idiopathic scoliosis followed to maturity. Spine 1997; 22:58–67.

Lenke LG, Bridwell KH, O'Brien MF, et al: Recognition and treatment of the proximal thoracic curve in adolescent idiopathic scoliosis treated with Cotrel-Dubousset instrumentation. Spine 1994;19: 1589–1597.

Lonstein JE: Salvage surgery. In Frymoyer JW, Wiesel SW (eds): The Adult and Pediatric Spine, 3rd ed. Philadelphia: Lippincott Williams and Wilkins, 2004, pp 505–525.

Lowe TG, Kasten MD: An analysis of sagittal curves and balance after Cotrel-Dubousset instrumentation for kyphosis secondary to Scheuermann's disease: A review of 32 patients. Spine 1994;19: 1680–1685.

Luk KD, Lee FB, Leong JC, Hsu LC: The effect on the lumbosacral spine of long spinal fusion for idiopathic scoliosis: A minimum 10-year follow-up. Spine 1987;12:996–1000.

McMaster MJ: A technique for lumbar spinal osteotomy in ankylosing spondylitis. J Bone Joint Surg Br 1985;67:204–210.

Papagelopoulos PJ, Klassen RA, Peterson HA, Dekutoski MB: Surgical treatment of Scheuermann's disease with segmental compression instrumentation. Clin Orthop Relat Res 2001:139–149.

Roberto RF, Lonstein JE, Winter RB, Denis F: Curve progression in Risser stage 0 or 1 patients after posterior spinal fusion for idiopathic scoliosis. J Pediatr Orthop 1997;17:718–725.

Sanders JO, Little DG, Richards BS: Prediction of the crankshaft phenomenon by peak height velocity. Spine 1997;22:1352–1356; discussion 1356–1357.

Sink EL, Newton PO, Mubarak SJ, Wenger DR: Maintenance of sagittal plane alignment after surgical correction of spinal deformity in patients with cerebral palsy. Spine 2003;28:1396–1403.

Smith-Petersen MN, Larson CB, Aufranc OE: Osteotomy of the spine for correction of flexion deformity in rheumatoid arthritis. Clin Orthop Relat Res 1969;66:6–9.

Suk SI, Lee SM, Chung ER, et al: Determination of distal fusion level with segmental pedicle screw fixation in single thoracic idiopathic scoliosis. Spine 2003;28:484–491.

Tveit P, Daggfeldt K, Hetland S, Thorstensson A: Erector spinae lever arm length variations with changes in spinal curvature. Spine 1994; 19:199–204.

Weatherley C, Jaffray D, Terry A: Vascular complications associated with osteotomy in ankylosing spondylitis: A report of two cases. Spine 1988;13:43–46.

Yang SH, Chen PQ: Proximal kyphosis after short posterior fusion for thoracolumbar scoliosis. Clin Orthop Relat Res 2003:152–158.

SUGGESTED READINGS

Balderston RA, Albert TJ, McIntosh T, et al: Magnetic resonance imaging analysis of lumbar disc changes below scoliosis fusions: A prospective study. Spine 1998;23:54–58; discussion 59.

Prospective study to evaluate the disks below long fusions for scoliosis terminating in the mid to lower lumbar spine, with outcomes of clinical pain symptoms and MRI grade of disc. At a 3-year follow-up from surgery, up to one third of patients demonstrated disc space narrowing and herniated discs one or two levels below their fusions, and up to 50% had decreased signal intensity on T2-weighted MRI. Patients with back or leg pain had worse imaging outcomes.

Boachie-Adjei O, Girardi FP: Surgical treatment of rigid sagittal plane deformity. In Margulies YJ (ed): Spine State of the Art Reviews, vol 12. Philadelphia: Hanley and Belfus, 1998, pp 65–72.

A review of the history of the eggshell procedure, indications for the osteotomy, surgical technique, and typical postoperative management of the patient.

Boachie-Adjei O, Girardi FP, Hall J: Posterior lumbar decancellation osteotomy. In Margulies JY, Aebi M, Farcy J-PC (eds): Revision Spine Surgery. St. Louis: Mosby, 1999, pp 568–575.

A review of the history of the decancellation osteotomy procedure, indications, preoperative planning, anesthesia, positioning, surgical technique, postoperative management, and complications.

Burton DC, Asher MA, Lai SM: Scoliosis correction maintenance in skeletally immature patients with idiopathic scoliosis: Is anterior fusion really necessary? Spine 2000;25:61–68.

Retrospective review of 18 Risser stage 0 patients, 7 with open triradiate cartilages, treated with isolated posterior fusion and assessed at follow-up for crankshaft phenomenon (progression of deformity of 10 degrees). One patient (with sublaminar wiring used as distal fixation) showed progressive deformity, but all others were controlled with segmental instrumentation. The authors suggest that anterior surgery can be avoided in young patients with the use of stiff segmental instrumentation constructs.

Buttermann GR, Glazer PA, Hu SS, Bradford DS: Revision of failed lumbar fusions: A comparison of anterior autograft and allograft. Spine 1997;22:2748–2755.

Retrospective study of patients treated with revision anterior-posterior spinal fusion, stratified according to use of femoral ring allografts or tricortical iliac autografts. Although numbers were limited, patients who received allografts used less pain medication, showed greater functional improvement, and had improved patient-perceived "success."

Dubousset J, Herring JA, Shufflebarger H: The crankshaft phenomenon. J Pediatr Orthop 1989;9:541–550.

A classic article describing the crankshaft phenomenon in 40 patients who received posterior spine fusions prior to Risser stage 1. Continued anterior growth of the spine was identified as a causative factor for the deformity, and anterior-posterior combined surgery in the younger patient population was suggested as a preventive measure.

Emami A, Deviren V, Berven S, et al: Outcome and complications of long fusions to the sacrum in adult spine deformity: Luque-Galveston, combined iliac and sacral screws, and sacral fixation. Spine 2002; 27:776–786.

A retrospective study comparing differing instrumentation techniques to the sacropelvis with radiographic, clinical, and Scoliosis Research Society outcomes assessed. Revision sugery was as safe as primary surgery but adversely affected self-image scores. Sagittal balance is a primary factor for success, and pelvic screws are recommended for long fusions unless anterior column support and triangulated screws are used at the lumbosacral junction.

Kim YJ, Bridwell KH, Lenke LG, et al: Pseudarthosis in primary fusions for adult idiopathic scoliosis: Incidence, risk factors, and outcome analysis. Spine 2005;30:468–474.

Retrospective study of primary surgery for adult idiopathic scoliosis to assess pseudarthrosis with radiologic and clinical outcomes. Pseudarthrosis rate was 17% and was more likely in patients older than 55 years, fusions of more than 12 segments, and fusions at the thoracolumbar junction, thoracolumbar kyphosis 20 degrees or greater being an independent negative predictor.

Lagrone MO, Bradford DS, Moe JH, et al: Treatment of symptomatic flatback after spinal fusion. J Bone Joint Surg Am 1988;70:569–580.

A retrospective case series of patients treated with osteotomies for sagittal plane imbalance assessed for radiographic and clinical outcomes. Sixty percent of patients had complications, and 50% reported being satisfied. Pseudarthrosis correlated with failure to restore sagittal balance, and combined anterior-posterior revision surgeries resulted in better maintenance of correction.

Lapp MA, Bridwell KH, Lenke LG, et al: Long-term complications in adult spinal deformity patients having combined surgery: A comparison of primary to revision patients. Spine 2001;26:973–983.

A minimum 2-year follow-up consecutive case series of anterior-posterior combined surgeries stratified by primary or revision status and assessed for complication and radiographic and clinical outcomes. Patients who underwent revision surgery had similar complication rates and better satisfaction but lower function scores postoperatively, possibly owing to relative preoperative debility.

Linville DA, Bridwell KH, Lenke LG, et al: Complications in the adult spinal deformity patient having combined surgery: Does revision increase the risk? Spine 1999;24:355–363.

A short-term follow-up (within 6 months of surgery) consecutive case series of anterior-posterior combined surgeries stratified by primary or revision status and assessed for major and minor complications. Complication rates were similar in the two groups. Nutrition appears to be important in preventing wound problems and infection, and the authors advocate total parenteral nutrition in patients who are thought to be at increased risk for wound problems.

Rinella A, Bridwell K, Kim Y, et al: Late complications of adult idiopathic scoliosis primary fusions to L4 and above: The effect of age and distal fusion level. Spine 2004;29:318–325.

A retrospective study of adult idiopathic scoliosis stratified by age, lowest instrumented vertebra, complications, and clinical outcomes, including the Scoliosis Research Society questionnaire. Higher rates of transition syndrome were seen with LIV at L3-4 than in higher LIV levels, but there was no change in pseudarthrosis rate, and there was no change in complications with age; SRS scores were lower when pseudarthrosis or revision surgeries were required.

Sanders JO, Little DG, Richards BS: Prediction of the crankshaft phenomenon by peak height velocity. Spine 1997;22:1352–1356; discussion 1356–1357.

A retrospective review of 40 patients who were managed with posterior spine fusion and Risser stage 0, stratified by open or closed triradiate cartilages and assessed for crankshaft deformity (10 degrees of progression) as an outcome. All patients with closed triradiates were beyond their peak height velocity, and only one of these patients demonstrated crankshafting. A recommendation was made for isolated posterior fusions to be performed after the peak height velocity has been reached.

Throckmorton TW, Hilibrand AS, Mencio GA, et al: The impact of adjacent level disc degeneration on health status outcomes following lumbar fusion. Spine 2003;28:2546–2550.

A retrospective review of patients who received limited lumbar fusions, stratified by fusion ending adjacent to an MRI diagnosed "normal" or "degenerated" disk. Patients were evaluated at a minimum 2-year follow-up with the SF-36 instrument. The authors found no difference in any of the eight SF-36 subgroups in the patients who were fused adjacent to a "degenerated" disk.

Voos K, Boachie-Adjei O, Rawlins BA: Multiple vertebral osteotomies in the treatment of rigid adult spine deformities. Spine 2001;26: 526–533.

A retrospective review of patients undergoing revision deformity surgery including osteotomies, assessed by radiography, clinical evaluation, and Scoliosis Research Society questionnaires. Use of osteotomies carried a 33% complication rate but provided good correction, balance, and patient satisfaction.

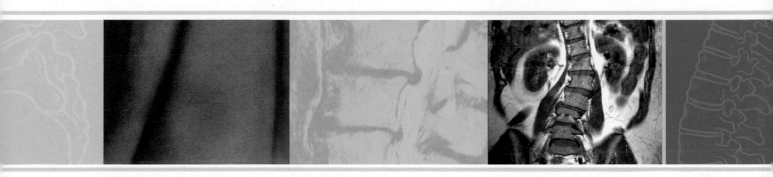

Perioperative Considerations

CHAPTER 26

Anesthesia for Spine Surgery and Management of Blood Loss

GEORGE J. SPESSOT *and* ANDREW D. ROSENBERG

PREOPERATIVE EVALUATION

Patients who undergo complex spine surgery face significant physiologic stress. Large blood loss, fluid shifts, and stress on the cardiovascular and pulmonary systems require that patients be properly evaluated prior to surgery to determine their physical status. The purpose of a thorough preoperative evaluation is to identify the patient's concurrent medical problems, address them, and optimize the patient's condition with the hopes of decreasing perioperative exacerbation of the coexisting disease and thus decreasing morbidity and mortality. In addition, special attention is given to those organ systems that could be affected by the corrective operation itself. Although the organ systems that are most commonly involved are the cardiovascular and pulmonary systems, evaluation must be thorough and must be tailored to the patient's individual medical state. Consultations and requests for optimization from other medical specialties are made as indicated, and additional testing is done on the basis of the patient's risk factors, the factors specific to the operation, and the patient's functional capacity.

Cardiac System

Patients are risk stratified for preoperative cardiac testing on the basis of their medical history. In addition to baseline studies such as electrocardiography, other studies might be indicated to evaluate the stability of the cardiac patient who is undergoing corrective spine surgery, in accordance with the American College of Cardiology/American Heart Association Guidelines on Perioperative Cardiovascular Evaluation for Noncardiac Surgery. A history of hypertension, angina pectoris, myocardial infarction, atherosclerotic heart disease, shortness of breath, congestive heart failure, or arrhythmia needs to be elicited, as it could prompt further testing. Consultation with cardiologists might be indicated on the basis of the patient's history to obtain the indicated test. An echocardiogram is an easily

tolerated, noninvasive procedure that can identify a spectrum of cardiac structural and functional abnormalities, such as valvular disease, effusions, and wall motion abnormalities, which might need to be addressed prior to corrective spine surgery. However, a resting echocardiogram is not a predictor of the ability of the heart to endure stress. A physical or chemical stress test might be indicated preoperatively, as the patient's physical status allows, to assess the exercise tolerance of the patient, as the operation is a "stress test" by itself. Stress echocardiography may also be performed. Data exist that the administration of perioperative beta blockers for cardioprotection may be indicated in the cardiac patient and perhaps even in the "suspected" cardiac patient undergoing noncardiac surgery. Mangano and colleagues demonstrated that beta-blocker administration instituted preoperatively and continued through the perioperative period was associated with decreased morbidity and mortality. Some in the medical field think the salutary effect of beta blockade so important that its effect is being monitored by researchers who study long-term outcome and complications in patients undergoing surgery. While some issues have arisen in the reported study and it is being repeated by others, there is most likely an advantage to the perioperative administration of beta blockers in high-risk patients who do not have contraindications to their administration. The patient's internist or cardiologist should use the preoperative evaluation period as the time to initiate the administration of these drug-eluting medications, if indicated. Patients who have had coronary artery stents placed in the past might present for corrective spine surgery. These patients might be taking potent antiplatelet medications such as clopidogrel (Plavix), which, as a result of its intended action, can result in significant intraoperative bleeding. Current thought indicates that patients should discontinue these platelet aggregation inhibitors at least 5 days prior to surgery, although some consensus studies suggest discontinuation 1 week prior to surgery. Because recommendations exist as to the amount of time that patients should remain on these medications following the particular type of stent placed, their discontinuation should be made in conjunction with the patient's cardiologist. In addition to their use following stent placement, platelet inhibitors have been administered to patients with cerebrovascular disease. If a patient is taking these medications, that could indicate that significant carotid or cerebrovascular disease might be present; these conditions would have to be evaluated and optimized as well. Additionally, consideration must be given to the potential postoperative cardiac changes that can occur following corrective thoracic procedures, especially in severe scoliosis.

Pulmonary System

Perhaps the organ system with the greatest potential alteration, the pulmonary system deserves the most attention preoperatively, intraoperatively, and postoperatively. Changes due to the disease process may be present within the lung parenchyma, as is seen, for example, in rheumatoid arthritis, with chronic diffuse interstitial pulmonary fibrosis, rheumatoid nodules, and cysts with honeycombing. Patients may present before surgery suffering from asthma or chronic obstructive pulmonary disease. These conditions need to be addressed and treated as necessary. Aggressive bronchodilator therapy may be indicated preoperatively. As the average weight of the general population increases, associated comorbidities such as sleep apnea become more prevalent among those who present for corrective spine surgery. This is commonly seen in the morbidly obese, and the administration of sedation and/or analgesia can result in airway obstruction and rapid desaturation. The patient might have to be placed on continuous positive airway pressure masks in the postoperative period, initiated as early as immediately following emergence from general anesthesia.

The musculoskeletal structural deformities that are to be corrected with surgery often compromise pulmonary function, and this must be addressed in the preoperative period. This is seen more frequently in patients who are undergoing corrective surgery for scoliosis secondary to a neuromuscular disorder. Patients who have muscle weakness and imbalance can have a higher incidence of aspiration pneumonia because of their inability to clear secretions effectively. Clinically, these patients may exhibit signs of respiratory insufficiency, such as baseline hypoxemia, tachypnea, use of accessory muscles, and coughing. Preoperative evaluation may include respiratory therapy, optimization of lung function with incentive spirometry, and identifying and treating any reversible component of bronchospasm. Preoperative testing may include pulmonary function studies, which can be valuable in the identification and reversal of bronchospasm. Additionally, forced vital capacity is also measured and is an excellent predictor of the need for postoperative ventilatory support. Generally, if vital capacity is greater than 70% of the predicted value,

the potential need for postoperative ventilatory support is low; if it measures between 35% and 70%, there is a moderate likelihood that the patient will need support; if it measures lower than 35% of predicted, then the chances are high that the patient will require ventilatory support. If there is a coexisting neuromuscular disorder, such as Duchenne's muscular dystrophy or Friedreich's ataxia, and the forced vital capacity is less than 30% of predicted, then the potential risks of the operation regarding postoperative ventilatory ability could outweigh the benefits, and serious consideration should be given as to whether or not the surgery can actually be performed safely for the patient. Other alterations in pulmonary lung function are decreased total lung capacity, decreased functional residual capacity, decreased residual volume, decreased chest wall compliance, increased pulmonary vascular resistance, and a ventilation/perfusion imbalance. Another condition that presents with potentially severe respiratory problems is Morquio syndrome, in which anatomic structural abnormalities compromise pulmonary function. In addition, these patients may present with markedly abnormal body habitus and difficult or impossible airways.

Other aggravating factors include history of smoking and coexisting asthma. However, cessation of smoking as little as 24 hours prior to surgery has been demonstrated to have beneficial effects. All patients are encouraged to stop smoking. Baseline arterial blood gas levels may be useful and can be used as a guide for postoperative respiratory management.

Airway

Evaluation of the airway is a high priority in the preoperative evaluation. Normal anatomic variations in the airway are considered, but since involvement of the airway in the spinal structural disease processes can be variable, it deserves special attention. Mouth opening is evaluated, as it can be limited by temporomandibular joint involvement with some disease processes. The normal three-fingerbreadth mouth opening is diminished, and intubating the patient can be problematic. Thyromental distance is also evaluated, and a receded chin might indicate a hypoplastic mandible, which results from early closure of the mandibular ossification centers. Usually, this is accompanied by protrusion of the upper teeth and an overbite appearance, and this may also be a warning sign of a difficult intubation. Rheumatic involvement of the cricoarytenoid joint is common, and it is clinically manifested by dysphagia, hoarseness, laryngeal tenderness, inspiratory stridor, and dyspnea. Since patients with this condition can present with life-threatening stridor and dyspnea several days postoperatively, a patient with cricoarytenoid arthritis should be evaluated by an otorhinolaryngologist, and in severe cases, elective preoperative tracheostomy could be considered.

In all patients, in particular those with rheumatoid arthritis and ankylosing spondylitis, the condition of the cervical spine and neck mobility are carefully evaluated. The greatest motion during maneuvering of the neck has been shown to be at the atlanto-occipital joint, followed by the atlantoaxial joint. The potential of neurologic injury in patients with a mobile neck and the inability to adequately extend the neck in those with a fixed deformity are taken into consideration as a plan for airway establishment is formulated. Cervical spine roentgenography in flexion and extension is useful in rheumatoid patients to assess atlantoaxial stability. Changes in the cervical spine that might be noted in patients with rheumatoid arthritis include atlantoaxial subluxation (from the destruction of the transverse axial ligament), subaxial subluxation, and the superior migration of the odontoid. Other conditions that may be coexisting and also affect the airway, such as Down syndrome, are also evaluated preoperatively. The potential for cervical spine compromise, if known preoperatively, is useful in the planning of a controlled intubation, perhaps with intubation-assist devices such as the fiber-optic bronchoscope. The patient's airway can be treated with topical anesthetics and appropriate nerve blocks so that the technique is performed in a less traumatic and less physiologically stressful fashion.

Other Systems

Patients with diabetes are assessed, and the adequacy of their therapeutic regimen is evaluated. Good control of blood glucose levels is important to avoid osmotic diuresis as well as to avoid infection. A perioperative blood sugar management plan can be formulated and includes management on the day of surgery when the patient is fasting. The entire musculoskeletal system is examined, as positioning can be affected by diseases in other joints. The neurologic system is evaluated to determine whether there are any deficits and the effect that positioning or surgery will have on them. The integument is examined, since intravenous access may be problematic, and friability of the skin can lead to avulsions. A routine hemogram and an electrolyte panel are ordered, and any other blood tests are ordered as indicated on the basis of clinical evaluation. In patients with cervical spine abnormalities, an evaluation of the vertebral artery is commonly done, as thrombosis can occur during surgery. Upward gaze can result in dizziness as flow through the vertebral arteries is compromised.

Finally, a review of medications and allergies is done, and implications for the anesthetic plan are considered. Patients who take medications such as nonsteroidal anti-inflammatory agents and anticoagulants are instructed to stop taking them ahead of time. For patients who take medications such as warfarin, bridging doses of shorter-acting anticoagulants such as heparin might be required to maximize the duration of anticoagulation, to be stopped at an allotted time before surgery to allow clotting for the operation.

Certain cardiac medications and antihypertensives should be continued prior to surgery; this should be determined in the preoperative period as well.

Additional Anesthetic Considerations in Rheumatoid Arthritis

Although mentioned elsewhere in this chapter, anesthetic consideration specific to patients with rheumatoid arthritis deserves reiteration. In addition to the findings described above in patients with rheumatoid arthritis, while it is a disease of joints and of adjacent connective tissue, it can manifest systemically as well. Pulmonary involvement may manifest as fibrosis or cysts with honeycombing. Renal involvement may occur from amyloidosis. Gastrointestinal problems may result from the various medications that the patient might be taking. Gastric irritation and/or bleeding ulcers can occur from steroidal and nonsteroidal anti-inflammatory agents. Suppression of adrenal function can occur if the patient is on steroid therapy. Peripheral intravenous access might be difficult owing to tissue damage in the blood vessels, and vasculitis is not uncommon. Neuropathy might be present and can affect positioning and spinal cord monitoring.

Rheumatoid arthritis can pose difficulties in airway establishment on several different levels, and affected patients should have their airways thoroughly examined as part of their preoperative evaluation. Preparing for a potentially difficult airway is perhaps the most important part of the anesthetic plan. Each area of involvement must be carefully considered and evaluated to maximize the success rate.

If the patient has a history of hoarseness, refractory "asthma," stridor, laryngeal tenderness, or difficulty breathing, the patient may have cricoarytenoid arthritis. This condition is of particular importance in that it can become manifest during induction of anesthesia, presenting as airway obstruction, but can also appear 4 to 6 days postoperatively. Patients can develop acute airway obstruction and require emergency tracheostomy. In severe cases that are identified preoperatively, elective preoperative tracheostomy can be considered.

Temporomandibular joint involvement can result in poor mouth opening and make direct laryngoscopy difficult. Similarly, micrognathia is also commonly seen, and this condition adds anatomic difficulty to those that are encountered as a result of the disease process itself. The structure of the larynx and trachea may also be altered as a result of the shortening in the cervical spine that occurs with the disease process.

The cervical spine in rheumatoid patients deserves special attention, as this is the root of the majority of the problems associated with the difficult airway. The destruction of the ligamentous structures in the cervical spine can cause instability and increase the chances of neurologic injury. Bony involvement may result in fixation and ankylosing of the cervical vertebrae and thus limitations in mobility of the neck.

Since most head extension occurs at the atlanto-occipital junction followed by the atlantoaxial junction, evaluation of the airway in rheumatoid arthritis should include X-ray films of the cervical spine in flexion and extension to assess atlantoaxial stability. Generally, if the C1–dens interval is greater than 4 mm in flexion, there is a risk of neurologic injury; the potential for injury is highest with the neck in flexion. During direct orotracheal instrumentation of the airway, the head is usually extended on the neck, and the neck is flexed on the chest; this position is usually safe for rheumatoid patients in whom airway difficulty has been deemed low. A high degree of suspicion and extreme care must be maintained, however, as many of these patients are asymptomatic in spite of a great deal of dens movement from flexion to extension. Symptoms and signs of cord impingement are continuously evaluated during the positioning of the patient in preparation for airway instrumentation.

If, after evaluation, the airway is deemed to be potentially difficult, then several nondirect intubation techniques may be considered. If an awake intubation is being contemplated, then the patient is fully instructed as to what to expect. The advantages of an awake intubation include the maintenance of spontaneous ventilation and upper airway tone and the ability to evaluate the patient neurologically on a continuing basis. Usually, the patient is given some mild sedation in the form of low-dose narcotics and diphenhydramine. The authors do not advocate deep sedation, as control of the airway in a sedated patient is not guaranteed. Furthermore, the authors do not advocate the use of benzodiazepines for sedation in these patients, as this class of medication suppresses somatosensory evoked potentials. The benefits of amnesia do not justify the suppression or loss of this valuable intraoperative monitor.

Fiber-optic–assisted oral or nasal intubation is commonly used for awake patients. As was mentioned previously, only light sedation and a drying agent should be administered. The mouth and oropharynx are topically anesthetized with either direct spray or nebulized local anesthetic. If a nasotracheal approach is considered, then intranasal cocaine 4% or a mixture of local anesthetic and oxymetazoline is given to provide topical anesthesia and vasoconstriction. Additional anesthesia can be accomplished by bilateral superior laryngeal nerve blocks at the hyoid bone, and transtracheal or transcricothyroid injections of local anesthetic will provide subglottic anesthesia to prevent coughing and the hemodynamic responses associated with an awake intubation. Some practitioners prefer to anesthetize the airway with a nebulized local anesthetic. Fiber-optic tracheobronchoscopy is performed by either the oral or the nasal route, and the glottic opening is identified and entered; when tracheal rings are identified, the endotracheal tube is advanced over the bronchoscope into the trachea. This technique is well tolerated by the awake patient.

Alternatively, an intubating laryngeal mask airway is placed blindly into the oropharynx, and the endotracheal tube is advanced through the lumen of the airway, entering the trachea. The laryngeal mask is then removed while the endotracheal tube stays in place. This technique is not well tolerated by the awake patient because the laryngeal mask is bulky and the manner of placement is uncomfortable. Other options include the use of a Bullard scope, a Wu scope, or an Airtraq laryngoscope. These are fiber-optic modifications of conventional laryngoscopes. Their advantage is that the head can be maintained in a neutral position while laryngoscopy and intubation are performed. The drawbacks are, as with the laryngeal mask airway, that they are more uncomfortable for an awake patient than is the fiber-optic–assisted approach and that there is limited availability and technical expertise in their use. Lighted wand/stylets have also generated interest, but as with the Bullard and Wu scopes, their use is limited. Other airway devices exist as well.

In extreme cases, a retrograde wire intubation technique can be considered. A 110-cm stiff wire guide is passed via the cricothyroid membrane through an introducer, directed cephalad through the trachea and out of the mouth. Then either a fiber-optic bronchoscope or a tapered guide catheter is advanced over the wire into the trachea. The guide wire is removed, and the endotracheal tube is then "railroaded" over the bronchoscope or catheter into the trachea. With topical oropharyngeal and transtracheal anesthesia and appropriate superior laryngeal nerve blocks, this procedure is usually well tolerated.

Extubation of rheumatoid patients requires as much diligence as does intubation. All considerations that were addressed have to be reconsidered during removal of the tube. The patient should be fully awake and able to sustain spontaneous respirations and airway tone. Following extubation, any excessive head or jaw manipulation should be avoided. As was mentioned earlier, the presence of cricoarytenoid arthritis may manifest itself after several days, so continued vigilance is important.

Although patients with atlantoaxial subluxation from rheumatoid arthritis tend to be more stable in extension, this is not always the case, as severe atlantoaxial subluxation can result in danger to the spinal cord whether there is movement into extension or flexion. Patients with subaxial subluxation must also be considered to be at risk for cervical spine injury if the degree of subluxation is significant. As with patients with atlantoaxial subluxation, care must be taken during extubation as well as during intubation so that rapid reintubation is not necessary.

Superior migration of the odontoid, as a result of cervical spine collapse and displacement of the odontoid through the foramen magnum and into the skull, presents a major challenge for both the surgeon and the anesthesiologist (Fig. 26-1). Patients with superior migration of the odon-

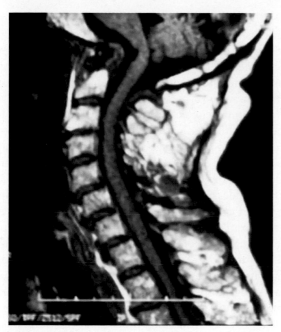

Figure 26-1. Superior migration of the odontoid as a result of cervical spine collapse and displacement of the odontoid through the foramen magnum and into the skull.

toid may present with signs of weakness or even quadraparesis. Compression relief is obtained by removal of the odontoid. However, access to the odontoid is difficult because it cannot be approached via a posterior approach, as one would have to go through the brain stem to reach the odontoid. Because a neck incision is too low to reach the odontoid, the best approach is transorally. The surgeon makes an incision in the retropharyngeal wall and then removes the cervical arch of C1 in order to have access to the odontoid. The odontoid is then carefully removed. After this decompression is complete, the patient is carefully rotated into the prone position, and a posterior cervical fusion is completed. One method for rotation includes utilizing a Jackson table and making a "sandwich" of the patient so that the patient does not have to be rotated off the table with an unstable cervical spine.

Important considerations for the anesthesiologist who is involved in caring for patients undergoing transoral odontoidectomy include understanding that intubating the patient can present considerable risk if there is impingement of the cord by the odontoid. Reviewing the radiologic studies with the surgeon is worthwhile to determine how much neck motion is allowed or whether, in fact, a fiber-optic intubation needs to be performed from the start. In the rheumatoid patient who is undergoing a transoral odontoidectomy, mouth opening is usually limited owing to temporomandibular arthritis, there is often an overbite, and the cervical spine may demonstrate effects of rheumatoid arthritis–related atlantoaxial and subaxial subluxation. These findings often necessitate a fiber-optic intubation from the start. In addition the endotracheal

tube, if placed orally, might infringe on the space needed by the surgeon who is operating transorally. A nasotracheal tube might be preferred. At the end of the procedure, there tends to be marked swelling in the posterior pharynx. This swelling can easily result in total obstruction of the airway, so the endotracheal tube must remain in place until swelling subsides. Some surgeons prefer to perform an elective prophylactic tracheotomy so that issues of swelling and potential airway obstruction are obviated, although others are concerned that a prophylactic tracheotomy can result in infection in the area.

Careful assessment prior to extubation is essential. There must be sufficient air leak around the cuff of the endotracheal tube to indicate that swelling in the glottic and subglottic areas has subsided before the tube is removed. Regression of swelling can take several days, and the patient should be informed of the possibility of prolonged postoperative intubation to avoid airway obstruction.

INDUCTION AND INTRAOPERATIVE MANAGEMENT ISSUES

The induction of general anesthesia in the patient undergoing corrective spine surgery ranges from the simple to the complex. The anesthetic plan and induction are formulated, taking into consideration all aspects of the patient's preexisting medical conditions, the airway status, the planned procedure and positioning for the operation, and the degree of neurophysiologic monitoring to be performed during the course of the operation. Invasive monitoring can be instituted either before or after induction at the discretion of the anesthesiologist.

In general, induction agents are selected on the basis of their lack of impact on somatosensory evoked potential monitoring. Preinduction sedation is not routinely utilized. In the circumstances in which sedation is indicated (e.g., planned awake intubation or poorly cooperative, overly anxious, or mentally challenged patients), an agent that does not have any adverse impact on somatosensory evoked potential monitoring, such as diphenhydramine or hydroxyzine, is usually selected. Because of its low impact on neurophysiologic monitoring, propofol is perhaps the most extensively used agent for induction of general anesthesia. Additionally, it is commonly used either alone as part of a total intravenous anesthesia technique or in conjunction with low-dose inhalation agents for maintenance of general anesthesia. We have found that a balanced technique of low-concentration desflurane or isoflurane in nitrous oxide/oxygen in combination with continuous propofol infusion and high-dose narcotics provides for the smoothest intraoperative course with the least chance of intraoperative recall. Because of its high degree of suppression of somatosensory evoked potentials even at low concentrations, the use of sevoflurane is limited to inhalation inductions in which preinduction intravenous access is not feasible or unobtainable. Once induction is complete, the inhalation agent is usually switched from sevoflurane to desflurane.

Ordinarily, selection of muscle relaxant is a personal preference, although for induction of anesthesia in a patient with a suspected difficult airway (if an awake intubation is not being considered), the first-line muscle relaxant is succinylcholine. In the initial exposure, muscle relaxation is often desirable to minimize blood loss and to facilitate surgical exposure. Once the exposure is completed and instrumentation of the spine has begun, however, muscle relaxation becomes less important, and indeed full recovery from neuromuscular blockade may be required if electromyographic stimulation of pedicle screws is going to be performed. Titration with a continuous drip in conjunction with a peripheral nerve stimulator placed at the wrist can provide better control than intermittent bolus administration.

The increased use of transcranial motor evoked potentials (TMEPs) monitoring during scoliosis correction has cast a different consideration on the use of muscle relaxants and the inhalation agents that enhance neuromuscular blockade. TMEPs are easily suppressed and may have a delayed or absent response in spite of excellent train-of-four peripheral nerve stimulation. Anecdotally, cisatracurium appears to provide the best degree of early muscle relaxation for exposure with the most rapid and complete return of TMEPs for monitoring, as compared to rocuronium, vecuronium, or mivacurium. In addition, for TMEP monitoring, the use of inhala-tional anesthetics is also avoided, and maintenance of anesthesia relies mostly on total intravenous anesthesia technique, with nitrous oxide in oxygen. Monitoring of the bispectral index may be useful in these patients, as there are no agents besides the nitrous oxide and propofol that can provide for amnesia.

In addition to basic monitoring (electrocardiography, pulse oximetry, blood pressure, and end-tidal carbon dioxide), continuous core temperature monitoring is also performed. Low core body temperature resulting from cold ambient temperature and infusion of cold intravenous fluids can adversely impact somatosensory evoked potentials and can delay emergence, should a wake-up test be necessary. The core temperature can be maintained by various methods, including raising the ambient room temperature, warming of intravenous and irrigation fluids, and using an external warming blanket (e.g., Bair Hugger).

As was mentioned previously, invasive monitoring such as arterial line placement or central venous line placement might be indicated on the basis of the operation being performed and the patient's history. Beat-to-beat monitoring of arterial blood pressure is important if a deliberate hypotensive technique is to be employed; and in patients who are undergoing thoracic procedures, intraoperative and postoperative blood gas sampling is facilitated if an arterial line is in place. Central venous catheterization can be useful for fluid resuscitation as an adjunct in the treatment of air embolism. Because of changes in positioning of patients during spine surgery, the exact numerical value for central venous pressure obtained through a central venous line might not be accurate in assessing volume status and therefore might be unreliable. Trend analysis, however, may be of greater benefit.

Transesophageal echocardiography may be employed in those institutions with such capabilities. Transesophageal echocardiography is useful in detecting cardiac alterations that occur during corrective thoracic surgery and in the detection of venous air embolism.

The bladder is catheterized for decompression during surgery and to monitor urine output during the operation. Careful attention to fluid balance is essential, as a hypovolemic state can increase the incidence of hypotension resulting from decreased intravascular volume, as well as venous air embolism. Overhydration can result in upper airway congestion and thus unanticipated postoperative ventilatory support. In addition, ocular venous engorgement can result in increased intraocular pressure and possible postoperative loss of vision.

Finally, antiembolic stockings or sequential pressure devices are placed on the lower extremities.

POSITIONING

Following induction of general anesthesia and intubation of the trachea, the patient is positioned according to the procedure to be performed. Procedures that are done on the spine may involve anterior, posterior, or combined approaches.

For a posterior lumbar or thoracic approach, the patient is anesthetized on a stretcher and is then placed prone on a frame that is designed to decrease intra-abdominal pressure and venous congestion in the vertebral venous plexus. Frames such as the Relton-Hall frame, the Wilson frame, and the Jackson cradle are all designed to support the upper body and the pelvis and leave the abdomen and the chest free. Proper support during the turning phase is imperative, as injury can occur to the patient as well as to those who are turning the patient. The anesthesiologist controls the endotracheal tube so as to avoid inadvertent extubation and also controls the intravascular lines. When the patient is placed in the prone position, the head is placed in a soft, contoured pillow such that no pressure is exerted on areas that are particularly vulnerable to injury from direct pressure and/or prolonged interruption of blood flow, such as the eyes, the malar eminences, and the nose. Prolonged direct pressure on the eyes can result in postoperative vision loss (see "Postoperative Visual Loss"), and the nose and malar eminences may be susceptible to skin necrosis and sloughing. The head and neck are examined and should be maintained in a neutral position. The head may be rotated to one side or placed directly prone, provided that all pressure points are checked and padded. The upper and lower extremities should be checked to ensure that blood flow is not interrupted to those parts because of the positioning. Also, all pressure points on the extremities should be checked and padded, with particular attention to the ulnar groove, the brachial plexus (arms should be flexed to less than 90 degrees in all angles), and the shoulders (which should be in neutral position).

For an anterior approach, the patient is positioned in accordance with the procedure. Anterior lumbar approaches may be done with the patient supine or in lateral tilt or lateral decubitus position. Anterior thoracic approaches may involve formal thoracotomy, thoracoscopic, or thoracoscopic-assisted techniques. In each case, the patient is induced on the operating room table and is then positioned following the completion of induction. Proper attention is paid to all pressure points, including the upper and lower extremities, as for the posterior approach. If the patient is in the lateral decubitus position, the lower extremities must be adequately protected against adduction and compression, and an axillary roll must be placed to protect the dependent arm. For thoracic procedures, the nondependent arm must also be protected and well padded, as movement of the upper torso can move the arm into a position where injury may occur.

For combined approaches, special care must be taken during the transfer from supine or lateral to prone. In addition to the considerations above, an anterior approach may involve the placement of drains or, in a thoracic approach, a chest tube. During the posterior procedure, the chest tube and drainage are monitored continuously to ensure the reexpansion of the lung as well as to identify any potential bleeding. In addition, the prone position is associated with alterations in pulmonary function by itself, so particular attention to the lungs is important following anterior thoracic approaches.

Positioning for procedures involving the cervical spine involve preparation for field avoidance and proper protection of the airway. In an anterior approach, a reinforced endotracheal tube is selected and protected alongside the face such that it is directed cephalad, away from the surgical field. To facilitate intraoperative radiographs of the cervical spine, the shoulders are often retracted downward, and the arms are tucked to the sides. Radial pulses are checked bilaterally to ensure that the retraction of the shoulders is not compromising blood flow. Great care is taken to tuck the arms in supination and external rotation, such that the ulnar groove is rotated to face medially instead of downward; this prevents inadvertent compression of the ulnar nerve against the edge of the operating room table. In a posterior cervical approach, the patient is often placed in a traction vise to maintain neck position. Considerations involving shoulder and arm placement are similar to those of the anterior cervical approach. Because of the nature of the vise device, the only concern regarding pressure points in the prone position is the tip of the nose, which may rest on a portion of the vise. As was mentioned previously, compression of this area can result in perfusion compromise, tissue ischemia, and sloughing. Care must be taken to pad the area or to manipulate the vise such that the nose does not rest on any portion of it.

THORACIC PROCEDURES

Anterior approaches to the thoracic spine may involve formal thoracotomy or thoracoscopic or thoracoscopic-assisted techniques. Consultation with the surgeon who will be performing the exposure will clarify the approach and identify the need for lung isolation. Open thoracotomies below T9 can often be performed without the need for one-lung ventilation; gentle lung retraction or packing does not usually result in significant alterations in lung function. Procedures above the T9 level frequently require one-lung ventilation and lung isolation techniques, and procedures involving thoracoscopy routinely require them.

Two different modalities are used to perform one-lung ventilation. The first involves placement of a double-lumen endobronchial tube. The longer lumen is directed toward the right or left main stem bronchus (depending on the tube selected), and the second lumen lies in the trachea above the carina. Since either lung can be inflated or deflated independently in this configuration, a left-sided endobronchial tube is commonly selected. One reason for this is the takeoff of the right upper lobe bronchus that occurs very shortly after bifurcation of the carina and thus can easily become obstructed by a right-sided tube. Another advantage to the endobronchial tube is that oxygen can be delivered to the collapsed lung, providing for additional oxygenation if one-lung ventilation proves to be inadequate. The biggest disadvantage to the endobronchial tubes is their size limitation because of the double lumen. They are poorly tolerated should postoperative ventilation be required, and their complexity is often intimidating. Although an exchange to a conventional tube is possible at the conclusion of the operation, this is not without risk and could result in airway trauma or loss of the airway because of difficulty reintubating the patient or from swelling in the airway from edema.

The other modality is a bronchial blocker tube. This consists of a single-lumen endotracheal tube, with an integrated balloon-tipped catheter in a casing alongside the tube (Fig. 26-2). The tube is placed conventionally, and then, with the use of a fiber-optic bronchoscope, the integrated catheter is advanced so that the bronchial blocker is placed in the main stem bronchus of the lung to be isolated and deflated. Once proper placement has been confirmed, the balloon on the catheter is inflated, and that lung is no longer ventilated. A proximal port of the balloon catheter is then opened, and the nonventilated lung is allowed to deflate. Once the procedure has been completed, the cuff on the occluder is deflated, the proximal cap is replaced, and the lung is ventilated. The biggest advantage is that if postoperative controlled ventilation is required, once the catheter is retracted into its integrated casing, the tube looks and behaves like a conventional single-lumen endotracheal tube. This modality has two

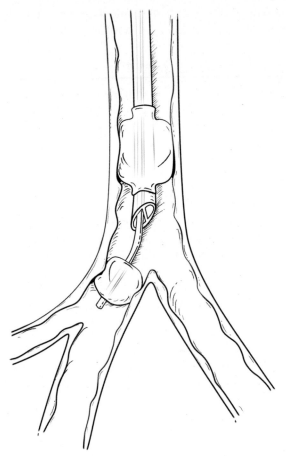

Figure 26-2. A bronchial blocker tube, consisting of a single-lumen endotracheal tube with an integrated balloon-tipped catheter in a casing alongside the tube. *(From Rosenberg AD: Current issues in the anesthetic treatment of the patient for orthopedic surgery. In Schwartz AJ (ed): ASA Refresher Courses in Anesthesiology. Philadelphia: Lippincott Williams & Wilkins, 2004, pp 155–164.)*

disadvantages. First, as with the endobronchial tubes, the tube diameter is much greater than that of the conventional endotracheal tube that would be appropriate for the patient, because of the integrated casing that houses the catheter. Second, administration of additional oxygen by insufflation or by continuous positive airway pressure to the collapsed lung is not possible.

In either case, adequate patient preparation for expectations, as well as education of the postoperative care team, is paramount for a successful postoperative experience.

POSTOPERATIVE VISUAL LOSS

A new phenomenon has been noted in patients who undergo spine surgery in the prone position: postoperative visual loss (POVL). Although the exact etiology of POVL is unknown, a combination of factors has been implicated. One predisposing factor is considered to be the variable blood supply to the optic nerve that arises from posterior ciliary arteries. These arteries are actually end arteries and supply the optic nerve in a watershed fashion. This water-

shed blood supply leaves areas that are at risk for decreased oxygen supply based on either decreased perfusion or increased resistance to arterial flow. In addition to the variable blood supply, other implicated predisposing factors include a small optic disc, a history of hypertension, smoking, diabetes, vascular disease, and morbid obesity. Perioperative factors include anemia resulting in decreased oxygen-carrying capacity, which can occur following major intraoperative blood loss, hypotension leading to decreased perfusion, prolonged surgery in the prone position, and increased resistance to blood flow. Increased resistance to blood flow can result from factors such as increased blood viscosity, local arterial disease, venous engorgement from infused fluids and Trendelenburg positioning, direct pressure, a small optic disc, or embolic disease. Despite all the possible potential causes, the etiology remains unclear. Ultimately, conditions that result in ischemic neuropathy of the optic nerve are considered to be the major causes of POVL. Ischemic optic neuropathy results from insufficient blood supply or inadequate ocular perfusion pressure (OPP) and is best understood by considering the relationship of mean arterial pressure (MAP) and intraocular pressure (IOP): OPP = MAP − IOP, such that a decrease in MAP or an increase in IOP will result in a decrease in OPP. If the blood pressure (MAP) is too low, then it can be seen how perfusion will be inadequate, just as if IOP is too high, there may be a significant resistance to blood flow. In an interesting study, Cheng and colleagues measured IOP in anesthetized patients in the prone position and were able to demonstrate that IOP increased over time. The addition of head-down tilt to the prone position can result in edema and venous engorgement, increased IOP, and an increase in the chance of POVL. Since the etiology of vision loss is unclear and in an attempt to better define the cause of POVL, the American Society of Anesthesiologists has established a national POVL registry to identify risk factors associated with postoperative vision loss. As of the summer of 2003, a total of 43 spine patients had been entered in the registry. Interestingly, no general conclusions can be made from the patient base. While the median age of patients suffering visual loss was 49 years, the age range was from 19 to 73 years. Prone time ranged from 3 hours to 24 hours, with a mean of 8 hours; estimated blood loss averaged 2.3 L, but the range was from 200 mL to 20 L; the lowest hematocrit was 25.5%, with a range of 19% to 40%; and the lowest blood pressure was a 37% decrease from baseline on average for patients suffering POVL, but the range was a 19% to 61% decrease. Deliberate hypotension was instituted in only 40% of the patients. More recently, during 2005, the postoperative visual loss registry issued an update. This update does not shed any significant new light on the etiology of POVL, as the patient population and relevant surgical data remained somewhat variable. The 2005 update demographics include a median patient age of 50 years, the age range being 16 to 73 years; median anesthetic duration was

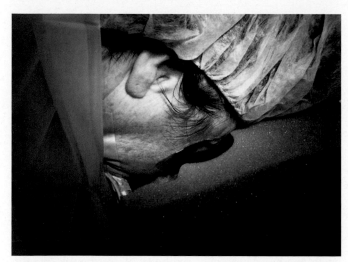

Figure 26-3. Positioning and padding to avoid pressure on the eyes.

10 hours, with a range of 3.5 to 18.7 hours; and there was blood loss of over 2 L in more than 54% of patients. However, 27.1% of patients had blood loss between 1 and 2 L, 10% had blood loss between 500 mL and 1 L, and 5.7% had up to a 499-mL blood loss. Recently published data point to ischemic optic neuropathy as the most common cause of POVL. Long procedures and large blood loss were associated with increased incidences of POVL. While this is a fairly new phenomenon, it is of major concern and devastating for the patient and the operative team. The POVL website can be accessed at http://depts.washington.edu/asaccp/eye. Remember to make certain that there is no pressure on the eyes (Fig. 26-3).

BLOOD TRANSFUSION IN THE SPINE SURGERY PATIENT

Many patients undergoing spine surgery experience significant blood loss during the course of the surgical procedure. While methods exist to minimize blood loss and avoid the need for allogeneic blood transfusion, it does at times become necessary to transfuse a patient. A number of factors must be considered in determining whether or not a patient requires a blood transfusion. For many years, the concept of a transfusion trigger was considered the standard for determining when a patient required a transfusion. Once the magic number of 10 g/dL of hemoglobin or a hematocrit of 30% was attained, the patient was considered to be adequately transfused. A number of factors have made this concept obsolete. First, it is now understood that the transfusion number for each patient has to be determined on the basis of the patient's physiology or pathophysiology. Many patients who undergo spine surgery are young, healthy patients with excellent compensatory reserves and therefore have the capability to withstand marked stress on their cardiopulmonary system. They can significantly increase both their cardiac output (mostly produced by an increase in heart rate) and their pulmonary

function (by increasing their respiratory rate) to supply sufficient oxygen to organs and tissues despite the lower concentration of blood in the circulating blood volume. In fact, it is now accepted in many healthy patients that transfusion not be given until hemoglobin levels fall below 7 g/dL. This criterion applies only to the patient who is not anticipated to sustain additional loss of blood. In a patient in the operating room who is expected to have continued ongoing blood loss, however, it is wise not to allow the blood level to decrease too much before starting a transfusion. Obviously, in an older patient or one who has any risk factors that would be adversely affected if the heart rate or respiratory function were to become stressed, transfusion should be instituted at a higher hemoglobin level or hematocrit. In a patient such as one who has coronary artery disease or chronic obstructive airway disease, the former transfusion trigger numbers of 10/30 probably still apply. So while most patients do not require a blood transfusion above 10/30 and most require one below 7/21, transfusion for patients in the intermediate range will depend on the factors outlined above: coexisting medical problems, ability to compensate for low blood counts, and ongoing and anticipated blood loss.

Factors that can be employed to decrease blood loss and minimize the need for blood transfusion can be divided into those that are addressed in the preoperative period and those that are addressed in the intraoperative period (Box 26-1). During preoperative preparation for surgery, the patient can donate autologous blood for reinfusion in the perioperative period as required. The patient should receive iron supplementation. If the patient has low weight, it is still possible to donate partial units. This has to be coordinated with the local blood predonation center. Limits for predonation have been liberalized as to both age and weight limits since they were first introduced, so it is worthwhile to contact the local predonation center to discuss the current criteria. In the patient who is anemic, erythropoietin might be a preoperative option. This has

---

BOX 26-1 Methods Used to Minimize Blood Loss and Avoid Allogeneic Transfusion

Preoperative
- Predonation of autologous blood
- Preoperative administration of erythropoietin

Intraoperative
- Proper patient positioning to minimize venous pressure
- Infiltration of incision with dilute epinephrine solution
- Intraoperative cell salvage techniques
- Hemodilution
- Controlled hypotension
- Lower the point at which a transfusion is initiated
- Pharmacologic means
   Tranexamic acid
   ε-Aminocaproic acid

gained some popularity, but the patient usually has to be anemic to achieve a significant response. Erythopoetin has been associated with thrombosis in some patients, so caution needs to be used so as not to increase the hematocrit too much.

In addition to meticulous and effective surgical hemostasis in the operating room, other maneuvers that can be instituted to decrease blood loss include positioning the patient properly, ensuring appropriate ventilator settings, maintaining adequate blood pressure control, infiltrating the incision site, utilizing red blood cell salvage reinfusion or hemodilution techniques, and possibly employing pharmacologic agents. In placing the patient on the operating table in the prone position, it is important to avoid pressure on the abdomen. Increased intra-abdominal pressure will be transmitted to the vertebral venous plexus and can result in increased intraoperative bleeding. If possible, a prolonged inspiratory pressure phase on the ventilator is avoided, as it will tend to decrease venous return and result in venous engorgement. Blood pressure control can play an important role in reducing intraoperative blood loss. While some physicians employ hypotensive anesthesia techniques, others decrease the blood pressure below the patient's baseline in an effort to minimize blood loss. True hypotensive techniques in which pharmacologic means are utilized to diminish blood pressure 30% from baseline have been used for many years. Although these are effective, it is important to consider the patient's baseline status and candidacy to have significant lowering of blood pressure. Patients with coronary or vascular disease may suffer ischemia in situations in which blood pressure is significantly decreased. It is imperative not to have the patient significantly hypotensive and very anemic at the same time, as this will contribute to inadequate oxygenation of important organs and tissues. Providing deeper anesthesia and muscle relaxation, if allowed by neurophysiologic monitoring techniques, also helps to diminish blood loss. At the beginning of surgery, infiltration of the wound with epinephrine 1 : 500,000 can decrease blood loss. Intraoperative use of a cell salvage device is important in avoiding allogeneic transfusions. The blood is collected in a reservoir, washed to remove debris, and reinfused into the patient. The blood that is reinfused from a cell saver device can have a hematocrit level in the 50% range, so it is very helpful in maintaining an adequate hematocrit level in the patient.

Pharmacologic means have been suggested for decreasing blood pressure. The use of aprotinin, a serine protease inhibitor, has been touted for its ability to decrease blood loss while at the same time preventing thrombosis. However, recent reports of renal complications associated with aprotinin use in the cardiac patient have led to a reevaluation for its indication in the spine patient.

Tranexamic acid and ε-aminocaproic acid are now used instead of aprotinin, which is no longer marketed by the manufacturer because of its negative side effects. In meta-analysis studies, tranexamic acid appears to be effective in decreasing blood loss during orthopedic surgery.

When indicated, blood transfusions should be administered. There are some risks associated with blood transfusion. In addition to the disaster associated with a mismatched transfusion, minor reactions such as fever and hives can occur with blood transfusion. There is a concern of transmission of infectious disease with the transfusion of blood. Human immunodeficiency virus, cytomegalovirus, and hepatitis B and C viruses as well as syphilis and other bacterial and parasitic diseases are some of the diseases that are potentially transmitted via transfusion. Although all blood is tested for infectious diseases prior to being released for transfusion, there is a time window for some infections in which the blood might test negative for antibodies but still be infectious. With new methods of testing blood, the window has been minimized but is still present. Another concern is that there has been an increased association with a general immunosuppression of the patient following transfusion. The thought is that, once transfused, a patient is faced with an antigenic overload and has difficulty mounting an immunologic response. This failure to mount an effective immunologic response is evidenced by the increased rate of cancer recurrence in transfused patients undergoing cancer surgery compared to nontransfused controls. Additionally, evidence exists that transfusion of allogeneic blood is associated with a higher infection rate. In separate studies Murphy and Triulzi and their colleagues demonstrated increased infection rates in patients who received allogeneic transfusions. In a study of 102 patients who underwent 109 spinal fusions, there was a 20.8% infection rate in those who received a transfusion compared to 3.5% in those who did not receive an allogeneic transfusion. Measurements of natural killer cell activity, a marker of immunologic function, decreased in patients who received transfusions.

Although these issues of immunosuppression and infection are real, a patient should receive a transfusion if it is indicated.

CONCLUSION OF THE SURGICAL PROCEDURE AND TRANSFER TO THE POSTANESTHESIA CARE UNIT

At the conclusion of the procedure, the patient will be returned to the supine position if the operation was not performed in this position. While everyone is relieved that the surgery is concluding, the operative staff cannot relax their vigilance at this time, as care must be taken in turning the patient. Injury to the patient and dislodgement of intravenous and arterial lines, drains, and the endotracheal tube can occur if movement is not coordinated.

The anesthesiologist needs to assess the patient, paying particular attention to fluid status, hemoglobin and hematocrit levels, pH, degree of fluid shifts, intraoperative blood loss, edema of the area of the airway, length and site of surgery, and the patient's temperature. These factors all play into consideration as to whether the patient should be extubated at the end of the procedure. One additional factor is the amount of pain relief the patient will require postoperatively. In patients who have undergone thoracic surgery and have a thoracic incision and chest tube placed, pain can result in splinting and an inadequate respiratory effort. This in turn results in a systemic acidosis as the patient's carbon dioxide level increases.

If extubated, the patient is observed prior to transfer to the postanesthesia care unit. Monitoring on transfer is usually at the discretion of the anesthesiologist, but the patient who might desaturate on the way to the postanesthesia care unit should be administered supplemental oxygen.

In the postanesthesia care unit, vital signs are obtained, a reassessment is performed, and information transfer is given to the postanesthesia care unit staff. If the procedure involved significant blood loss, hemoglobin and hematocrit levels should be obtained, as well as appropriate metabolic assays.

Illustrative Case Presentation

CASE 1. Hemangioma of the Eye

A patient with a hemangioma of the eye presented for anterior-posterior spine surgery. MRI demonstrated that the hemangioma tethered the optic nerve in its course to the globe (Fig. 26-4). After consultation with an ophthalmologist, the patient's surgery was modified to just performing the posterior approach. The patient was kept normotensive during the surgical procedure. Positioning was carefully performed, ensuring that there was no direct pressure on the eye. Additionally, no head-down tilt was allowed during the procedure. In the early postoperative period, the patient had only minor visual complaints and tolerated the procedure well.

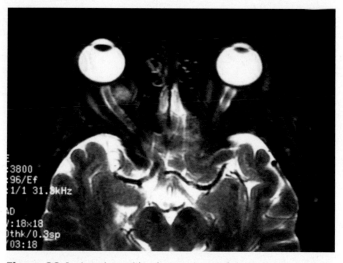

Figure 26-4. A patient with a hemangioma of the eye who presented for anterior-posterior spine surgery. MRI demonstrated that the hemangioma tethered the optic nerve in its course to the globe.

REFERENCES

Murphy P, Heal JM, Blumberg N: Infection or suspected infection after hip replacement surgery with autologous or homologous blood transfusions. Transfusion 1991;31:212–217.

Triulzi DJ, Vanek K, Ryan DH, Blumberg N: A clinical and immunologic study of blood transfusion and postoperative bacterial infection in spinal surgery. Transfusion 1992;32:517–524.

SUGGESTED READINGS

Bernstein RL, Rosenberg AD: Manual of Orthopedic Anesthesia and Related Pain Syndromes. New York: Churchill Livingstone, 1993.

This book provides many of the basic considerations that are important for the physician's care of the patient who is undergoing spine surgery. There are chapters on scoliosis spine surgery and the rheumatoid patient undergoing surgery.

Cheng MA, Todorov A, Tempelhoff R: The effect of prone positioning on intraocular pressure in anesthetized patients. Anesthesiology 2001;95:1351–1355.

The increase in the incidence of postoperative visual loss has initiated a search for its etiology. Although many factors have been implicated, no clear-cut etiology has been identified. One cause is thought to be increased intraocular pressure. These articles demonstrate the increase in intraocular pressure as a result of the patient's being in the prone position.

Glassman SD, Rose SM, Dimar JR, et al: The effect of postoperative nonsteroidal anti-inflammatory drug administration on spinal fusion. Spine 1998;23:834–838.

This article addresses the concern that anti-inflammatory medications can result in preventing spinal fusion. Anything that could interfere with spine fusion is of major concern to those who are caring for the patient who is undergoing spine surgery.

Mangano DT, Tudor IC, Dietzel C, et al: The risk associated with aprotinin in cardiac surgery. N Engl J Med 2006;354:353–365.

This article questions the use of aprotinin in patients. The study demonstrates that there is an incidence of renal failure in patients who receive this medication in an attempt to decrease the incidence of blood loss.

Rosenberg AD: Current issues in the anesthetic management of the patient for orthopedic surgery. In Schwartz AJ (ed): ASA Refresher Courses in Anesthesiology. Philadelphia: Lippincott Williams & Wilkins, 2004, pp 155–164.

This article reviews many of the considerations of spine surgery, including anterior-posterior cases, thoracic procedures, the concern of postoperative visual loss, and the question of bone fusion being affected by nonsteroidal anti-inflammatory medications.

Williams EL: Postoperative blindness. Anesthesiol Clin North Am 2002; 20:367–384.

This article reviews the issue of postoperative blindness.

CHAPTER 27

Bone Graft and Fusion Enhancement

ELLIOT R. CARLISLE *and* JEFFREY S. FISCHGRUND

Spinal fusion is a very commonly performed and well-accepted procedure for the treatment of spinal disorders, including degenerative, traumatic, deformity, tumor, infection, and other spinal pathologies. The goal of these spinal fusions is to eliminate the instability of the spine caused by the above-noted pathologies. Spinal fusion by definition refers to the achievement of a bony union between the involved vertebrae. This chapter will discuss the currently available types of bone grafting and spinal fusion enhancement that are commonly used to achieve spinal fusion.

Bone tissue has the capacity for repairing itself without scarring. Bone grafting makes use of this core characteristic. To achieve optimal use of the clinically available graft options, the biology of bone, as well as its capacity for remodeling and self-repair, must be utilized and understood.

EXTRACELLULAR MATRIX

The mineralization of osteoid, which consists primarily of collagen and ground substance, begins approximately 2 weeks after its formation. Early mineral content rises rapidly to approximately 70% of its final amount; the final 30% is deposited over a period of several months. Even after complete mineralization, bone continues to have 25% organic matrix, including cells. Hydroxyapatite, the bone mineral, accounts for 70% of its final weight, while water accounts for the remaining 5%. Bone morphogenetic proteins (BMPs), proteins, growth factors, and cytokines are imbedded in the remaining extracellular matrix and play an important role in the bone marrow stabilization process.

BONE ARCHITECTURE

Mature cortical and cancellous bone has a matrix of lamellated structure. The lamellae run parallel to the trabeculae of cancellous bone or concentrically surround the haver-

sian canal and cortical bone, which forms an osteon, which is the functional unit of cortical bone. Modeling is the process whereby bone is laid down onto a surface without necessarily being preceded by resorption. Remodeling is the osteoblastic activity that fills voids following osteoclastic activity. In the adult skeleton, remodeling is the more active process and gives bone capacity to adapt to changes and loading as well as metabolic stimuli. Bone tissue is able to adapt to mechanical stimuli such as compression and bending moments, according to Wolff's Law, which states that bone is laid down where stresses require its presence and bone is absorbed where the stresses do not require it.

OSTEOINDUCTION

Osteoinduction is a process whereby less differentiated, pluripotent cells are stimulated and develop into cells of the bone-forming lineage. A great deal of research is focused on BMPs as inducing agents. BMPs are soluble glycoproteins that are released in response to a fracture or some type of physical stimuli such as mechanical, electrical, or magnetic alterations. While osteoblasts at the site of an injury participate in healing of a fracture, bone and soft tissue injuries are the primary trigger for the transformation of undifferentiated cells into osteoblasts. The response to this injury involves coordinated involvement of vascular and nervous tissue as well as a sensitization to precursor cells, leading to the production of growth factors by these cells and their differentiation into actively remodeling cell types. Because bone formation requires an adequate blood supply, bone growth factors are also angiogenic.

OSTEOCONDUCTION

Osteoconduction is the appositional growth of bone onto a three-dimensional surface of suitable scaffold. This includes capillary ingrowth, perivascular tissue ingrowth, and development of osteoprogenitor cells and follows a highly organized, predictable spatial pattern.

OSTEOGENESIS

Osteogenesis is the process of bone formation through cellular osteoblastic activity. Osteogenesis is dependent on osteoconduction as a matrix for the delivery of the osteoinductive factors that are necessary for the differentiation of osteoprogenitor stem cells.

AUTOGRAFT

Autografts are grafts that have been harvested from the patient at the time of surgery and are the "gold standard" by which the success of other grafting techniques is assessed. While the main source of autograft is the iliac crest, other sources, such as the proximal tibia, the fibula, or a rib, can be used as well. Iliac crest tends to be harvested in the form of cancellous bone chips, respecting the inner and outer tables of the crista, or as tricortical strut grafts (Fig. 27-1), providing bone that is capable of structural support.

Autografts maintain viable osteoblasts and osteoprogenitor cells and also confer osteoconductive and osteoinductive potential. The calcified matrix of mature bone, as well as its organic components such as collagen and ground substance, supplies the graft with biocompatible osteoconductive properties. Bone growth factors, such as the BMPs, are primarily responsible for the osteoconductive capacity of autograft.

The trabeculae, highly porous structures of autogenous cancellous bone, promote ingrowth of blood vessels that are necessary for bone growth and reduces the risk of complications from hypoxia. Importantly, autograft does not pose a risk of disease transmission. Autograft proce-

dures show a high rate of success for certain spinal fusions, such as anterior and posterior cervical arthrodesis.

However, autograft has several drawbacks, including both surgical complications and its limited supply. Although transplanted donor cells most likely contribute to new bone graft, most of the osteogenic cells that repopulate the graft are thought to migrate from the fusion bed. While transplanted cells are initially active, graft viability is diminished when graft tissue is separated from its blood supply, leading to ischemic or apoptotic cell death and leaving behind only a mineral scaffold. Surviving cells receive their oxygen and nutrients by diffusion only, and for this reason, the cells are likely to die from ischemia before the graft is vascularized. Rapid vascularization of the graft may be impeded by fibrin formation in the autograft and by the packing procedure that is used to place a graft into the surgical site. Autogenous bone viability can be further complicated by variables such as donor age, gender, genetic makeup, and physical health of the patient.

Autograft harvest is associated with high donor site morbidity, estimated to occur in 10% to 39% of patients. Donor site morbidity is common and dependent on the surgical approach; for example, sacroiliac subluxation and dislocation have been reported more frequently with a posterior approach, while infection occurs more frequently following the anterior approach. Complications may occur, including superficial infections, temporary sensory impairment, and milder transient pain. Acute and chronic pain at the donor site is commonly reported, and chronic pain may occur in over 25% of patients who undergo an autograft procedure for spinal fusion.

Major complications associated with bone graft harvest from the iliac crest have been reported to be as high as 0.7% to 25%. These include severe catastrophic bleeding, herniation, serious infection, scarring, hematoma formation, injury to nervous or vascular tissue, pelvic fracture,

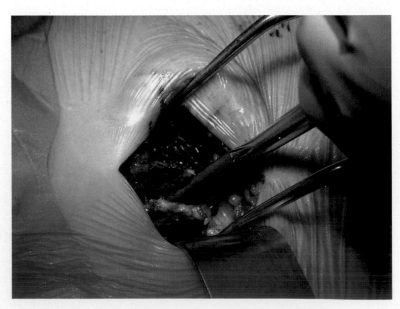

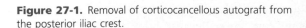
Figure 27-1. Removal of corticocancellous autograft from the posterior iliac crest.

and chronic pain at the procurement site. Skaggs and colleagues reported that 15% of pediatric patients had complications that affected daily living activities after autogenous bone graft harvest.

ALLOGRAFT

Allografts are grafts that have been harvested from a cadaver. Allografts were originally used only when the amount of bone graft material that was required for a procedure exceeded the amount of autogenous bone that could be harvested. Recent improvements in the safety, quality, and availability of allogenic materials have resulted in substantial increases in the use of allograft. In the mid-1990s, allograft made up nearly 35% of all bone grafts performed in the United States. Advantages of allograft include avoidance of donor site morbidity, the potential for providing immediate mechanical support, and availability in a variety of forms for customized applications. Allograft can be used as either a particulate or a structural material.

Allografts can have variability in bone quality and may pose a small but definite risk of disease transmission and immunogenic reactions. Processing techniques to reduce these risks involve the loss of osteogenic potential, due to the lack of donor cells, and reduced osteoinductive potential, presumably due to inactivation or removal of osteotropic factors such as BMPs, as well as cells. Risks of disease transmission are related to the rigor with which the allograft tissue was processed. For example, transmission of human immunodeficiency virus has been documented in fresh-frozen allograft but not in freeze-dried allograft. Transmission of human immunodeficiency virus and hepatitis is also dependent on the way in which donors are screened. For orthopedic applications, freezing, freeze-drying, and irradiation, sometimes followed by demineralization, are commonly used methods for processing and preserving allograft materials. In addition, freeze-dried grafts are incorporated into host tissue less completely and retain BMPs less efficiently than fresh-frozen grafts do. Graft strength, immunogenicity, risks for transmission of disease, and capacity for incorporation at the host site can vary widely with the technique that is used for allograft preparation. An additional disadvantage of allograft is its expense.

Allograft has been used successfully in posterior cervical, thoracic, and interbody fusion procedures. Indeed, successful fusion occurs in over 90% of patients following anterior cervical fusions. The success rate for posterolateral lumbar fusion is lower when allograft is used alone or in combination with autograft. High rates of success have also been reported for allograft posterior lumbar interbody fusion procedures. Allograft has been shown to be useful as bone void filler, since it provides early structural support without donor-site morbidity. Perhaps the best indication for allograft is in adolescent patients who have undergone

scoliosis correction and fusion. In one study, 40 patients with idiopathic scoliosis who underwent corrective surgery were treated with either femoral head allograft or autograft from the iliac crest. Successful unions were obtained for all patients in both groups. Interestingly, the group that was treated with allograft experienced reduced postoperative pain relative to the group that was treated with autograft.

In spite of improvements in modern technology and instrumentation, the rate of failure with nonunion of spinal arthrodesis remains relatively high, particularly in cases involving multilevel fusions. Improvements in fusion may depend on further innovations in bone graft technology, including the use of autograft/allograft combinations, as well as the development of composite materials that provide scaffold and biologic stimuli necessary for successful bone remodeling.

CERAMICS

The mineral phase of bone makes up approximately 60% to 70% of its dry weight. This carbonated calcium phosphate apatite mineral, termed *dahllite*, contains 46% carbonate by weight and small amounts of sodium, magnesium, and other trace elements. The structural integrity of bone, especially its compressive strength, depends directly on the state of the mineral phase. It has been demonstrated that the chemical structure of the substrate is vital to its observed osteoconductive properties. Ideally, bone graft substitute would have a similar mineral composition structure.

Because ceramics do not normally exhibit osteogenic or osteoinductive properties, when used alone they are dependent on local host tissues for osteoprogenitor cells and osteoinductive factors. Ceramic scaffolds facilitate cellular adhesion and vascular ingrowth and promote new bone formation when loaded with a source of osteogenic cells, such as autogenous bone or bone marrow.

The advantages of biodegradable osteoconductive ceramic bone graft substitutes include the availability and unlimited quantity and no donor site complications or infection risks. For synthetic materials to be useful in vivo, they must be compatible with surrounding tissues, be chemically stable in body fluids, have compatible mechanical and physical properties, be able to be produced in functional shapes, be able to withstand sterilization processes, have reasonable cost, and have reliable quality control. Calcium phosphate possesses many of these properties. Bone forms directly on the surface and chemically binds to bioactive osteoconductive ceramics. Moreover, the bone grows three-dimensionally along the ceramic surface.

Calcium phosphates, the most commonly used ceramics in bone surgery, include coral-based or synthetic hydroxyapatite (HA) and tricalcium phosphate (TCP) (Fig. 27-2). These have a high degree of biocompatibility with host tissue. Optimal interconnection between pores (connective

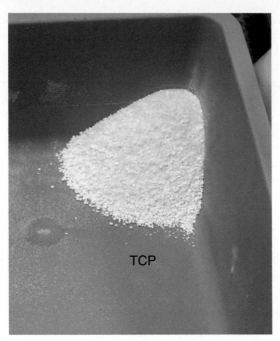

Figure 27-2. Pure tricalcium phosphate granules. This osteoconductive material has no inherent strength.

porosity greater than 100 μm) and pore size of 100 to 500 μm have been demonstrated to be essential for osteoconductivity.

Commercially available HA is relatively inert and biodegrades poorly. Nonresorbing materials may interfere with remodeling, create stress risers, and impede the accretion of strength of the fusion mass. Conversely, ceramic TCP undergoes biodegradation within 4 to 8 weeks of implantation, which might be too early for optimal fusion mass healing. Biphasic ceramics with an optimized ratio between HA and TCP may increase the mechanical strength or the degree and rate of resorption.

Emery and colleagues studied anterior interbody fusion in the thoracic spine of dogs using autologous tricortical iliac crest bone graft, HA ceramics, calcium carbonate, and a mixture of HA and TCP. All fusions were performed with anterior spinal instrumentation. Autologous bone graft was found to be most effective biomechanically and histologically. In another study, the same authors found that autologous bone graft was significantly better than calcium carbonate ceramics when combined with internal fixation. Although fixation did not statistically improve the biomechanical properties of ceramic fusion segments, it did have a profound beneficial effect on the ability of the ceramic to be revascularized and remodeled.

Toth and colleagues studied the effect of ceramic porosity in a goat anterior cervical spine fusion model. Autograft was compared to 30%, 50%, and 70% porosity implants of 50:50 HA:TCP. All of the tested ceramic implants were equal to or better than the autograft iliac crest bone at 3 and 6 months. There were more porous implants with a higher union rate early on but also at a higher incidence of graft

fracture. Overall fusion rates were 67% for the ceramic implants and 50% for autograft. The relatively low fusion rates in all groups were thought to be due to excessive neck motion in the goat; however, these low fusion rates called into question the ability of this model to be validly extrapolated into human anterior cervical fusions.

Posterior lateral intertransverse lumbar fusion has been studied in the sheep model. Some authors have demonstrated better results with autologous bone than with different ceramics, while others found similar results in terms of fusion rate when using coral *Porites* (calcium carbonate), a combination of HA and TCP, or resorbable coralline HA.

The efficacy of porous HA granules in achieving posterior lateral lumbar fusion in a sheep model was studied by Baramki and colleagues. Bisegmental instrumentation was performed using either no graft material, autologous bone, HA alone, or an HA/autograft composite in a 1:1 ratio. According to mechanical stability criteria, the fusion rates for the different groups were 100% (14 of 14) for the autologous bone group, 72% (10 of 14) for the bone/interconnected porous HA group, 50% (7 of 14) for the pure interconnected porous HA group, and 15% (2 of 14) for the sham group. Delecrin and colleagues studied the influence of the fusion site microenvironment on incorporation of ceramic and new bone formation in a canine posterior lumbar fusion model. Bone growth into a macroporous ceramic implant in an interlaminar fusion site and a posterolateral intertransverse fusion site, using block HA/TCP (60%/40%) composite as a graft material, was evaluated. The percentage of newly formed fusion bone was significantly higher in the interlaminar fusion site than in the intertransverse site, where decorticated bone in the fusion bed was scarce. For both locations, the highest amount of newly formed bone was observed in the area of close contact between the ceramic and decorticated bone. The lowest was observed in the central areas. This demonstrated a deficiency of osteoinduction properties of the graft and a consequent reliance on bone growth induction, with the decorticated bleeding bone and the fusion bed serving as a source of stem cells, as well as osteogenic factors.

Zdeblick and colleagues evaluated the efficacy of porous coralline HA as a substitute for autogenous or allogeneic bone graft following multilevel anterior cervical discectomy in a goat cervical spine fusion model. Significant rates of implant collapse with the bone graft substitute at 12 weeks were noted, but there was an excellent biologic compatibility with good early creeping substitution of the graft by host bone. The concomitant use of an anterior cervical plate with a graft prevented extrusion and led to graft incorporation rates that were comparable to those of the autogenous bone group and superior to those of the allograft bone results. However, mechanically, while the HA and allograft groups were compatible, they were significantly inferior to the autogenous graft group, leading to early collapse of the fusion mass.

Ceramics have mainly been used as bone graft extenders with autologous bone clinically, especially in fusion with long instrumentations. Ransford and colleagues compared 170 cases of posterior spinal fusion to treat idiopathic scoliosis using a synthetic porous ceramic (Triosite; Zimmer SAS, Swindon, UK) with 171 cases of autogenous bone graft in a prospective, randomized study. Their results indicated no significant difference between the two groups. In a prospective study of 32 patients who were treated with single-level posterolateral fusion using a biphasic calcium phosphate ceramic implant mixed with locally harvested bone, the overall rates of solid construct were 97% with clinical improvement in all but one case. There was a high rate of graft resorption, and poor fusion mass was noted on radiographs. The authors believe that the reason for a small fusion mass could be the tensile forces placed across the graft and the inferior supply of osteogenic factors as compared with massive autologous graft.

In patients who underwent anterior cervical interbody fusion using cages filled with Coral HA, Thalgott and colleagues demonstrated high fusion. McConnell and colleagues compared tricortical iliac crest bone graft to ProOsteon 200 (coralline HA) in a prospective, randomized study of 29 patients with anterior cervical interbody fusion with plating. There was no significant difference in clinical outcome and fusion rate. However, significant graft settling occurred in 50% of HA grafts and in 11% of autografts ($P < 0.009$).

Medical-grade calcium sulfate is in the form of regularly shaped crystals of similar size and shape. It produces slower, more predictable solubility and resorption. It has been shown to possess an osteoconductivity equal to that of autogenous iliac crest marrow/bone, with a rate of absorption that is equal to the rate at which new bone is formed. OsteoSet (Wright Medical Technology, Arlington, TN) is available in 3- to 4-mm pellets that dissolve in vivo within 30 to 60 days. The pellets are packaged in vials and are sterilized by gamma irradiation. Cunningham and colleagues showed OsteoSet to be comparable to autograft in a sheep posterolateral spinal fusion model. OsteoSet is also available in a powdered form, thus maximizing the surgical options for adding antibiotics and filling defects with custom-molded beads or shapes. The chief advantage is that it can be used in the presence of infection.

The effectiveness of calcium sulfate was compared with that of other graft materials (autogenous iliac crest, frozen allogenetic bone, ProOsteon 500 coralline graft, osteoinductive demineralized sheep bone preparation, and admixtures of autogenous iliac crest bone with calcium sulfate and coralline graft) in achieving lumbar interbody fusion in mature sheep. The substrates were placed into titanium mesh cages, which were implanted intervertebrally and recovered after 4 months. The histomorphology showed that the different graft types were equally effective at producing bone and that the effects were not different from the outcome of the empty control cages. However, biomechanically, the behavior of the control fusion masses (with no graft material) was inferior to that of the fusion masses with other graft materials. The demineralized sheep bone preparations were noted to be the least effective of the different substrates in achieving a solid interbody fusion. With regard to torsional strain, volume of tensile failure, and volume of bone formed within the titanium cages, the effects of calcium sulfate and autogenous bone were indistinguishable from each other; similarly, the effect of calcium sulfate was indistinguishable from that of ProOsteon and 1:1 admixtures of those substrates with autogenous bone.

Allergy to calcium sulfate, although rare and related to minor additives, should be considered in assessing the risk-to-benefit ratio of using it as a bone graft substitute. In one series of 15 implantations of calcium sulfate pellets (OsteoSet) used for bone reconstruction after resection of bone tumors, three cases of inflammatory reactions were noted. However, other investigators have noted that calcium sulfate is innocuous in terms of producing a local soft-tissue chemical or pyogenic inflammatory reaction.

COLLAGEN

The most abundant protein in the extracellular matrix of bone is type I collagen. Type I collagen has a structure that is conductive for mineral deposition, growth factor binding, and vascular ingrowth and provides a favorable physical and chemical environment for bone regeneration. It binds to noncollagenous matrix proteins, which initiates and controls mineralization. Collagen is a poor bone graft material by itself; however, when combined with BMPs, HA, or osteoprogenitor precursors, it may enhance the incorporation of grafts.

Collagraft (Zimmer, Warsaw, IN) is a composite of fibrillar collagen from bovine dermis and a porous calcium phosphate ceramic (65% HA and 35% TCP) in a ratio of 1:1. Although it does not provide structural support by itself, it is commonly mixed with autologous bone as a bone graft extender or with autologous bone marrow aspirate. The collagen serves as a carrier for the ceramic and the autogenous marrow. Appositional new bone is formed directly on the calcium phosphate surfaces. Walsh and colleagues evaluated the use of this composite in a posterolateral intertransverse lumbar fusion in the sheep model, which supported the use of Collagraft. A separate study by Zerwekh and colleagues showed that the use of Collagraft and autogenous bone mixture in a 3:1 ratio for lumbar interbody fusion in the canine model provided a suitable osteoconductive alternative to autogenous bone and resulted in the formation of a mechanically competent fusion mass that was similar to that obtained with autogenous bone alone.

Healos (Orquest, Mountain View, CA) is a mineralized collagen sponge. Each microscopic type I collagen fiber is coated with HA. By itself, it is osteoconductive, but it can be mixed with a bone marrow aspirate to provide osteogenic and osteoinductive potential. In a study of posterolateral intertransverse lumbar spine fusion in the New Zealand white rabbit model, Tay and colleagues showed that Healos could be used in combination with an osteoinductive or osteogenic agent to ensure reliable fusion rates.

OSTEOINDUCTIVE MATERIALS

Marshall Urist and colleagues first showed that demineralized bone matrix induces ingrowth of connective tissue cells and differentiation of cartilage and bone, and this was a great breakthrough in biologic bone graft substitute technology. Advances in isolation of proteins have yielded evidence of a series of osteoinductive glycoproteins, including BMPs, transforming growth factor-β, platelet-derived growth factor, and epidermal growth factor, as well as others. Extracts of bone containing the above growth factors produce new bone in ectopic sites in animal trials. Of all of these osteoinductive proteins, the most important for bone formation has been shown to be BMPs, which stimulate osteoblastic differentiation of pluripotent stem cells in vitro and are the only bioactive molecules capable of inducing ectopic bone production in vivo.

DEMINERALIZED BONE MATRIX

Demineralized bone matrix (DBM) is an osteoconductive scaffold that is manufactured by acid extraction of allograft bone. While it provides no structural support, it contains noncollagenous proteins, osteoinductive growth factors, and type I collagen. DBM is a mixture of BMPs and immunogenic, noninductive proteins. It has greater osteoinductive potential than allograft, owing to enhanced bioavailability of growth factors secondary to the demineralization.

The osteoinductive potential of DBM is subject to a great deal of variability and depends on a number of factors, such as processing solution, temperature extremes, demineralization time, DBM particle size, and method of terminal sterilization.

The variability in osteoinductive potential DBMs may reflect differences in BMP content, although the absolute concentration of BMP within the preparation does not necessarily correlate with its clinical efficacy. Also, DBM acquired from young donors has been shown to have greater osteoinductive potential than that taken from older donors.

Because DBM lacks an osteogenic potential, it is most effective when implanted in environments that offer sufficient vascularity and an adequate supply of osteoprogenitor cells. DBM has been shown to promote successful arthrodesis of the spine when used alone or in conjunction with autograft, bone marrow, or ceramics. In humans, DBM is mainly indicated as a bone graft extender when used in spinal fusion and is not thought to be sufficient for complete substitution for autogenous bone grafts in these more challenging healing environments.

Several DBMs are now commercially available. Grafton (Osteotech, Inc., Eatontown, NJ) consists of DBM combined with a glycerol carrier and is available in the form of gel, malleable putty, or flexible sheets. Opteform (Medtronic Sofamor Danek, Memphis, TN), a multiple bone paste, contains cortical bone chips. Osteofil (Medtronic Sofamor Danek) is an injectable bone paste that combines DBM with thermoplastic, collagen-based hydrogel carrier matrix. This nonwater soluble composite is easily extruded through a syringe when warmed to 46 to 50°C and becomes firm when cooled to body temperature. DynaGraft (Regeneration Sciences, Inc., Irving, CA) combines DBM with a pleuronic reverse-phase copolymer carrier that becomes firmer as it warms to body temperature. Both the DynaGraft and Osteofil products were reported to contain greater amounts of DBM per unit volume than did the glycerol-containing composites.

BONE MORPHOGENETIC PROTEINS

In 1965, Marshall R. Urist made the seminal discovery that the extracellular matrix of bone has materials that contain the capacity to induce new bone formation by implanting a substance into extraskeletal sites in a host. At a later date, this substance was named *bone morphogenetic protein*. Since that time, BMPs have become a subject of intensive research aimed at developing treatment strategies for skeletal conditions resulting from trauma and degenerative diseases. By 1988, the molecular clones had been characterized, along with the activities associated with this protein, and the amino acid sequence from a highly purified preparation from bovine bone was derived. This led to the isolation and expression of human complementary DNAs (cDNAs), which were recognized as members of the transforming growth factor-β supergene family. Over the next 15 years, investigators have determined the molecular genetics of BMP biology and have identified more than 15 individual human BMPs that possess varied degrees of bone or cartilage inductive activities, which have led to the development of therapeutic preparations for specific clinical applications.

Clinical Uses for Bone Morphogenetic Proteins

It is estimated that approximately 1.5 million bone-grafting operations are performed annually in the United States. These include a multitude of procedures such as spinal fusion, internal fixation of fractures, and treatment of bone defects. Autologous bone graft is usually the preferred material for these procedures, owing to its known osteogenic properties as well as a significant compliment of live cells. Autologous bone graft contains other essential properties, including osteoconduction and osteoinduction, which have formed the basis for the development of the field of bone graft substitutes. Osteoconduction is the process that supports the ingrowth of sprouting capillaries and perivascular tissues as well as osteoprogenitor cells into the three-dimensional structure of an implant or graft. Synthetic osteoconductive materials, including calcium phosphate, calcium sulfate, and calcium hydroxyapatite as well as composites of collagen and calcium salts, have been developed to mimic the properties of autologous bone graft. The osteoconductive properties are believed to be a result of a substance's architecture and chemical structure as well as its surface charge.

Osteoinduction, which is attributed to BMPs, supports the proliferation of undifferentiated mesenchymal cells and the formation of osteoprogenitor cells with the capacity to form bone. Harvesting autologous bone graft from a patient is well known to have associated morbidity, including postoperative pain at the donor site, potential injury to local nerves and/or vessels, postoperative infection or hematoma formation, as well as disturbances in gait. It follows that development of synthetic materials containing both osteoconductive and osteoinductive properties would be beneficial by limiting the need of harvesting autograft bone.

In the past 20 years, investigators have evaluated the principles of bone induction with the treatment of musculoskeletal conditions in a variety of uncontrolled case reports or series. Reports have suggested the potential clinical efficacy of a variety of preparations of demineralized bone matrix or purified human BMPs. Randomized clinical trials have supported the use of recombinant and have led to various regulatory agency approvals for specified indications of recombinant human BMPs in the United States and abroad.

Bone Morphogenetic Protein-2

Recombinant human bone morphogenetic protein-2 (rhBMP-2) has been tested for use in spinal fusion in several completed, prospective, randomized clinical trials beginning in 1997. A preliminary report by Boden and colleagues demonstrated that rhBMP-2 was equivalent to autogenous iliac crest bone graft in regard to both fusion rate and clinical outcome. Subsequently, a scientific advisory panel of the Food and Drug Administration (FDA) advised that rhBMP-2 be approved for the first complete bone graft substitute for anterior interbody spinal fusion. Currently, rhBMP-2 carried on a type I collagen sponge is approved for use in conjunction with a tapered, threaded intervertebral cage (LT-Cage; Medtronic Sofamor Danek, Minneapolis, MN) for the treatment of degenerative lumbar disc disease. Preclinical proof-of-concept, feasibility, and efficacy studies laid the foundation that established parameters for the clinical use of rhBMP-2. Successive spinal fusion studies contributed to the evolution of the design and dose of the carrier-protein combination.

Animal Studies of rhBMP-2

The first preclinical study of the use of an interbody cage with rhBMP-2 augmentation was through single-level anterior lumbar interbody fusions performed through a retroperitoneal approach in a sheep model. Cylindrical threaded fusion cages were filled with either autologous iliac crest bone graft or rhBMP-2 on type I bovine absorbable collagen sponge carrier. At 6 months after surgery, all animals appeared to have achieved fusion on radiographs; however, there were significant differences histologically. Thirty-seven percent of the animals that were treated with autograft-filled cages had a histologic union, compared to 100% of the animals that were treated with rhBMP-2/collagen-filled cages. Sidhu and colleagues used a goat model to study whether tantalum with and without rhBMP-2 can facilitate bony ingrowth and arthrodesis. Eight goats underwent single-level anterior cervical discectomy and stabilization with a porous tantalum implant, four of which had rhBMP-2 added. The goats were sacrificed at 12 weeks; three of four with BMP-2 demonstrated bony ingrowth (average 12.5%), while only one of four goats without BMP-2 had any bony ingrowth (average 2.5%).

Boden and colleagues used rhBMP-2 with the same collagen carrier contained in a titanium lumbar interbody fusion cage in rhesus monkeys. Two different concentrations of rhBMP-2 (0.75 and 1.50 mg/mL) were inserted into tapered titanium cages. All animals that were treated with either concentration of rhBMP-2 achieved fusion. A dose-response phenomenon was observed (bone formation associated with higher concentration was denser and quicker than that associated with a lower concentration). Subsequent human clinical trials used these results to define the 1.5 mg/mL dose for interbody fusion in subsequent human clinical trials.

Hecht and colleagues studied the use of rhBMP-2–loaded threaded cortical allograft dowels in the interbody environment of the rhesus monkey. Six months following single-level interbody fusion, all animals that were treated with allograft bone dowels filled with rhBMP-2 on a collagen sponge had solid fusion, whereas only one of three animals that were treated with allograft bone dowels filled with autologous bone graft had fusion. Of note, the allograft dowels containing rhBMP-2 had undergone complete resorptive remodeling, suggesting that the presence of rhBMP-2 accelerated not only osteoblastic bone formation but also osteoclastic remodeling. In the control group, no bone remodeling was observed (Fig. 27-3A–D).

Numerous authors have performed preclinical studies using BMP-2 in the posterolateral spine. Sandhu and colleagues reported a 100% fusion rate in a canine posterolateral fusion model within 12 weeks after the implantation

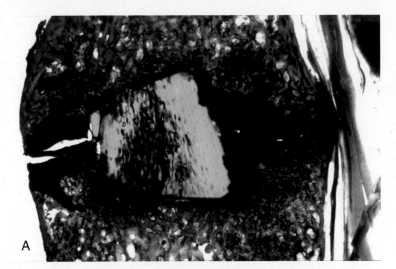

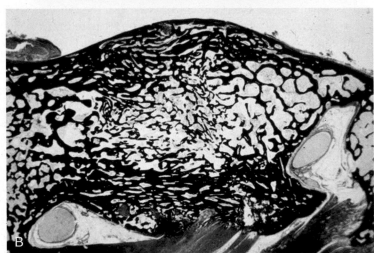

Figure 27-3. A, Six-month histology demonstrating minimal incorporation of the allograft cortical dowel. (No rhBMP-2). **B,** Allograft + rhBMP-2. The allograft has completely resorbed, with solid interbody fusion present.

of rhBMP-2 on a collagen sponge. Decortication was later found to be unnecessary for fusion in the presence of rhBMP-2 by the same authors. Fischgrund and colleagues used rhBMP-2 in a canine posterolateral fusion model to enhance the effects of autogenous bone graft, by applying it directly onto the autograft or by applying it on a collagen sponge and then adding the combination to the autograft. Larger fusion mass volumes were noted with rhBMP-2/ autograft combination.

Martin and colleagues found that rhBMP-2 concentrations that were effective in posterolateral fusions in lower animals (0.43 mg/mL) were not effective in primates. It was thought that overlying muscles caused compression of the collagen sponge carrier. A porous polyethylene shield was designed and placed over the collagen sponge carrier across the transverse processes for protection from muscle compression, which led to successful fusion with a lower rhBMP-2 concentration. Boden and colleagues developed a highly porous biphasic calcium phosphate ceramic carrier consisting of 60% hydroxyapatite and 40% tricalcium phosphate for use in posterolateral fusions in nonhuman primates. The biphasic calcium phosphate composition

allowed resorption while maintaining the residual scaffold of hydroxyapatite on which new bone could be deposited. All three rhBMP-2 concentrations (1.4, 2.1, and 2.8 mg/mL) resulted in solid fusions, whereas fusion was not achieved in animals in which autograft had been implanted.

Human Trials of rhBMP-2

In March 1996, an investigational device exemption was filed with the FDA to study the use of rhBMP-2 in patients with symptomatic degenerative disc disease. The rhBMP-2 was combined with Helistat absorbable collagen sponge (Integra Life Sciences, Plainsboro, NJ) as a carrier. The composite was placed into a lumbar tapered titanium interbody fusion device (LT-Cage; Medtronic Sofamor Danek). This was a prospective, nonblinded, randomized, controlled trial. Fourteen patients were approved for entry into the study and were enrolled at four investigational centers. An LT-Cage filled with rhBMP-2 was implanted in 11 of these patients. Three patients were enrolled in the control group, in which an LT-Cage filled with autograft

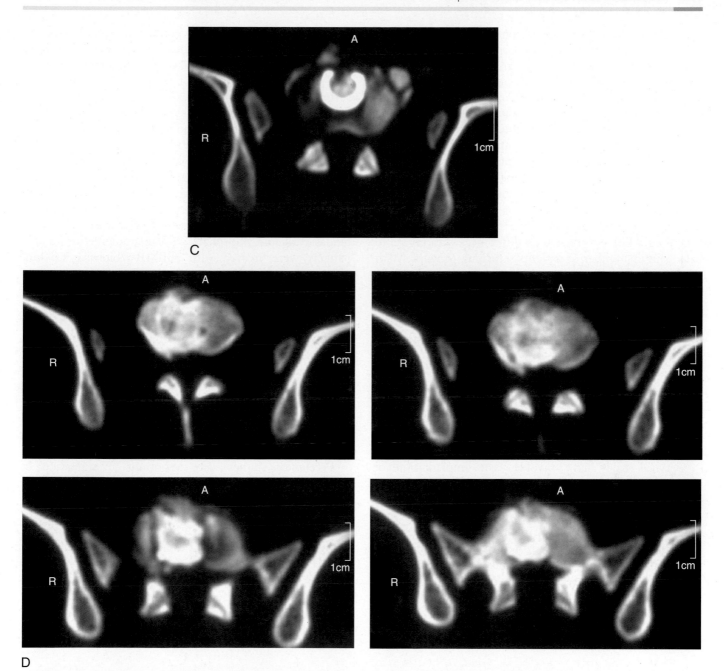

C

D

Figure 27-3, cont'd. C, Three-month postoperative CT scan demonstrating minimal incorporation of the allograft cortical dowel (no rhBMP-2). **D,** Allograft + rhBMP-2. CT scan demonstrating that the allograft has completely resorbed, with solid interbody fusion present.

from iliac crest was implanted. The composite device consisting of rhBMP-2 carried by the absorbable collagen sponge was trademarked as INFUSE (Medtronic Sofamor Danek, Memphis, TN). The primary objectives were to compare fusion by fine-cut computed tomography (CT) scans and to establish the safety of rhBMP-2 in humans. A secondary objective was to evaluate patient-driven outcomes for assessment of the effectiveness of treatment with regard to pain and function. All 11 patients who were treated with rhBMP-2 had successful fusion as determined by thin-cut CT scans. One control patient had a pseudoarthrosis and required supplemental posterior fixa-

tion and fusion 18 months after the index procedure. The experimental cohort had superior Oswestry scores at each of the follow-up time points; however, with the small numbers of patients enrolled, the differences were not significant. Serum samples were analyzed for the presence of antibodies to rhBMP-2 and bovine type I collagen, because Helistat collagen sponge is derived from bovine collagen. None of the study patients had rhBMP-2 antibody titers, but three patients had increased antibovine type I collagen titers; however, no clinical sequelae were noted, and all three of these patients had successful spine fusions.

The safety and efficacy data from the pilot clinical trial were used for initiation of a larger pivotal trial; 143 patients were enrolled in the experimental group, and 136 patients were enrolled in the control group. This study was designed as a prospective, multicenter, randomized trial. The experimental group was treated with the LT-Cage with INFUSE for a single-level anterior lumbar interbody fusion. The control group was treated with the same cage filled with iliac crest autograft. Operative time and blood loss were significantly less in the experimental group. Donor site pain was noted by over one third of the patients in the control group 2 years following surgery. Oswestry outcome scores showed no differences at any follow-up time point. There were also no differences with regard to back pain or number of patients returning to work. With the use of a 15-point improvement in the Oswestry score for criterion for success with regard to pain and function, the success rate at 24 months postoperatively was 84.4% in the experimental group compared with 82.4% in the control group. Successful radiographic fusion was noted in 99.2% in the experimental group (Fig. 27-4) compared to 96.7% in the control group at 6 months. At 24 months' follow-up, 100% of the experimental group was noted to have radiographic fusion, compared to 95.7% in the control group. Overall, clinical fusion was noted to be 94.5% in the experimental group, compared to 88.7% in the control group.

Cervical trials have involved the implantation of machined fibular ring grafts (Cornerstone; Medtronic Sofamor Danek) filled with autograft or INFUSE for anterior cervical discectomy and fusion. This was a prospective, randomized, controlled study involving 33 patients. Eighteen patients were enrolled in the experimental group, of whom 10 underwent a single-level fusion and 8 underwent a two-level fusion. Fifteen patients were enrolled in the control group and were treated with machine fibular ring filled with autograft from iliac crest. In this group, 8 underwent single-level fusion, and 11 underwent two-level fusion. Blood loss was less in the INFUSE single-level

cervical fusion cohort: 91 mL compared with 123.3 mL in the control group. Donor site pain was negligible by 3 months postoperatively in the control cohort. All patients had radiographic evidence of fusion by 6 months after surgery.

Posterolateral lumbar fusion trials have also been performed. A prospective, randomized clinical pilot trial evaluated the use of rhBMP-2 with a biphasic calcium phosphate carrier in single-level posterolateral lumbar fusion. The follow-up averaged 17 months. There were three cohorts in this study: 5 patients were treated with iliac crest bone graft with posterior instrumentation (control group), 11 patients were treated with rhBMP-2/biphasic calcium phosphate with instrumentation, and 9 patients were treated with rhBMP-2/biphasic calcium phosphate without instrumentation. At 17 months, only two of five control patients exhibited fusion, compared with all of the patients who were treated with rhBMP-2. Clinical success, according to the Oswestry scores for pain and function, was equivalent among the three groups. The study also included two additional patients who were treated with rhBMP-2/biphasic calcium phosphate without posterior instrumentation and were diagnosed with grade II spondylolisthesis. Only one of these patients achieved fusion, which indicates the importance of mechanical stability in providing a favorable environment for successful fusion.

Preclinical studies were important in evaluation of effectiveness and limitations of rhBMP-2 in various spinal fusion environments. Proof-of-concept as well as feasibility studies in lower animals led to data including carrier kinetics, dose-response, site of fusion, and response in higher animals. Important studies demonstrated that rhBMP-2 carried on an absorbable collagen sponge consistently produced higher fusion rates in interbody fusion cages. New rhBMP-2 carriers, including biphasic calcium phosphate ceramic granules and the compression-resistant matrix sponge, have been found to be superior to autogenous bone graft in posterolateral fusions. A review of the

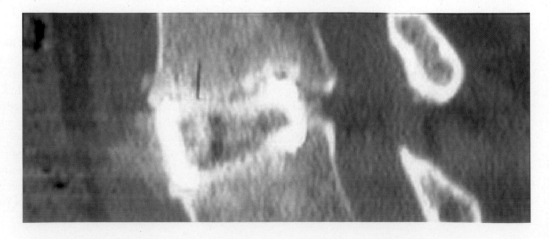

Figure 27-4. CT scan demonstrating bone formation through an LT cage. INFUSE was placed inside the cage prior to implantation.

clinical trials shows that inclusion of INFUSE bone graft with machined allografts for anterior lumbar interbody fusion is associated with improved fusion rates, improvement in pain and function scores, and greater likelihood of patients returning to work. All clinical trials of spinal fusion with INFUSE have shown a decrease in blood loss when compared to iliac crest autograft. Also, there was significant prevalence of iliac crest donor site pain, which was noted to be 30% to 40% at 2 years following surgery.

Currently, INFUSE is approved by the FDA for anterior interbody lumbar fusion, when used with an LT cage (see Fig. 27-4). Many surgeons have taken this opportunity to use the product for off-label indications. At this time, however, there are only limited clinical data regarding dose and carrier recommendations for use in the posterior lumbar and anterior cervical spines. There have been numerous anecdotal reports of bone formation adjacent to the neural elements when INFUSE is placed in the interbody space via a transforaminal interbody approach. It is likely that these areas of unintended bone formation are due to technical factors that are directly related to the surgical procedure and improper placement of the INFUSE-soaked sponge.

Of more concern is the off-label use of INFUSE in the anterior cervical spine. To date, several events have been reported regarding postoperative cervical soft-tissue swelling after the use of INFUSE. The cause of the generalized "edema" remains unknown, but it might be due to hyperconcentration of the product and/or placement of the INFUSE-soaked sponge adjacent to the anterior cervical soft tissues.

At this time, surgeons should be cautious regarding the use of this product for off-label indications. Further clinical studies are needed (and are currently under way) to determine the appropriate concentration and carrier for these off-label indications.

Bone Morphogenetic Protein-7 (BMP-7)

Recombinant human osteogenic protein-1 (rhOP-1), also known as bone morphogenetic protein-7 (BMP-7) was isolated by molecular cloning techniques and subsequently introduced into a Chinese hamster ovarian cell line that was able to express rhOP-1. The protein product is a homodimer that is purified by column chromatography to greater than 97% purity. Commercially available rhOP-1 is marketed by Stryker Biotech (Hopkinton, MA). Clinically, 3.5 mg of lyophilized rhOP-1 is combined with a carrier containing 1 g of type I bovine bone collagen for a final rhOP-1 concentration of 0.875 mg/mL. The carrier serves to deliver and contain the osteogenic molecules at the site of fusion and acts as a resorbable matrix for bone growth. This OP-1 implant is currently approved by the FDA for treatment of nonunions of long bone fractures. The addition of 230 mg of carboxymethylcellulose to the

OP-1 implant forms OP-1 putty. This product is currently being used in clinical trials of spinal fusion.

Animal Studies of OP-1

Cook and colleagues studied posterolateral fusions in the dog model using autograft bone or OP-1. Nine dogs were divided into groups of three and subjected to posterolateral fusion using four implant substances: OP-1 with collagen carrier, bovine collagen (type I) carrier alone, autologous iliac crest bone, or no implant material. The implants were randomized to various vertebral locations such that each animal received all four types of implants. The animals were sacrificed at 6, 12, and 26 weeks. Evaluations were done, including CT imaging, MRI imaging, mechanical testing, and histology. All OP-1-treated levels showed stable fusion by 6 weeks and complete fusion by 12 weeks. Autologous bone graft levels showed slower progression to fusion by 26 weeks. No fusion was noted at levels that were treated with either collagen carrier alone or no implant. Histology was consistent with radiologic results: OP-1 induced bone formation faster than autograft did.

Magin and Delling studied a sheep interbody fusion model by comparing OP-1 (3.5 mg of rhOP-1 to 1 g of bovine bone collagen) with an osteoconductive hydroxyapatite bone graft substitute or autograft bone. Thirty sheep underwent interbody fusion via posterolateral approach and supplemental transpedicular instrumentation. At 6 months after the surgical procedure, the animals were sacrificed, and the spines were subjected to mechanical testing and histology. The amount of bone formation was statistically higher in the OP-1-treated animals than in either the autograft-treated or hydroxyapatite-treated animals by 4 months ($P < 0.05$). Mechanical testing and histology confirmed the maturity and stiffness of fusion in the OP-1–treated animals, which were significantly improved in comparison to those qualities in the hydroxyapatite group ($P < 0.05$). Bone scintigraphy demonstrated significantly less activity in the OP-1 group at the 6-month time interval than in any other groups, signifying a more mature fusion mass.

Grauer and colleagues used a rabbit posterolateral fusion model to compare rhOP-1 with autograft or collagen-carboxymethylcellulose carrier alone. Posterolateral fusion was performed in 31 rabbits at the L5-6 level using one of the three substances. At 5 weeks, the spines were evaluated by manual palpation, biomechanical testing, and histology. Seven animals (23%) were sacrificed early because of complications and were excluded from the analysis. By manual palpation, all 8 rabbits (100%) in the OP-1 group achieved a solid fusion compared to 5 of 8 (63%) in the autograft group and 0 of 8 (0%) in the carrier group. This was statistically significant in both autograft and OP-1 groups, as compared to the carrier-alone group ($P < 0.05$). Flexion stiffness was greatest in the OP-1 group and least in the carrier-alone group ($P < 0.05$). Histology showed that

OP-1 sites demonstrated mature trabecular bone surrounded by a cortical shell compared to predominant fibrocartilage observed at the autograft fusion sites.

Cunningham and colleagues studied the fusion time course in a skip-level posterolateral dog model using autograft alone, autograft and OP-1, or OP-1 alone. Thirty-six animals were divided into four groups, which were sacrificed at 4, 8, 12, and 24 weeks postoperatively. Fusion was performed at L3-4 and L5-6. Evaluation was performed on the dog spines by radiography and biomechanical testing to determine fusion status. At 4 weeks, radiographic fusion was noted in 0 of 18 (0%) of autograft sites, 7 of 18 (38%) of autograft and rhOP-1 sites, and 4 of 18 (22%) rhOP-1 sites. At 8 weeks, 4 of 18 (22%) autograft sites, 16 of 18 (88%) autograft and rhOP-1 sites, and 12 of 18 (66%) rhOP-1 sites demonstrated fusion. At 12 weeks, 5 of 18 (28%) autograft sites, 15 of 18 (83%) autograft and rhOP-1 sites, and 13 of 18 (72%) of rhOP-1 sites demonstrated fusion. The difference between autograft-alone- and OP-1-containing sites was statistically significant ($P < 0.01$) at each time point. Mechanical testing demonstrated significantly increased stiffness in the OP-1 sites compared to the autograft-alone sites at the 8- and 12-week time points.

The toxicity of OP-1 was studied by Paramore and colleagues by intentionally placing OP-1 into the subarachnoid space during a lumbar laminectomy and fusion in a dog model. Three dogs underwent posterior L2 laminectomy and durotomy. Four control animals underwent dural closure and autologous posterolateral fusion using bone from the laminectomy site. The study animals underwent implantation of OP-1 (3.5 mg of rhOP-1 to 1 g of bovine bone collagen) with and without 230 mg of carboxymethylcellulose within the dural sac followed by dural closure. Posterolateral fusion was performed by placing the remaining OP-1 mixture in autograft from the laminectomy site between the decorticated transverse processes. The animals were sacrificed at 16 weeks, and assessment was carried out by palpation for fusion, as well as CT scanning and histology of the spine and spinal cord. Two animals in the OP-1 group were sacrificed early because of paraplegia from epidural hematoma. Eighty percent of the OP-1 animals and 25% of the autograft animals achieved solid fusion ($P < 0.05$) according to palpation criteria. Bone formation adjacent to the spinal cord causing mild spinal cord compression was noted in the animals that were subjected to OP-1 in the subarachnoid space. Spinal cord histology demonstrated inflammation adjacent to the newly formed bone; however, no evidence of spinal cord inflammation or neuronal cell death was noted.

Patel and colleagues studied a rabbit posterolateral lumbar fusion model to evaluate the ability of OP-1 to overcome the inhibitory effect of nicotine. Eighteen rabbits underwent L5-6 posterolateral intertransverse fusion with either autograft or OP-1. Nicotine was administered through subcutaneous miniosmotic pumps. Animals were sacrificed at 5 weeks postoperatively. Two of eight (25%) autograft rabbits and all OP-1 rabbits (100%) achieved fusion; this correlated with biomechanical testing. Histologic studies showed autograft fusion zones to be distinctly less mature than were OP-1 fusion masses. The researchers concluded that OP-1 was able to overcome the inhibitory effects of nicotine in a rat model.

Human Trials of OP-1

An FDA-approved human pilot study evaluating safety and efficacy of OP-1 has been completed, which compared autograft with OP-1 for posterolateral spinal arthrodesis. Thirty-six patients with degenerative lumbar spondylolisthesis and spinal stenosis underwent laminectomy and partial medial facetectomy and were randomized to uninstrumented posterolateral fusion with OP-1 putty (3.5 mg of rhOP-1 to 1 g of bovine bone collagen to 230 mg of carboxymethylcellulose) or autograft alone. Independent, blinded neuroradiologists reviewed static and dynamic radiographs to determine fusion status. Fusion was determined by bilateral bridging bone between the transverse processes, less than or equal to 5 degrees of angular motion, and less than or equal to 2 mm translation (all three criteria being required for fusion success). At the 24-month time point, clinical success, as determined by 20% improvement in Oswestry score, was achieved in 17 of 18 (94%) OP-1 putty patients and 6 of 10 (60%) autograft patients. SF-36 scores showed similar improvement in the two groups. Successful posterolateral fusion was achieved in 11 of 17 (65%) OP-1 putty patients (Fig. 27-5) and 4 of 10 (40%) autograft patients. No toxicity, ectopic bone formation, or adverse events were related to use of OP-1.

This challenging clinical model was chosen owing to the known high rate of pseudoarthrosis in this patient population. This uninstrumented scenario allows for evaluation of the product in an environment in which the fusion mass alone provides clinical stability. Postoperative evaluation of the flexion-extension radiographs would reveal no motion only if the fusion was "solid." It was thought that the use of transpedicular screws would make radiographic evaluation of the fusion mass more difficult and that it might give the impression of a "solid fusion" even if there is minimal bone between the transverse processes.

On the basis of the successful results of the pilot study, an FDA-approved pivotal study was begun in 2001 using the identical study protocol and the enrollment of nearly 300 patients. The final 2-year follow-up of all patients was completed in 2005.

The FDA recently approved OP-1 as a substitute for autogenous bone in attempting revision posterolateral lumbar fusions. This approval is under a humanitarian device exemption. The use of OP-1 putty is considered an on-label use in situations in which there has already

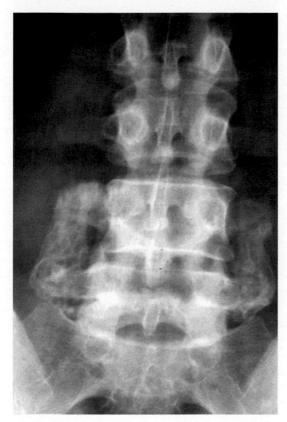

Figure 27-5. Two-year postoperative radiograph demonstrating solid bilateral intertransverse fusion with OP-1 putty.

been a failed attempt at posterolateral fusion (Fig. 27-6) and the patient is considered to be at risk for further pseudoarthrosis.

Animal studies and early human clinical trials have shown the efficacy of OP-1 as an alternative as well as an enhancer to autologous bone graft for spinal fusion. To date, no serious adverse side effects of OP-1 have been noted in these trials. Continued work is under way to help optimize the dose and carrier to improve results. OP-1 could replace and/or augment autograft bone in the wide spectrum of spinal pathology encountered in clinical practice.

Current Challenges and Limitations

Clinical trials have shown promising results and do provide insight that this new technology could enhance the treatment of skeletal injuries and conditions. However, various animal studies have shown more impressive bone formation and healing. This might be due to the nature of the host but might also be related to the need for improved methods of BMP delivery. Multiple factors might be necessary, including possible introduction as a "cocktail" with simultaneous and/or sequential activity; indeed, there might be a need for sufficient numbers of responding cells at the site of implantation in the host.

The ideal BMP delivery system could be dependent on multiple factors, including anatomic location, local soft-tissue envelope, and the mechanical strain environment provided by the fixation or reconstructive system involved

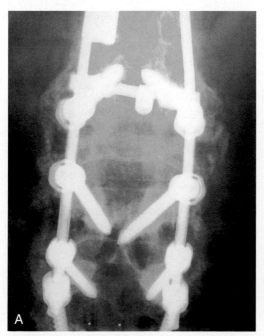
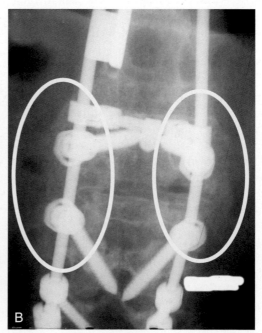

Figure 27-6. A, Six-week postoperative radiograph following a pedicle subtraction osteotomy. This revision fusion attempt was performed with OP-1 putty combined with TCP. Note the punctuate calcifications over the transverse processes. **B,** Six-month radiograph showing excellent consolidation of the fusion mass.

in the surgical treatment. Other conditions that should be considered include the possible timed release of BMP from the delivery system, the ability of the delivery system to control and maintain a proper dose of BMP, and the presence of the proper substrate that will enhance cell recruitment and/or attachment. It is also important for the delivery system to refrain from generating some type of immune and/or inflammatory response that could inhibit the reconstructive process.

There might also be financial restraints on the quantities of affordable BMP, which can in some situations become prohibitively expensive. In these situations, it may be necessary to combine rhBMPs with other grafting materials. A recent economic model was developed to compare the cost of stand-alone anterior lumbar fusion with rhBMP-2 on an absorbable collagen sponge versus autogenous iliac crest in a tapered cylindrical cage or a threaded cortical bone dowel. The upfront price of BMP ($3380) was likely to be offset by reductions in the use of other medical resources, particularly if costs incurred during the 2-year time period after the index hospitalization are considered.

The currently available delivery systems for recombinant BMPs include demineralized bone matrix, synthetic polymers, type I collagen, hyaluronic acid gels, and a variety of bone graft substitutes, including hydroxyapatite, coralline hydroxyapatite, and alpha-BSM (Extex, Cambridge, MA). An alternative approach that might in the future allow BMPs to produce even greater therapeutic effects could be achieved with gene therapy. In this situation, the genetic information would be transferred to a host cell such that the host cell would express and produce endogenous BMP protein. Gene therapy could offer several advantages, including possible control of the timing as well as the duration and quantity of BMP production.

Future Directions of BMPs

While a variety of BMPs are being investigated for their therapeutic potential, a combination of different BMPs and other growth factors might prove to be more effective in bone formation. The use of BMP-2/7 and BMP-4/7 heterodimers have shown increased bone formation in comparison to their homodimer counterparts alone. Because endochondral bone formation requires angiogenesis within newly formed tissue, upregulation of vascular endothelial growth factor or basic fibroblast growth factor might also improve efficacy of BMP gene therapy. Boden and colleagues have discovered an osteogenic protein (LMP-1) that appears to work through different mechanisms. BMPs function as secreted ligands, while LMP-1 functions intracellularly by upregulating the expression of several other osteogenic growth factors. Boden and colleagues found that this protein induces bone formation in several different experimental models with a relatively low transfection rate.

Growth factors with osteogenic activity have been shown in a variety of basic research studies, as well as human clinical trials, to have beneficial effects on bone repair and regeneration. The genetic overexpression of BMP could have some role in the future treatment of these difficult clinical problems. However, advances must be made in the field of vector design, gene regulation, and tissue targeting before clinical trials in humans can be conducted safely.

In the near future, additional clinical trials and case series will have been completed to determine the efficacy of BMPs in a variety of conditions. There will likely be continued development of putties, injectable formulations, and other materials with bone-inductive properties. Gene therapy might one day help to regenerate bone or assist in spinal arthrodesis. Increasing the host's responsiveness to BMPs, such as increasing the number of cells at the site of treatment that respond to BMP, could be equally important in clinical situations. It has been 40 years since the landmark discovery of bone induction by Marshall Urist, and we are now beginning to use this technology to treat pathologic conditions directly with BMPs. As these growth factors become more readily available clinically, they will likely have an increasing role in the future of spinal surgery.

PEARLS & PITFALLS

PEARLS

- Autograft has both osteoconductive and osteoinductive properties and is the gold standard for bone grafting.
- Adolescent scoliosis surgery is one of the best indications for allograft.
  - Same union rate as autograft, but less pain
- DBM may be used as a bone graft extender.
- BMPs with machined allograft for anterior lumbar interbody fusion have higher fusion rates, decreased blood loss, and less iliac crest donor site pain.
  - BMP-2 (INFUSE) and BMP-7 (OP-1) are the two commercially available BMPs.

PITFALLS

- Iliac crest autograft has a major complication rate of 0.7% to 25%, including chronic pain.
- Allograft has a small risk of disease transmission, especially with fresh frozen allograft.
- DBM is not for use as a stand-alone graft.
  - Variable quality and osteoinductive properties depending on source and processing
- BMP must be used with caution in anterior cervical procedures where there might be more swelling.
  - Pay attention to good biomechanical technique and support to achieve fusion.

REFERENCES

Baramki H, Steffen T, Lander P, et al: The efficacy of interconnected porous hydroxyapatite in achieving posterior lumbar fusion in sheep. Spine 2000;25:1053–1060.

Boden SD: Biology of lumbar spine fusion and use of bone graft substitutes: Present, future, and next generation. Tissue Eng 2000;6: 383–399.

Boden S, Martin G, Morone M, et al: Posterolateral lumbar intertransverse process spine arthrodesis with recombinant human bone morphogenetic protein-2/hydroxyapatite-tricalcium phosphate after laminectomy in the nonhuman primate. Spine 1999;24: 1179–1185.

Boden SD, Martin GJ Jr, Horton WC, et al: Laparoscopic anterior spinal arthrodesis with rhBMP-2 in a titanium interbody threaded cage. J Spinal Disord 1998;11:95–101.

Boden SD, Titus LP, Hair GP, et al: Lumbar spine fusion by local gene therapy with cDNA encoding a novel osteoinductive protein (LMP-1): 1998 Volvo Award Winner in Basic Science Studies. Spine 1998;23:2486–2492.

Cook SD, Dalton JE, Tan EH, et al: In vivo evaluation of recombinant human osteogenic protein (rhOP-1) implants as a bone graft substitute for spinal fusion. Spine 1994;19:1655–1663.

Cunningham BW, Sefter JC, Buckley R, et al: An investigational study of calcium sulfate for posterior spinal arthrodesis: An in vivo animal model. Paper presented at Scoliosis Research Society Meeting, New York, September 16–19, 1998.

Cunningham BW, Shimanoto I, Sefter JC, et al: Posterolateral spinal arthrodesis using osteogenic protein-1: An in vivo time-course study using a canine model. Paper presented at NASS, New Orleans, 2000.

Delecrin J, Aguado E, Nguyen JM, et al: Influence of local environment on incorporation of ceramic for lumbar fusion: Comparison of laminar and intertransverse sites in a canine model. Spine 1997;22: 1683–1689.

Emery S, Fuller D, Stevenson S: Ceramic anterior spinal fusion: Biologic and biomechanical comparison in a canine model. Spine 1996;21: 2713–2719.

Fischgrund JS, James SB, Chabot MS, et al: Augmentation of autograft using rhBMP-2 and different carrier media in the canine spinal fusion model. J Spinal Disord 1997;10:467—472.

Fuller D, Stevenson S, Emery S: The effects of internal fixation on calcium carbonate: Ceramic anterior spinal fusion in dogs. Spine 1996;21:2131–2136.

Grauer JN, Patel TC, Erulkar JS, et al: Evaluation of OP-1 as a graft substitute for the intertransverse process lumbar fusion. Spine 2000;6:127–133.

Hecht BP, Fischgrund JS, Herkowitz HN, et al: The use of recombinant human bone morphogenetic protein 2 (rhBMP-2) to promote spinal fusion in a nonhuman primate anterior interbody fusion model. Spine 1999;24:629–636.

Heise U, Osborn J, Duwe F: Hydroxyapatite ceramic as a bone substitute. Int Orthop 1990;14:329–338.

Magin M, Delling G: Improved lumbar vertebral interbody fusion using rhOP-1. Spine 2001;26:469–478.

Martin TJ Jr, Boden SD, Marone MA, Moskovitz PA: Posterolateral intertransverse process spinal arthrodesis with rhBMP-2 in nonhuman primate: Important lessons learned regarding dose, carrier and safety. J Spinal Disord 1999;12:179–186.

McConnell JR, Freeman BJC, Debnath UK, et al: A prospective randomized comparison of coralline hydroxyapatite with autograft in cervical interbody fusion. Spine 2003;28:317–323.

Paramore CG, Lauryssen C, Rauzzino J, et al: The efficacy of OP-1 for lumbar fusion with decompression: A canine study. Neurosurgery 1999;44:1151–1156.

Ransford AO, Morley T, Edgar MA, et al: Synthetic porous ceramic compared with autograft in scoliosis surgery: A prospective, randomized study of 341 patients. J Bone Joint Surg 1998;80B:13–18.

Sandhu HS, Kanim LE, Kabo JM, et al: Effective doses of recombinant human bone morphogenetic protein-2: An experimental spinal fusion. Spine 1996;21:2015–2022.

Sidhu KS, Prochnow TD, Schmitt P, et al: Anterior cervical interbody fusion with rhBMP-2 and tantalum in a goat model. Spine J 2001;1: 331–340.

Skaggs DL, Samuelson MA, Hale JM, et al: Complications of posterior iliac crest bone grafting in spine surgery in children. Spine 2000;25: 2400–2402.

Tay BK, Le AX, Heilman M, et al: Use of a collagen-hydroxyapatite matrix in spinal fusion: A rabbit model. Spine 1998;23:2276–2281.

Thalgott J, Fritts K, Ginffre J, et al: Anterior interbody fusion of the cervical spine with coralline hydroxyapatite. Spine 1999;24: 1295–1299.

Toth JM, An Hs, Lim TH, et al: Evaluation of porous biphasic calcium phosphate ceramics for anterior cervical interbody fusion in a canine model. Spine 1995;20:2203–2210.

Urist M, Silverman B, Buring K, et al: The bone induction principle. Clin Orthop 1967;53:243–228.

Walsh WR, Harrison J, Loefler A, et al. Mechanical and histologic evaluation of Collagraft in a bovine lumbar fusion model. Clin Orthop 2000;375:258–266.

SUGGESTED READINGS

Boden SD, Hair G, Viggeswarapu M, et al: Gene therapy for spine fusion. Clin Orthop Relat Res 2000;379(suppl):S225–S233.

This article reviews the current local gene therapy and highlights specific issues that must be addressed in pursuing a gene therapy program. The authors suggest that the most critical step in gene therapy for bone formation might be choosing an appropriate osteoinductive gene. The choice of delivery vector is also thought to be important and depends on the potency of the gene and the specific application that is intended. Establishing the effective dose and the transduction time and determining the gene transfer method are important decisions, as is the choice of carrier material to form the scaffold for the new bone formation. Also, a strategy for in vitro and in vivo testing must be developed to maximize the chances of success in human trials.

Boden SD, Kang J, Sandhu H, Heller JG: Use of recombinant bone morphogenetic protein-2 to achieve posterolateral lumbar spine fusion in humans: A prospective randomized clinical pilot trial: 2002 Volvo Award and Clinical Studies. Spine 2002;27:2662–2673.

A prospective randomized clinical pilot study was conducted to determine whether the dose and carrier of rhBMP-2 that were successful in rhesus monkeys could induce consistent radiographic spine fusion in humans. Twenty-five patients undergoing lumbar arthrodesis were randomized (1:2:2 ratio) on the basis of the arthrodesis technique: autograft/pedicle screw instrumentation, rhBMP-2/pedicle screw instrumentation, and rhBMP-2 only without internal fixation. The radiographic fusion rate was 40% (2 of 5) in the autograft/pedicle screw group and 100% (20 of 20) with rhBMP-2 group with or without internal fixation (P = 0.004). This pilot study was the first with at least 1 year of follow-up evaluation to demonstrate successful posterolateral spine fusion using a BMP-based bone graft substitute, with radiographs and CT scans as the determinant.

Boden S, Schimandle J: Biologic enhancement of spinal fusion. Spine 1995;20:113S–123S.

This is a historical review of spinal arthrodesis and pseudoarthrosis. It notes that internal fixation has not eliminated the problem of nonunions and reviews the biologic enhancement of spinal fusion and its early research.

Boden SB, Zdeblick TA, Sandhu HS, Heim SC: The use of rhBMP-2 in interbody fusion cages. Definitive evidence of osteoinduction in humans: A preliminary report. Spine 2000;25:376–381.

This is a prospective randomized human pilot trial to determine use of rhBMP-2/collagen as a substitute for autogenous bone graft inside interbody fusion cages to achieve arthrodesis. Fourteen patients were randomized to receive lumbar interbody arthrodesis with a tapered cylindrical threaded fusion cage filled with rhBMP-2/collagen sponge or autogenous iliac crest bone. The arthrodesis was found to occur more reliably in patients who were treated with rhBMP-2-filled fusion cages. This is one of the first studies to show consistent osteoinduction by a recombinant growth factor in humans.

Burkus JK, Transfeldt EE, Kitchel SH, et al: Clinical and radiographic outcomes of anterior lumbar interbody fusion using recombinant human bone morphogenic protein-2. Spine 2002;27:2396–2406.

This is a prospective, multicenter study of 46 patients undergoing single-level anterior lumbar interbody fusion with rhBMP-2 (INFUSE Bone Graft). They were randomly assigned to one of two groups, and the results in the investigational patients who received threaded cortical allograft dowels with INFUSE Bone Graft were compared with the results of those who received threaded allograft dowels with autogenous iliac crest bone graft. At 12 and 24 months, the investigational group showed higher rates of fusion and improved neurologic status and back and leg pain when compared to the control group, and there were no unanticipated adverse events related to the use of INFUSE Bone Graft.

Patel TC, Erulkar JS, Grauer JN, et al: Osteogenic protein-1 overcomes the inhibitory effect of nicotine on posterolateral lumbar fusion. Spine 2001;26:1656–1661.

A rabbit posterolateral lumbar fusion model was studied to evaluate the ability of OP-1 to overcome the inhibitory effect of nicotine. Eighteen rabbits underwent L5–L6 posterolateral intertransverse fusion with either autograft or OP-1. Nicotine was administered subcutaneously, and animals were sacrificed at 5 weeks. Two of eight (25%) autograft rabbits and all OP-1 rabbits (100%) achieved fusion; this correlated with biomechanical testing. Histology showed autograft fusion zones to be less mature than OP-1 fusion masses. The authors concluded that OP-1 was able to overcome the inhibitory effects of nicotine in a rat model.

Polly DW, Ackerman SJ, Shaffrey CI, et al: A cost analysis of bone morphogenetic protein versus autogenous iliac crest bone graft in single-level anterior lumbar fusion. Orthopaedics 2003;26: 1027–1037.

An economic model was developed to compare the costs of anterior lumbar interbody fusion with rhBMP-2 on an absorbable collagen sponge versus autogenous iliac crest bone graft in a tapered cylindrical cage or a threaded cortical bone dowel. The economic model was developed from clinical trial data, peer-reviewed literature, and clinical expert opinion. The cost of bone morphogenetic protein ($3380) was thought likely to be offset to a significant extent by reductions in the use of other medical resources, particularly if costs incurred during the 2-year period following the index hospitalization are taken into account.

Schimandle JH, Boden SD, Hutton WC: Experimental spinal fusion with recombinant human bone morphogenetic protein-2. Spine 1995; 20:1326–1337.

Recombinant human bone morphogenetic protein-2 successfully and reliably achieved lumbar intertransverse process fusion in a validated rabbit model for posterolateral spinal fusion. Radiographically and histologically, greater and more rapid bone formation, consolidation, and remodeling were shown with recombinant human bone morphogenetic protein-2 compared to autogenous bone graft. Fusions that were achieved with recombinant human bone morphogenetic protein-2 were biomechanically stronger and stiffer than autograft fusions.

Urist M: Bone: Formation by autoinduction. Science 1965;150: 893–899.

This is a historical reference to the first study in which demineralized bone matrix was shown to induce ingrowth of connective tissue cells and differentiation of cartilage and bone. It has been credited as a major breakthrough in the advancement of biologic bone graft substitute technology.

Vaccaro AR, Patel T, Fischgrund J, et al: A pilot safety and efficacy study of OP-1 putty (rh-BMP-7) as an adjunct to iliac crest autograft in posterolateral lumbar fusions. Eur Spine J 2003;12:495–500.

This is an FDA-approved human pilot study evaluating safety and efficacy that compares autograft to OP-1 for posterolateral spinal arthrodesis in a challenging clinical model of uninstrumented posterolateral fusion. Thirty-six patients with degenerative lumbar spondylolisthesis and spinal stenosis underwent laminectomy and were randomized to posterolateral fusion with OP-1 putty or autograft alone. At 24 months, clinical success was achieved in 17 of 18 (94%) OP-1 putty patients and in 6 of 10 (60%) autograft patients. Successful posterolateral fusion was achieved in 11 of 17 (65%) OP-1 putty patients (see Fig. 4 in the article) and in 4 of 10 (40%) autograft patients. No toxicity, ectopic bone formation, or adverse events were related to use of OP-1.

CHAPTER 28

Complications in Spinal Deformity Surgery

Frank Schwab, Matías G. Petracchi, *and* Jean-Pierre Farcy

Prior to a review and discussion on surgical complications in spinal surgery, it is important to define the term *surgical complication*. In the literature, a *complication* has been defined as a morbid process or event occurring during a disease that is not an essential part of the disease, although it may result from it or from independent causes. While this definition covers the broad spectrum of complications across the medical field, it appears poorly suited to the "complications" that can arise during or after a surgical procedure. Perhaps it would be more helpful to narrow the definition of surgical complication to the following: an unfavorable, unexpected event involving the interruption, cessation, or disorder of one or more bodily functions, systems, or organs related directly or indirectly to a surgical intervention. The term *unfavorable* is applied because the event is deleterious to the patient's health. The event is *unexpected* because the surgeon did not plan to generate it. The event may be related directly to an intervention because during the surgery, an action or a maneuver produced the untoward event, (e.g., dural tear, great vessel injury). An event that is related indirectly to an intervention can mean that the secondary effects of performing a surgery lead to the untoward event (complication). For example, bed rest and limited activity of the patient during the postoperative period can lead to atelectasis, pulmonary infection, or a deep venous thrombosis.

According to the above proposed definition, it should be noted that a specific surgical secondary medical issue could be termed a complication in one setting while being considered merely a side effect in another, depending on whether it was expected or not. For example, a blood loss of 2000 mL might well be expected (side effect) in a revision surgery when a pedicular subtraction osteotomy has been performed but is not expected (complication) after a thoracoscopy for an anterior release and discectomy of three levels in a patient who is being treated for a thoracic scoliotic curve.

PATIENT PREPARATION: COMPLICATIONS, EXPECTATIONS, CONSENT PROCESS, AND DOCUMENTATION

It is important to underline that prior to the planning of any surgical intervention, the patient should understand all treatment options available and comprehend the basic plan and implications of the operation and its probable side effects, risks, and potential complications. Ensuring a proper understanding by the patient and answering all questions related to the surgical procedure are essential parts of the consent process (informed consent). Within this process, the surgeon may deliberate on how much the patient should be told and whether the consent form should cover all the possible complications. There is no clear answer to these important questions, and common sense might be the best guideline. As part of the consent process, the patient is provided with a consent form, which must include a description of the procedure, who will perform the procedure, a statement that the risks and complications have been discussed, and a statement that alternative treatments have been reviewed. The latter should be explained to the patient in plain language (the patient's own language or via a translator) so that the patient can understand what he or she is reading. The surgeon must be able to answer all questions and explain points that the patient might not understand. The patient should be given the time to read and understand the form and then formulate questions. In addition to the surgeon's and patient's signatures, a third person should witness the signing of the consent form.

COMMON COMPLICATIONS

It is essential to understand, and to make patients understand, that complications, even very serious ones, can and do happen, even in the best hospitals and with the best medical teams at hand. Given this fact, the goal of this chapter is to help anticipate potential problems that could arise, plan surgery optimally to minimize risk of complications, and be prepared to face a complication when it arises.

Complications related to surgery can occur at various points along a patient's treatment spectrum: during an operation, during the early postoperative time, or late (months or years following surgery). It should be noted, though, that in some cases, the worst complications are already set to occur, owing to a suboptimal surgical plan and strategy before surgery has even begun. Detailed preoperative planning is necessary in each case. It is important to define the approach or approaches, the positioning required, the exposure to the spine, and the details of each surgical step. For more complex cases, the need for osteotomies, the levels to fuse, the type and sequence of instrumentation, and the type of bone graft or biologic agents to employ must all be reviewed. Surgery related to spinal deformity treatment is complex and requires proper training and experience of the surgical team. It is important to accept that every surgeon who performs this type of surgery has encountered complications. Working as part of an experienced team and paying attention to proper planning can help to reduce complications.

Risks of surgically related complications are not entirely in the hands of the surgeon, and associated medical morbidities play a significant role. The impact of cardiac conditions, pulmonary conditions, mental status, hypertension, diabetes, coagulopathy, malnutrition, age, smoking history, previous surgery, bone quality, length of the procedure, and previous infection have all been noted to affect the risk of developing a complication and impact the outcome of operative intervention. Age, independent of overall health and medical issues, is a consideration but rarely a true contraindication to surgery. It is remarkable that patients who have already undergone several procedures to treat pain or deformity are nevertheless willing to endure more surgery to improve their condition, particularly revision surgery, which carries a significant risk of complications for the adult patient. Some series report very high complication rates, the more serious complications occurring in 35% of cases. Although meticulous preoperative planning and careful patient selection can decrease risks of significant problems, the risks remain relatively high in this type of revision surgery. Among the intraoperative complications, blood loss is high on the list. Complication rates for tissue problems and infection may increase with each subsequent procedure. Poor bone quality, in addition to fusion concerns, poses significant challenges in instrumentation anchorage. The length of a surgical procedure has been listed as a risk factor, given that it affects several parameters, including blood loss, third space fluid balance, pulmonary edema, and surgical team fatigue. Decision on stages (one, two, or three) as well as time for anesthesia and time to position or turn the patient must be added. Beyond a certain operative time, it can be better for the patient if the team plans for staging, owing to physiologic considerations and surgical team exhaustion. For complicated cases, at least two fully trained spine surgeons should work together. This can markedly reduce surgical time and increase patient safety.

Intraoperative Complications

As was noted earlier, complications are often related to numerous factors. Patient medical issues, the procedure at hand, and the physician's surgical expertise are all important. A review of common complications will be presented.

Neurologic Injury (Cord or Nerve Root)

The incidence of neurologic complications is rare in spinal deformity surgery. Qiu and colleagues did a retrospective study in 1373 scoliosis patients treated surgically at one institution. The total incidence of neurologic deficits was 1.89%, and that of serious and mild ones was 0.51% and 1.38%, respectively. They found the following risk factors for neurologic deficits: congenital scoliosis, scoliosis with hyperkyphosis, scoliosis correction by combined procedures, scoliosis with a Cobb's angle more than 90 degrees, and a revision surgery. Complications can develop because of direct injury, such as a trauma of the neural elements, or indirectly, such as through edema or compromised blood supply. Traumatic lesions commonly result from contusion, laceration, compression, electrocauterization, or traction. The neurologic complications can be acute or delayed, incomplete or complete, transient or permanent. In the setting of a complete injury (cord or root), the probability of full recuperation is very low. In general, the spinal cord is less forgiving to manipulation than are the nerve roots, and spinal nerves are more likely to recover than are the intradural nerve roots, probably because of the protection of the perineurium and epineurium.

A variety of tools have been developed to evaluate neurologic function (discussed in Chapter 29). Somatosensory evoked potentials, motor evoked potentials, free-running electromyelographic potentials, and direct implant monitoring by electromyelographic potential and Stagnara wake-up test are the most commonly employed. Each test has its limitations, but in concert, these tests complement each other and offer essential information on neurologic structures and pathways. Baseline waveforms for somatosensory evoked potentials and motor evoked potentials should be obtained prior to any osteotomy or realignment maneuver in the setting of spinal deformity. In some cases, intraoperative monitoring might not be reliable. In those cases, when a cooperative patient is involved, a wake-up test should be considered. Collaboration between the anesthesia team and neurophysiology team is crucial to ensure the ability to properly monitor potentials throughout the procedure (e.g., the use of muscle relaxants).

Operative positioning requires great care, owing to the length of spinal deformity corrective procedures. Pressure points or stretching can cause permanent neurologic damage. The surgical team must ensure meticulous positioning of the arms, legs, and head, protecting the bony areas to avoid nerve compression and skin pressure lesions. Particular attention must be paid to areas where the nerves are poorly protected by soft tissue, such as the ulnar nerve at the elbow and the peroneal nerve near the knee. It is important to pad vulnerable areas with foam, pillows, or silicone pads. In positioning the arms, special attention should be taken to avoid stretching the brachial plexus, by limiting positioning of the shoulder to no more than 40 degrees of abduction, 90 degrees of flexion, and 0 degrees of external rotation.

During revision procedures, operative exposure is more demanding than it is in primary cases, with more chances for a neurologic complication. Special care should be taken because scar can be adherent to nerve tissue, limiting its identification and safe retraction. We recommend pursuing the exposure from a safe (virgin) area to the high-risk area. Dissecting with a sharp wide Cobb elevator in the initial muscular planes helps to gain rapid and safe exposure to the bone elements posteriorly and can reduce the risk of cauterization near the dura with attendant complications. When working in narrow spaces, one should consider use of thin-foot kerrisons and consider unroofing posterior bone elements with a burr, peeling the last shell of bone with a curette.

Neurologic dysfunction related to spinal deformity surgery might be detected during the surgery, in the early postoperative period, or in the late postoperative period. When a neurologic deficit develops, numerous options may be available.

Intraoperative: If signal deterioration is related to placement of instrumentation, then remove the latter. If the reduction maneuvers lead to signal deterioration (somatosensory evoked potential, motor evoked potential), then release and undo the corrective action. Pedicle screws can be monitored by electromyelographic potential. If a change in potential occurs apart from instrumentation or manipulation, raise blood pressure (MAP > 90 mm Hg), give steroids, and observe.

Early postoperative: Steroids and imaging might be warranted. Consider a reoperation if the complication is caused by a new compression. Hematoma formation may be treated by percutaneous drainage or aspiration.

Delayed postoperative: Consider ischemia, swelling, or hematoma. Imaging is important for progressive deficit. Laboratory tests include hematocrit and coagulation studies. If hematoma is detected, urgent decompression or drainage is necessary in the setting of progressive deterioration.

Blood Loss

Surgery related to spinal deformity generally entails marked intraoperative bleeding. Although blood loss can be reduced through careful technique and recycling (cell saver), preparation for potential significant loss is important. Weeks prior to elective surgery, arrangements can be made to send the patient to a blood bank for autologous transfusion preparation. If the patient has a coagulation defect or is anemic, this must be treated prior to surgery. Before starting an operation, it is important to ensure that packed red blood cells and any other necessary products are available (compatible) for the patient. To limit blood transfusion requirements, lengthy and complex surgeries might warrant the use of tranexamic acid, Amicar, hemodilution, and hypotension (during exposure and closure). Complications related to injury of major vessels are rare, but anterior approaches to the spine require assistance of a surgeon who is trained in the required exposure, and potential repair, of vascular structures. Much more common are complications related to prolonged intraoperative and postoperative bleeding with delayed or incomplete reconstitution.

The extent of operative blood loss is commonly elevated in the setting of revision surgery related to spinal deformity due to neovascularization in scarred tissue. Bone bleeding, elevated in revision surgery but also common in primary deformity surgery, can be difficult to control with only limited success of cautery. Bone wax, thrombin-soaked Gelfoam, topical collagen (FloSeal), and packing techniques are helpful. When an osteotomy is performed, sudden and substantial blood loss can ensue, particularly in the setting of pedicle subtraction osteotomy and vertebral column resection. For that reason, the surgical team must have all spinal fixation elements in place and a contoured rod (or proximal/distal constructs with connectors) prepared for possible immediate realignment and closure following osteotomy. The anesthesia team must be aware of the timing around the osteotomy to prepare blood products as necessary in advance. (As a guideline, we are used to transfusing 1 unit of fresh frozen plasma for 2 L of blood loss compensated by transfusion and add platelets if the blood loss is more than 2500 mL.)

Ischemia of the spinal cord or optic nerves can develop after acute blood loss or low blood pressure. Additionally, the kidneys, brain, and intestinal tract can be affected. Utilizing cell saver is helpful to diminish or avoid allogenic blood transfusions. However, retransfusion can cause coagulation problems, particularly if more than 3 units are utilized (loss of coagulation factors). Diffuse intravascular coagulation is a clear risk with significant blood loss combined with retransfusion of blood that lacks clotting factors and platelets. If coagulopathy develops or is likely to occur, blood products such as fresh frozen plasma, cryoprecipitate, and platelets should be administered urgently. It is important to discuss preoperatively with the patient and family the potential need to use such products, which are pooled from multiple donors.

Dural Tear

During surgical lumbar spine surgery, incidental tear of the dural sac and subsequent cerebrospinal fluid leak constitute a rather frequently occurring complication. On a multicenter prospective study, Tafazal and Sell evaluated the incidence of dural tears. The rate was 3.5% for primary discectomy, 8.5% for spinal stenosis, and 13.2% for revision discectomy. One can expect a higher percentage in adult scoliosis surgery associated with spinal stenosis decompression or in complex deformity spine pathology, in which osteotomies around the spinal canal are necessary. Tafazal and Sell found a wide variation in the rates of dural tears among spine surgeons. This can be explained by variations in surgical technique. Meticulous exposure of neurologic structures, use of cottonoids, and coagulation of the peridural vessels with bipolar electrocautery can help to avoid complications. Tears of the dura are common and must be identified. Primary repair of a dural lesion consists of closure of the dural edges without tension. We recommend using a small stitch and needle such as a 6-0 Prolene or silk suture. A running locking stitch is usually placed. If a simple closure is not possible, a patch with fascia, muscle, or fat graft and fibrin glue can be utilized. At the close of the case, a Valsalva maneuver can verify the seal that was obtained. If an adequate closure is not achieved, it might be necessary to utilize a subarachnoid drain (with the assistance of a neurosurgical colleague).

Unrecognized or inadequately repaired tears during surgery can result in the formation of a fistula with a continuous cerebrospinal fluid leak or pseudomeningocele. A fistulous tract is a conduit for infection and should be repaired immediately. Although they are often asymptomatic, pseudomeningoceles can cause low-back pain, headaches, and even nerve root entrapment. Diagnosis can be confirmed on clinical examination or imaging studies, including magnetic resonance imaging (MRI) and computed tomography (CT) myelography. The initial management for lumbar symptomatic pseudomeningocele entails the closed external drainage of cerebrospinal fluid with or without blood patch application. The failure of nonoperative measures could necessitate surgery. Ideally, the procedure should involve repairing the dural defect, removing the encapsulated cavity of the pseudomeningocele, and obliterating the extraspinal dead space to minimize the recurrence of the problem.

Creating Imbalance, Insufficient Correction

Proper spinal alignment is critical for a long-term preservation of pain-free spine function. The ability for some adaptation to occur depends on the length of fusion, the area of fusion, and the degree of imbalance. Alignment in the setting of spinal deformity must be addressed three dimensionally, and particular attention should be paid to the sagittal plane. In general, long fusions into the lower lumbar spine with poor sagittal alignment are least well tolerated. Loss of physiologic lumbar lordosis has been associated with flat-back syndrome, also termed *fixed sagittal imbalance*. Proper freestanding anteroposterior and lateral X-ray films on which the sacrum, hips, and C2 odontoid can be clearly seen are mandatory. Measurement on the lateral film of the thoracolumbar kyphosis if present, the lumbar lordosis, and the pelvic parameters (incidence and sagittal pelvic tilt index) is mandatory. Evaluation on the anteroposterior film of the deformity, the obliquity of the lumbar end plates, and the closure of the iliosacral notch is also mandatory. In the frontal plane, it is important to achieve a plumbline that is centered within 2 cm of the central sacral vertical line (midpelvis). Causes of early imbalance are mostly related to strategic problems and suboptimal intraoperative assessment of balance. Spinal imbalance after surgery in a patient who is being treated for deformity can be due to a number of conditions, such as poor initial correction, imbalanced correction in the setting of multiple curves (usually lumbar more corrected than thoracic), and fusions to the pelvis, permitting limited accommodation to even moderate malalignment within the fusion. Crankshaft phenomenon, adding-on, and decompensation are late imbalance issues, which can be progressive in skeletally immature patients. Loss of balance around the fusion, accelerated degeneration above or below a fusion, and exhaustion of compensatory mechanisms (e.g., pelvic retroversion, hip hyperextension) are problems that are more commonly seen in adult patients following long spinal fusions for deformity, particularly when suboptimal spinal alignment is created by an operative intervention.

At this point, it is extremely helpful to do a preoperative plan on tracing paper or with digital software (e.g., Surgimap-Spine) to prepare the level of osteotomy and the amount of degrees required to obtain an acceptable final alignment.

Surgery related to spinal deformity often involves complex realignment across multiple vertebral levels. The positioning of a patient prior to the start of such a procedure will markedly affect the ability to achieve a desired alignment. This concept is particularly important to consider when surgery includes a lumbar fusion of multiple levels and even more so with fusions to the sacrum. Posterior spinal fusions are commonly performed with the patient prone on a Jackson frame or cushioned rolls. It is important to ensure hip extension and a support at the chest level. In such a position, optimal lordotic alignment of the lumbar spine can be ensured. In the setting of sagittal malalignment/imbalance (e.g., flat back), some surgeons place the patient onto a standard electric table with flexion that can be removed once an osteotomy is complete. Our preferred position has been on the Jackson table with eggcrate padding over the iliac positioners such that once an osteotomy has been completed, the spine will sink in a controlled fashion to the desired lordosis (controlled by instrumentation adjustments).

Assuming proper patient positioning, good surgical strategy, and skill in placing instrumentation, careful planning of the instrumentation assembly becomes the next important step. A good understanding of the flexibility of spinal segments and obtained mobility (through facet resection, osteotomies, etc.) is crucial. When it is necessary to obtain fixation at the cranial level of the thoracic spine, we implant screws in the pedicles of T2 and T4 and pass cables under the lamina of T3; the cables will be reflected and tied up on a cross-link at the level of T3, balancing stress forces and decreasing the pullout force. When the fixation is extended to the sacrum, supplementation of fixation to the pelvis is indicated. This will permit planning of the number of rods and the necessary corrective maneuvers to be exerted at each level. This in turn will dictate the contour of each rod and the sequence of attachment to the spine as well as adjustments in spinal alignment. Generally, the more rigid the deformity, the more attachment points and separate rod constructs are necessary to permit controlled correction. It is often desirable to consider proximal and distal constructs (two rods each), which can then be adjusted in respect to one another for fine-tuning the correction of complex deformity. A failure to do so could limit the ability to properly balance the spine once long rods have been seated. Intraoperative long-cassette (36-inch) films will help to determine spinal alignment but are limited in the ability to assess final pelvic and lower-extremity position (standing alignment).

Treatment for imbalance that is noted early after deformity surgery is prompt revision surgery. Delaying treatment can lead to consolidation of the fusion, which then requires osteotomy to properly correct spinal balance. Aside from modifying existing instrumentation, there might be a need to extend fusion levels if a suboptimal initial strategy is evident.

Approach-Related Complications of Anterior Spinal Surgery

Depending on the anatomic area, complications related to an anterior, anterolateral, or lateral surgical approach to the spine can occur. These include injury to blood vessels, nerves, lungs, ureters, the gastrointestinal system, and other anatomic features. Particular expertise or assistance by a colleague in thoracic, general, and vascular surgery might be necessary for these cases.

An anterior approach via a thoracotomy or thoracoscopy can cause thoracic nerve lesions (postthoracotomy pain), lung lesions (pneumothorax, atelectasis, mucous plugging) and possibly vascular or thoracic duct lesions. During the surgical approach, meticulous attention to the intercostal neurovascular bundle is important, and padding with soft trocars for endoscopic surgery or with lap pads for open procedures is important. During closure, entrapment of the bundle during thoracic reconstruction should be avoided (suture to include the pleura and rib periosteum/muscle but passed around the intercostal nerve). Careful identification of local anatomy is essential prior to

TABLE 28-1. Complications of the Anterior Approach: Relationship between the Spine Level and Adjacent Structure Lesion

Approach	Structure Lesion
Thoracotomy	Lung (pneumothorax, atelectasis)
	Vessel (hemothorax)
	Thoracic duct laceration (chylothorax)
	Thoracic nerve (neuroma, paresthesias)
Lumbotomy/anterior	Bowel
	Ureter injury
	Sympathic chain
	Great vessel

spinal work, and protection of soft tissues with malleable retractors and abundant lap pads is important. Full lung expansion prior to final thoracic closure (and after chest tube placement) is recommended.

An anterior approach of the lumbar or thoracolumbar spine can cause abdominal wall weakness, hernia, and lesion of the abdominal and thoracic organs and structures (ureters, great vessels, intestine, sympathic chain, nerves, thoracic duct). Experience in the surgical exposure, careful identification of the salient anatomy (e.g., ureters), and retraction can reduce the risks of complications. In the revision setting, the risks are markedly elevated, owing to altered anatomy and adherence of tissues. Primary repair of lacerated structures such as the ureter, major vessels, and bowel is necessary and requires specialized assistance. We therefore do not recommend undertaking surgical procedures in which such complications can arise without having proper backup specialists in proximity. Injury to structures such as smaller vessels (e.g., segmentals), the thoracic duct, and the peritoneum (not intestines) is often easy for experienced spine surgeons to treat. Segmental vessel bleeding requires proper exposure of both ends of the vessel followed by clamping and ligature placement (clips can be less reliable). Peritoneal sac openings should be carefully reconstructed with a purse-string suture (e.g., chromic gut) (Table 28-1).

Short-Term (Early) Postoperative Complications

Early postoperative complications in a patient who is being treated for spinal deformity may result from aggravation of comorbid conditions (e.g., infarct in the setting of cardiovascular disease), operative events (major blood loss), or indirect organ system compromise or dysfunction (e.g., pulmonary embolus). Early postoperative complications commonly include urinary tract infections, atelectasis, pneumonia, deep venous thrombosis, anemia requiring transfusion, cardiac ischemia, and wound infection. The usual clinical signs of a particular disorder or pathologic process can become blurred in the postoperative period.

Early detection of the complications requires repeated evaluation of the patient by the operating surgeon and other team members. Early detection of a postoperative complication is essential such that rapid treatment and optimal outcome can be ensured for the patient.

Wound Hematoma

Development of large hematomas in a surgical area following spine surgery can be concerning when compression of neurologic structures occurs, persistent drainage develops, or seeding by organisms and potential serious infection ensues. To minimize these potential problems, meticulous wound closure is essential, and avoidance of large dead spaces must be ensured. We therefore recommend preparing for closure during the initial surgical approach by carefully exposing the fascial layers with a small margin that will permit good visualization in reconstruction at the conclusion of the operation.

Unfortunately, the literature is not fully convincing on the need for postoperative wound drainage after spinal procedures. We utilize drains when the patient is obese (large dead space, fat necrosis, etc.) or when significant bleeding was observed during the surgery. The drain is preferably inserted above the fascia. If a dead space cannot be eliminated with a simple closure, one can consider creating a local muscle flap to fill the void. A simple lateral release of the posterior fascia can help markedly in the medial mobilization of the posterior muscle groups. At the conclusion of surgery, bulky dressings and adherent plastic films (e.g., Ioban) may help to protect the wound from pathogens and keep the dead space collapsed. To maintain sterility at the surgical site, dressings are preferably not changed in the first 48 hours. Drains are often removed when the output is less than 30 mL per shift.

Wound Infection

Early postoperative infections after spine surgery are uncommon. Fortunately, prophylactic antibiotics have led to a marked reduction in this challenging complication. There are a great number of variables that affect the probability of developing a postoperative infection. A literature review reveals surgical infection rates from 0.1% to 15% depending on numerous parameters, including primary or revision status, idiopathic versus neuromuscular spinal deformity, nonfusion or fusion procedure, fusion with or without instrumentation, healthy or unhealthy patient, anterior, posterior, or combined approach, operating time, and blood loss. Deep infection after spinal surgery is a devastating complication, increasing the risk for pseudarthrosis, poor outcome, adverse neurologic sequelae, and death. The medical, economic, and social costs of such infections are enormous. Despite advances in prophylactic antibiotic therapy, surgical techniques, and postoperative care, wound infection continues to compromise patient outcomes following spinal surgery.

The most important patient risk factors for developing a postoperative infection include the following:

- Malnourishment
- Neuromuscular deformities
- Immunocompromise
- Diabetes
- Rheumatoid arthritis
- Long-term steroid use
- Prolonged preoperative hospitalization
- Obesity
- Smoking
- Revision surgery

A number of these factors can be optimized, which underlines the importance of proper preoperative planning and teamwork with other medical services.

During surgery, several factors can affect the probability of a postoperative infection developing. The role of the surgeon can directly affect these factors through prophylactic antibiotic use, proper scrub technique, soft-tissue management, reduced operating time, limited blood loss, reduced operating room traffic, abundant wound irrigation, and meticulous wound closure. All the team members in the operating room (e.g., physicians, nurses, medical students, instrumentation company representatives) should be keenly aware of sterile technique and factors that influence the risk of infection.

Brown and colleagues have offered a literature review relating to antibiotic prophylaxis, wound irrigation, and wound drainage in patients undergoing spinal surgery. On the basis of their findings, a recommendation was made to utilize first- or second-generation cephalosporins as prophylaxis. Patients who are allergic to cephalosporins and those who are known to be either colonized or infected with methicillin-resistant *Staphylococcus aureus* should receive a combination of a glycopeptide (vancomycin or teicoplanin) and gentamicin. Further recommendations included frequent irrigation of the surgical field in patients who are undergoing prolonged spinal surgery.

Irrigation of surgical wounds with antibiotics and antiseptics has been used for decades to decrease infection rates. Numerous in vitro and animal studies have demonstrated the effectiveness of topical antibiotics (neomycin, bacitracin, polymyxin) in eliminating causative organisms that are encountered during surgery. Most clinical studies of topical antibiotics were performed in the field of general surgery. Cheng and colleagues performed a prospective, randomized study to evaluate the clinical effectiveness of dilute (3.5%) betadine solution irrigation for prevention of wound infection following spinal surgery. They found fewer wound infections in the group of patients irrigated with dilute betadine solution before wound closure. The authors recommended dilute betadine irrigation in patients with accidental wound contamination and marked risk factors for wound infection.

In a patient who is developing a postoperative infection, clinical signs may include fever, with associated findings of wound erythema, tenderness, fluctuance, and drainage. However, in some cases, diagnosis can be difficult when it is based on only limited clinical findings. In all suspected infections, laboratory tests are required to assist in the diagnosis. The C-reactive protein (CRP) analysis has been shown to be well suited in the setting of establishing a diagnosis of infection. Although elevated in the first days following surgery, the CRP value gradually diminishes and tends to normalize after 2 weeks postoperatively. The plotting of daily CRP values will establish whether normalization is occurring or whether there is an increase, which would suggest an inflammatory reaction such as an infection. The erythrocyte sedimentation rate is a more long-term indicator of inflammation and will not respond promptly to changes in clinical status. Likewise, the white blood cell count is not reliable in the setting of acute inflammatory changes and postoperative infection.

In the setting of suspected wound infection and drainage, sterile preparation and culture should be considered. This must be performed with the utmost diligence to ensure proper superficial sterilization and culture of only expressed fluid from within the wound area. In collaboration with an infectious disease specialist, antibiotic treatment can then be started. However, as the time course from surgery is prolonged, wound colonization will occur, and inaccurate culture results might be obtained. If the wound area is fluctuant but no apparent drainage is present yet other signs of infection have developed, then imaging by CT or MRI followed by sterile aspiration could be considered. If the suspicion is very high for a deep infection (or superficial infection continuous with deep tissues), then surgical débridement should be performed, and cultures should be obtained. Any previously started antibiotics should be discontinued, preferably with a 48-hour window, to optimize the yield of cultures. In the setting of early postoperative infection, spinal instrumentation should be kept in place to maintain stability. Following copious irrigation with saline solution, large-bore drains (to minimize clotting and collapse) are placed and hermetic wound closure is pursued. For repeated infections and poor response to previous irrigation or débridement, we consider application of a continuous aspiration system. The use of a commercially available system such as the vacuum-assisted closure device has been shown to be an effective way to accelerate healing of various wounds. Animal studies have demonstrated that this technique optimizes blood flow, decreases local tissue edema, and removes excessive fluid from the wound bed. These physiologic changes facilitate the removal of bacteria from the wound. Sometimes repeated débridements are necessary until the infection is controlled and an elective definitive reconstructive wound surgery is pursued.

In some instances, postoperative infections remain deep, and clinical symptoms may be less evident than is the case with superficial infections. If the patient presents with pain and systemic signs following a procedure such as a discectomy, a diagnosis of postoperative spondylodiscitis should be considered. Patients may report fever, chills, sweats associated with nocturnal pain, or an increasing lumbar pain after a period of relief. The surgical incision may seem quite unremarkable. Usually CRP and erythrocyte sedimentation rate levels are elevated. MRI is the first choice in terms of imaging to assist in diagnosis (Fig. 28-1). If it is not possible to obtain an MRI, then sequential technetium-99 and gallium-67 scanning should be considered. For a confirmed disc space infection but without neurologic compromise, sepsis, or peridural abscess, antibiotic therapy is the treatment of choice. Biopsy of the disc space is essential to determine the organism at hand and to guide proper antibiotic therapy. If the patient presents with neurologic compromise, sepsis, peridural abscess, or failure of the nonsurgical treatment, a surgical débridement with complete discectomy should be considered.

Instrumentation Failure or Displacement

Failure or unplanned displacement of instrumentation can occur at any point following surgery for spinal deformity. In the short term following an operation, common causes include poor anchorage at time of surgery, suboptimal strategy with excessive mechanical load on the instrumentation, injury (e.g., patient fall), or excessive motion (particularly twisting or bending) postoperatively. Poor instrumentation anchorage may be related to reduced bone quality and fracture or avulsion in the area of instrumentation. The most common cause for late or long-term instrumentation failures is failure of proper fusion (pseudarthrosis).

Poor bone quality can present a significant challenge in instrumentation anchorage during deformity surgery. A number of different devices and implants have been developed to address the needs of attachment to the vertebral anatomy. While there are trends in which type or system of instrumentation is utilized for deformity correction, commonly applied devices include pedicle screws, hooks, cables, wires, and combinations of all of these. When poor anchorage is achieved with any given device, alternate strategies should be considered. In general, augmenting the number of attachment sites to the spine will reduce the stress at any one level; therefore, this approach is commonly applied when poor local bone quality is detected. Unfortunately, all implants carry risks of loosening or failure of fixation.

Use of hook implants remains common in spinal deformity surgery. It is rare for hook dislodgement to occur. However, on occasion, particularly in distraction mode, these implants displace postoperatively. Most likely, this is a result of patient flexion and rotation movements causing vertebral displacement in relation to the foot of an incompletely seated hook. Hook dislodgement is most commonly observed at the ends of an instrumentation construct where significant forces and displacement can occur. The techniques of claw-hook (two hooks compressed against one another on the same or adjacent vertebral segments) con-

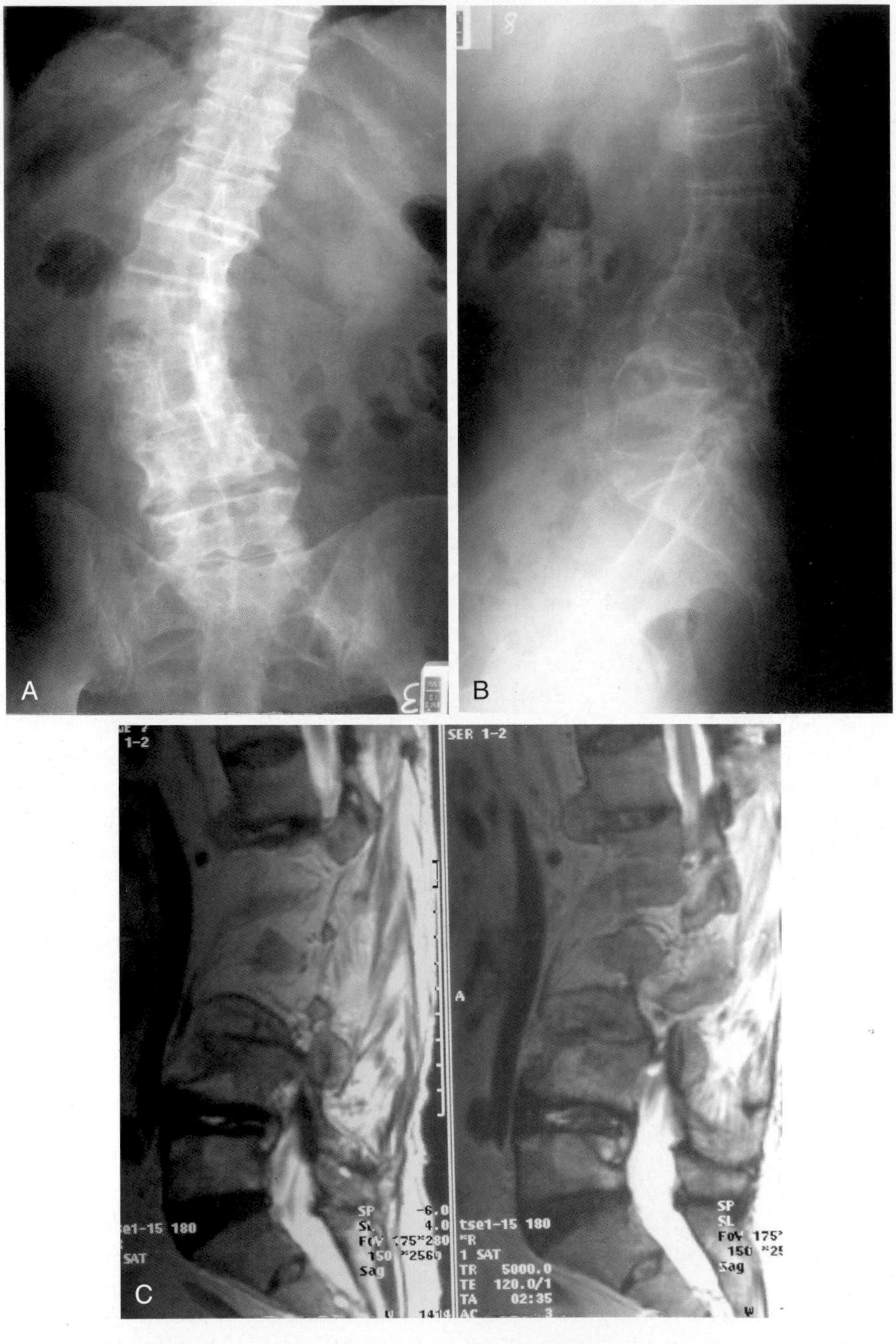

Figure 28-1. **A** and **B,** Anteroposterior and lateral radiographs of a 68-year-old man with scoliosis and stenosis of the lumbar spine that underwent decompression surgery. After the surgery, he complained of increasing back pain. **C,** MRI shows hyperintensity of L4-5 disc in T2-weighted image. Laboratory tests, CT-guided biopsy, and cultures confirmed a postoperative discitis.

figurations and segmental fixation have diminished the incidence of hook dislodgement. Additionally, augmentation of a construct with sublaminar cables in the top segments can help to avoid this complication.

Sublaminar wiring, while still commonly applied in the setting of neuromuscular (and some cerebral palsy) deformities, has seen limited application in idiopathic and adult deformities owing to complications that were noted in the past in the Luque technique. The latter have included neurologic sequelae as well as wire breakage, dural tears, and difficulty of removal. A cable system con-

sisting of two 49-stranded stainless steel cables connected to a common malleable leader was designed to overcome these shortcomings. We have utilized these cables in combination with screws and hooks with good results and no neurologic issues to date. A hybrid implant strategy can be particularly helpful in revision surgery with associated thoracic kyphosis or sagittal imbalance. Cables are helpful in those settings in the upper thoracic segments to prevent the pullout of the top screws or hooks. The sublaminar cables can be looped around a rod or the cross-link connecting two rods. It is important to be very careful during passage of the cables in the sublaminar tunnel, given the described neurologic complications, particularly in passing them at the extreme kyphotic or lordotic portions of a deformity.

Pedicle screw spinal implants are widely used in the operative treatment of spinal deformity. While they provide potentially excellent anchorage and control over vertebral positioning, their use has been associated with potential injury of structures in the vicinity of the pedicle and more generally the spinal column (dura, spinal cord, nerve root, great vessel, bowel). Risk factors for dislodgement of a pedicle screw, once seated, include poor insertion (partial or no pedicle anchorage), insufficient length, insufficient diameter (more important than length), pedicle fracture during insertion, and poor bone stock (e.g., osteoporosis). In addition to meticulous insertion technique, bone cement augmentation for screw anchorage and sublaminar cables should be considered when the patient has severe osteoporosis.

Instrumentation utilized after an anterior approach for correction of the deformity or to augment the chances of fusion, such as cages, structural allograft, screws, and rods, can also fail or be inserted in a wrong position with potential injury of relevant structures (Fig. 28-2).

The proper treatment for failure or unplanned displacement of instrumentation depends on the underlying reason for the failure. Early failures are usually addressed by revision instrumentation and supplemental fixation techniques (e.g., cables in addition to hooks or screws). Late failures, if not associated with pain or infection, are sometimes treated nonoperatively. There are cases of delayed fusion that go on to consolidation, once "distractive" instrumentation fails and permits compression in the arthrodesis area. If infection is suspected, prompt removal of instrumentation and exploration are essential.

Venous Thromboembolism

Deep vein thrombosis (DVT) and pulmonary embolism are well-known complications of orthopedic procedures. A combination of individual predisposing factors and the specific type of surgery determines the risk of developing venous thromboembolism in surgical patients. Few studies have evaluated DVT incidence and prophylactic protocols in the setting of spinal surgery for deformity. Incidence rates have ranged from 0.9% to 14%, depending on the investigating team and the prophylactic method utilized. The most common prophylactic protocol involves mechanical methods such as thigh-high elastic compression stockings and/or intermittent pneumatic compression stockings. The latter have been shown to be the most effective. The general consensus is that anticoagulation should not be used routinely following spinal surgery owing to potential complications such as epidural hematoma formation.

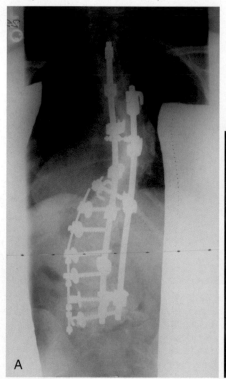
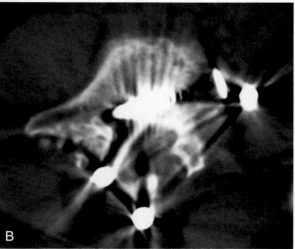

Figure 28-2. A, Standing radiograph of an adult patient who was treated by anterior and posterior surgery for severe scoliotic deformity. Back and leg pain were present. Imbalance in the frontal plane associated with anterior instrumentation failure (cable dislodgement) and pseudarthrosis is noted. **B,** CT scan reveals a malpositioned screw producing impingement of the L5 right root.

The placement of an inferior vena cava filter (IVCF) is an approach that should be considered in patients who are at high risk for venous thromboembolism following major spinal reconstruction. Leon and colleagues studied 74 patients undergoing spinal surgery with contraindication to anticoagulation who received prophylactic IVCFs. Criteria for filter placement included history of thromboembolism, diagnosed thrombophilia, malignancy, being bedridden for more than 2 weeks prior to surgery, staged procedures or multiple levels, combined anterior-posterior approaches, expected need for significant iliac vessel manipulation during exposure, and single-stage surgery with anesthesia time exceeding 8 hours. Twenty-seven limbs in 23 patients developed DVT. Five limbs had isolated calf DVT, and 22 had proximal vein involvement. Insertion-site DVT for IVCF placement accounted for nearly one third of the thrombi. The authors concluded that prophylactic IVCF placement protects patients who are in a high-risk category from pulmonary embolism.

Superior Mesenteric Artery Syndrome or Cast Syndrome

A rare complication of spinal surgery relates to an upper gastrointestinal obstruction syndrome originating from extrinsic compression of the third portion of the duodenum as it crosses between the superior mesenteric artery (SMA) (anterior), the abdominal aorta, and the upper levels of the lumbar spine (posterior). The SMA arises from the anterior aspect of the aorta at the level of the L1 and L2 vertebral bodies and descends downward and anteriorly, generating the aortomesenteric angle. The aortomesenteric angle normally ranges between 20 and 50 degrees and is filled by the duodenum, fat, and lymphatic tissue. The retroperitoneal fat and lymphatic tissues act as a cushion, protecting the duodenum from compression of the "nutcracker" arteries. Any factors that increase contact between the aortomesenteric structures and the duodenum can lead to an extrinsic compression. A number of variables may play a role in generating the SMA syndrome. In the setting of spinal deformity surgery, a sudden correction of a kyphoscoliotic spinal column, producing upward tension on the SMA, can lead to narrowing of the aortomesenteric angle and resultant clinical manifestations.

Historically, the incidence of SMA syndrome was noted to be a complication of casting and Harrington instrumentation placement when applied for spinal correction of deformities. The incidence is between 0.5% and 2.4%, according to two recent retrospective studies in which third-generation instrumentation was used. Zhu and Qiu reported seven cases of SMA syndrome in a prospective study of 640 patients with adolescent scoliosis. The main risk factors for this complication appear to be very thin body build, sagittal kyphosis correction with a distraction maneuver, and abrupt postoperative weight loss.

Signs and symptoms of SMA syndrome generally appear between the 4th and 14th days after spinal surgery but can develop before or after that period. Abdominal pain, nausea, and vomiting are common, as well as abdominal distention, although bowel sounds are usually present (normal to hyperactive). Differential diagnosis should include the common postoperative paralytic ileus, in which the bowel sounds are diminished or absent, particularly in cases in which high doses of narcotics were given for pain. The diagnosis of SMA syndrome is confirmed by gastrointestinal contrast radiographic evaluation with demonstration of contrast material cutoff in the distal part of the duodenum (Fig. 28-3).

Treatment of SMA syndrome varies from nonoperative to operative procedures. The most significant adverse sequelae from SMA syndrome include aspiration pneumonia, acute gastric rupture, and cardiovascular collapse with resultant death. If nonoperative treatment is started early in the clinical picture, the likelihood for the need of opera-

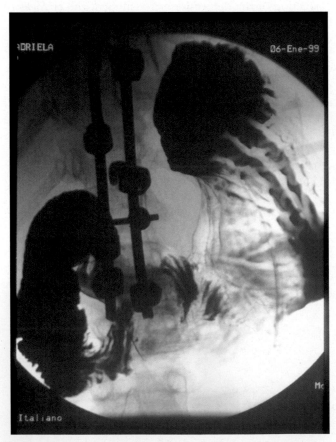

Figure 28-3. An 11-year-old patient was treated with a double approach to correct her idiopathic scoliosis. During the second postoperative day, the patient started with an upper gastrointestinal obstruction syndrome. An upper gastrointestinal series was performed that revealed a superior mesenteric artery syndrome. Enlargement of the proximal duodenum is noted, with apparent blockage in the third portion. The patient was treated with a nasogastric tube, parenteral nutrition, and positional modifications and was discharged from the hospital on the seventh postoperative day. *(Courtesy of Dr. R. Maenza, Italian Hospital of Buenos Aires, Argentina.)*

tive intervention is very low. It is therefore important to identify at-risk patients prior to the development of a complication. If a diagnosis of SMA syndrome is made, treatment begins with intravenous replacement of fluid and electrolytes to avoid hypovolemia, hypokalemia, and metabolic alkalosis. A nasogastric tube should be inserted to drain gastric fluids and diminish duodenal edema. A consult with the general surgeon and gastroenterologist should be considered. Placement of a nasojejunal or jejunostomy tube is generally recommended to permit enteral alimentation distal to the obstruction. Parenteral feeding is rarely necessary. Ensuring continued nutrition can help the patient gain weight and promote increased volume of retroperitoneal fat. For patient comfort, positional modifications may also be helpful: left lateral decubitus, seated leaning forward, or prone positioning to permit opening of the aortomesenteric angle.

Long-Term Complications

Pseudarthrosis

Surgery related to spinal deformity correction commonly involves planned arthrodesis across several levels of the spinal column. To obtain a solid arthrodesis (or fusion), transplantation of bone is commonly performed. However, in adult patients, locally harvested autologous bone graft material is frequently insufficient and needs to be augmented with allograft material and osteoinductive or osteoconductive products. Bone quality in children and adolescents is rarely an issue of concern, and fusion rates with locally transplanted bone are usually very high. Exceptions are patients with underlying neuromuscular conditions, cerebral palsy, and metabolic bone disease.

Pseudarthrosis following deformity surgery is suspected when, after a reasonable postoperative period (9 to 12 months), pain persists and loss of correction and/or instrumentation failure is observed. Not all of these findings may be present in cases of failed fusion, making proper diagnosis a challenge. Dynamic radiographs (flexion/extension), oblique radiographs, CT scans with reconstruction images, tomograms, and bone scans may contribute in confirming a pseudarthrosis. Given the diagnostic difficulty, in some cases only surgical exploration will confirm incomplete bone healing.

The rates of fusion failure reported in the literature vary widely depending upon the population studied: from 2% in adolescent scoliosis to 45% in the adult population with fusions extended to the sacrum. In a recent article, Kim and colleagues published an incidence of 17% of pseudarthrosis in the surgical treatment of adult idiopathic scoliosis. Failed fusion was most likely to occur at the thoracolumbar junction. Older patients (>55 years), patients with longer fusion (>12 vertebrae), and patients with thoracolumbar kyphosis (≥20 degrees) demonstrated increased risk for pseudarthrosis.

The complication of failure of intended fusion can be related to local parameters or global mechanical or stability issues. Local factors that can lead to pseudarthrosis include poor preparation or decortication of the fusion area, insufficient viable graft material, vascular insufficiency, effects of smoking or medication (e.g., certain nonsteroidal anti-inflammatory drugs), nutritional and metabolic problems, poor bone quality, or infection. Meticulous surgical preparation and adequate-quality bone graft (or use of extenders/factors) will help to reduce the chances of fusion failure.

Global parameters that can contribute to fusion failure include malalignment of the spine with poor sagittal and/or frontal balance, insufficient compression forces (or a fusion area under tension), and inadequate stability at the fusion site. Mechanical concerns become increasingly significant with the length of fusion and extension across transition zones, particularly the lumbosacral junction (Fig. 28-4).

We have found in the adult population a significant correlation between pseudarthrosis and sagittal malalignment. Pseudarthrosis in the pediatric population is rare in the setting of idiopathic scoliosis and is therefore seen mostly in high-risk patients for spinal fusion. This group of patients includes those with neuromuscular deformities or neurofibromatosis, nonambulators with porotic bone, patients with poor nutritional profiles (e.g., cerebral palsy with significant retardation), and cases of metabolic bone disease.

The treatment of pseudarthrosis (as in a primary procedure for high-risk patients) might require circumferential fusion with abundant autologous bone and, if necessary, augmentation with osteoconductive and osteoinductive bone materials. Anchorage for implants must be solid. Osteoporotic bone requires segmental fixation, and when fusion extends to the sacrum, supplemented instrumentation (in addition to pedicle screws) with iliac screws or nails (or other sacral anchorage) should be strongly considered. Delayed fusion with no evidence of instrumentation loosening may be treated with bracing, activity limitation, and observation. Once evidence of true pseudarthrosis has been established, treatment is almost always surgical. In rare cases of nonfusion without progressive deformity or pain, the treatment may be observational with close follow-up.

When surgical treatment for symptomatic pseudarthrosis is undertaken, aggressive removal of fibrous tissues, renewed grafting with autologous bone, and revision instrumentation are necessary. Circumferential fusion is usually recommended. Evaluation of sagittal alignment and pelvic retroversion must be completed and presence of poor alignment must be addressed. In the latter situation, osteotomies are commonly necessary to ensure satisfactory balance and contact between viable, bleeding bone to increase fusion success. The importance of proper alignment rises with the length of fusion and extension across junctional zones, such as the lumbosacral junction. The results of pseudarthrosis treatment in the pediatric population and adolescents are good. However, in our experience, the adult success rate is only around 60% with a "gray zone" of tolerated fibrous unions, which might enhance the clinical success rate to 80%.

Junctional Failure or Adjacent Segment Failure after Spinal Fusion

The term *junctional failure* in the setting of spinal fusion refers to structural incompetence or accelerated degeneration with associated instability and stenosis in levels above or below the fusion. The combination of mechanical stress and individual predisposition plays an important role in the junctional failure. Altered mechanical stress in the zone adjacent to fusion is explained by the adaptation, or imposed demands, of the unfixed segments to maintain global prearthrodesis movement and sagittal alignment.

Kumar and colleagues have shown the importance of obtaining physiologic segmental lordosis in performing fusion of the lower lumbar or lumbosacral areas. The authors performed a retrospective review of 83 consecutive patients who underwent fusion for degenerative disc disease with a mean follow-up period of 5 years. The association between two parameters of sagittal configuration (C7 plumbline offset, sacral inclination) and postoperative adjacent segment degeneration was analyzed. Patients with normal sagittal balance in the immediate postoperative radiographs had the lowest incidence of adjacent level changes. Patients with alteration of at least one of the two parameters that were analyzed demonstrated a 49% to 53% rate of adjacent segment degeneration (Fig. 28-5).

The thoracolumbar and lumbosacral junctional zones are particularly prone to the problem of junctional failure.

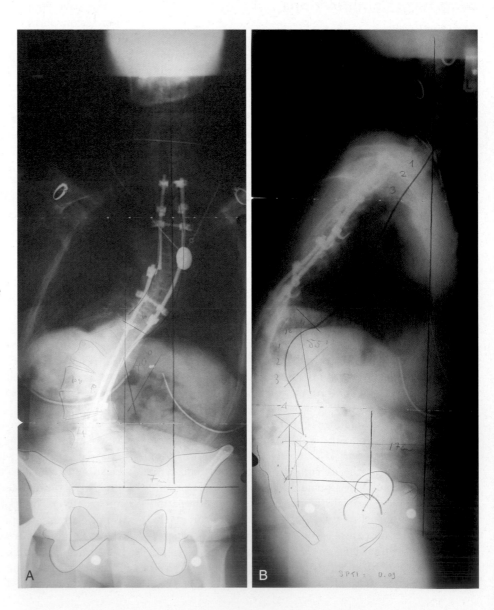

Figure 28-4. Images of a 66-year-old woman with marked imbalance of the spine after multiple surgeries. The patient complained of pain and increasing deformity. Notice a broken rod at the T6-7 level, which suggests a pseudarthrosis.

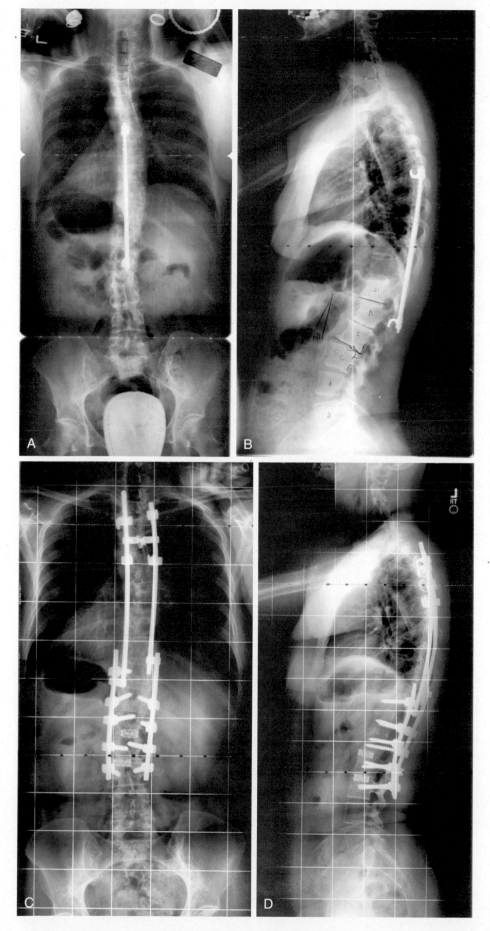

Figure 28-5. A and **B,** Full-length spine radiographs showing degeneration in the adjacent distal level of a T6-L1 fusion. The patient complained of lower-back pain and claudication symptoms. **C** and **D,** A circumferential fusion was done distally and connected to the previous fusion. Notice the restoration of balance.

Poorly aligned fusions that leave a junctional segment in marked deviation from normal anatomic position appear to pathologically load this segment to such a degree that eventual failure can be anticipated. To get a correct diagnosis of this complication requires a thorough evaluation, including dynamic radiographs, CT studies, and, if possible, MRI.

The treatment approach for junctional failure is greatly dependent on the driving force behind this complication. When conservative measures fail to provide relief, surgical treatment can be considered but must address local stability (by fusion) in addition to treatment of associated stenosis and, in some cases, a proper realignment of the fusion mass.

Deformity Progression after a Fusion on a Growing Spine

Spinal deformity progression after an apparent solid posterior fusion can occur in a growing spine. This usually occurs in a young child well before skeletal maturity (Risser 0) and often occurs in a gradual but progressive manner following an initial posterior surgical correction for scoliosis. Progressive deformity may develop in the segments of previous fusion (crankshaft phenomenon) or adjacent to it (adding-on phenomenon or decompensation).

Crankshaft Phenomenon: Deformity Progression in the Fusion. This phenomenon has been described as a complication following spinal fusion in skeletally immature patients. Crankshaft phenomenon occurs in the segments of the spine that, despite posterior arthrodesis, maintain significant anterior growth. Owing to disproportionate growth of the fused vertebrae, a progressive rotation and lateral deviation arise with a subsequent clinical manifestation of progressive deformity. Marked truncal asymmetry and imbalance may develop after an initial apparently acceptable correction of scoliosis. Crankshaft phenomenon is confirmed radiographically by evaluation of sequential films in the postoperative period. The patients who are most at risk for this complication are the skeletally immature: prior to the adolescent growth spurt, open triradiate cartilages, Risser stage 0 or 1. Given the risks of crankshaft phenomenon, it is thus important to identify when the growth spurt will start and when it is likely to end, as this can influence optimal surgical approach and timing. Avoidance of crankshaft phenomenon requires careful evaluation of the real growth potential at the time of initial spine surgery (hand films and elbow films for pre-Risser 1), and when necessary the judicious use of an anterior fusion in addition to a posterior procedure. When a patient presents with congenital problems, such as a cardiac malformation for which he or she underwent surgery in infancy, we must keep in mind that a growth delay is going to modify the usual growth pattern. These patients are candidates for spine deformity, and they are often at risk for crankshaft phenomenon.

The treatment approach for a crankshaft deformity will depend on severity, progression, and risk for further progression (skeletal maturity). The cases that require surgical management are those with severe imbalance and progressive deformity, which carry significant concerns that are functional, cosmetic, and vital. Dubousset has recommended a three-stage procedure under the same anesthesia to address this complication. Posterior instrumentation is nearly always extended cranially or caudally, if not at both ends. The goal is to achieve proper spine balance in all planes. In dealing with adults who present late with crankshaft deformity, we have found that at surgery, if a three-stage approach is applied, there are significant risks of spine instability between the second and third stages. The instability is impossible to fully control while turning the patient for the last stage. An alternative approach in these complex deformities, if they involve long fusions into the lower lumbar spine, might therefore be to address the sagittal and frontal planes separately. A first surgery can focus on sagittal balance by a low lumbar osteotomy, and after recovery, a second procedure addresses the frontal and transverse deformity in performing the necessary wedge osteotomy in the transverse/frontal plane. Instrumentation is placed after the first procedure, which can then be revised for the second procedure.

Adding-on Phenomenon: Deformity Progression Adjacent to the Fusion. Adding-on phenomenon is a progressive spinal deformity after spinal arthrodesis that becomes evident in the unfused levels. It appears to occur due to the choice of an inferior end segment and is most commonly noted in the treatment of adolescent idiopathic scoliosis, especially in treating major thoracic-compensatory lumbar curve, in which the goal is to obtain a balanced spine and perform a selective thoracic fusion to preserve motion segments in the lumbar area (Fig. 28-6). Ideally, after selective thoracic fusion, the unfused lumbar curve will spontaneously accommodate to the corrected position of the thoracic curve. However, with the use of segmental spinal instrumentation systems, postoperative coronal decompensation after selective posterior thoracic fusion in this type of deformity has been an unsolved postoperative complication. Selecting the ideal inferior fusion level in idiopathic scoliosis can be challenging. It is accepted that ending a fusion caudally at the stable vertebra, as noted by standing radiograph, is reasonable. The concept of a stable zone was defined by Harrington and is a useful guide; however, it is crucial to also consider the sagittal plane prior to selecting the end vertebra. If the "stable" vertebra that is selected on the posteroanterior radiograph falls in the apical region of a junctional kyphosis, then this is an unacceptable level to end fusion. In such a case, the fusion must be extended caudally to the next stable vertebra. Dobbs and colleagues analyzed different preoperative radiographs (36-inch posteroanterior radiograph taken with the patient standing, a supine posteroanterior radiograph, a supine right and left side-bending posteroanterior

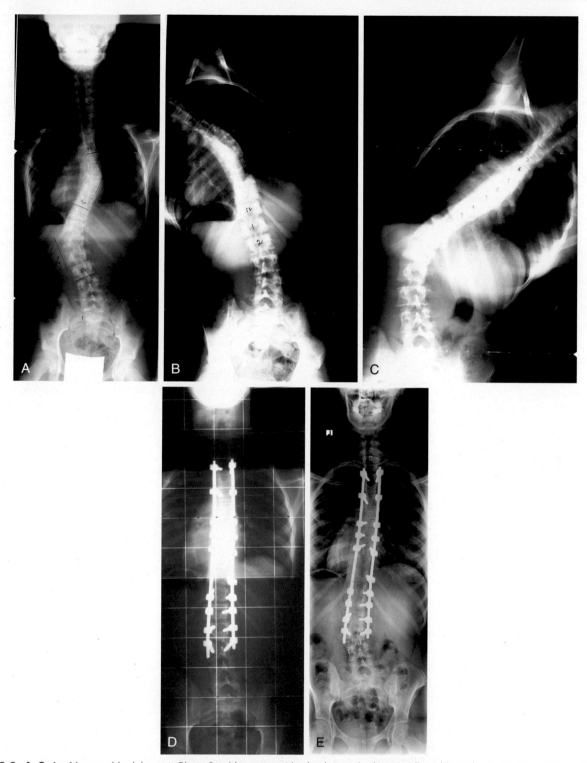

Figure 28-6. A–C, An 11-year-old adolescent, Risser 0, with a progressive lumbar–main thoracic idiopathic scoliosis. **D,** He was treated by a posterior approach with pedicle screws in both curves. **E,** Notice the curve progression below the fusion 2 years after surgery. This is a case of adding-on phenomenon.

radiograph of the spine, and a push-prone radiograph). They found that the preoperative push-prone radiograph is the best preoperative flexibility radiograph to predict the final lumbar curve measurement and, along with other factors, can be used to formulate a model that will help the treating surgeon to more confidently predict the final lumbar curve response in patients undergoing a selective thoracic fusion. Selection of the inferior end vertebra should also consider the bending films. The disc below the inferior vertebral fusion level should open on both sides on these films.

Using posteroanterior radiographs as a guide without attention to the lateral radiograph (which could reveal slight kyphosis between the curves) can lead to an inappropriate selective fusion. A tendency to fuse short in addition to this oversight will set the stage for decompensation and adding-on phenomenon, with a progressive deformity below the fusion. Decompensation can also occur above a fusion for deformity. In the upper thoracic levels, a structural curve might be mistaken for a compensatory curve. If this curve is not included in the fusion, it can progress significantly, creating a combined kyphotic and rotational deformity.

The treatment for significant decompensation or adding-on phenomenon requires an extension of fusion with planned realignment through the deformity. Early detection is essential. If initial postoperative films after primary deformity correction reveal a poor fusion level, then repeat assessment within a few months is important. When progression is noted and decompensation is anticipated, revision surgery should not be delayed.

Flat Back and Other Sagittal Late Imbalance Issues

Spinal imbalance after surgery in a patient who is being treated for deformity can be due to a number of conditions (Fig. 28-7). Early or delayed causes of imbalance were discussed earlier in the chapter and include poor initial correction, crankshaft phenomenon, and adding-on phenomenon. Late imbalance issues include those that arise several years after deformity surgery. This category includes progressive loss of balance around the fusion, accelerated degeneration below a fusion, and loss of compensatory mechanisms in the setting of residual deformity. Cases of late imbalance are most commonly due to lack of proper anatomic alignment at the time of initial surgery (Fig. 28-8). Global imbalance of the spinal column places elevated demands on remaining mobile segments and compensatory mechanisms (e.g., hip hyperextension/flexion, pelvic retroversion, knee flexion) to maintain balance and function. The most common late balance problems or complications of spinal deformity surgery include progressive kyphosis over a hypolordotic or kyphotic lumbar or lumbosacral fusion, flat-back deformity (fixed sagittal imbalance), swan neck deformity with long fusions ending proximally in a thoracic

kyphosis, and failure and instability of segments adjacent to a fusion (Fig. 28-9).

The treatment approach to late sagittal spinal imbalance after deformity surgery is based on symptoms, degree of imbalance, and levels of previous fusion. A conservative treatment approach in cases of mild or moderate symptoms can be considered in fusion ending at L4 or L5, absence of severe disc degeneration, and limited gravity line or plumbline offset from S1. An initial approach in these cases might consist of intensive physical therapy with strengthening and aerobic conditioning. However, in cases of severe malalignment, repeated attempts at physical therapy and pain management might not yield good results, and surgical realignment might be a good option. In some cases, early intervention (realignment) can avoid inevitable degeneration of disc levels caudal to a poorly aligned fusion.

Poor balance in the frontal plane, when mild, can be partially compensated by a shoe lift and a physical therapy approach. However, surgery might be necessary if there is poor sagittal and/or frontal imbalance in a patient in whom the lumbosacral junction has degenerated or fusion extends to the sacrum. In such cases, the treatment options include surgical realignment by means of osteotomies and revision instrumented fusion. The extent of revision fusion is determined by the status of the discs below the previous fusion. When possible, particularly in younger adults, distal segments should be spared to permit some degree of compensation and mobility. Extending a long fusion across the lumbosacral junction involves a high risk of pseudarthrosis (interbody fusion and iliac fixation are important) and is sometimes poorly tolerated by young patients.

The timing of realignment surgery poses an additional challenge. If balance is very poor, it is only a matter of time before the discs below the previous fusion fail. It might be in the best interest of the patient to proceed with surgical realignment (and avoid extension of the fusion) before further disc degeneration and failure set in. If extension of fusion is inevitable, then surgical treatment timing can be less critical, although the goal of obtaining optimal frontal and sagittal plane alignment remains the same.

Essential considerations in planning surgical correction of malalignment by osteotomies include the level of osteotomy (consider the hazards of osteotomy at the conus level or above), the type of osteotomy, the degree of frontal and sagittal realignment required, and the need for spinal stability during the procedure. Preoperative planning utilizing tracing paper cuttings or digital image manipulations is of great help in determining the ideal location of osteotomies and the degree of correction necessary. At the time of operation, exacting technique is essential; instrumentation must provide solid anchorage but avoid impingement or injury to unfused facet joints and supportive ligaments. Intraoperative stability and controlled correction through osteotomies may require the use of a four-rod technique or multiple exchanged rods of varying correction (Fig. 28-10). The four-rod technique has been our preferred approach, as it offers a distinct advantage over

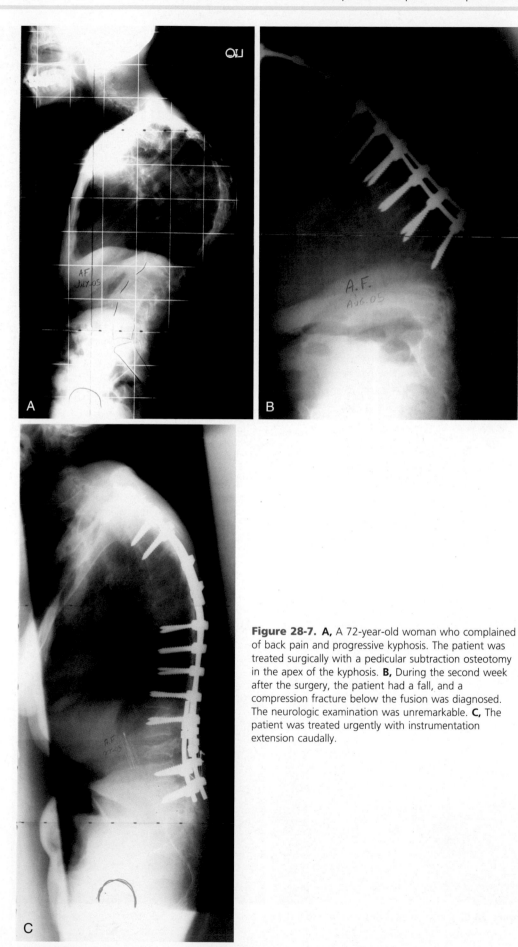

Figure 28-7. A, A 72-year-old woman who complained of back pain and progressive kyphosis. The patient was treated surgically with a pedicular subtraction osteotomy in the apex of the kyphosis. **B,** During the second week after the surgery, the patient had a fall, and a compression fracture below the fusion was diagnosed. The neurologic examination was unremarkable. **C,** The patient was treated urgently with instrumentation extension caudally.

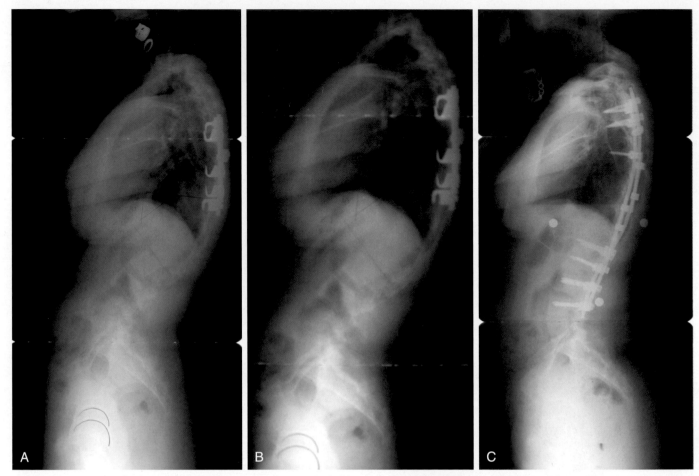

Figure 28-8. A, A 35-year-old woman who was treated surgically for thoracolumbar kyphosis with insufficient initial correction. **B,** Because of continued pain localized in the thoracolumbar junction, the surgeon interpreted the problem as an instrumentation prominence in the lower level, and a distal part of the construction was removed. Notice the progression of the kyphosis. **C,** Revision surgery with extension of the fusion below the thoracolumbar kyphosis to the horizontal vertebra was done to correct the deformity and avoid further progression.

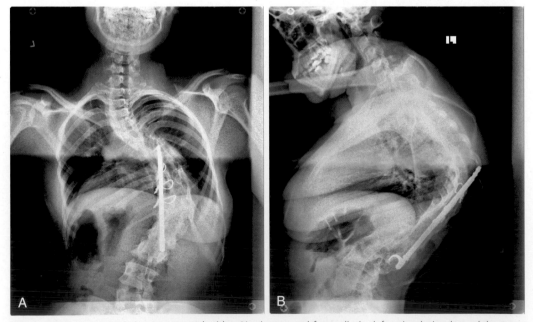

Figure 28-9. A woman who was treated with a Harrington rod for scoliotic deformity during her adolescence.

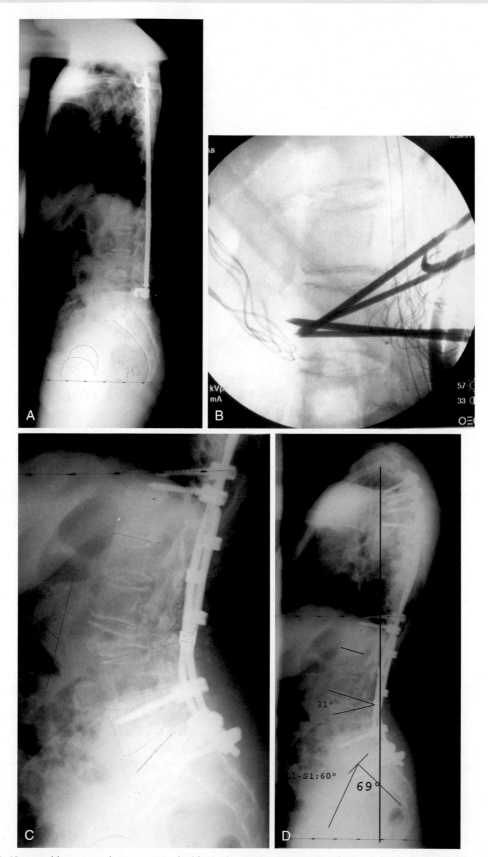

Figure 28-10. A, A 48-year-old woman who was treated with Harrington instrumentation during puberty. Notice the loss of lumbar lordosis (flat back or fixed sagittal imbalance) with compensatory pelvic adaptation (vertical sacrum/pelvic retroversion) and L5-S1 junctional failure with degenerative spondylolisthesis. The patient complained of typical symptoms of flat-back syndrome. **B–D,** Surgical correction with a single posterior approach, including a pedicular subtraction osteotomy at L2 and a transforaminal lumbar interbody fusion at L5-S1.

other techniques through controlled correction via proximal and distal constructs. The correction of complex deformities can be more safely undertaken, avoiding sudden translational or rotational movements that can jeopardize neurologic structures.

CONCLUSION

The risks inherent in spinal deformity surgery are significant and well established. Unfortunately, complications are not entirely avoidable and occur at the finest institutions and in the best teams. This chapter has attempted to provide an overview of the common complications and strategies that is intended to help in reducing their occurrence.

A common thread seen in many complications (short, middle, and long term) of deformity surgery is the concept of alignment. Iatrogenic spinal malalignment can be the consequence of numerous factors, of which surgical strategy is an essential one. Unfortunately, complete three-dimensional evaluation of the spine and the pelvis is not always easily obtained, and the precise optimal alignment for a given patient still remains poorly defined. It is now increasingly evident that pelvic parameters (e.g., pelvic incidence) are instrumental in the appreciation of patient-specific spinal alignment and balance. While marked advances in spinal care are certain to occur, as long as most spinal deformity operations involve fusion of multiple segments, the importance of balance must continuously be emphasized, given that even apparently small errors can lead to long-term complications.

PEARLS & PITFALLS

- Use of the bipolar electrocautery for homeostasis near neurologic structures
- Adequate magnification and illumination (sometimes consider loupes or a microscope)
- Sufficient exposure of neural elements in the field (usually a greater exposure is needed)
- Abundant use of cottonoids in working around nerve tissue
- Avoidance of excessive retraction of the neural elements; use of frequent breaks to release tension

- Use of thin-foot plate kerrisons and burrs in working in stenotic areas
- Performance of corrections slowly (discuss with monitoring team)
- Provisional instrumentation of the spine prior to destabilizing maneuvers (e.g., pedicle subtraction osteotomy)
- Avoidance of impingement after a correction (undercut all osteotomy bone edges)
- Consider aminocaproic acid (Amicar), or tranexamic acid when heavy blood loss (e.g., osteotomies of fusion mass) is anticipated.
- Keep the field as dry as possible early on, using powdered Gelfoam, Gelfoam with thrombin (FloSeal), bone wax, or packing gauze. Work in segments of the spine, and pack other areas. Consider segmental exposure instead of exposing the spine all at once.
- A vascular surgeon should be involved during anterior approaches in revision surgeries.
- For sequential surgery (anterior/posterior), do not hesitate to stage. Warn the patient ahead of time that two stages might be necessary.
- Discuss the sequence of surgery with the anesthesia team. Be particularly prepared around the time of osteotomy. Do not wait for hematocrit results.
- Expose properly to be certain that you know where the dura and nerve structures are.
- Use cottonoids as protection when working around the dura.
- Identify and expose dural tears so that they can be safely repaired.
- In addition to suture, use a patch or sealant (e.g., fibrin glue).
- Plan complex deformity surgery with the potential for staging, and advise the patient of this possibility.
- Ensure careful attention to the lumbar sagittal plane position on the operating table.
- Consider multirod constructs to optimize the fine-tuning of alignment and global balance.
- Properly evaluate spinal alignment with freestanding films preoperatively.
- Have a clear plan regarding the alignment that is to be obtained.
- Intraoperative radiographs (preferably long cassette) are better than fluoroscopy to determine alignment.
- Plan realignment surgery with paper tracings or digital image software (e.g., Surgimap-Spine, Photoshop).

Illustrative Case Presentation

CASE 1. A 68-Year-Old Female Who Had Six Prior Surgeries for Lumbar Scoliosis*

The last operation extended the fusion higher after a decompression for symptomatic thoracic scoliosis. The two rod systems were left unconnected, and the patient unfortunately developed a severe compression fracture, resulting in a severe kyphotic deformity (Fig. 28-11). She presented with severe back pain and inability to lie supine. She had difficulty walking and looking forward. There was a past medical history of Parkinson's disease treated with medications. On physical examination, she had a severe thoracolumbar kyphotic deformity. The skin was intact over the gibbus. She also had a 30-degree contracture of the left hip. She was neurologically intact (Figs. 28-12 and 28-13).

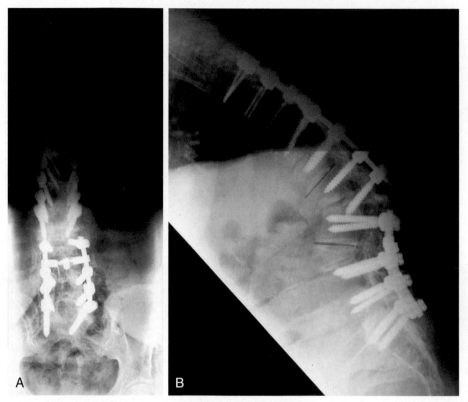

Figure 28-11. Anteroposterior and lateral radiographs showing acute 55-degree kyphosis over the compression fracture between the two instrumentation systems.

*Case courtesy of Thomas J. Errico, MD

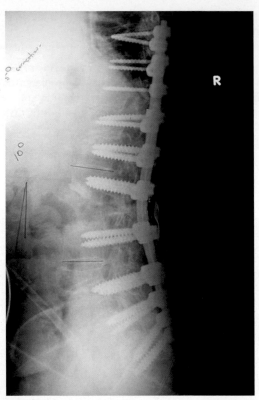

Figure 28-12. The correction obtained through a pedicle subtraction osteotomy through L1. The 55-degree kyphotic deformity was converted to 10 degrees of lordosis.

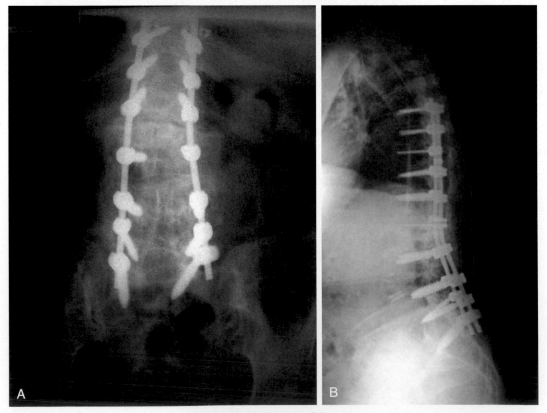

Figure 28-13. One-year follow-up.

REFERENCES

Aaron AD, Wiedel JD: Allograft use in orthopedic surgery. Orthopedics 1994;17:41–48.

Albert TJ, Pinto M, Denis F: Management of symptomatic lumbar pseudarthrosis with anteroposterior fusion: A functional and radiographic outcome study. Spine 2000;25:123–129; discussion 130.

Altiok H, Lubicky JP, DeWald CJ, Herman JE: The superior mesenteric artery syndrome in patients with spinal deformity. Spine 2005;30: 2164–2170.

Arlet VB: Revision pediatric spine surgery: Success and failures. In Margulies JY, Aebi M, Farcy JPC (eds): Revision Spine Surgery. St. Louis: Mosby, 1999, pp 439–465.

Been HD, Kalkman CJ, Traast HS, et al: Neurologic injury after insertion of laminar hooks during Cotrel-Dubousset instrumentation. Spine 1994;19:1402–1405.

Belmont PJ Jr, Klemme WR, Robinson M, Polly DW Jr: Accuracy of thoracic pedicle screws in patients with and without coronal plane spinal deformities. Spine 2002;27:1558–1566.

Benazet JP, Thoreux P, Saillant G, Roy-Camille R: Neurologic complications of surgery of the spine in adults. Chirurgie 1994;120: 39–42.

Benfanti PL, Geissele AE: The effect of intraoperative hip position on maintenance of lumbar lordosis: A radiographic study of anesthetized patients and unanesthetized volunteers on the Wilson frame. Spine 1997;22:2299–2303.

Bernhardt M, Bridwell KH: Segmental analysis of the sagittal plane alignment of the normal thoracic and lumbar spines and thoracolumbar junction. Spine 1989;14:717–721.

Boachie-Adjei O, Girardi FP, Bansal M, Rawlins BA: Safety and efficacy of pedicle screw placement for adult spinal deformity with a pedicle-probing conventional anatomic technique. J Spinal Disord 2000;13: 496–500.

Boden SD, Kang J, Sandhu H, Heller JG: Use of recombinant human bone morphogenetic protein-2 to achieve posterolateral lumbar spine fusion in humans: A prospective, randomized clinical pilot trial: 2002 Volvo Award in Clinical Studies. Spine 2002;27:2662–2673.

Boden SD, Schimandle JH, Hutton WC: The use of an osteoinductive growth factor for lumbar spinal fusion. II: Study of dose, carrier, and species: 1995 Volvo Award in Basic Sciences. Spine 1995;20: 2633–2644.

Boden SD, Schimandle JH, Hutton WC, Chen MI: The use of an osteo-inductive growth factor for lumbar spinal fusion. I: Biology of spinal fusion: 1995 Volvo Award in Basic Sciences. Spine 1995;20: 2626–2632.

Brambilla S, Ruosi C, La Maida GA, Caserta S: Prevention of venous thromboembolism in spinal surgery. Eur Spine J 2004;13:1–8.

Bridwell KH, McAllister JW, Betz RR, et al: Coronal decompensation produced by Cotrel-Dubousset "derotation" maneuver for idiopathic right thoracic scoliosis. Spine 1991;16:769–777.

Brown EM, Pople IK, de Louvois J, et al: Spine update: Prevention of postoperative infection in patients undergoing spinal surgery. Spine 2004;29:938–945.

Chanda A, Smith DR, Nanda A: Autotransfusion by cell saver technique in surgery of lumbar and thoracic spinal fusion with instrumentation. J Neurosurg 2002;96:298–303.

Chapman JR, Mirza SK: Neurologic deficits following surgery. In Margulies JY, Aebi M, Farcy JPC (eds): Revision Spine Surgery. St. Louis: Mosby, 1999, pp 271–284.

Cheng MT, Chang MC, Wang ST, et al: Efficacy of dilute betadine solution irrigation in the prevention of postoperative infection of spinal surgery. Spine 2005;30:1689–1693.

Crowther MA, Webb PJ, Eyre-Brook IA: Superior mesenteric artery syndrome following surgery for scoliosis. Spine 2002;27: E528–E533.

Curylo LJ, Johnstone B, Petersilge CA, et al: Augmentation of spinal arthrodesis with autologous bone marrow in a rabbit posterolateral spine fusion model. Spine 1999;24:434–438; discussion 438–439.

Dawson EG, Clader TJ, Bassett LW: A comparison of different methods used to diagnose pseudarthrosis following posterior spinal fusion for scoliosis. J Bone Joint Surg Am 1985;67:1153–1159.

Dearborn JT, Hu SS, Tribus CB, Bradford DS: Thromboembolic complications after major thoracolumbar spine surgery. Spine 1999; 24:1471–1476.

DiCindio S, Theroux M, Shah S, et al: Multimodality monitoring of transcranial electric motor and somatosensory-evoked potentials during surgical correction of spinal deformity in patients with cerebral palsy and other neuromuscular disorders. Spine 2003;28:1851–1855; discussion 1855–1856.

Dobbs MB, Lenke LG, Walton T, et al: Can we predict the ultimate lumbar curve in adolescent idiopathic scoliosis patients undergoing a selective fusion with undercorrection of the thoracic curve? Spine 2004;29:277–285.

Eck KR, Bridwell KH, Ungacta FF, et al: Complications and results of long adult deformity fusions down to L4, L5, and the sacrum. Spine 2001;26:E182–E192.

Epstein JA, Epstein BS, Jones MD: Symptomatic lumbar scoliosis with degenerative changes in the elderly. Spine 1979;4:542–547.

Erstad BL: What is the evidence for using hemostatic agents in surgery? Eur Spine J 2004;13(suppl 1):S28–S33.

Farcy JC, Schwab FJ: Limits of lumbosacral fusion. In Margulies J, Floman Y, Farcy JPC, Neuwirth M (eds): Lumbosacral and Spinopelvic Fixation. Philadelphia: Lippincott-Raven, 1996, pp 795–804.

Farcy JP, Schwab F: Posterior osteotomies with pedicle substraction for flat back and associated syndromes: Technique and results of a prospective study. Bull Hosp Jt Dis 2000;59:11–16.

Farcy JP, Schwab FJ: Management of flatback and related kyphotic decompensation syndromes. Spine 1997;22:2452–2457.

Ferree BA, Wright AM: Deep venous thrombosis following posterior lumbar spinal surgery. Spine 1993;18:1079–1082.

Finnegan WJ, Fenlin JM, Marvel JP, et al: Results of surgical intervention in the symptomatic multiply-operated back patient: Analysis of sixty-seven cases followed for three to seven years. J Bone Joint Surg Am 1979;61:1077–1082.

Gersin KS, Heniford BT: Laparoscopic duodenojejunostomy for treatment of superior mesenteric artery syndrome. J Soc Laparoendosc Surg 1998;2:281–284.

Goll SR, Balderston RA, Stambough JL, et al: Depth of intraspinal wire penetration during passage of sublaminar wires. Spine 1988;13: 503–509.

Goshi K, Boachie-Adjei O, Moore C, Nishiyama M: Thoracic scoliosis fusion in adolescent and adult idiopathic scoliosis using posterior translational corrective techniques (ISOLA): Is maximum correction of the thoracic curve detrimental to the unfused lumbar curve? Spine J 2004;4:192–201.

Gruenberg MF, Campaner GL, Sola CA, Ortolan EG: Ultraclean air for prevention of postoperative infection after posterior spinal fusion with instrumentation: A comparison between surgeries performed with and without a vertical exponential filtered air-flow system. Spine 2004;29:2330–2334.

Holland NR, Kostuik JP: Continuous electromyographic monitoring to detect nerve root injury during thoracolumbar scoliosis surgery. Spine 1997;22:2547–2550.

Kalen V, Conklin M: The behavior of the unfused lumbar curve following selective thoracic fusion for idiopathic scoliosis. Spine 1990; 15:271–274.

Kassam A, Nemoto E, Balzer J, et al: Effects of Tisseel fibrin glue on the central nervous system of nonhuman primates. Ear Nose Throat J 2004;83:246–248, 250, 252 passim.

King HA: Analysis and treatment of type II idiopathic scoliosis. Orthop Clin North Am 1994;25:225–237.

Knapp DR Jr, Jones ET, Blanco JS, et al: Allograft bone in spinal fusion for adolescent idiopathic scoliosis. J Spinal Disord Tech 2005;18 (suppl):S73–S76.

Knapp DR Jr, Price CT, Jones ET, et al: Choosing fusion levels in progressive thoracic idiopathic scoliosis. Spine 1992;17: 1159–1165.

Kokoszka A, Kuflik P, Bitan F, et al: Evidence-based review of the role of aprotinin in blood conservation during orthopaedic surgery. J Bone Joint Surg Am 2005;87:1129–1136.

Kumar MN, Baklanov A, Chopin D: Correlation between sagittal plane changes and adjacent segment degeneration following lumbar spine fusion. Eur Spine J 2001;10:314–319.

Lapp MA, Bridwell KH, Lenke LG, et al: Long-term complications in adult spinal deformity patients having combined surgery: A comparison of primary to revision patients. Spine 2001;26:973–983.

Lauerman WC, Bradford DS, Ogilvie JW, Transfeldt EE: Results of lumbar pseudarthrosis repair. J Spinal Disord 1992;5:149–157.

Lauerman WC, Bradford DS, Transfeldt EE, Ogilvie JW: Management of pseudarthrosis after arthrodesis of the spine for idiopathic scoliosis. J Bone Joint Surg Am 1991;73:222–236.

Lee HM, Suk KS, Moon SH, et al: Deep vein thrombosis after major spinal surgery: Incidence in an East Asian population. Spine 2000; 25:1827–1830.

Lenke LG, Betz RR, Bridwell KH, et al: Spontaneous lumbar curve coronal correction after selective anterior or posterior thoracic fusion in adolescent idiopathic scoliosis. Spine 1999;24:1663–1671; discussion 1672.

Lenke LG, Bridwell KH, Baldus C, Blanke K: Preventing decompensation in King type II curves treated with Cotrel-Dubousset instrumentation: Strict guidelines for selective thoracic fusion. Spine 1992;17: S274–S281.

Lenke LG, Edwards CC 2nd, Bridwell KH: The Lenke classification of adolescent idiopathic scoliosis: How it organizes curve patterns as a template to perform selective fusions of the spine. Spine 2003;28: S199–S207.

Lentschener C, Cottin P, Bouaziz H, et al: Reduction of blood loss and transfusion requirement by aprotinin in posterior lumbar spine fusion. Anesth Analg 1999;89:590–597.

Leon L, Rodriguez H, Tawk RG, et al: The prophylactic use of inferior vena cava filters in patients undergoing high-risk spinal surgery. Ann Vasc Surg 2005;19:442–447.

Liljenqvist U, Lepsien U, Hackenberg L, et al: Comparative analysis of pedicle screw and hook instrumentation in posterior correction and fusion of idiopathic thoracic scoliosis. Eur Spine J 2002;11: 336–343.

Linville DA, Bridwell KH, Lenke LG, et al: Complications in the adult spinal deformity patient having combined surgery: Does revision increase the risk? Spine 1999;24:355–363.

Lonstein J, Winter R, Moe J, Gaines D: Wound infection with Harrington instrumentation and spine fusion for scoliosis. Clin Orthop Relat Res 1973:222–233.

Maenza R, Segal E, Hokama J, Malvárez H: Superior mesenteric artery syndrome in scoliosis surgery: Case report and literature review. Poster presentation at the XXXVIII Annual Meeting of the Argentine Orthopedic Association. Buenos Aires, Argentina, 2001.

May VR Jr, Mauck WR: Exploration of the spine for pseudarthrosis following spinal fusion in the treatment of scoliosis. Clin Orthop Relat Res 1967;53:115–122.

McNeill TW, Anderson GBJ: Complications of Degenerative Lumbar Spine Surgery, 2nd ed. Philadelphia: Lippincott-Raven, 1997.

Misra SN, Morgan HW, Sedler R: Lumbar myofascial flap for pseudomeningocele repair. Neurosurg Focus 2003;15:E13.

Munns SW, Morrissy RT, Golladay ES, McKenzie CN: Hyperalimentation for superior mesenteric-artery (cast) syndrome following correction of spinal deformity. J Bone Joint Surg Am 1984;66:1175–1177.

Muschler GF, Nitto H, Matsukura Y, et al: Spine fusion using cell matrix composites enriched in bone marrow-derived cells. Clin Orthop Relat Res 2003:102–118.

Myers MA, Hamilton SR, Bogosian AJ, et al: Visual loss as a complication of spine surgery: A review of 37 cases. Spine 1997;22:1325–1329.

Newton PO, Faro FD, Lenke LG, et al: Factors involved in the decision to perform a selective versus nonselective fusion of Lenke 1B and 1C (King-Moe II) curves in adolescent idiopathic scoliosis. Spine 2003;28: S217–S223.

Noonan KJ, Walker T, Feinberg JR, et al: Factors related to false- versus true-positive neuromonitoring changes in adolescent idiopathic scoliosis surgery. Spine 2002;27:825–830.

O'Brien MF, Lenke LG, Mardjetko S, et al: Pedicle morphology in thoracic adolescent idiopathic scoliosis: Is pedicle fixation an anatomically viable technique? Spine 2000;25:2285–2293.

Oda T, Fuji T, Kato Y, et al: Deep venous thrombosis after posterior spinal surgery. Spine 2000;25:2962–2967.

Parke WW, Watanabe R: The intrinsic vasculature of the lumbosacral spinal nerve roots. Spine 1985;10:508–515.

Peterson MD, Nelson LM, McManus AC, Jackson RP: The effect of operative position on lumbar lordosis: A radiographic study of patients under anesthesia in the prone and 90–90 positions. Spine 1995;20: 1419–1424.

Qiu Y, Wang S, Wang B, et al: Incidence and risk factors of neurological deficits of surgical correction for scoliosis: Analysis of 1373 cases at one Chinese institution. Spine 2008;33:519–526.

Ray JM, Flynn JC, Bierman AH: Erythrocyte survival following intraoperative autotransfusion in spinal surgery: An in vivo comparative study and 5-year update. Spine 1986;11:879–882.

Reitman CA, Watters WC 3rd, Sassard WR: The cell saver in adult lumbar fusion surgery: A cost-benefit outcomes study. Spine 2004; 29:1580–1583; discussion 1584.

Richards BS: Lumbar curve response in type II idiopathic scoliosis after posterior instrumentation of the thoracic curve. Spine 1992;17: S282–S286.

Rinella A, Bridwell K, Kim Y, et al: Late complications of adult idiopathic scoliosis primary fusions to L4 and above: The effect of age and distal fusion level. Spine 2004;29:318–325.

Rittmeister M, Leyendecker K, Kurth A, Schmitt E: Cauda equina compression due to a laminar hook: A late complication of posterior instrumentation in scoliosis surgery. Eur Spine J 1999;8:417–420.

Rokito SE, Schwartz MC, Neuwirth MG: Deep vein thrombosis after major reconstructive spinal surgery. Spine 1996;21:853–858; discussion 859.

Rosner MK, Kuklo TR, Tawk R, et al: Prophylactic placement of an inferior vena cava filter in high-risk patients undergoing spinal reconstruction. Neurosurg Focus 2004;17:E6.

Roy-Camille R, Saillant G, Mazel C: Internal fixation of the lumbar spine with pedicle screw plating. Clin Orthop Relat Res 1986;(203):7–17.

Schwab F, Farcy JPC: Rationale for realignment surgery of the spine. In Margulies J, Aebi M, Farcy JPC (eds): Revision Spine Surgery. St. Louis: Mosby, 1999, pp 746–751.

Shah MA, Albright MB, Vogt MT, Moreland MS: Superior mesenteric artery syndrome in scoliosis surgery: Weight percentile for height as an indicator of risk. J Pediatr Orthop 2003;23:665–668.

Songer MN, Spencer DL, Meyer PR Jr, Jayaraman G: The use of sublaminar cables to replace Luque wires. Spine 1991;16:S418–S421.

Southern EP, Hammerberg KW, Dewald R: Complex spinal deformities in severe spinal infection. Paper presented at GICD-USA meeting on "The Surgical Management of Complex Spinal Deformity," Ottawa, Ontario, September 25, 1996.

Stagnara P: Experience with the wake up test in 623 cases (1970–1977). Paper presented at the conference of the Italian Society for Spinal Deformity, 1977.

Stedman TL: Stedman's Medical Dictionary, 26th ed. Baltimore, MD: Williams & Wilkins, 1995.

Steinmann JC, Herkowitz HN: Pseudarthrosis of the spine. Clin Orthop Relat Res 1992;(284):80–90.

Stephens GC, Yoo JU, Wilbur G: Comparison of lumbar sagittal alignment produced by different operative positions. Spine 1996;21: 1802–1806; discussion 1807.

Tafazal SI, Sell PJ: Incidental durotomy in lumbar spine surgery: Incidence and management. Eur Spine J 2005;14:287–290.

Thompson JP, Transfeldt EE, Bradford DS, et al: Decompensation after Cotrel-Dubousset instrumentation of idiopathic scoliosis. Spine 1990; 15:927–931.

Tribus CB, Belanger TA, Zdeblick TA: The effect of operative position and short-segment fusion on maintenance of sagittal alignment of the lumbar spine. Spine 1999;24:58–61.

Vauzelle C, Stagnara P, Jouvinroux P: Functional monitoring of spinal cord activity during spinal surgery. Clin Orthop Relat Res 1973;(93): 173–178.

Wenger DR, Mubarak SJ, Leach J: Managing complications of posterior spinal instrumentation and fusion. Clin Orthop Relat Res 1992;(284): 24–33.

West JL 3rd, Anderson LD: Incidence of deep vein thrombosis in major adult spinal surgery. Spine 1992;17:S254–S257.

Whitecloud TS 3rd, Davis JM, Olive PM: Operative treatment of the degenerated segment adjacent to a lumbar fusion. Spine 1994;19: 531–536.

Will SC, Nagan J: Legal medicine for the surgeon. In Way LW, Doherty GM (eds): Current Surgical Diagnosis & Treatment, 11th ed. New York: McGraw-Hill, 2003, pp 80–81.

Wilson-Holden TJ, VanSickle D, Lenke LG: The benefit of neurogenic mixed evoked potentials for intraoperative spinal cord monitoring during correction of severe scoliosis: A case study. Spine 2002;27: E258–E265.

Winter RB, Denis F, Lonstein JE, Dezen E: Salvage and reconstructive surgery for spinal deformity using Cotrel-Dubousset instrumentation. Spine 1991;16:S412–S417.

Wood KB, Kos PB, Abnet JK, Ista C: Prevention of deep-vein thrombosis after major spinal surgery: A comparison study of external devices. J Spinal Disord 1997;10:209–214.

Yuan-Innes MJ, Temple CL, Lacey MS: Vacuum-assisted wound closure: A new approach to spinal wounds with exposed hardware. Spine 2001;26:E30–E33.

Zhu ZZ, Qiu Y: Superior mesenteric artery syndrome following scoliosis surgery: Its risk indicators and treatment strategy. World J Gastroenterol 2005;11:3307–3310.

Zindrick MR, Knight GW, Bunch WH, et al: Factors influencing the penetration of wires into the neural canal during segmental wiring. J Bone Joint Surg Am 1989;71:742–750.

SUGGESTED READINGS

Behrman MJ, Keim HA: Perioperative red blood cell salvage in spine surgery: A prospective analysis. Clin Orthop Relat Res 1992; (278):51–57.

Reinfusion of perioperative blood loss was studied in 150 spinal surgery patients to evaluate its efficacy in reducing transfusion requirements. The authors concluded that the combination of intraoperative and postoperative blood salvage was highly effective in reducing the need for transfused blood.

Bitan FD: Aprotinin in spine surgery: Review of the literature. Orthopedics 2004;27:S681–S683.

Based on a literature review, this article evaluates the efficacy of aprotinin to limit blood transfusion during spine surgery. Most prospective studies confirm this effect. However, broader studies are required to evaluate adverse effects. Severe complications are rarely, if ever, reported. Given the small size of most samples, complications are expected because of the widespread use of the drug. The cost of the medication has to be balanced with the cost of blood transfusion. A careful use of aprotinin allows a surgeon who deals with high-risk patients to avoid or limit the use of transfusions. For patients who are not at high risk, aprotinin should be avoided until other questions have been answered.

Brown CW, Orme TJ, Richardson HD: The rate of pseudarthrosis (surgical nonunion) in patients who are smokers and patients who are nonsmokers: A comparison study. Spine 1986;11:942–943.

The aim of this study was to investigate the relationship of smoking with the rate of pseudarthrosis (surgical nonunion). In this study, 50 patients who were smokers and 50 patients who were not and who had had a two-level laminectomy and fusion during 1977 and 1978 were randomly selected. Examination 1 to 2 years after surgery revealed that 40% of the smokers had developed a pseudarthrosis, whereas among nonsmokers, the rate was 8%. The authors hypothesized that the higher incidence of surgical nonunion among smokers could be related to blood gas levels.

Couture D, Branch CL Jr: Spinal pseudomeningoceles and cerebrospinal fluid fistulas. Neurosurg Focus 2003;15:E6.

Spinal pseudomeningoceles and cerebrospinal fluid fistulas are rare extradural collections of cerebrospinal fluid that result following a breach in the dural-arachnoid layer. They may occur because of an incidental durotomy, during intradural surgery, or from trauma or congenital abnormality. In this article, the authors review the diagnosis and treatment of spinal pseudomeningoceles and cerebrospinal fluid fistulas.

Esses SI, Sachs BL, Dreyzin V: Complications associated with the technique of pedicle screw fixation: A selected survey of ABS members. Spine 1993;18:2231–2238; discussion 2238–2239.

This survey of 617 surgical cases, in which pedicle screw implants were used, was undertaken to ascertain the incidence and variety of associated complications. The authors concluded that pedicle screw placement may be associated with significant intraoperative and postoperative complications. This information is of value to surgeons using pedicle implant systems as well as to their patients. Repeat surgery is associated with greater numbers of complications.

Glassman SD, Dimar JR, Puno RM, Johnson JR: Salvage of instrumental lumbar fusions complicated by surgical wound infection. Spine 1996;21:2163–2169.

This study retrospectively reviewed instrumented lumbar fusions complicated by surgical wound infection and managed by a protocol including antibiotic impregnated beads. Although wound infection is a significant complication, this study suggests that aggressive surgical management can result in preservation of an adequate fusion rate and maintenance of an acceptable postoperative outcome.

Jones AA, Stambough JL, Balderston RA, et al: Long-term results of lumbar spine surgery complicated by unintended incidental durotomy. Spine 1989;14:443–446.

Unintended incidental durotomy is a not infrequent complication of spinal surgery (reported incidence: 0.3% to 13%). This retrospective review of 450 patients undergoing lumbar spine surgery revealed 17 cases (4%) of incidental durotomy, recognized intraoperatively and repaired primarily. These patients were evaluated at long-term follow-up (mean: 25.1 months). The study concluded that incidental durotomy, when recognized and repaired intraoperatively, does not increase perioperative morbidity or compromise the final result.

Kim YJ, Bridwell KH, Lenke LG, et al: Pseudarthrosis in primary fusions for adult idiopathic scoliosis: Incidence, risk factors, and outcome analysis. Spine 2005;30:468–474.

This is a retrospective study that analyzes the incidence, characteristics, risk factors, and Scoliosis Research Society Instrument-24 (SRS-24) outcome scores of pseudarthrosis in adult idiopathic scoliosis primary fusions. The incidence of pseudarthrosis following adult idiopathic scoliosis primary fusion was 17%. The pseudarthrosis was most likely to occur at the thoracolumbar junction. Older patients (>55 years), longer fusion (>12 vertebrae), and those with thoracolumbar kyphosis (≥20 degrees) demonstrated increased risk for pseudarthrosis. Patients' outcomes as measured by the SRS-24 were negatively affected by the pseudarthrosis.

Lonstein JE, Denis F, Perra JH, et al: Complications associated with pedicle screws. J Bone Joint Surg Am 1999;81:1519–1528.

The safety and the effectiveness of pedicle-screw instrumentation in the spine have been questioned, despite its use worldwide to enhance stabilization of the spine. This review was performed to answer questions about the technique of insertion and the nature and etiology of complications directly attributable to the screws. It concluded that few problems are associated with the insertion of screws, provided that the surgeon is experienced and adheres to the principles and details of the operative technique.

Mehbod AA, Ogilvie JW, Pinto MR, et al: Postoperative deep wound infections in adults after spinal fusion: Management with vacuum-assisted wound closure. J Spinal Disord Tech 2005;18:14–17.

Vacuum-assisted wound closure exposes the wound bed to negative pressure, resulting in removal of edema fluid, improvement of blood supply, and stimulation of cellular proliferation of reparative granulation tissue. This study concluded that vacuum-assisted wound closure therapy is an effective adjunct in closing complex deep spinal wounds with exposed instrumentation.

Padberg AM, Wilson-Holden TJ, Lenke LG, Bridwell KH: Somatosensory- and motor-evoked potential monitoring without a wake-up test during idiopathic scoliosis surgery: An accepted standard of care. Spine 1998;23:1392–1400.

This was a retrospective study of 500 patients who underwent corrective surgery between 1987 and 1997 for spinal deformity caused by idiopathic scoliosis. The objective was to report the sensitivity and specificity of somatosensory evoked and neurogenic motor-evoked potentials monitoring and the requirements for an intraoperative wake-up test for all idiopathic scoliosis surgeries at a single institution. The study concluded that a combination of somatosensory evoked and neurogenic motor-evoked potential monitoring during idiopathic scoliosis surgery represents a standard of care that obviates the need for an intraoperative wake-up test when reliable data are obtained and maintained.

Smith MD, Bressler EL, Lonstein JE, et al: Deep venous thrombosis and pulmonary embolism after major reconstructive operations on the spine: A prospective analysis of three hundred and seventeen patients. J Bone Joint Surg Am 1994;76:980–985.

In this study, the author performed a prospective study of 317 patients to determine the prevalence of deep venous thrombosis after reconstructive operations on the spine. The study concluded that routine screening for the detection of asymptomatic thrombosis in patients who have had a procedure on the spine is unwarranted.

Stevens WR, Glazer PA, Kelley SD, et al: Ophthalmic complications after spinal surgery. Spine 1997;22:1319–1324.

This is a retrospective review of 3450 spinal surgeries with the objective of reviewing ophthalmic complications and their etiologies, as well as treatments and outcomes, in patients who have undergone spinal surgery. It concluded that the risk of ophthalmic complications with spinal surgery has not been fully appreciated. Because ophthalmic complications in spinal surgery can be reversed with prompt recognition and intervention, it is important for clinicians to be aware of their possible occurrence.

Tsirikos AI, Jeans LA: Superior mesenteric artery syndrome in children and adolescents with spine deformities undergoing corrective surgery. J Spinal Disord Tech 2005;18:263–271.

Obstruction of the third part of the duodenum by the superior mesenteric artery (SMA) is associated with spinal manipulation in the surgical or conservative management of scoliosis. The purpose of the present study was to investigate the prevalence of SMA syndrome in a cohort of 165 consecutive pediatric patients who underwent spine deformity surgery and had minimum 2-year follow-up. This work draws attention to the significance of the prevention of the condition by recognizing patients who are at a higher risk. An early diagnosis of SMA syndrome will allow for application of conservative methods and will increase the chances for a successful outcome.

Zheng F, Cammisa FP Jr, Sandhu HS, et al: Factors predicting hospital stay, operative time, blood loss, and transfusion in patients undergoing revision posterior lumbar spine decompression, fusion, and segmental instrumentation. Spine 2002;27:818–824.

This is a retrospective chart review that was conducted for 112 patients who underwent revision posterior lumbar spine decompression, fusion, and segmental instrumentation. The main objective was to ascertain factors predicting hospital stay, operative time, blood loss, and transfusion in patients undergoing revision posterior lumbar spine decompression, fusion, and segmental instrumentation. It concludes that number of levels fused and age seem to be the most significant predicting factors.

CHAPTER 29

Neuromonitoring for Scoliosis Surgery

DAVID S. WEISS

INTRODUCTION TO INTRAOPERATIVE SPINAL CORD AND NERVE ROOT MONITORING

Intraoperative neuromonitoring provides the surgical team with real-time information about the status of the patient's nervous system during ongoing surgical manipulation. The objective of monitoring is to protect the patient from iatrogenic injury. The intent of this chapter is to provide the surgeon with a fundamental understanding of the neuromonitoring tests that are used during spinal deformity surgery. The chapter will highlight some of the variables that can lead to false-positive and false-negative outcomes. This understanding will help the surgeon to formulate the most appropriate questions to ask of the neuromonitoring team during critical phases of the procedure. Figure 29-1 presents an overview of the basic electrophysiologic approach to monitoring spine surgery.

The first intraoperative test of spinal cord function was the Stagnara wake-up test. The first electrophysiologic test of intraoperative spinal cord function was the somatosensory evoked potential (SSEP). Recent additions include the transcranial motor evoked potential (TcMEP) and intraoperative electromyography (EMG). Taken together, these tests provide full coverage of the patient's sensory and motor functions during the surgical procedure. The dermatomal somatosensory evoked potential tends to be unreliable in the operating room and is not recommended for monitoring surgical procedures.

THE STAGNARA WAKE-UP TEST

The Stagnara wake-up test provides direct evaluation of the patient's motor functions without depending on computers or specialized equipment. The wake-up quickly became the "gold standard" measure of spinal cord integrity. In today's operating room, the wake-up test is used less often than it was in the past. However, it does make good sense to perform a wake-up test when questions or doubts about the integrity of the motor pathways remain

after a neuromonitoring change has been detected and reported to the surgical team.

Clearly, the wake-up test puts the patients at risk for surgical recall and increased apprehension about surgery. However, careful planning and control of the situation can help to alleviate patients' fears. Preparation for the wake-up test will help to reduce the chance of an adverse reaction. Before surgery, the surgeon and anesthesiologist should explain the reasons for the test and the conditions under which the test would occur. This includes implanting the idea that at some point during the surgical procedure, patients might have to respond to a voice asking them to move their arms and legs, hands and feet, and fingers and toes. The patients should be reassured that they will not feel any pain during the test and might not remember the test after surgery is over. The patients should be instructed to respond to the verbal commands even if they think the test is a dream. The patients should be reassured that they will go back to sleep after the test is finished.

The anesthesiologist should be experienced in setting up and performing the wake-up test. It is difficult to perform a wake-up test on short notice, especially if the technique of total intravenous anesthesia is being used to facilitate the acquisition of motor evoked potentials. If possible, providing at least 45 minutes' advance warning will help the anesthesiologist control the level of central nervous system depression more reliably. Attempting to accelerate the wake-up by reversing surgical muscle relaxant or narcotics is discouraged, as this can result in violent movements that could be harmful to the patient. The patient typically remains pain-free through continued use of narcotic. Amnesia can be maintained through administration of midazolam or another benzodiazepine. The surgeon should inform the anesthesiologist if a second wake-up test will be required at a later point during the surgery.

The wake-up test is monitored by an individual who lifts the surgical drapes to observe the movement of the lower extremities. The anesthesiologist can observe move-

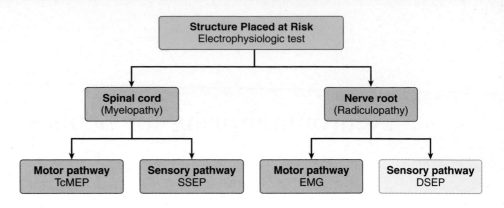

Figure 29-1. Electrophysiologic tests used to monitor spinal deformity procedures are organized according to the structures they protect and the neural injuries they help to prevent. DSEP, dermatomal somatosensory evoked potential; EMG, intraoperative electromyography; SSEP, somatosensory evoked potential; TcMEP, transcranial motor evoked potential.

ments of the upper extremities. Strong upper- and lower-extremity movements should be observed. The wake-up test is negative when patients are observed moving their legs, feet, and toes on direct command and positive when patients fail to move their lower extremities. Directed movements of the upper extremities (hands and fingers) are control measures that ensure that the patients are able to respond to verbal commands. If the patients move appropriately, they are put back to sleep, and surgery continues. In case of a positive test, the spinal instrumentation is loosened or removed immediately. In most situations, reducing the correction or removing the instrumentation will remedy the situation. Standard nerve or spinal cord injury protection protocols can be instituted at the discretion of the surgeon.

Complications of the wake-up test are infrequent. Surgical recall is rare. If necessary, the medical professional team should be ready to arrange psychological counseling. Another potential complication is dislodgement of the endotracheal tube. This is unlikely if the tube is properly secured and the patient's head movements are controlled.

The wake-up test is not a continuous measure of spinal cord function; it evaluates spinal cord integrity at one discrete point during surgery and assesses only gross motor function. There have been anecdotal reports of patients who moved their lower extremities during the intraoperative wake-up test yet emerged from the procedure with motor deficits.

THE SOMATOSENSORY EVOKED POTENTIAL

In the early 1970s, the SSEP was introduced. The SSEP is the second component in the multimodal approach to monitoring spinal cord function. It was recognized that the SSEP did not directly monitor the motor pathways, the anterior blood supply to the spinal cord, or the motor nerve roots. Nonetheless, it was also recognized that gross mechanical injury to the spinal cord would affect both ascending sensory and descending motor pathways. Numerous scientific studies demonstrated that the SSEP was a viable test of overall spinal cord function. The SSEP

was convenient and easy to perform and avoided interrupting the procedure to wake the patient. The SSEP test provided continuous assessment of the patient's neurophysiologic status before, during, and after placement of spinal instrumentation and correction of deformity. The SSEP evolved into the next "gold standard" test of spinal cord function and remains a stable and reliable technique for monitoring spinal cord function.

Interpreting Change in the Somatosensory Evoked Potential

To understand and interpret the significance of SSEP changes that can occur during surgery, it is important for the surgeon to have a basic understanding of the evoked potential signal. The SSEP is the summation of inhibitory and excitatory postsynaptic potentials generated in response to repetitive electrical stimulation of a mixed peripheral nerve. The SSEP is embedded within the patient's naturally occurring electroencephalogram (EEG). However, the amplitude of the somatosensory response is minuscule in comparison with the EEG signal. Therefore, the SSEP is derived by averaging together single trial epochs (sweeps) of EEG data that contain the somatosensory response to repetitive peripheral nerve stimulation. The averaging process continues until EEG and other background noises cancel out, leaving only the characteristic deflections of the SSEP.

Each sweep in the ensemble average is triggered by the onset of the sensory stimulus. Each sensory response is time-locked (stationary) in relation to the stimulus. Unless a change in the patient's neurophysiologic status occurs, the waveforms of each sensory response in the ensemble will remain consistent from each single trial to the next, resulting in a well-formed and replicable set of evoked potential data. However, changes or instabilities in nervous system function that occur during the sampling period will alter the averaging process and affect the formation of the evoked potential waveforms. For example, a consistent change in amplitude or latency during the sampling period will be reflected as a well-defined change in the averaged evoked response (e.g., increased latency, decreased amplitude, loss of signal). An inconsistent or variable change can lead to poorly formed, diffuse, or blunted signals. A set of extremely weak somatosensory responses might not have sufficient energy to withstand the averaging process and might cancel out along with the background noise, leaving only a low-amplitude signal that does not replicate well. Several iterations of the data might be required to determine whether a signal is really present. The sudden loss of an otherwise strong somatosensory response will result in a rapid decrease in signal amplitude, often leading to a diminished response and then a flat line response.

A typical SSEP can take from several seconds to several minutes to acquire, depending on the number of sweeps required to summate the data. Improvements in neuromonitoring equipment, amplifiers, filters, and software have enhanced the data acquisition process such that reliable signals can be recorded with fewer sweeps per average than was previously possible. This is an important consideration because rapid findings are essential to avoid an impending or ongoing spinal cord injury.

As part of the neuromonitoring protocol, the surgeon should be kept informed about the quality of the SSEP signals and whether there are any difficulties in obtaining good-quality, reproducible data. One of the more common "freshman" errors in neuromonitoring is the failure to distinguish a real SSEP from regularly occurring noise. This problem can be exacerbated by neuromonitoring software that automatically detects and labels waveform features and assigns numeric values to the results. A signal that contains mostly noise will average out into a flat line response when the number of sweeps is increased beyond the "usual and customary" amount. Conversely, a real SSEP will remain relatively unchanged as the number of sweeps is increased.

Both upper- and lower-extremity somatosensory evoked potentials are monitored during spinal deformity procedures. The lower-extremity SSEP monitors the function of the sensory system along the entire length of the patient's neuroaxis, from the peripheral nerve at the lower extremity through the sciatic nerve, sacral plexus, cauda equina, dorsal columns of the spinal cord to the patient's brain stem and, finally, cerebral cortex. The posterior tibial nerve at the medial aspect of the ankle is the most commonly used site for eliciting a lower-extremity SSEP; additional sites include the common peroneal nerve at the fibular head and the tibial nerve at the popliteal fossa. The upper-extremity SSEP is used to assess the function of the patient's cervical spine, brachial plexus, and ulnar nerve as well as to provide a control measure for physiologic and technical factors that can adversely affect the lower-extremity signals. The upper-extremity SSEP is elicited by stimulating the ulnar nerve at the medial aspect of the wrist.

Figure 29-2 depicts the general characteristics of the evoked potential and waveform features that are used to evaluate changes in the status of the patient's somatosensory pathways. The evoked potential waveform is displayed as a function of voltage over time. The waveform is characterized by upward- and downward-moving biphasic or triphasic deflections that are "V" or "W" shaped. Depending on the nature of the patient's disease process, the deflections may be sharp and well formed or diffuse and poorly formed. The primary latency marker for the posterior tibial nerve SSEP is the P37 deflection, and the primary latency marker for the ulnar nerve SSEP is the N20 deflection. Waveform characteristics that are monitored during surgery are peak latency from stimulus onset, peak-to-peak amplitude, and overall signal morphology.

The most commonly accepted SSEP warning criteria are a 10% increase in latency (measured from stimulus onset) and a 50% decrease in amplitude (measured peak-to-peak). The application of these criteria is somewhat flexible and often will be interpreted in relation to normal variations in the patient's signals (see "Importance of Preoperative Baseline Data"). Subtle changes in SSEP waveform morphology may also signify a change in the patient's neurophysiologic status (see Case 2). The onset of SSEP change can be rapid or delayed. In general, sudden changes tend to have vascular origins, while changes that result from mechanical trauma usually take longer to develop. However, this is not always the case. Every change in the monitored signals poses an immediate cause for concern. Changes in signal latency accompanied by significant decreases in signal amplitude can be misinterpreted as a reversal in signal polarity. Once defined by the neuromonitoring technician, the SSEP waveforms should be labeled consistently.

Figure 29-3 provides samples of SSEP waveforms recorded during an uneventful procedure. SSEP neuro-

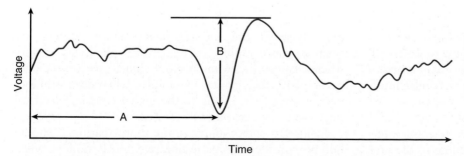

Figure 29-2. The evoked potential waveform is a function of voltage over time. Waveform characteristics that are used to evaluate change in evoked potential signals are (A) latency in milliseconds from stimulus onset and (B) peak-to-peak amplitude in microvolts. The most commonly accepted SSEP warning criteria are a 10% increase in latency and a 50% decrease in amplitude.

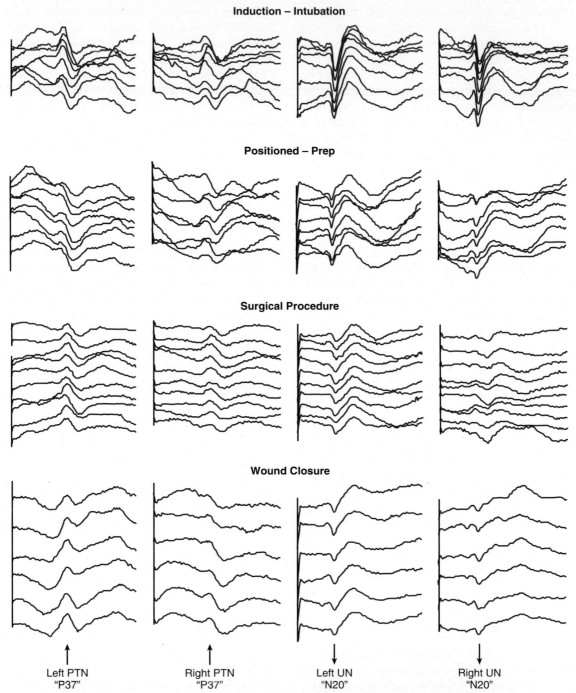

Induction – Intubation

Positioned – Prep

Surgical Procedure

Wound Closure

Left PTN
"P37"

Right PTN
"P37"

Left UN
"N20"

Right UN
"N20"

Figure 29-3. An uneventful set of SSEP data recorded during spine surgery. The latency marker for the posterior tibial nerve somatosensory evoked potential is the P37 deflection. The latency marker for the ulnar nerve somatosensory evoked potential is the N20 deflection. In this example, the polarity of the P37 is upward, and that of the N20 is downward. PTN, posterior tibial nerve; UN, ulnar nerve.

monitoring began immediately after induction of anesthesia and continued through wound closure to assess all critical periods when changes in nervous system function are likely to occur. The studies were run at regular intervals during surgery, typically at a rate of once per minute during acquisition of baseline data and once every 2 or 3 minutes during the operation itself. In practice, the interval between SSEP studies will vary according to the pre-

dicted risk of the surgical manipulation. Studies are acquired more rapidly during critical phases of surgery when changes in the monitored signals are expected to occur. SSEP data cannot be sampled when electrocautery devices are in use, owing to the high-frequency electrical interference emitted by such devices.

Failure to detect injury to the motor pathways should not be considered a false-negative SSEP finding when motor system neuromonitoring is being performed during the procedure. As with all monitored signals, the surgical team must be informed immediately when a change in the status of the SSEP waveforms occurs. The reason for the change should be identified and remedied. All efforts should be made to validate the findings. It is essential to rule out physiologic, technical, and other extraneous factors that can mimic or mask a surgically related change and lead to a false-positive or a false-negative interpretation, respectively. The neuromonitoring technician must remain cognizant of these factors so that rapid and accurate assessment can be made without hesitation. A certain amount of variation in the SSEP waveforms is expected to occur during the surgical procedure. Given the inherent variability in the signals, false-positive SSEP outcomes are not uncommon. False-negative SSEP events rarely occur when the extraneous factors that influence SSEP interpretations are well controlled.

A frequently observed and potentially dangerous error in neuromonitoring is the failure to report an uncertain finding to the surgeon. The significance of an uncertain change can be debated, but the change itself must be reported as soon as it is detected. The surgeon should encourage good communication with the technician. The technician should be able to convey the appropriate information to the surgeon in a concise yet thorough manner, even under stressful circumstances.

In the event of a significant or almost significant SSEP change, a motor evoked potential study should be performed, and the surgeon should consider ordering a wake-up test. Immediate counteractive measures are required, especially if changes in both sensory and motor signals occur following placement of spinal instrumentation and/or correction of the spine. Identifying and remedying the cause of the change should result in recovery of the monitored signals. Return of the signals to baseline following ameliorative action validates the change. Should the surgeon choose to go forward with the procedure, this should be done very slowly and under constant neuromonitoring control. The limits of the patient's tolerance to the correction will be reached at the point at which changes in the neuromonitoring signals suggest motor or sensory system dysfunction. Do not ignore significant SSEP changes if there are no changes in the motor evoked potentials. The patient could be experiencing somatosensory system dysfunction.

Factors That Affect the Somatosensory Evoked Potential

Most surgical maneuvers with potential for incurring trauma to the spine, dural sac, and cauda equina will affect the SSEP. The most obvious examples are placement of instrumentation, distraction, compression, performing cantilever maneuvers during osteotomy, applying corrective force, and spinal ischemia. Other events can result in SSEP changes as well: peripheral ischemia, neck manipulation during intubation and positioning of the patient, position of the patient's arms and legs on the operating table, localized swelling, and epidural hematoma. Care must be taken during all phases of surgery. The neuromonitoring technician should always be on the alert for changes in the monitored signals. Reviewing the patient's history prior to surgery will help the technician to identify aspects of the patient's disease process that could engender a change in the signals.

Figure 29-4 illustrates a significant change in left side posterior tibial nerve SSEP function during distraction of the left L4-5 interspace. The responses improved following release of the distraction. The signals remained stable through wound closure, and the patient emerged from anesthesia without deficit. Another common surgical manipulation that will affect the SSEP is occlusion of the great vessels during exposure of the anterior spine. Figure 29-5 shows sudden loss and recovery in the left-side posterior tibial nerve SSEP during mobilization of the left iliac artery. The etiology of this change was most likely loss of distal perfusion to the left femoral artery affecting peripheral nerve function. The signal recovered immediately after the vessel was released and repositioned. The patient emerged from anesthesia without deficit.

The most common technical factors that affect electrophysiologic signals during surgery are incorrectly placed stimulating and recording electrodes, electrode dislodgement, loose wires or connections, unbalanced or excessively high electrode impedances, ground problems, 60-Hz noise from operating room equipment, and incorrect equipment settings. The neuromonitoring technician should be proficient in identifying, isolating, and repairing technical problems. The operating room staff must be willing to assist the technician in locating and removing sources of electrical noise; powering-down, unplugging, and replugging equipment; and relocating devices, wires, electrical extensions, and the like.

The most common physiologic factors that affect SSEP signals are the concentration of potent inhalational anesthetic agent, hypotension, and hypothermia. The effects of anesthetic agents on SSEP signals are well known and documented. To prevent false-positive errors, it is essential that the anesthesiologist maintain steady-state concentrations of potent inhalation agents and nitrous oxide within the limits established for SSEP neuromonitoring. Significant increases in SSEP latency and/or significant decreases in SSEP amplitude are observed when the concentration of a potent inhalational agent exceeds 50% of the minimum alveolar concentration recommended for the particular agent: isoflurane (0.5%), desflurane (3.0%), or sevoflurane (0.8%). Nonsignificant SSEP changes may be noted with lower concentrations of gas. Nitrous oxide administered in concentrations greater than 70% is known to cause significant decreases in SSEP amplitude. Nitrous oxide has an agonist effect on halogenated agents.

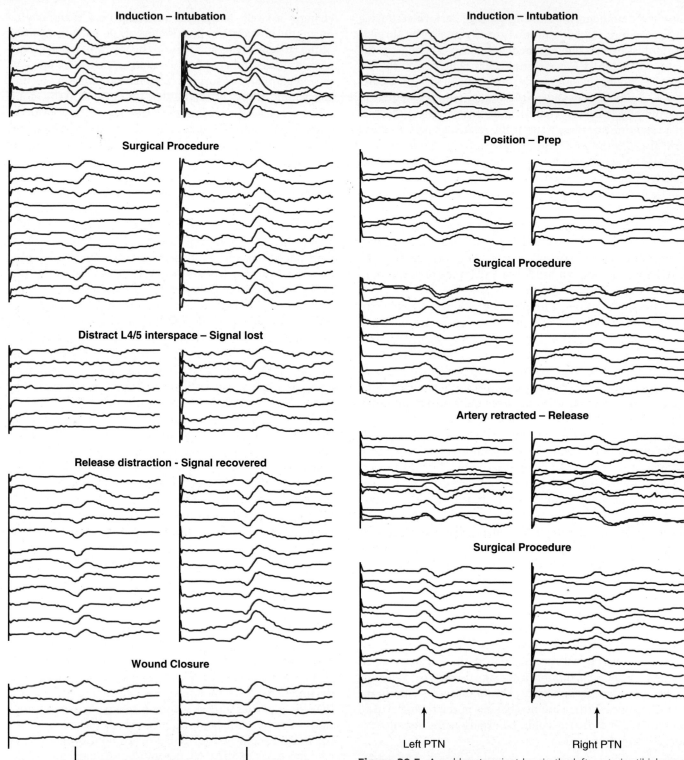

Figure 29-4. A significant change in the left posterior tibial nerve SSEP occurred during distraction of the lumbar spine at the L4-5 interspace. The signals recovered after the distraction was released. In this example, the polarity of the P37 is downward. PTN, posterior tibial nerve.

Figure 29-5. A sudden, transient loss in the left posterior tibial nerve SSEP occurred during mobilization of the left common iliac artery. The signals recovered immediately after the vessel was released. In this example, the polarity of the P37 is upward. PTN, posterior tibial nerve.

Spinal cord neuromonitoring signals are very responsive to sudden or gradual changes in the patient's blood pressure. Both the sensory and motor pathways are sensitive to the perfusion of the patient's cerebral cortex and spinal cord. Blood pressure–related changes are likely to occur if the surgeon prefers the patient in a hypotensive state in order to control blood loss. SSEP signal amplitude will decrease proportionally with increased hypotension. Motor evoked potential signals might disappear altogether. The neuromonitoring technician should pay close attention to variations in the patient's blood pressure and the status of the neuromonitoring signals. The anesthesiologist and surgeon should be kept informed about changes in the monitored signals as a result of a labile blood pressure. The signals should improve as the patient's mean arterial blood pressure is increased to 70 mm Hg or greater. Hypertensive patients who have upward modulation at the lower level of autoregulation might require a higher mean pressure. Careful monitoring of the SSEP can help the anesthesiologist to determine the limits of controlled hypotension.

SSEP latency will increase in direct proportion to a decrease in the patient's core body temperature. This usually does not pose a problem during surgery, as the patient's core temperature is maintained with a warming blanket. However, localized cooling at the surgical site will also affect the SSEP signals. A certain amount of variability in SSEP latency is expected to occur during and after exposure of the spine as the patient's tissues begin to cool. Application of warm irrigation can help to alleviate the situation.

An uneventful somatosensory study does not guarantee an intact motor system (see Case 1). Several incidents of postoperative motor deficit with unchanged intraoperative SSEP function have been reported both in the literature and anecdotally. With the advent of reliable motor system neuromonitoring, the necessity for combining somatosensory and motor evoked potential studies into a single protocol is well established. The TcMEP is the third component in the multimodal approach to monitoring spinal cord function. However, one should not dismiss the SSEP outright in favor of the TcMEP (see Case 2). Moreover, there will be instances when motor system neuromonitoring is unavailable, contraindicated, or unobtainable, so the need for good-quality SSEP data acquisition and interpretation will always remain.

THE TRANSCRANIAL MOTOR EVOKED POTENTIAL

Early on, the monitoring community recognized the need to augment SSEP-based neuromonitoring with motor pathway studies. Paraplegia is the most feared neurologic complication of spine surgery. Both anterior and posterior aspects of the spine are affected by the procedures that are used to correct a deformity. Blood flow to the anterior cord can be disrupted very easily by various surgical manipulations. The thoracic spine is particularly vulnerable to manipulation, distraction, compression, and perfusion-related injuries. Various spinal reconstruction techniques can place the anterior and posterior cord at great risk for injury.

Over the years, many diverse techniques for monitoring the motor pathways have been developed, some with greater success than others. The initial applications were limited to facilities and surgical neuromonitoring teams with independent research board approval. This restricted the scope of motor system neuromonitoring to a small number of research hospitals and medical centers. Gradually, the many variations in motor system neuromonitoring were reduced to a few techniques, most notably neurogenic motor evoked potentials and transcranial electrical stimulation of the motor cortex. In 2003, the U.S. Food and Drug Administration (FDA) approved the first transcranial stimulation device for intraoperative assessment of acute dysfunction in corticospinal motor pathway function. Since then, several manufacturers have received FDA approval for similar devices, leading to a widely expanded presence of motor system neuromonitoring in the operating room. The suggested electrophysiologic replacement for the Stagnara wake-up test is the TcMEP.

Interpreting Change in the Transcranial Motor Evoked Potential

Transcranial stimulation of the motor cortex generates well-defined compound muscle action potentials (CMAPs) at contralateral musculature in the upper and lower extremities. The motor response is an almost instantaneous EMG potential, an all-or-nothing signal, either present or absent following electrical stimulation of the cortex. Stimulation is delivered by using subdermal needle electrodes placed into the scalp over the left and right motor cortices. CMAPs are recorded distally by using needle electrodes placed into the skin over the target muscles of interest. The CMAP response is characterized by complex polyphasic deflections.

A common error in motor system neuromonitoring (TcMEP or EMG) is relying on a single muscle to cover distal myotomes. It is difficult to predict exactly which muscles will be activated by transcranial stimulation of the cerebral cortex. Insufficient coverage of the distal musculature can result in a failure to detect motor system dysfunction, leading to a false-negative finding. It seems prudent to monitor as many lower-extremity muscles as possible and to maximize the opportunity for capturing a distal TcMEP or EMG response. The limiting factor is the availability of data channels on the monitoring equipment, a serious concern with older equipment.

TcMEP studies are performed at regular intervals during surgery, notably before, during, and after any surgical manipulation that can potentially injure the spinal cord. The onset of motor system dysfunction can be very rapid. The interval at which TcMEP data are collected should be adjusted accordingly. Figure 29-6 provides an example of an uneventful motor evoked potential study. The patient, a 16-year-old male, was admitted to the operating room with a diagnosis of Scheuermann's kyphosis. The patient underwent posterior spinal fusion with instrumentation, T4-L1, for correction of the spinal deformity. Baseline TcMEP data were acquired as soon as repetitive muscle action potentials could be recorded. CMAP activity was noted at the left and right abductor pollicis brevis, tibialis anterior, and gastrocnemius muscles. This presentation uses the "waterfall" display to show the progression of the motor trials over time. Each line in the display represents the CMAP response to a single presentation of transcranial stimulus. At least three to five replications were required to validate a study. No changes in the motor responses were noted before, during, or after correction of the kyphosis. The patient emerged from anesthesia without deficit.

The current methods for assessing significant change in the TcMEP are stimulus threshold, loss of signal, and change in morphology. In the stimulus threshold technique, the minimum stimulus intensity required to elicit a CMAP at contralateral distal musculature is determined and established as a baseline threshold. The outcome criterion is the presence or absence of the CMAP at the target

muscle(s) in relation to the predetermined stimulus threshold. A significant change in motor function is said to occur when an increase of 100 or more volts is required to elicit the same response at the target muscle(s). In children, an increase of less than 100 volts may be clinically significant. The threshold technique is based on the assumption that additional electrical stimulation is required to elicit a distal CMAP after a significant number of descending motor tract fibers have been compromised by the surgical manipulation. The second method for assessing change in the TcMEP considers the loss of signal as measured against a suprathreshold stimulus value. The sudden loss of signal suggests impending motor system dysfunction. Proponents of the loss of signal technique believe that there is too much inherent variability in potentials elicited by a threshold stimulus intensity for a reliable assessment of motor system function. Finally, the change in morphology technique uses the shape and patterning of the CMAP waveforms as criteria for assessing motor system dysfunction. For example, a significant event may be occurring when the complexity of the CMAP waveform changes from a polyphasic to a biphasic signal.

The reader should be aware that controversy exists within the monitoring community regarding the validity of each technique. No one disputes the necessity for motor system neuromonitoring. Practical experience suggests that elements of all three methods should be considered when following the progression of TcMEP data. The initial

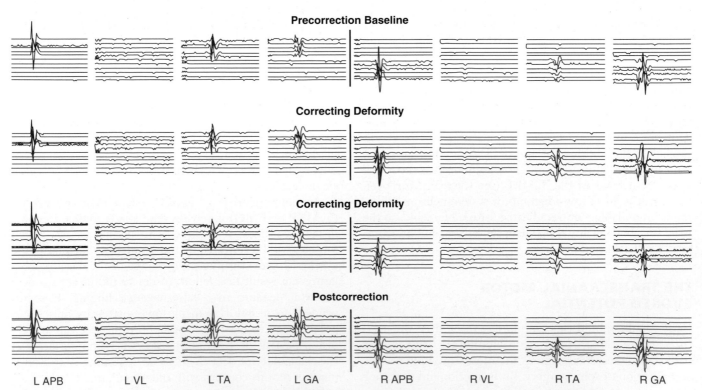

Figure 29-6. Stable, unchanged upper- and lower-extremity TcMEPs were recorded before, during, and after correction of the spine for Scheuermann's kyphosis. APB, abductor pollicis brevis; GA, gastrocnemius; L, left; R, right; TA, tibialis anterior; VL, vastus lateralis.

warning might be the need to increase stimulation voltage or the sudden loss of TcMEP signal. Variation in waveform morphology or pattern of muscle response might follow the initial change (see Case 2). Other warning criteria include sudden changes in SSEP function and sudden onset or offset of EMG activity. The surgeon should be aware of the warning criteria that are used to determine the significance of a potential motor system change.

Significant changes in the TcMEP require immediate action. There is no margin of error when changes in motor potentials occur. The response is the same as that with significant SSEP changes: The surgeon must be informed immediately, the exact nature of the change must be reported, and the cause of the change must be identified and remedied. A wake-up test may be ordered at the discretion of the surgeon. The neuromonitoring literature and practical experience suggest that false-negative errors are rare with TcMEP neuromonitoring.

Recovery of the motor signals following remedial action validates the significance of the event. An immediate recovery suggests temporary motor system dysfunction. A delayed recovery is troublesome. Return of motor signals by the end of the procedure is a good sign. However, continued absence of the TcMEP to the end of the procedure is a very bad indication. Examples of significant changes in motor evoked potentials are illustrated in Cases 1 and 2.

Factors That Affect the Transcranial Motor Evoked Potential

Prior to surgery, the neuromonitoring technician should consult with the surgeon and anesthesiologist regarding the risks and contraindications of transcranial motor stimulation. The exclusion criteria for transcranial stimulation of the motor cortex are (1) head injury, stroke, seizures, epilepsy, neurologic or psychiatric disorders, cerebral aneurysm; (2) any type of implanted biomedical device; or (3) metallic fragments or plates in the head. As reported in the literature, the likelihood of seizure activity induced by transcranial stimulation of the motor cortex is very low when an FDA-approved device is used. This is due to the brief pulse trains, low repetition rates, and low number of stimuli delivered to the patient.

As with the SSEP, it is important to rule out extraneous factors that can influence the interpretation of the motor evoked signals. First, the TcMEP appears to be highly sensitive to changes in the patient's blood pressure and to hypotension in particular. The patient's blood pressure should be maintained at a normal level if possible. Second, the integrity of the neuromonitoring equipment, including the placement of the recording and stimulating electrodes, should be verified. In surgeries involving the thoracic and lumbar spines, the loss of upper- and lower-extremity motor responses suggests a technical or physiologic explanation. Third, techniques of general anesthesia that combine inhalational agents, nitrous oxide, and surgical muscle relaxants suppress the TcMEP. One solution is to administer total intravenous anesthesia, in which, in the absence of any inhalational agent, the nitrous oxide to oxygen mixture is maintained at 50%. A second approach is a partial intravenous technique in which sevoflurane is maintained at 0.8% (50% minimal alveolar concentration) in 100% oxygen. The addition of nitrous oxide to the sevoflurane/oxygen mixture will result in a potential loss of the TcMEP. The use of surgical muscle relaxation is obviously restricted, as with all EMG-based modalities. The surgeon should be aware that requesting surgical muscle relaxant during exposure of the spine can interfere with the neuromonitoring.

Patients may jump and their faces may move during transcranial stimulation. Patient movements may impede the surgical procedure and pose a risk for inadvertent neural injury. The neuromonitoring technician should determine the extent of patient movement and, if necessary, warn the surgeon before initiating a TcMEP study. Patients might bite down on the endotracheal tube and/or damage their tongue or lips as a consequence of the transcranial stimulation. The anesthesiologist should place a soft bite block to protect the endotracheal tube and prevent soft-tissue damage from occurring. A hard bite block alone might not provide sufficient protection. The bite block should be routinely monitored during the surgery to prevent misplacement or total displacement. Patient movement is hardly noticeable when TcMEP stimulation electrodes are placed into the scalp exactly over the motor cortices.

Intravenous agents take longer to wear off than inhalant anesthesia. Additional time is usually required to prepare the patient for a wake-up test. Similarly, the emergence of the patient from general anesthesia at the end of surgery might be delayed. The anesthesiologist should keep the surgeon informed of the status of the anesthesia regimen. The surgeon might have to adjust the procedure accordingly.

INTRAOPERATIVE ELECTROMYOGRAPHY

The final component in the multimodal approach to neuromonitoring is intraoperative EMG. The first intraoperative applications of EMG were neurosurgeries for resection of brain stem, spinal cord, and cauda equina tumors. The technique was applied to spine surgery in the early 1990s, when scientific studies suggested that EMG monitoring could help to prevent injuries incurred by a misplaced pedicle screw or other spinal implant. The role of EMG has now expanded beyond spinal instrumentation cases to include decompressive techniques for excision of disc herniation, spinal stenosis, and degenerative disc disease and techniques for minimally invasive exposure, endoscopic instrumentation, total disc replacement, and intraspinous decompression devices.

It is not uncommon for the surgeon, surgical assistant, or scrub nurse to be aware of muscle activity beneath the surgical drapes. However, most myogenic activities are occult and can be detected only by intraoperative EMG. Muscle potentials are recorded by using paired needle electrodes inserted into the skin over the muscles of interest. EMG volume conducts through the muscle tissue to be recorded by the subdermal electrodes. Target muscles are selected according to the specific nerve roots that are placed at risk by the surgical manipulation and the disease process that is afflicting the patient.

Not every muscle within a distal myotome will respond to manipulation or stimulation of the associated spinal nerve root. A serious error in neuromuscular monitoring is to rely on a single target muscle within a particular myotome. To avoid a false-negative outcome, it is prudent to monitor as many muscles as possible. If necessary, two muscles can be linked together to provide greater coverage. This technique can result in a loss of nerve root specificity; the neuromonitoring technician might not be able to differentiate between surgical levels as precisely as would be the case if the muscles were monitored individually. Table 29-1 lists muscles that are used to monitor spinal nerve roots and the cauda equina. Monitoring the external anal sphincter is especially important to help prevent loss of bowel and bladder function.

Two variations of EMG neuromuscular monitoring are free-running and stimulated EMG. Free-running EMG monitors ongoing surgical maneuvers. The free-running technique provides continuous, real-time assessment of spinal nerve roots and the cauda equina during all phases of the surgical procedure. Although the obvious example is a misplaced pedicle screw, any surgical technique that has the potential for affecting spinal nerve roots will elicit EMG at distal muscle groups. The presence of activity implies manipulation and potential for injury. The absence of activity suggests that nerve roots are unaffected by surgery. The absence of otherwise expected EMG activity should be questioned. It might be the case that the surgeon is being exceptionally gentle. It might also be the case that the nerve root is nonresponsive or damaged. In addition, as was mentioned previously, the patient might be relaxed. The anesthesiologist can control the dosage and timing of surgical muscle relaxation quite accurately. The surgeon can also adjust portions of surgery to accommodate EMG neuromonitoring.

Stimulated EMG is an all-or-nothing response, a CMAP in response to directed electrical stimulation of a nerve fiber, motor nerve root, or surgical implant. Stimulated EMG tests the integrity of the bony elements of the spine in relation to implanted devices and nerve root impingement. Stimulated EMG can prove useful during revision surgery when it becomes necessary to separate viable nerve from embedded scar tissue. The techniques of free-running and stimulated EMG are used to safely guide minimally invasive approaches to the spine.

Interpreting Free-Running Electromyographic Potentials

EMG activity is specific to the particular root or roots that are affected by the surgical manipulation. Once the pattern of the muscle response has been determined, it is not unusual for the neuromonitoring technician to inform the surgeon as to the exact level of the spine where he or she is working. Activity noted at multiple sites can help to reveal conjoined nerve root innervations. The EMG response to the surgical manipulation is usually immediate; however, delayed reactions to surgical stimulation might also be observed. The neuromonitoring technician is obligated to inform the surgeon of all EMG activities as soon as they occur in real time. The surgeon can correlate the EMG events with ongoing or recent surgical manipulations.

A certain amount of EMG activity is expected to occur; however, every EMG event should be considered a cause for concern. Even potentially benign episodes of EMG activity can help to map the anatomy of the nerve root and bony elements of the spine so that the surgeon learns where the root might be at greater risk for irritation and injury. The intensity and pattern of free-running EMG responses will vary depending on the sensitivity of the root to manipulation and the extent and type of the surgical manipulation that elicits the activity. For example, a sudden burst of intense muscle activity might be the first and only warning that the surgeon receives of a misdirected pedicle screw or probe. Early warning and immediate redirection of the probe or implant can prevent a breach of the pedicle wall and potential injury to the affected nerve root.

The most common types of free-running EMG that are observed during spine surgery are bursting, sustained, tapping, and waking EMG. As is shown on the left side of Figure 29-7, bursting is characterized by a high-frequency EMG discharge of relatively short duration. A transient

TABLE 29-1. Muscles Used to Monitor Spinal Motor Nerve Roots and Motor Pathways During Electromyographic and Transcranial Motor Evoked Potential Studies

Surgical Level	Muscle
C8, T1	Hand intrinsics (abductor pollicis brevis, lumbricals)
T8-12	Rectus abdominis
Conus, cauda equina	External anal sphincter
L1-3	Sartorius, adductor magnus, vastus lateralis
L4, L5	Tibialis anterior
L5	Peroneus longus
L5, S1	Biceps femoris
S1, S2	Gastrocnemius
S1, S2, S3	External anal sphincter
S1, S2, S3	Foot intrinsics

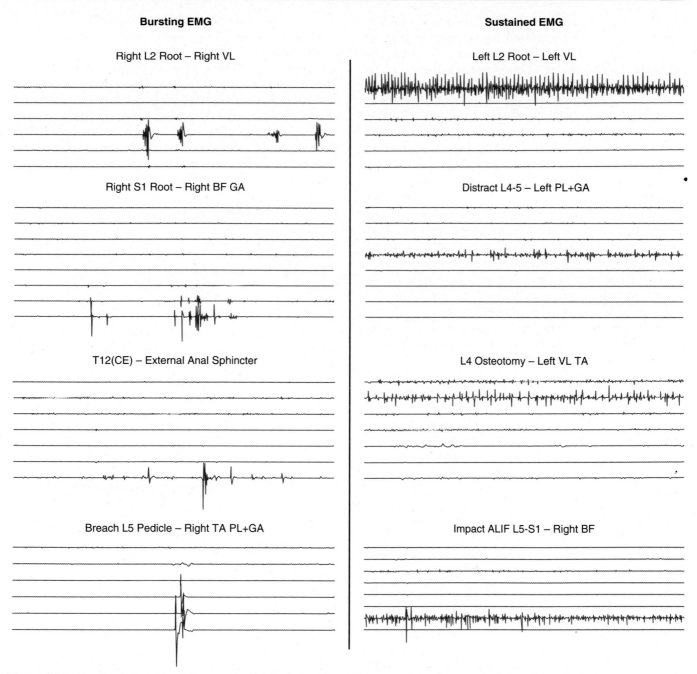

Figure 29-7. Bursting and sustained, free-running EMG events were noted in response to direct manipulation of the spinal nerve roots or cauda equina. Muscle activity is specific to the radicular distribution of the affected nerve root or fiber. ALIF, anterior lumbar interbody fixation; BF, biceps femoris; CE, cauda equina; GA, gastrocnemius; PL, peroneus longus; TA, tibialis anterior; VL, vastus lateralis; the plus sign indicates linked muscles.

episode of bursting activity usually follows a single, isolated manipulation of the root or cauda equina. Clusters of bursting suggest a more forceful manipulation. As is shown on the right side of Figure 29-7, sustained EMG is characterized by a regular train of neurotonic activity, similar in appearance to bursting but of longer duration. Sustained EMG can continue for several minutes. Sustained EMG, especially of longer duration, can indicate potential nerve root irritation. Sustained activities are typically observed during exploration, decompression, or

manipulation at very tight, stenotic levels of the spine. Sustained activity has also been observed following blunt trauma to a nerve root or when a nerve root is stretched. High-amplitude bursting can often lead to a bout of sustained activity.

Examples of tapping EMG are shown in Figure 29-8. Tapping is elicited when the surgeon strikes the bony elements of the spine with an osteotome, pedicle probe, spacing device, or other surgical device or tool. Impacting a graft plug, disc prosthesis, or other implant into the disc interspace will also generate a response. Tapping EMG is characterized by biphasic or triphasic deflections similar to a CMAP. Impact maneuvers can also elicit episodes of bursting or sustained activity.

Tapping EMG is not artifact. As is shown in Figure 29-8, tapping EMG follows the radicular distribution of the affected nerve roots. Moreover, the amplitude of the response is directly proportional to the percussive force directed against the bone. A strong impact will elicit a large-amplitude spike. The etiology of tapping EMG may be the mechanical depolarization of the nerve root or roots in question.

Alerting the surgeon to tapping EMG during an impact maneuver affords the opportunity to use minimal force while limiting the exposure of the nerve root to potential injury. Tapping responses may indicate sensitive regions of local anatomy. Tapping activity may forewarn the surgeon of nerve root sensitivity or the possibility of a double crush effect. Tapping seems to be more pronounced when the surgeon is using an osteotome whose edge has become dull. Although tapping is specific to the level where the surgeon is operating, it can be referred to sites beyond the primary point of impact, suggesting transmission of mechanical force to distal nerve roots. Referred activity can indicate levels of the spine where nerve roots are susceptible to irritation, thus alerting the surgeon to potential injury later on during the surgery.

An example of waking EMG is shown in Figure 29-9. The electrodes monitoring EMG also record changes in the patient's muscle tone. Waking EMG is observed when the depth of anesthesia becomes insufficient to prevent movement in a nonrelaxed patient. The onset of waking EMG can be quite sudden. The surgeon and anesthesiologist should be informed immediately of the change in muscle tension. Often, sudden patient movement can occur without the anesthesiologist's being alerted to a change in the status of the patient's hemodynamics and other monitored parameters. Waking EMG activity may precede or coincide with patient movement. Waking EMG can prove useful during the administration of total intravenous anesthesia with limited doses of surgical muscle relaxant. The neuromonitoring technician should discuss the waking EMG phenomenon with the anesthesiologist prior to surgery so that the anesthesiologist will be familiar with the monitoring information that may be provided during the case.

Interpreting Stimulated Electromyographic Potentials

A sterile probe placed onto the surgical field is used to deliver pulses of electrical current to the structure in question. The level of stimulus intensity that is required to elicit a CMAP at the appropriate distal musculature is determined. Directly stimulating an exposed nerve fiber or

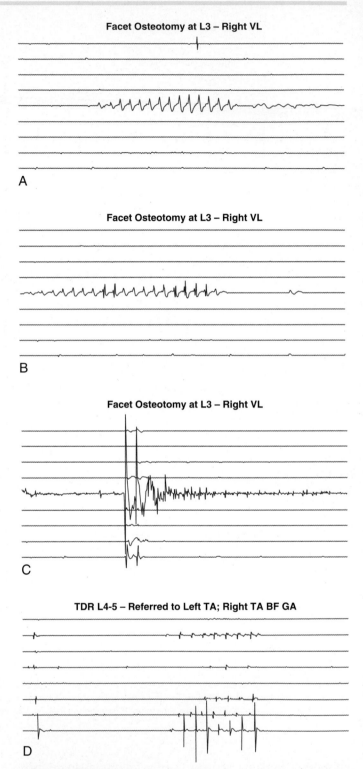

Figure 29-8. Striking bony elements of the spine with a surgical instrument, graft plug, implant, or other device elicits tapping EMG. **A,** Facet osteotomy at L3 elicited tapping activity at the right vastus lateralis muscle. EMG amplitude is directly proportional to the force of impact. **B,** Small bursts of EMG embedded within a tapping response. **C,** Bursting followed by sustained EMG elicited by a single tap. **D,** Impacting a total disc replacement prosthesis into the L4-5 interspace elicited EMG at the left tibialis anterior and the right tibialis anterior, biceps femoris, and gastrocnemius muscles. BF, biceps femoris; GA, gastrocnemius; TA, tibialis anterior; TDR, total disc replacement; VL, vastus lateralis.

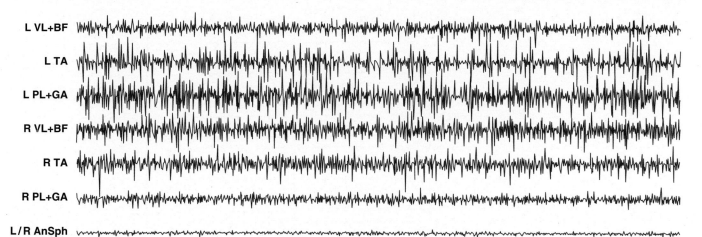

Figure 29-9. Monitoring free-running EMG can alert the surgeon and anesthesiologist to changes in the patient's muscle tone. Ongoing EMG is observed at multiple sites when the level of surgical anesthesia becomes insufficient to prevent patient movement. BF, biceps femoris; AnSph, external anal sphincter; GA, gastrocnemius; L, left; PL. peroneus longus; R, right; TA, tibialis anterior; VL, vastus lateralis; the plus sign indicates linked muscles.

filament will elicit a CMAP using very low stimulus intensities (0.1 to 1.5 mA). Stimulation of scar or nonviable nerve tissue will fail to elicit a response. In the lumbar spine, when pedicle screw placement is being monitored, a stimulus intensity of less than 3.0 mA signifies direct contact with a nerve root. Stimulus intensities between 3.0 and 8.0 mA are marginal and might require further investigation. Often, electrical current will leak through a small hole in the pedicle wall, or a small portion of the screw thread is impinging on the root. Values between 8.0 and 11.0 mA usually indicate an intact pedicle wall. It is useful to increase stimulus intensity well beyond the minimum range for determining a safe implant. This technique usually provides the actual stimulus intensity for eliciting a distal CMAP. The surgeon should observe movements of the paraspinal muscles during the increase in stimulus intensity.

The quality of the patient's bone can play a role in determining the significance of the findings. Osteoporotic bone may transmit electrical current differently than normal bone. Determine the threshold values for all implants first, and then look for outliers in the data. If the surgeon has any doubts, the implant may be temporarily removed. The pedicle wall is palpated for a breach. If necessary, the implant can be redirected, and a new threshold can be acquired. The revised value might not reflect an improvement over the original finding. This could be due to a leak of current through the original breach in the pedicle wall. In other instances, the revision might push bone fragments into the breach and seal the defect. The surgeon may opt to forgo placing an implant into a compromised pedicle.

An example of a left side, lumbar pedicle screw study is illustrated in Figure 29-10. Stimulated EMG was observed at the left vastus lateralis muscle (L2, L3) and the left tibi-

alis anterior muscle (L4). Threshold intensities were 44, 27, and 35 mA, at the L2, L3, and L4 pedicles, respectively. These values suggest that the implants did not breach the pedicle walls or impinge on the motor nerve roots.

THE IMPORTANCE OF PREOPERATIVE BASELINE DATA

Electrophysiologic data are subject to naturally occurring variability over the course of a surgical procedure. The acquisition of baseline data from induction of anesthesia onward will give the monitoring technician a solid foundation on which to gauge the significance of neuromonitoring changes that may occur later on during surgery. Because so many extraneous variables affect monitored signals, the technician should have a good understanding of the patient's data trends prior to any manipulation that can adversely affect the patient's nervous system. Patients with previously operated spines (i.e., laminectomy, pseudarthrosis, failed back syndrome), rigid spinal deformities, degenerative sagittal imbalance, and the like may be at greater risk for intraoperative neurologic deficit. Good-quality baseline data from one modality can help to compensate for poor-quality data from another modality (see Case 2). The surgeon should be informed about the quality of the preoperative baseline data before surgery begins. Patients with peripheral neuropathy, radiculopathy, myelopathy, neuromuscular disease, or other neurologic comorbidities might not generate well-formed and reproducible signals. SSEPs might be diffuse, variable, or erratic. TcMEP signals might be difficult to obtain, require a very high stimulus level, or be absent altogether. EMG might demonstrate ongoing motor unit activity. Understanding the baseline trends will help the surgeon to assess

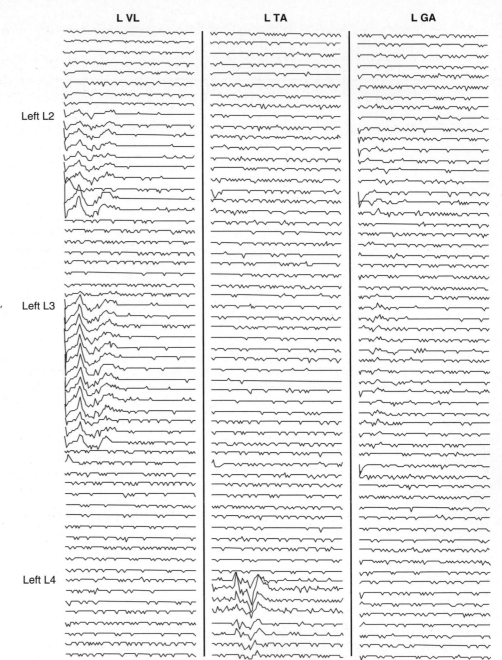

L VL   L TA   L GA

Left L2

Left L3

Left L4

Figure 29-10. Stimulation of the left L2, L3, and L4 pedicle screws generated CMAPs at the left vastus lateralis and tibialis anterior muscles. GA, gastrocnemius; L, left; R, right; TA, tibialis anterior; VL, vastus lateralis.

the potential value that neuromonitoring will provide during the case.

Baseline SSEP data should be acquired immediately after induction of anesthesia, before the surgical muscle relaxant that is used for intubation has taken effect. This allows the technician to determine the stimulus thresholds that are required to generate the SSEP as well as to elicit movement at the distal extremities. Moreover, early acquisition of SSEP data allows neuromonitoring through laryngoscopy, insertion of the endotracheal tube, and positioning of the patient onto the operating room table. Modern neuromonitoring equipment can acquire SSEP data far more rapidly than older instruments could. The technique of interleaving stimuli permits almost simulta-

neous sampling of left and right, upper- and lower-extremity SSEP data. In a patient with well-formed and reproducible signals, rapid acquisition makes it possible to collect sufficient baseline data during the time it takes to induce, mask, and intubate the patient. In circumstances in which the SSEP signals are poorly formed or not very reproducible, the anesthesiologist can cooperate with the neuromonitoring technician to allow additional time for the technician to maximize the signals.

Baseline neuromuscular data are collected as soon as the surgical muscle relaxant that is used for intubation of the trachea has worn off enough to permit distal EMG activity. Depending on the dose of neuromuscular blockade that is used at intubation, the TcMEP can be examined before final positioning of the patient onto the operating room table. Movements of the arms, legs, hands, and feet in response to transcranial stimulation can be observed visually even if the EMG electrodes have not yet been attached to the monitoring amplifier.

TECHNIQUES FOR IMPROVING THE QUALITY OF NEUROMONITORING DATA

Several techniques can be used to improve the quality of baseline SSEP and TcMEP data. For example, the average number of sweeps can be increased to improve the signal-to-noise ratio of the SSEP signal. Stimulus parameters such as intensity, rate, duration, and polarity can be adjusted to maximize the SSEP responses. The arrangement of recording electrodes at the scalp can be varied to locate sites where the SSEP signals are strongest. Stimulating electrodes used to deliver TcMEP pulses can be relocated along the medial-to-lateral and anterior-to-posterior axes to maximize stimulation of the motor cortex and not just induce a diffuse spread of current across the scalp. The number of pulses in the stimulus train and the width of the interstimulus interval that is used to elicit the TcMEP can be varied to generate a more focused transcranial stimulation. Obviously, the best time to maximize neuromonitoring parameters is during the presurgical acquisition of baseline data. Sometimes, it becomes necessary to troubleshoot or repair a technical fault during the case. Under these circumstances, the surgeon should not be surprised to see the neuromonitoring technician checking the recording or stimulating electrodes, perhaps under the drapes. The technician should always inform the surgical and operating room staff if it becomes necessary to enter within close proximity to the surgical field. Obviously, the technician must inform the surgeon if monitoring is suspended because of a technical issue.

PREPARING THE PATIENT FOR NEUROMONITORING

Patient preparation should be quick and not interfere with the regular operating room routines. Application of the neuromonitoring electrodes should not cause patient discomfort. Surface electrodes at the ankles and wrist that are used to elicit SSEP responses can be applied while the patient is awake, usually in the holding area or when the patient first enters the operating room. Ulnar nerve electrodes can be placed medially on the wrist so as to avoid interfering with the insertion of a radial artery catheter. Subdermal needle electrodes used to record the SSEP signals at the scalp are applied after the patient has been sedated. This permits acquisition of baseline SSEP data immediately following induction of anesthesia. Subdermal needle electrodes used to record muscle activity for the EMG tests are applied after the patient has been anesthetized. The surgeon should wait until the EMG needles are fixed in place before initiating positioning of the patient for the surgical procedure. The subdermal needle electrodes at the scalp used to elicit the TcMEP are also applied after the patient is anesthetized. In children, the acquisition of baseline data should be delayed until the child has been anesthetized and, if necessary, intubated. The electrodes can then be applied without causing the patient or the patient's family undue distress.

CONCLUDING COMMENTS

Neuromonitoring spinal deformity surgery requires protecting the patient's spinal cord and nerve roots. This is accomplished with the Stagnara wake-up test, the somatosensory evoked potential, the transcranial motor evoked potential, and techniques of free-running and stimulated electromyography. The Stagnara wake-up test provides a good measure of motor system function but also requires substantial preparation; moreover, the wake-up test occurs after spinal instrumentation is in place. The SSEP test provides a reliable and continuous measure of the patient's spinal cord function throughout all phases of surgery but does not monitor motor function directly. The TcMEP test assesses the function of the patient's motor system without monitoring the integrity of individual motor nerve roots. EMG neuromuscular monitoring protects the motor nerve roots from excessive surgical manipulation. Taken together, these tests provide coverage of the patient's spinal cord and nerve root function during the surgical procedure. These tests are considered the standards of care for monitoring spinal deformity surgery.

In a typical multimodal monitoring protocol for spinal deformity surgery, SSEP and free-running EMG studies are run continuously during the procedure. Transcranial motor evoked potential studies are performed at regular intervals, notably before, during, and after any manipulation that places the spine at risk. Stimulated EMG studies are available when needed to guide the probing and placing of pedicle screws and other spinal implants. At the surgeon's discretion, a wake-up test can be performed to confirm motor system function.

Given a well-controlled environment, it is reasonable to assume that all neuromonitoring changes that occur during the surgical procedure are real events. The surgeon should understand that changes in the monitored signals do not always correlate with immediate surgical events. Some changes will be a consequence of the administration of anesthesia or other physiologic factors that affect monitoring signals. Other changes might be a delayed reaction to a surgical manipulation. The surgeon should be able to use available information to help discern real monitoring events from false-positive and false-negative events. The surgeon should question the neuromonitoring technician regarding the outcomes of the tests being performed. Having established the basis for the change, the surgeon can begin remedial action as soon as possible. Ideally, recovery of changed signals back to baseline will reflect improvement in the patient's status.

The coming years should see advances in the field of clinical intraoperative neuromuscular monitoring. This is due in part to recent FDA approval for transcranial motor stimulation devices and the subsequent increase in the clinical applications of motor system neuromonitoring in the operating room. Topics of interest might include clinical comparisons between somatosensory and motor evoked potentials, explorations into the etiology of neuromonitoring changes in relation to vascular and mechanical insults to the cord, resolution of the debate between various warning criteria for TcMEP changes, improvements in "monitoring-friendly" anesthetic techniques, and development of more reliable techniques for monitoring pedicle screw implantation in the thoracic spine. Different patterns of EMG activities have been observed during monitoring of spine procedures. Research correlating these activities to patient outcome should be forthcoming within the next few years.

Finally, intraoperative neurologic deficits are still common following deformity surgery. The risk increases when techniques such as pedicle subtraction osteotomy are used to restore lumbar lordosis and correct sagittal imbalance. Widespread utilization of multimodal neuromonitoring protocols can help to change the defined standards of care at an increasing number of health care institutions. Neuromonitoring techniques and protocols will come under greater scrutiny with respect to hospital standards and practices and, of course, legal discovery. Hospitals and surgeons that do not currently require or use neuromonitoring might begin to do so. Each neuromonitoring practice will have to develop well-defined and established protocols that cover all aspects of the surgical procedure. It is hoped that the continued application of good neuromonitoring practices will further reduce the risk of iatrogenic injury and the incidence of postoperative neurologic deficits. This chapter concludes with two case presentations that illustrate the importance of monitoring both the sensory and the motor pathways during spinal deformity surgery.

PEARLS & PITFALLS

PEARLS

- A signal that contains mostly random noise will average out into a flat line response when the number of sweeps is increased beyond the "usual and customary" amount. Conversely, a real SSEP will remain relatively unchanged as the number of sweeps is increased.
- Failure to detect injury to the motor pathways should not be considered a false-negative SSEP finding when motor system neuromonitoring is being performed during the procedure.

- Care must be taken during all phases of surgery. The neuromonitoring technician should always be on the alert for changes in the monitored signals.
- The suggested electrophysiologic replacement for the Stagnara wake-up test is the TcMEP.
- It seems prudent to monitor as many lower-extremity muscles as possible and thus maximize the opportunity for capturing a distal TcMEP or EMG response.
- No one disputes the necessity for motor system neuromonitoring. Practical experience suggests that elements of all three methods should be considered in following the progression of TcMEP data.
- The neuromonitoring literature and practical experience suggest that false-negative errors are rare with TcMEP neuromonitoring.
- Patient movement is hardly noticeable when TcMEP stimulation electrodes are placed into the scalp exactly over the motor cortices.
- Alerting the surgeon to tapping EMG during an impact maneuver affords the opportunity to use minimal force while limiting the exposure of the nerve root to potential injury.
- Often, sudden patient movement can occur without the anesthesiologist being alerted to a change in the status of the patient's hemodynamics and other monitored parameters.
- The surgeon should observe movements of the paraspinal muscles during the increase in stimulus intensity.
- Determine the threshold values for all implants first, and then look for outliers in the data.
- The surgeon should be informed about the quality of the preoperative baseline data before surgery begins.

PITFALLS

- One of the deepest fears that patients bring to the operating room is the possibility of waking up during the procedure.
- The wake-up test is not a continuous measure of spinal cord function.
- The SSEP is not an instantaneous measure of spinal cord function.
- One of the more common "freshman" errors in neuromonitoring is the failure to distinguish a real SSEP from regularly occurring noise.
- Changes in signal latency accompanied by significant decreases in signal amplitude can be misinterpreted as a reversal in signal polarity.
- A frequently observed and potentially dangerous error in neuromonitoring is the failure to report an uncertain finding to the surgeon.
- Do not ignore significant SSEP changes if there are no changes in the motor evoked potentials. The patient could be experiencing somatosensory system dysfunction.
- An uneventful somatosensory study does not guarantee an intact motor system.

- A common error in motor system neuromonitoring (TcMEP or EMG) is relying on a single muscle to cover distal myotomes.
- Controversy exists within the monitoring community regarding the validity of each technique.
- The surgeon should be aware that requesting surgical muscle relaxant during exposure of the spine can interfere with the neuromonitoring.
- Intravenous agents take longer to wear off than inhalant anesthesia does.

- Not every muscle within a distal myotome will respond to manipulation or stimulation of the associated spinal nerve root.
- The absence of otherwise expected EMG activity should be questioned.
- The quality of the patient's bone can play a role in determining the significance of the findings.

Illustrative Case Presentations

CASE 1. Significant Deterioration in the Motor Potentials During the Application of Corrective Force to the Spine

The patient, a 17-year-old male, was admitted to the operating room with a diagnosis of idiopathic scoliosis. The surgical procedure was a T2-L4 posterior spinal fusion with instrumentation to correct a right-side 65-degree thoracic curve. The monitored signals included left and right upper- and lower-extremity SSEPs, left and right lower-extremity TcMEPs, and EMG studies of the L1-S3 spinal nerve roots and cauda equina.

Figure 29-11 provides examples of the neuromonitoring data sampled during the critical phases of the procedure. Baseline TcMEP signals were recorded at the left tibialis anterior and gastrocnemius muscles in response to stimulation of the right motor cortex (235

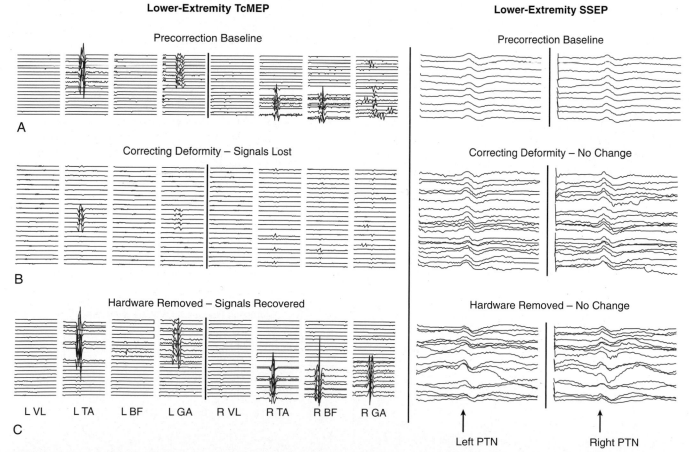

Figure 29-11. A significant change in the right-side TcMEP occurred during correction of the spine for idiopathic scoliosis. SSEP data remained unchanged. **A,** Baseline TcMEP noted at the left tibialis anterior and gastrocnemius muscles and at the right tibialis anterior, biceps femoris, and gastrocnemius muscles. Baseline posterior tibial nerve SSEPs were well formed and reproducible bilaterally. **B,** A significant change in right-side TcMEP signals occurred when corrective forces were applied to the spine. Left-side motor responses were attenuated. No changes in left- or right-side SSEPs were observed. **C,** TcMEP signals recovered immediately after the rod was removed. SSEP data remained unchanged. In this example, the polarity of the posterior tibial nerve "P37" is upward. BF, biceps femoris; GA, gastrocnemius; L, left; PTN, posterior tibial nerve; R, right; SSEP, somatosensory evoked potential; TA, tibialis anterior; TcMEP, transcranial motor evoked potential; VL, vastus lateralis.

volts) and at the right tibialis anterior, biceps femoris, and gastrocnemius muscles in response to stimulation of the left motor cortex (235 volts). Baseline posterior tibial nerve SSEP data were well formed, stable, and reproducible bilaterally.

A significant change in the patient's right-side motor function, characterized by a loss of all muscle potentials, was noted immediately after corrective force was applied to the spine. Attenuation in the amplitude of the left-side muscle responses also occurred. Stimulus intensity was increased from 235 volts to over 350 volts with only a sporadic improvement in the right-side muscle potentials. The SSEP waveforms remained unchanged during the event. The rod was removed, and the corrective forces on the spine were released. Left- and right-side motor responses began to recover immediately. Threshold stimulus intensities gradually returned to baseline levels at 235 volts bilaterally. The SSEP signals remained stable and unchanged.

On the basis of the findings of the TcMEP studies, it was determined that the patient's nervous system would not tolerate further attempts at manipulation of the spine. The surgery was therefore canceled. The patient emerged from anesthesia without neurologic deficits. The patient was brought back to the operating room at a later date for a successful and event-free partial correction of his curve. This case provides a convincing example of the need to monitor both SSEP and TcMEP during surgery to correct spinal deformity.

CASE 2. Significant Change in Both the Somatosensory and Motor Evoked Potentials During the Application of Corrective Force to the Spine

The patient, a 17-year-old female, was admitted to the operating room with a diagnosis of idiopathic scoliosis. The surgical procedure was a T6-L3 posterior spinal fusion with instrumentation to correct a right-side, 30-degree thoracic/42-degree lumbar curve. The monitored signals included left and right upper- and lower-extremity SSEPs, left and right lower-extremity TcMEPs, and electromyographic studies of the L1 to S3 spinal nerve roots and cauda equina.

Figure 29-12 provides examples of the neuromonitoring data that were sampled during the critical phases of the procedure. Preoperative assessment of bilateral SSEP function indicated poorly formed, diffuse signals that were characterized by variable amplitudes

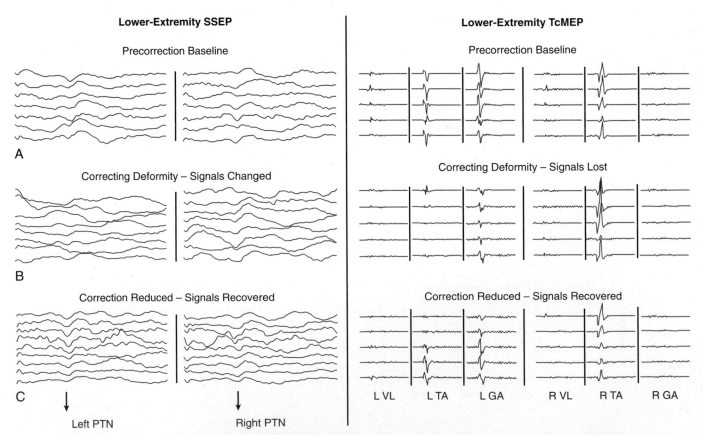

Figure 29-12. Significant changes in both SSEP and TcMEP signals noted during correction of the spine for idiopathic scoliosis. **A,** Baseline SSEP data indicated poorly formed signals bilaterally. Good-quality baseline TcMEP signals were noted at the left tibialis anterior and gastrocnemius muscles and at the right tibialis anterior muscle. **B,** Significant deterioration in the left posterior tibial nerve SSEP waveform occurred as the surgeon began to correct the deformity. A loss in the left tibialis anterior TcMEP was then observed. The left gastrocnemius response was attenuated but still within baseline limits. **C,** SSEP and TcMEP signals recovered immediately after the correction was reduced. The wake-up test was negative. In this example, the polarity of the posterior tibial nerve P37 is downward. GA, gastrocnemius; L, left; PTN, posterior tibial nerve; R, right; SSEP, somatosensory evoked potential; TA, tibialis anterior; TcMEP, transcranial motor evoked potential; VL, vastus lateralis.

and latencies. The SSEP waveforms did not replicate well. Left-side responses were worse than right-side responses. These findings suggested that monitoring spinal cord function using only SSEP data would prove difficult at best. Fortunately, good-quality, baseline TcMEP signals were recorded at the left tibialis anterior and gastrocnemius muscles in response to stimulation of the right motor cortex (306 volts) and at the right tibialis anterior muscle in response to stimulation of the left motor cortex (310 volts).

Interestingly enough, the first indication of nervous system dysfunction was a change in the status of the left-side posterior tibial nerve SSEP. The change occurred when the surgeon first began to apply corrective force to the spinal column. Left-side SSEP waveforms became even more diffuse, with a loss of signal characterized not by a flat line response but rather by irregular waveforms that failed to replicate consistently. Right-side responses were only moderately affected. The deterioration in evoked potential morphology satisfied the warning criteria for a significant change in spinal cord function. A series of TcMEP studies was initiated immediately, and a change in the overall patterning of the left-side motor potentials was noted. Transcranial stimulation at the baseline intensity of 306 volts failed to elicit a consistent response at the left tibialis anterior muscle, even though an attenuated response at the left gastrocnemius muscle was still present. Increasing the stimulus intensity beyond 306 volts failed to elicit a consistent response at the left tibialis anterior muscle. The rod was removed; corrective forces on the spine were released; and both the SSEP and TcMEP signals recovered. Surgery was continued, and the patient tolerated a lesser degree of correction with no changes observed in the monitored signals. A negative wake-up test was performed after the final construct was in place. The patient emerged from anesthesia without neurologic deficit. The surgical team was informed of all changes in the monitored signals as they occurred in real time. In this example, taken together, both sensory and motor signals provided warning of a change in the patient's neurophysiologic status.

ACKNOWLEDGMENTS

The author would like to thank Paul Alfano, MD; David Berger, MD; Fabien Bitan, MD; Robert Chuda, MD; Anthony Giordano, MD; Scott Hanan, MD; John Ho, MD; Oswald Jules, MD; Edward Lang, CST; Robert LaPorta, MD; Vincent Leone, MD; Gregory Lollo, MD; Baron Lonner, MD; Miguel Maranan; Sean McCance, MD; Joseph Moreira, MD; Patrick O'Leary, MD; Roland Rizzi, MD; Dariuz Rudz, MD; Bobby Taskey, R EEG T, CNIM; and Mark Winik, MD, for their help in preparing this manuscript.

SUGGESTED READINGS

Buchowski JM, Bridwell KH, Lenke LG: Neurologic complications of lumbar pedicle subtraction osteotomy: A ten year assessment. Spine 2007;32:2245–2252.

The authors report a high rate of significant neurologic complications following pedicle subtraction osteotomy. The techniques of intraoperative neuromonitoring that were used during these surgeries failed to warn the surgical team of changes in the patients' nervous system function.

Calancie B, Harris W, Brindle GF, et al: Threshold-level repetitive transcranial electrical stimulation for intraoperative monitoring of central motor conduction. J Neurosurg Spine 2001;95:161–168.

The authors discuss the threshold technique for determining significant change in the transcranial motor evoked potential.

Calancie B, Madsen P, Lebwohl N: Stimulus-evoked EMG monitoring during transpedicular lumbosacral spine instrumentation: Initial clinical results. Spine 1994;19:2780–2786.

The authors suggest that EMG is a sensitive and reliable technique for monitoring lumbar pedicle screws.

Dawson EG, Sherman JE, Kanim LE, Nuwer MR: Spinal cord monitoring: Results of the Scoliosis Research Society and the European Spinal Deformity Society survey. Spine 1991;16(8 suppl):S361–S364.

This review article suggests that false-positive and false-negative outcomes are not uncommon when SSEPs are used to monitor spinal deformity surgery.

Lewis SJ, Lenke LG, Raynor B, et al: Triggered electromyographic threshold for accuracy of thoracic pedicle screw placement in a porcine model. Spine 2001;26:2485–2489; discussion 2490.

The authors suggest that techniques of stimulated EMG developed for monitoring lumbar pedicle screws might not be appropriate for monitoring thoracic pedicle screws.

Lotto ML, Banoub M, Schubert AL: Effects of anesthetic agents and physiologic changes on intraoperative motor evoked potentials. J Neurosurg Anesthesiol 2004;16:32–42.

The authors review the effects of anesthetic agents and physiologic factors on the motor evoked potential.

Nuwer MR, Dawson EG, Carlson LG, et al: Somatosensory evoked potential spinal cord monitoring reduces neurologic deficits after scoliosis surgery: Results of a large multicenter survey. Electroencephalogr Clin Neurophysiol 1995;96:6–11.

This review paper discusses SSEP monitoring during spinal surgery. Apparently better patient outcomes were obtained when more experienced neuromonitoring teams provided the monitoring.

Padberg AM, Wilson-Holden TJ, Lenke LG, Bridwell KH: Somatosensory- and motor-evoked potential monitoring without a wake-up test during idiopathic scoliosis surgery: An accepted standard of care. Spine 1998;23:1392–1400.

The authors suggest that monitoring somatosensory and motor evoked potentials results in a sensitive and specific method for predicting postoperative outcomes with low rates of false-positive and false-negative events.

Quinones-Hinojosa A, Lyon R, Zada G, et al: Changes in transcranial motor evoked potentials during intramedullary spinal cord tumor resection correlate with postoperative motor function. Neurosurgery 2005;56:982–993.

The authors suggest that the complexity of the TcMEP waveform, along with the stimulus threshold and loss of signal techniques, correlates well with postoperative motor system outcome.

Shi YB, Binette M, Martin WH, et al: Electrical stimulation for intraoperative evaluation of thoracic pedicle screw placement. Spine 2003; 28:595–601.

The authors suggest that stimulated EMG may be applied to the placement of thoracic pedicle screws.

Slimp JC: Electrophysiologic intraoperative monitoring for spine procedures. Phys Med Rehabil Clin N Am 2004;15:85–105.

The author discusses multimodal applications of somatosensory, motor, nerve root, and H-reflex neuromonitoring.

Slimp JC, Rubner DE, Snowden ML, Stolov WC: Dermatomal somato-sensory evoked potentials: Cervical, thoracic, and lumbosacral levels. Electroencephalogr Clin Neurophysiol 1992;84:55–70.

This review article describes techniques for monitoring dermatomal somatosensory evoked potentials.

Sloan TB: Anesthesia and motor evoked potential monitoring. Intraoperative Neurophysiological Monitoring in Neurosurgery 2004, IV International Symposium, pp 88–102.

The author explains the effects of anesthetic agents on motor evoked potentials.

Tsai RY, Yang RS, Nuwer MR, et al: Intraoperative dermatomal evoked potential monitoring fails to predict outcome from lumbar decompression surgery. Spine 1997;22:1970–1975.

The authors conclude that dermatomal somatosensory evoked potentials are not reliable.

Weiss DS: Spinal cord and nerve root monitoring during surgical treatment of lumbar stenosis. Clin Orthop Relat Res 2001;384: 82–100.

The author reviews multimodal neuromonitoring techniques for surgical treatment of spinal stenosis, with emphasis on EMG.

CHAPTER 30

A Modified Anterior Muscle-Sparing Retroperitoneal Approach to the Lumbar Spine: Technique and Outcomes

Matthew M. Nalbandian *and* Bart E. Muhs

Anterior exposures to the lumbar spine have rapidly gained in popularity in recent years for surgical decompression and reconstruction of the spine. This chapter describes approaches to the lateral lumbar spine proximally and the anterior lumbar spine distally. Various anterior exposure techniques have been described in the literature for accessing the anterior lumbar spine. Ito and colleagues first reported anterior exposure to the lumbar spine for the treatment of spondylolisthesis and Pott's disease in the 1930s. A vertical, paramedian incision through the abdominal wall was utilized to gain access to the retroperitoneal space. In 1964, Harmon described a simplified technique for anterior lumbar discectomy and fusion, using hypogastric and paramedian vertical incisions with mobilization of the rectus abdominis muscle laterally. In 2002, Brau described an approach for anterior lumbar interbody spinal fusions using a transverse incision with mobilization of the rectus abdominis muscle both medially and laterally.

LUMBOSACRAL SPINE EXPOSURE: ANTEROLATERAL APPROACH

The anterolateral approach to the lumbar spine is used for best access to multiple lumbar levels from T12 to L4. In contrast, the anterior techniques are most helpful at L4-S1. Both approaches can be extended to include upper or lower levels. Incisions are made between the 12th rib and the superior iliac crest and are localized over the vertebral levels to be exposed.

Patient Position

Patients are positioned on their right side in a modified lateral decubitus position, with hips rotated 45 degrees (Fig. 30-1). In addition, the kidney rest is raised, and the operating table is adjusted or flexed to enhance the exposure between the 12th rib and the iliac crest.

Operative Exposure

For exposure to levels L1 and L2, an incision is begun over the 12th rib and is continued in an oblique direction from the lateral border of the quadratus lumborum muscle to the lateral border of the rectus abdominis muscle (see Fig. 30-1A). Exposures to L3 through L5 are created through a like incision but are placed approximately 2 cm below the costal margin. Underlying subcutaneous tissues, including fasciae of the external and internal oblique, transversus abdominis, and transversalis muscles, are then divided by electrocautery. The retroperitoneal space is entered from the lateral aspect.

To improve the exposure for a left-sided approach, an Omni retractor is attached to the right side of the table and positioned across the incision. Various wide- and right-angle retractors are applied to further open the field. The peritoneum and kidney are retracted medially and protected by a wide retractor, which also serves to shield the aorta. Several right-angle retractors are placed to reposition the psoas muscle posteriorly and the iliac vessels inferiorly. The diaphragm is moved superiorly with a single additional right-angle retractor.

The peritoneal sac is carefully separated from the anterior and lateral aspects of the abdominal wall, using blunt dissection. All precautions are taken not to penetrate the peritoneum. The peritoneum, with the kidney, is then reflected anteriorly and medially while being held by a retractor. With the use of blunt dissection, the peritoneum is detached from the posterior rectus sheath, and, working in a medial direction, from the sheath of the psoas muscle, Gerota's fascia being kept intact and retracted medially.

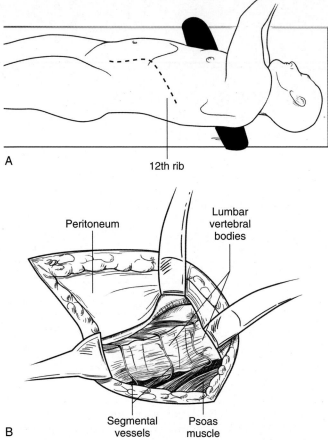

Figure 30-1. The anterior approach for lumbosacral exposure. **A,** For exposure to levels L1 and L2, an incision is begun over the 12th rib and continued in an oblique direction from the lateral border of the quadratus lumborum muscle to the lateral border of the rectus abdominis muscle. **B,** Using blunt dissection and starting at the "hills" (the discs), the psoas muscle is elevated off the lumbar vertebrae and then retracted posterolaterally. At the bottommost point of the "valleys" (the vertebral bodies) are the lumbar segmental vessels, which might need to be ligated. *(Redrawn from Saltzberg S, Nalbandian MM: Spine exposure for the vascular surgeon. In Moore WS [ed]: Vascular and Endovascular Surgery: A Comprehensive Review. Philadelphia: Saunders [Elsevier], 2006, pp 929–934.)*

The ureter can be expected to move anteriorly with the peritoneum, although care must be taken to ensure that it has not been inadvertently left behind. The iliac vessels are exposed and protected by using renal vein retractors. At this point, it is important to appreciate the "hills and valleys" of the lumbar spine. The "hills" represent the discs, and the "valleys" represent the lateral aspects of the vertebral bodies. By using blunt dissection and starting at the "hills" (the discs), the psoas muscle is elevated off the lumbar vertebrae and then retracted posterolaterally. At the bottommost point of the "valleys" (the vertebral bodies) are the lumbar segmental vessels, which might need to be ligated (see Fig. 30-1B).

Reapproximation of fasciae is performed in two layers. Subcutaneous tissue is closed with an absorbable suture, while the skin is closed with clips or subcuticular stitching.

During the exposure procedure, if the pleura has been violated, a chest tube should be appropriately placed and monitored.

Complications

Preoperative complications are similar to those described for the thoracolumbar approach to the spine. Care should be taken to avoid injury to the diaphragm, vessels, ureter, and sympathetic chain. Inadvertent entry into the pleural space can result in a pneumothorax or lung injury. Violation of the peritoneum can result in unrecognized visceral injuries. Preoperative and postoperative pulses should be obtained to evaluate for a missed arterial injury, thrombosis, or embolus.

LUMBOSACRAL SPINE EXPOSURE: ANTERIOR APPROACH

The retroperitoneal exposure of the lumbar spine benefits from the relatively avascular plane existing in the retroperitoneal space. Although this exposure can be performed through the flank with relative ease, flank exposure requires division of the external and internal oblique muscles as well as the transversus abdominis muscle. We utilize a modified anterior muscle-sparing retroperitoneal approach to expose the lumbar spine for all anterior spinal reconstructions (Fig. 30-2).

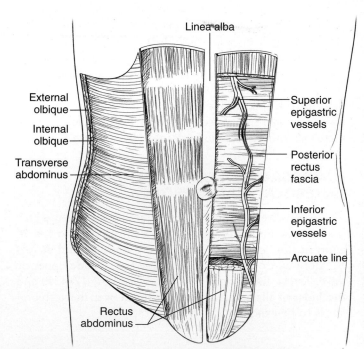

Figure 30-2. Muscles of the abdominal wall. Note the plane between the rectus muscle and the posterior rectus fascia. This plane is utilized to gain retroperitoneal access from a midline incision. The superior and inferior epigastric vessels provide circulation to the rectus muscle. These vessels enter the rectus muscle laterally.

Operative Exposure

An incision is made through the skin at the level of spine to be reconstructed (Fig. 30-3). The incision can be a transverse incision or a small vertical incision, depending on the level(s) being accessed (Fig. 30-4). The incision can be facilitated by anatomic landmarks. The L5-S1 disc space is usually directly beneath the midpoint between the umbilicus and the symphysis pubis. The L4-5 disc space is approximately 2 inches higher. In thin patients, the lumbosacral promontory can often be palpated. Alternatively, a guidewire or clamp placed lateral to the patient can be seen with a fluoroscope and can accurately position the incision over the correct disc space. Confirmation of the vertebral level that is to be approached by the planned incision can be especially important in cases of spondy-

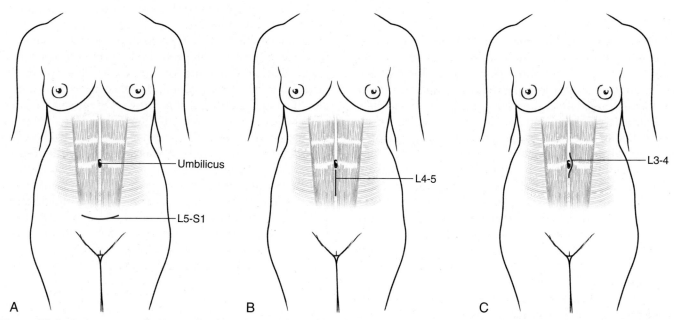

Figure 30-3. **A,** A transverse incision made above the symphysis pubis. This incision is best used for exposure of the L5-S1 disc space. **B,** A small vertical midline incision, which can be used for exposure of the L4-5 disc space. **C,** A small vertical incision extended above the umbilicus. This incision is utilized to expose the L3-4 disc space.

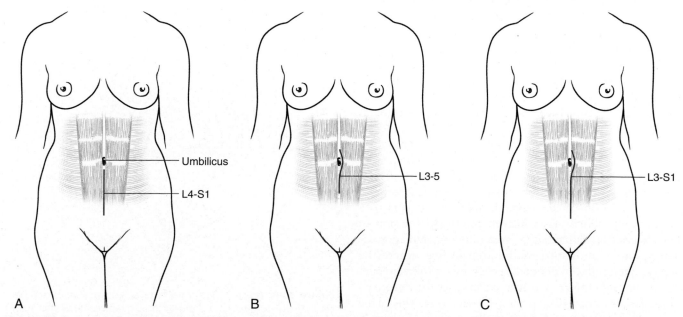

Figure 30-4. **A,** A small vertical midline incision used for multilevel exposures from L4 to S1. **B,** A vertical midline incision used for exposures of the L3-5 disc spaces. **C,** A vertical midline incision used for exposures of the L3-S1 disc spaces.

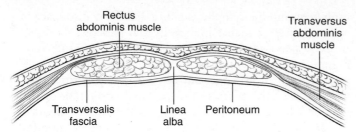

Figure 30-5. Axial view of the anterior abdominal wall. Note the relationships of the rectus abdominis muscle, linea alba, transversus abdominis muscle, and peritoneum.

lolisthesis, in which the lumbosacral slippage can present approach difficulties if the incision is too cranial. The skin incision is carried down through the subcutaneous tissue to the abdominal wall fascia. Prefascial planes are developed along the midline, superiorly and inferiorly, to allow a generous fascial incision in the anterior fascia of the rectus abdominis muscle. Placement of the skin incision to facilitate adequate fascial exposure of the proper spine levels is critical. On the basis of the lateral radiographs of the spine, the disc or discs to be exposed can be correlated to the iliac crest. Also, the angle of the disc, whether cephalad or caudad, can be estimated. Although a transverse incision can often be utilized with good cosmetic results, proper exposure of the spine is paramount. For this reason, a vertical midline incision can be used to provide better exposure.

A left paramedian incision is made in the anterior leaf of the fascia of the rectus abdominis muscle. The medial border of the left rectus abdominis muscle is then mobilized off the median raphe and is retracted laterally. Dissection deep to the left rectus abdominis muscle and superficial to the deep fascia exposes branches of the inferior epigastric vessels (see Fig. 30-2). The dissection, as it extends laterally, is performed in a manner such that the inferior epigastric vessels are maintained on the posterior aspect of the rectus abdominis muscle. As the dissection is extended laterally along this fascial plane using blunt dissection, the invagination of the abdominal wall fascia with the musculature and fascia of the flank becomes evident. This posterior fascia of the abdominal wall is then incised laterally, adjacent and just medial to this area of invagination (Fig. 30-5). The arcuate line is evident in the dissection at the L4-5/L5-S1 level. Often, the arcuate line is not a strict inferior border of this posterior fascia but rather a distinct transition of the fascia as it quickly tapers to a progressively thinner fascial layer, inferiorly. Incision of this posterior fascia laterally is generally initiated approximately 2 to 3 cm cranial to the arcuate line, where the fascia is thick and well defined. Incision with Metzenbaum scissors through this posterior fascia exposes the retroperitoneal fat adjacent to the peritoneal sac. Once this plane has been entered, the posterior fascia is incised further in a craniocaudal fashion, freeing it laterally. The range of

incision on the posterior fascia should mimic that on the rectus abdominis fascia and be generous enough to allow adequate exposure of the retroperitoneal space. Incision of this thin, often transparent fascia caudad to the identifiable arcuate line is performed to mobilize the peritoneal sac medially.

Once the retroperitoneal space is widely exposed, the retroperitoneal fat is bluntly dissected off of the peritoneal sac. The peritoneal sac is then retracted medially. This plane is followed down to the iliopsoas muscle and then medially to the left iliac artery and vein. The ureter will be adherent to the posterior peritoneal sac and will be swept medially. Once this level of exposure has been obtained, an Omni retractor system is used with four fixed renal blades to maintain exposure into the retroperitoneal space. During dissection of the L5-S1 disc space, the medial border of the left common iliac artery and vein is identified and mobilized (Fig. 30-6). Often, small venous branches are present along the medial border of the left common iliac artery and vein and must be divided between ligatures. Once the medial border of the vein is mobilized fully, the renal blade retractors are placed so that the vein and artery can be retracted laterally. On the anterior L5-S1 disc, the middle sacral artery and one to three middle sacral veins are often identified and should be divided between ligatures. Once this has been accomplished, blunt dissection allows the soft tissue on the anterior aspect of the spine to be swept off the disc to the patient's right. The

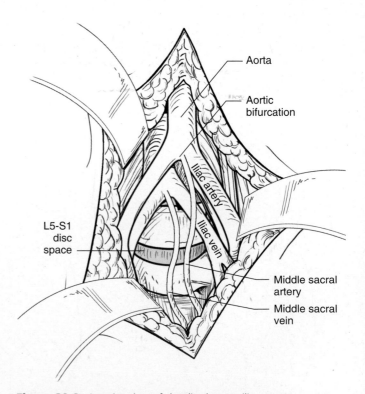

Figure 30-6. Anterior view of the distal aorta, iliac arteries, and iliac veins. The L5-S1 disc space is usually located between the bifurcation of the iliac vessels. Ligation of the middle sacral vessels is usually necessary to mobilize the iliac vessels and expose the L5-S1 disc space.

left iliac artery and vein are retracted to the patient's left. This will allow complete exposure of the L5-S1 disc. It is important not to excessively dissect the soft tissue off the sacrum caudally, because bleeding will result from perforators into the bone. If presacral bleeding does occur, compression and thrombotic agents such as thrombin and Gelfoam will generally be adequate to control this bleeding.

If the L4-5 disc is to be exposed, dissection along the lateral aspect of the left iliac vessels is performed. The left common iliac artery is mobilized and retracted medially. The left common iliac vein is identified deep to the artery. The iliolumbar vein is then sought. The iliolumbar vein (sometimes multiple veins are found) joins with the left common iliac vein from a lateral and posterior position at the level of the L5 vertebral body. Once the iliolumbar vein has been identified, it is doubly ligated and divided. The left common iliac vein is then mobilized toward the midline. We then identify the segmental artery and vein relative to the aorta and inferior vena cava at the level of the L4 vertebral body and divide these vessels between ligatures. The anterior soft tissues can be bluntly dissected off the L4-5 disc and retracted to the patient's right along with the left iliac artery and vein (Fig. 30-7). If exposure of lumbar discs superior to this level is required, the next segmental artery and vein are divided between ligatures so that the soft tissue anterior to the spine can be easily dissected off the spine to allow retraction of the aorta and vena cava to the patient's right. This action exposes the anterior disc at multiple levels. It is important to note that for male patients, we never use a cautery in the area of the iliac vessels, to avoid injury to the sympathetic nerves, possibly resulting in retrograde ejaculation. The use of metal clips for ligating small vessels or lymphatics is preferred to cautery.

On completion of the disc resection and reconstruction, abdominal wall closure consists of approximation of the anterior fascia of the rectus abdominis muscle. The laterally incised posterior fascia is not reapproximated, unless it was opened for a long distance (>4 cm). The superficial Scarpa's fascia is closed with a nonabsorbable suture, and the skin is closed in a subcuticular fashion. At the end of the anterior spinal reconstruction, examination of the pedal pulses is performed to confirm that there have been no changes during surgery to suggest arterial dissection, thrombosis, or embolus.

Clinical Application

A retrospective review of the medical records of 179 patients (between August 1999 and November 2002) who had anterior exposures for lumbar spine surgery performed by a fellowship-trained vascular surgeon for four fellowship-trained orthopedic spine surgeons was completed. Of the 179 patients, 105 patients had a modified anterior muscle-sparing retroperitoneal approach performed through a small transverse (5- to 8-cm) midabdominal incision. The remaining patients had standard thoracoabdominal or flank incisions. These approaches were chosen for the 74 patients before the anterior approach was widely adopted or because of the need to expose three or more levels for fusion. The data that were collected included diagnosis, age, gender, height, weight, levels exposed, smoking history, comorbid conditions, previous abdominopelvic procedures performed, vascular injuries, technique of vascular repair, and estimated blood loss related to vascular injury.

VASCULAR INJURIES

Inadvertent vascular injury is a potential complication of anterior retroperitoneal spine exposure. Although arterial injury is possible, it is less common than is injury to the iliac vein. Arterial injuries are repaired by using standard vascular techniques. Injury to the iliac vein can occur from direct laceration or through avulsion of a branch. Avulsion of the middle sacral veins, the iliolumbar vein, or other unnamed branches is the most common. Careful ligation of small venous branches precludes this in most circumstances. Double ligation of the iliolumbar vein should be performed. Should an iliac vein injury occur, we have found the following approach to be useful with minimal morbidity. First, immediate tamponade of the bleeding

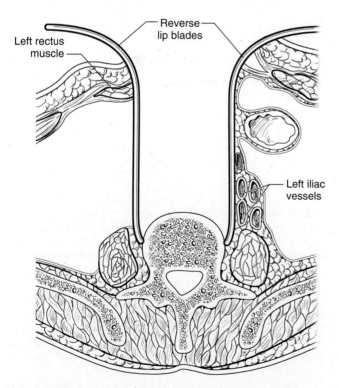

Figure 30-7. Axial view of the abdomen with placement of the reverse lip renal vein retractors. The iliac vessels, along with the ureter and peritoneum, are retracted to the patient's right for exposure of the disc space of L4-5 and higher.

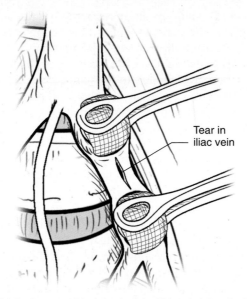

Figure 30-8. Sponge stick control of the iliac vein injury both proximal and distal to the tear. This maneuver can be helpful to control bleeding in order to repair the iliac vein. When necessary, the skin incision and exposure can be enlarged to facilitate this type of repair. Iliac vein injuries can usually be repaired primarily with 5-0 Prolene sutures.

vein is performed. This can be either with a finger or with a lap pad. Alternatively, compression of the iliac vein proximal and distal to the site of injury with sponge sticks will allow control of bleeding (Fig. 30-8). At this point, preparation for repair includes the following:

1. Adequate visualization of the vein might require increasing the size of the abdominal skin and fascial wound.
2. Anesthesia should be instructed to obtain a rapid infusion if blood loss becomes uncontrolled. Blood products should be brought to the room.
3. In our experience, as many as three experienced surgeons might be necessary for repair. One surgeon controls hemorrhage with sponge sticks, with compression of the vein proximal and distal to the injury or ultimately through vessel loop control of the iliac veins. A second surgeon performs suction of any blood. The third surgeon performs a lateral venorraphy repair of the vein. Once anesthesia has adequate intravenous access to provide a high volume of fluids and blood, the iliac vein is controlled proximally and distally with sponge sticks or with vessel loops, and then the laceration is visualized within the iliac vein. The lacerated vein is then repaired, restoring hemostasis. For very small bleeding points, thrombin-soaked Gelfoam may be used over the bleeding point. Once this has been completed, any further manipulation of the vein is avoided.
4. Postoperatively, sequential pneumatic compression devices are used in the lower extremities. We obtain a venous duplex scan 24 hours after surgery to ensure that the iliac vein has not thrombosed. Anticoagulation

drugs are not used routinely unless a deep vein thrombosis is diagnosed. If the patient has a deep vein thrombosis and is not thought to be a candidate for anticoagulation, an inferior vena cava filter should be placed to protect against a pulmonary embolism.

RESULTS

A total of 105 patients was identified who underwent this modified anterior muscle-sparing retroperitoneal approach to the lumbar spine. There were 48 males and 57 females. The average height was 5′ 7″ (range: 4′ 11″ to 6′ 2″), and the average weight was 174.9 pounds (range: 112 to 270 pounds). There were 33 smokers. The average age was 41 years. There were 15 (14%) isolated exposures of L4-5 and 71 (68%) isolated exposures of L5-S1. Nineteen (18%) patients had both L4-5 and L5-S1 exposed. Twenty-one patients had a total of 40 previous abdominopelvic surgeries (Table 30-1). Four (3.8%) vascular injuries occurred that required repair. There were two (50%) vascular injuries during L4-5/L5-S1 exposures, one (25%) during an L4-5 level exposure, and one (25%) during an L5-S1 level exposure (Table 30-2). Of the four vascular injuries, three were repaired with lateral venorraphy, and one was controlled with pressure and application of a hemostatic agent. The average estimated blood loss for all vascular injuries was 225 mL (range: 150 to 300 mL). No late vascular sequelae of the repairs were noted, such as swelling of the leg, deep vein thrombosis, or ischemia.

SUMMARY

In our retrospective review of vascular complications utilizing this modified anterior muscle-sparing retroperitoneal approach to expose the lumbar spine, we observed a vascular complication rate of 3.8%. All vascular injuries were promptly repaired, and no adverse outcomes were identified postoperatively in these patients. We believe that this exposure allows the spine surgeon complete visu-

TABLE 30-1. Previous Abdominopelvic Surgeries in a Series of 105 Patients Who Underwent the Modified Anterior Muscle-Sparing Retroperitoneal Approach to the Lumbar Spine

Surgery	Previous Surgeries (N = 40)	Percentage
Caesarean section	16	15
Small bowel resection	1	1
Hysterectomy	4	4
Cholecystectomy	5	5
Appendectomy	3	3
Pelvic laparoscopy	3	3
Abdominal hernia	2	2
Tubal ligations	3	3
Multiple abdominal surgeries	3	3

TABLE 30-2. Vascular Injuries Occurring in a Series of 105 Patients Who Underwent the Modified Anterior Muscle-Sparing Retroperitoneal Approach to the Lumbar Spine

Age/Sex	Tobacco	Height/Weight	Level	Complication	Estimated Blood Loss/Repair
45/female	Yes	5' 3"/165 lb	L4-5	Traction tear of branch of common iliac vein	300 mL/venorraphy
48/male	No	5' 5"/200 lb	L5-S1	Tear of small branch of common iliac vein	150 mL/venorraphy
49/female	No	5' 6"/160 lb	L4-5/L5-S1	Tear of branch of common iliac vein	150 mL/hemostatic agent/pressure
34/female	No	5' 4"/220 lb	L4-L5/L5-S1	Laceration of common iliac vein	300 mL/venorraphy

alization of the anterior lower lumbar disc spaces for reconstruction or arthroplasty. The direct anterior exposure to the lumbar spine facilitates proper positioning of either interbody grafts or the newer prosthetic disc replacements. Furthermore, the direct anterior working pathway afforded by the midline approach is desirable for the newer implant instrumentation that is used for proper positioning of interbody grafts. By avoiding division of the muscles of the abdominal wall, abdominal closure is facilitated, bleeding is decreased, postoperative pain appears to be decreased, and vascular complications are low. Moreover, the anterior spine exposure is more than adequate. Finally, the skin incision is cosmetically better than with a large flank, midline, or paramedian abdominal wall incision.

PEARLS & PITFALLS

- During exposure of the L4-5 level, it is almost always necessary to ligate the iliolumbar vein to avoid avulsion. The proximal side of the iliolumbar vein is best ligated with silk sutures to avoid inadvertent avulsion of a metal clip during retraction of the iliac vein.
- Isolated exposures of L5-S1 can be performed by using a right-sided retroperitoneal approach. This will allow the left retroperitoneal plane to remain undisturbed in case a revision is required or an adjacent level breaks down, requiring a second anterior approach.
- Anterior approaches in patients with spondylolisthesis can often be facilitated by placing a roll underneath the patient's lower lumbar spine. This is especially helpful in patients with spondylolisthesis at L5-S1.
- During mobilization of the peritoneum, it is important not to dissect the ureter from the peritoneum. This can cause an ischemic stricture if the blood supply to the ureter becomes compromised. It is best to keep the ureter intact with the peritoneum and to move them together for optimal exposure.
- Always confirm the spine level to be operated on by checking an intraoperative radiograph with needle localization.
- Intraoperative venous injuries are best treated initially with topical pressure. Utilizing topical agents and direct pressure will often eliminate the need for a vascular repair in small injuries to the vein. Larger injuries to the iliac vein should be treated with suture repair. It is important to utilize cell-saver during this portion of the

surgery as well as having blood products available in the operating room, as venous blood loss can be substantial even in the best of circumstances.
- Always confirm that preoperative and postoperative pulses have remained the same.

CONCLUSIONS

The role of the vascular surgeon has undergone substantial evolution. Vascular surgeons have become needed specialists during procedures that were formerly performed by orthopedic or other types of surgeons. As a result, vascular surgeons can find themselves inadequately trained in regard to orthopedic spine procedures. That having been said, although spine access surgery might be unfamiliar to trained vascular surgeons, their training and expertise in thoracoabdominal and retroperitoneal aortic surgery, also prepare them for the techniques of anterior spine exposure. A most frequent complication, hemorrhage from iliac artery and vein injuries, is typically managed by vascular surgeons. It stands to reason that vascular surgeons should be proactive and prepared in the management of spine patients. It is by applying a team perspective to spine surgery that vascular surgeons can best contribute to reducing the morbidity and mortality of spine procedures.

SUGGESTED READINGS

Baker JK, Reardon PR, Reardon MJ, Heggeness MH: Vascular injury in anterior lumbar surgery. Spine 1993;18:2227–2230.
Some of the potential vascular complications involved in anterior lumbar surgery are discussed.

Brau SA: Mini-open approach to the spine for anterior lumbar interbody fusion: Description of the procedure, results and complications. Spine J 2002;2:216–223.
This is an excellent summary of a mini-approach to the lumbar spine. The article outlines the technique and results as well as the potential complications.

Cavallieri S, Riou B, Roche S, et al: Intraoperative autologous transfusion in emergency surgery for spine trauma. J Trauma 1994;36:639–643.
The use of cell-saver therapy during emergency spine surgery is described.

Flynn JC, Hoque MA: Anterior fusion of the lumbar spine: End-result study with long-term follow-up. J Bone Joint Surg Am 1979;61:1143–1150.
A long-term follow-up (up to 15 years) of 50 patients who underwent anterior lumbar spine fusion with autogenous fibular and iliac crest grafts. It

reveals a high nonunion percentage (44%) and longer healing time for nonunion patients with fibular grafts than patients with iliac crest grafts.

Franzini M, Altana P, Annessi V, Lodini V: Iatrogenic vascular injuries following lumbar disc surgery. J Cardiovasc Surg 1987;28:727–730.

This article describes an iatrogenic injury during a posterior discectomy. The vascular injury was treated successfully.

Fraser RD: A wide muscle-splitting approach to the lumbosacral spine. J Bone Joint Surg Br 1982;64:44–46.

A muscle-splitting approach to gain access to lumbosacral spine by the retroperitoneal route is described. It carries specific surgical and tissue advantages over approaches that employ dividing the rectus muscle.

Harmon PH: Anterior extraperitoneal lumbar disc excision and vertebral body fusion. Clin Orthop Relat Res 1960;18:169–198.

A two-part article with extensive discussion. The first part is a literature review of intervertebral disc surgery and a presentation and analysis of the author's own operative experience (250 patients). The second part describes the author's operative "uniform" technique using an extraperitoneal approach with special modifications and comment to variations of the left common iliac vein and instrument.

Harmon PH: A simplified surgical technique for anterior lumbar diskectomy and fusion; Avoidance of complications; anatomy of the retroperitoneal veins. Clin Orthop Relat Res 1964;37:130–144.

This article describes a midrectus anterior surgical access technique and anterior discectomy using surgical modifications that reduce surgical length and estimated blood loss. Anatomic surgical safeguards that avoid retroperitoneal venous complications are emphasized.

Ito H, Tsuchiya V, Asami G, et al: A new radical operation for Pott's Disease. J Bone Joint Surg 1934;16:499–515.

This is a historical article describing the first "radical" surgical management technique for Pott's disease. Reasons for the difficulties in devising an effective surgery are described. It also describes a new anterior surgical approach with a pararectal incision and retraction of peritoneum in order to access the retroperitoneum. The authors describe their experience with 10 different patients.

Oskouian R, Johnson P: Vascular complications in anterior thoracolumbar spinal reconstruction. J Neurosurg 2002;96(1, suppl):1–5.

The vascular complications from thoracic spine approaches are described. There is very little discussion regarding lumbar spine approaches and complications.

Rajaraman V, Vingan R, Roth P, et al: Visceral and vascular complications resulting from anterior lumbar interbody fusion. J Neurosurg 1999;19(1, suppl):60–64.

The potential complications resulting from an anterior lumbar interbody fusion are described.

Raugstad TS, Harbo K, Hogberg A, Skeie S: Anterior interbody fusion of the lumbar spine. Acta Orthop Scand 1982;53:561–565.

The article reports on 47 patients with either spondylolisthesis or disc degeneration who received anterior interbody fusion of the lumbar spine (the majority were one-level fusions) for incapacitating low-back pain. Although they found a nonunion of 20%, the authors believe that the technique provides a generally positive outcome with a need for careful patient selection.

Saltzberg S, Nalbandian MM: Spine exposure for the vascular surgeon. In Moore WS (ed): Vascular and Endovascular Surgery: A Comprehensive Review. Philadelphia: Saunders (Elsevier), 2006, pp 929–934.

This chapter provides an excellent summary of the technique for the anterior, lateral, and thoracolumbar approaches to the spine. The chapter also describes the complications associated with the approach.

Tsai YD, Yu PC, Lee TC, et al: Superior rectal artery injury following lumbar disc surgery. J Neurosurg 2001;95(1, suppl):108–110.

This article describes the case of a patient who had a posterior discectomy and developed a rectal artery injury during the discectomy. This injury was treated successfully.

Watkins R: Anterior lumbar interbody fusion surgical complications. Clin Orthop Relat Res 1992;284:47–53.

This is a very good review article describing the operative technique. The author also discusses patient selection as well as the complications associated with the anterior lumbar fusion.

CHAPTER 31

Thoracic Exposures for Spinal Deformity Surgery

BERNARD K. CRAWFORD *and* JEFFREY A. MORGAN

OVERVIEW

Exposure of the anterior thoracic spine and the thoraco-lumbar spine is utilized in the corrective surgery performed for many spinal deformities as well as for more limited intervention on localized neoplastic, structural deformities and infectious diseases that affect the stability and function of the vertebral column and the spinal cord. This chapter will review the various approaches in use today that allow intervention on the anterior spine from the cervicothoracic to the thoracolumbar areas.

Although classic thoracotomy and thoracolumbar ap-proaches are still used in some centers, advances in tech-nology over the past 2 decades have significantly affected the surgeon's ability to see and manipulate intrathoracic structures with less invasive and therefore less morbid interventions. Particularly the development of fiber-optic thoracoscopes and high-definition digital imaging com-bined with sophisticated anesthetic management have enabled the thoracic and spine surgeon to accomplish complex surgical interventions with a significant reduction in patient morbidity.

The thoracic surgeon is a consultant for the patient. His role is to provide the necessary exposure of the spine as needed to allow the orthopedic surgeon to safely and effec-tively intervene with the resection of the intervertebral discs, manipulation, and if necessary instrumentation of the vertebral bodies of the spine. Simply put, the thoracic surgeon moves everything out of the way to allow ma-nipulation of the spine. He ensures that no structures are inadvertently injured during the surgical intervention. Ultimately, the thoracic surgeon returns the structures of the thorax to their normal anatomic positions on comple-tion of the corrective surgery.

CLASSIFICATION

Anterior Spine Exposure Techniques

There are three basic techniques to expose the anterior spine. An open technique involves an incision in the skin taken down to the chest wall, where an intercostal incision or sternotomy is performed to access the pleural cavity. The incision with this open approach can be extensive, and the spreading of the ribs must be adequate to allow visu-alization and manipulation of the spine. This approach allows the surgeon to work with direct visualization of the spine with truly hands-on capability with regard to resec-tion and manipulation of the spinal elements. The disad-vantage is for the patient, as this is the most painful technique. This method is associated with the greatest morbidity because of the extensive tissue damage to the musculoskeletal chest wall.

At the other end of the spectrum is the "closed" tech-nique, in which a thoracoscope is inserted through a small intercostal incision. The underlying lung is collapsed as selective ventilation of the opposite lung is accomplished by utilizing a double-lumen or bronchial blocking endo-tracheal tube, thereby allowing visualization of the intra-thoracic structures. Through additional small intercostal incisions, instruments are inserted into the pleural space to perform the surgery. The surgeons who are involved must be adept at performing the operation while viewing the spine on the monitor in two dimensions rather than directly. Three-dimensional robotic surgical intervention is not yet widely available. The loss of three-dimensional presentations can be disadvantageous for some surgeons. However, the experienced surgeon can accomplish ante-rior release maneuvers, discectomies, and even instru-mentation of the anterior spine thoracoscopically. The advantage of this technique is for the patient, as the peri-operative pain is diminished because there is essentially no rib spreading and much less in the way of musculoskeletal trauma to the chest wall. The use of the thoracoscope has become routine in the hands of most thoracic surgeons, and selective lung ventilation is also commonly utilized by the experienced anesthesiologist.

The third method of anterior spine surgical interven-tion developed by Errico and the author is the minithora-cotomy with video assistance. In this technique, a limited, nearly vertical incision in the skin, usually 3 inches in length, is positioned over the level of operative intent in approximately the posterior axillary line. The incision is taken down to the chest wall, and mobilization of the muscular layer overlying the ribs allows movement of the skin and soft-tissue incision in a cephalad or caudad direction to move one or two interspaces up or down the chest wall. The movement of the incision allows two or three short segments of ribs, for example, the third, fifth, and seventh rib segments (for bone grafting), to be excised and the pleural space to be accessed through the bed of each resected rib. The thoracoscope is inserted through an anterior incision, providing excellent optics and light while the operating surgeon is also able to look directly onto the spine through the beds of the resected ribs without significant rib spreading. The advantage of this technique is to both the operating surgeon, whose depth of field is restored for perhaps more accurate intervention, and to the patient, who has minimal scar and musculoskeletal damage.

Techniques of Exposure

Cervicothoracic Exposures

Exposure of the anterior spine from C7 to T3 is only occasionally necessary in cases of spinal deformity. Diseased vertebral bodies in this area are more likely to be involved with a neoplastic, infectious, or degenerative process. When exposure of this area of the spine is necessary, it is usually accomplished by a lateral cervical incision taken to the midline at the top of the manubrium with the addition of an upper sternal incision taken to the second or third intercostal space as needed.

The patient is positioned in the supine position. General anesthesia and single-lumen endotracheal intubation are utilized. Extension of the neck and caudal traction on the arms can be helpful, depending on the exposure needed. Dissection through the cervical incision is taken down medial to the sternocleidomastoid muscle. The omohyoid and sternohyoid muscles are divided, reflecting the trachea and esophagus medially and the carotid sheath and internal jugular vein laterally. The plane of the anterior vertebral bodies is identified. In entering the mediastinum along the anterior longitudinal ligament in the prevertebral plane, great care is taken not to injure the thoracic duct as it leaves the prevertebral plane and courses to the left subclavian vein. Whether approaching from the left or right side of the neck, the recurrent laryngeal nerves must be considered. From the right side, a traction injury to the nerve can occur in retracting the innominate artery in a caudal direction. From a left-sided approach, the recurrent nerve is in the tracheoesophageal groove and is less likely to be injured during dissection but can be damaged by pressure from a retractor blade. The parietal pleura overlying the lateral aspects of the vertebral bodies is gently reflected bluntly with a peanut sponge, and deep-bladed retractors are then carefully placed to maintain appropriate exposure on the anterior aspects of the vertebral bodies.

The midline incision in the manubrium and upper sternal body with retraction and separation of the sternal tables does allow an appropriate angle of incidence for the instruments and direct visualization of the vertebral bodies, allowing resection, debridement, and reconstruction of T1 and T2. To intervene at the level of the second and third thoracic vertebral bodies, the great vessels must be mobilized and carefully retracted. In elderly patients with atherosclerotic disease in the great vessels, embolic complications can occur, and manipulation of these arteries is to be avoided whenever possible in this population.

On completion of the spinal intervention, a drain is usually not necessary. However, if the pleural space has been entered or if there is any question of bleeding or lymphatic drainage in the area of operative exposure, a Jackson-Pratt or similar suction drain should be left in the base of the wound until minimal daily volumes are noted. A sternal incision is reapproximated with wire in standard fashion, while closure of the soft tissues is accomplished with absorbable suture material in anatomic layers.

Thoracic Anterior Spine Exposures

The anterior spine from T2 to T12 can be exposed for intervention on the spine by utilizing a transpleural approach. For a short segment of spinal intervention, an extrapleural approach can also be accomplished, but there is no significant advantage to this approach over the intrapleural exposure.

Most cases of scoliosis involving the thoracic spine are convex to the right in the midthoracic region. The entire length of the spine is generally better seen from the right chest, owing to the presence of the thoracic aorta in the left chest, which overlies the anterior and lateral aspects of the spine in the midthoracic region. This convexity also brings the area of operative intent closer to the surgeon when the approach is from a posterolateral thoracotomy incision.

The patient is placed under general anesthesia and turned to the lateral decubitus position with appropriate care taken to protect areas of bony prominence and the axillary vessels. Double-lumen endotracheal tubes or single-lumen endotracheal tubes with bronchial blocking balloon catheters are of benefit in providing exposure and are essential if a thoracoscopic technique is to be utilized.

Open Technique

Upper Thoracic Spine Exposures

A single thoracotomy incision is utilized for the classic open technique. The patient is positioned in the lateral decubitus posterolateral thoracotomy position. The incision is placed to provide exposure of the entire area of intervention. To expose a single vertebral body in the upper spine, the patient is rotated slightly more to the prone position, and a vertical incision midway between the spinous processes and the medial edge of the scapula is performed. The incision is taken to the chest wall with division of the trapezius and rhomboid muscles. Palpation allows accurate counting of the ribs, and the rib above the vertebral body or disc to be resected is removed in a subperiosteal fashion. The rib is saved for grafting as needed. A small Finochetto retractor is utilized. The parietal pleura is incised and reflected, and the segmental vessels are taken if necessary to provide adequate exposure or if instrumentation is to be utilized. Radiographic confirmation at this level (T2-4) is difficult, owing to patient positioning, but direct visualization is confirmatory.

On completion of the intervention on the spine, hemostasis is assured, the parietal pleura is closed, and a thoracostomy drain is placed in the paravertebral groove and brought out through the skin in the posterior axillary line in the sixth intercostal space. There might be no need for paracostal sutures if there has not been significant spreading of the intercostal space. Intercostal muscles above and below the resected rib are closed with running absorbable suture material, as are the muscular layers of the chest wall, subcutaneous tissue, and skin.

Midthoracic Spine Exposures

A classic posterolateral thoracotomy incision is utilized for exposure of the midthoracic spine for intervention on three to seven spinal segments. This incision begins vertically midway between the spinous processes and the medial border of the scapula, is extended caudally and curves two fingerbreadths around the inferior tip of the scapula, and extends anteriorly into the inframammary groove. The incision is taken down to the chest wall with division of the underlying trapezius, latissimus dorsi, rhomboid, and serratus anterior muscles as needed. This incision allows entry into the chest through the fourth, fifth, sixth, or seventh interspace. A rib can be resected for improved exposure or for use as bone-grafting material. Significant spreading of the interspace with a Finochetto retractor can provide exposure from one or two levels below the resected rib to the lower thoracic spine. Posterior segmental resection of the rib above (shingling) can improve the angle of incidence for intervention on the upper vertebral body without a significant increase in morbidity. The lung is retracted with a malleable retractor or is simply reflected passively if selective ventilation of the opposite lung is utilized. The parietal pleura is incised over the lateral aspect of the vertebral bodies and bluntly reflected anteriorly to beyond the anterior longitudinal ligament and posteriorly to the rib heads. Care is taken not to injure the azygos vein and thoracic duct. The segmental vessels are ligated, divided, and reflected off the vertebral bodies with mobilization of the azygos vein if necessary for exposure

of the discs or vertebral bodies or for the placement of instrumentation.

On completion of the spinal intervention, hemostasis is assured. The pleura is closed over the area of operation if possible, but it is not essential to do so. The pleural cavity is irrigated and drained with a tube thoracostomy placed in the paravertebral groove adjacent to the area of operative intent and brought out through the skin in the posterior axillary line in the eighth intercostal space.

Paracostal ligatures are needed for reapproximation of the large intercostal incision. In adults, the ribs might be broad enough to allow drilling of the lower ribs and passage of the paracostal ligature through the lower rib, thereby avoiding entrapment of the intercostal nerve on the inferior margin. This maneuver is of significant benefit in postoperative pain management. The muscular layers of the chest wall are closed anatomically with running absorbable suture material, as are the subcutaneous tissues and skin.

Lower Thoracic Spine Exposures

Open exposure of the lower thoracic spine is initiated in a fashion similar to that noted above with anesthetic induction and positioning in the lateral decubitus position. A single-lumen endotracheal tube can be used if the area of the spine to be exposed is at T9 or below or if intrapleural retraction of the lung is to be used.

Because we are below the level of the scapula, the open posterolateral thoracotomy incision is made directly over the interspace to be entered with division of the skin, soft tissues, latissimus dorsi muscle, and deep fascia. The interspace that is entered should be two levels above the area of operative intent. Owing to the caudal angulations of the ribs, this approach will put the surgeon directly over the objective. Additional spreading of the retractor and lengthening of the incision will provide additional exposure.

The lung is reflected, and, if necessary, a malleable retractor can be employed to maintain its position. The parietal pleura is incised over the length of spine to be manipulated, and the segmental vessels are divided if necessary. The parietal pleura is reflected anteriorly to beyond the anterior longitudinal ligament and posteriorly to the rib heads. On completion of the spinal procedure, the drainage and closure are as described previously.

Thoracolumbar Spine Exposures

When exposure of the lower thoracic as well as lumbar spine is required, an intercostal, flank, and diaphragmatic incision is utilized (see Fig. 31-1). Exposure of the thoracolumbar spine is generally best accomplished by resection of the 10th rib and reflection of the diaphragm to expose the retroperitoneal plane.

General anesthesia and single-lumen intubation are utilized. Lateral decubitus positioning with the patient slightly supinated to allow exposure of the anterolateral abdominal wall is accomplished. The skin incision for the full open technique is performed directly over the 10th rib and anteriorly curved inferiorly lateral to the rectus sheath. The 10th rib is excised in a subperiosteal fashion. The pleural space is entered with extension of the incision to the posterior angle of the resected 10th rib. The retroperitoneal plane can be identified beneath the anterior tip of the 10th rib. The fatty tissues of the retroperitoneum are then reflected away from the undersurface of the diaphragm. The diaphragm is then incised in a circumferential manner, leaving a 2-cm margin peripherally for later repair.

Retroperitoneal fat is then reflected off the quadratus and psoas muscles. The fascia overlying the muscles should not be disturbed. The peritoneum is reflected off the underside of the lateral and anterior abdominal wall musculature to allow transfascial extension of the skin incision and retraction of peritoneal as well as retroperitoneal structures off the lumbar vertebral bodies.

To expose the lumbar discs and vertebral bodies, the psoas muscle must be reflected, and the segmental vertebral arteries and veins must be ligated and transected. This is best accomplished by beginning at the T12-L1 level and working in a caudad direction, identifying the discs, reflecting the muscle, and ligating the segmental vessels over each body sequentially. The use of an Omni retractor is of great benefit in the maintenance of exposure in this circumstance.

On completion of the spinal corrective procedure, care is taken to ensure that there is no hemorrhage or lymphatic leakage. Repair of the diaphragm is performed in two layers of nonabsorbable suture material. The pleural cavity is drained in a routine fashion, and the flank and chest wall incision is closed with absorbable suture material in anatomic layers.

Closed Thoracoscopic Technique

Exposure of the thoracic vertebral column from T2 to T12 can be accomplished by utilizing thoracoscopic techniques. Preoperative evaluation and management are similar to what is performed for any exposure procedure. Anesthetic management for a thoracoscopic approach requires the use of either a double-lumen endotracheal tube or a bronchial blocking balloon through a single-lumen tube to allow single lung ventilation.

After induction of general anesthesia, the patient is positioned in the lateral decubitus position with the right side or side of operative intent upward. Isolation of the lung ventilation is accomplished, and an initial incision in the anterior axillary line at the fifth intercostal space, about 1 inch in length, is used. A segment of rib can be resected through this incision for bone grafting. The pleural space is entered by using sharp and blunt dissection, and a thoracoscope is inserted. The authors prefer the 10-mm, 30-degree scope, as it provides excellent optics and versatility. Carbon dioxide insufflations can be utilized to improve exposure.

Thoracoscopic evaluation of the pleural space reveals the spinal deformity as well as any adhesions that require pneumonolysis for exposure of the spine. Placement of additional thoracoports for instruments and retraction is dictated by the specific intervention. Generally, four to six ports are necessary to accomplish multiple discectomies. Additional ports located more posteriorly will be necessary if instrumentation is to be utilized.

It is usually beneficial for exposure of the discs to divide the segmental vessels overlying the vertebral bodies and then to reflect the soft tissues away from the anterolateral aspect of the spine. The exposure obtained is generally excellent, and the optics display the spine well for the intervention of an experienced orthopedic surgeon. The present videoscopic systems that are in general use provide only two-dimensional viewing of the operative area, and herein lies the difficulty for the surgeon who is inexperienced in thoracoscopic techniques.

The primary benefit provided by this technique is decreased perioperative pain for the patient. The numerous incisions that are necessary for the performance of the intervention might or might not be more cosmetically appealing.

Mini Open Video-Assisted Technique

This method of exposure of the thoracic spine has been developed over the past 10 years and is essentially a combination of a limited thoracotomy incision and a single port site for a thoracoscope that is ultimately used as the chest tube drainage incision.

Preparation of the patient for surgery is similar to that which is necessary for any spine intervention. General anesthesia is induced, and a selective ventilation endotracheal intubation is carried out if possible. It is of assistance but not essential to isolate the ventilation to the nonoperated pleural cavity.

The patient is positioned in the lateral decubitus position, and a posterior thoracotomy incision is performed, usually about 3 inches in length in an adult patient. The incision is generally slightly medial and inferior to the tip of the scapula and nearly vertical in orientation. The incision is taken down to the chest wall with division of the underlying latissimus dorsi muscle and deep fascial layer. The soft tissues overlying the ribs are then bluntly mobilized extensively, allowing movement of the skin incision, soft tissue, and muscle up and down the chest wall. This mobility allows exposure of five or more ribs along the posterior chest wall. By resecting segments of the fourth, sixth, and eighth ribs, for example, three separate entries through the beds of the resected ribs into the pleural space can be accessed. The rib segments resected are usually 4 or 5 cm in length and are set aside for use as bone graft. A small rib retractor is moved from one interspace to the next as work progresses. The surgeon can sequentially intervene from the 5th thoracic vertebral body to the 9th or 10th vertebral body with direct visualization of each area as well as an enhanced view of the anterior aspect of each dissection by reference to the thoracoscopic image.

On completion of the surgical intervention on the spine, the intercostal incisions might not require paracostal ligatures, depending on how much spreading of the ribs took place. The periosteum of the resected ribs and intercostal muscles should be reapproximated, and the remaining closure of the soft tissues of the chest wall is performed in routine fashion.

Mini Open Thoracolumbar Exposure

Exposure of the lower thoracic and lumbar spine requires an extensive intervention. In an attempt to create a more cosmetic final result for the patient, Dr. Joseph Dryer proposed a new orientation for the skin incision. A nearly vertical incision in the midaxillary line is performed, beginning just above the ninth rib and extending caudally as necessary for the exposure of the lowest lumbar segment to be operated. The incision is taken down through the latissimus muscle and deep fascia to the chest wall. The soft tissues are mobilized extensively to expose the 10th rib from the posterior angle to its anterior tip. The 10th rib is then resected in standard fashion. The remaining dissection and exposure of the spine are accomplished in standard fashion. Care should be taken not to transect the 10th intercostal nerve, as this can result in partial paresis of the flank and rectus muscles postoperatively with resultant asymmetry of the anterior abdominal wall.

ROLE OF THE THORACIC SURGEON IN ANTERIOR SPINE SURGERY

The decision to operate on a patient to correct a spinal deformity or to decompress the spinal cord by the resection of a protruding disc or cancerous vertebral body is made by the orthopedic surgeon or neurosurgeon. The thoracic surgeon as a consultant is of value as a facilitator in the preoperative, intraoperative, and postoperative phases.

Patients with severe spinal deformities of scoliosis or kyphosis can demonstrate impairment of pulmonary function. Additionally, older patients might have acquired pulmonary compromise or cardiac conditions due to smoking or other cardiopulmonary disease processes. The preoperative evaluation of these conditions can significantly affect the operative approach. These conditions clearly affect the risk to the patient and therefore must be noted, evaluated, and discussed preoperatively. Ideally, all patients should be seen preoperatively by the consulting thoracic surgeon and evaluated with an understanding of the orthopedic intervention to be performed. This interaction will allow proper counseling of the patient as well as

ensuring that the best approach is utilized for the intended procedure.

Invariably, radiographs, and at times a magnetic resonance image, of the spine will have been performed, as these studies dictate the area of deformity and need for intervention. In addition, routine tests that are of value in the preoperative appraisal include chest radiograph, computed tomography scan of the involved area (neck, chest, and abdomen), pulmonary function tests, and, when indicated, cardiac stress testing. In addition to other routine presurgical testing, other evaluations by a pediatrician, neurologist, endocrinologist, oncologist, cardiologist, and other specialists might be indicated by concomitant medical conditions. The majority of patients who undergo corrective surgery for a spinal deformity are young and otherwise healthy, but they are by definition not normal. Appropriate evaluation will avert misadventure.

Intraoperative involvement by the thoracic surgeon is primarily to provide the necessary exposure for the intervention. The type of exposure is dictated not only by the orthopedic procedure to be accomplished, but also by the needs of the orthopedic surgeon. Some surgeons will prefer the open technique, while others will utilize some degree of minimally invasive technology. During the performance of the orthopedic portions of an operation, the thoracic surgeon assists by ensuring the safety of vital structures.

Postoperatively, the patient is monitored in a routine fashion, with particular attention to cardiac stability and respiratory function. Atelectasis from mucous plugging and the associated hypoxia and arrhythmias are best treated by aggressive pulmonary toilet. Chest physical therapy and timely removal of chest drainage tubes are essential. Bronchoscopy might occasionally be indicated to remove secretions and to reexpand atelectatic lung.

PEARLS & PITFALLS

- In performing reoperative anterior spine surgery, it is important to intervene from the same side as the previous encounter. Although the adhesions will necessitate additional time to create the required exposure, the approach is dictated by the significant risk of paraplegia if a contralateral approach is used. Ligation of bilateral segmental vessels can result in significant ischemia to the spinal cord with resultant irreversible neurologic dysfunction.
- Surgical techniques to minimize perioperative pain result in fewer postoperative complications. Minimizing trauma and attention to safeguarding against nerve compression and entrapment are paramount.
- In children with small airways and main stem bronchi, the use of double-lumen endotracheal tubes is to be avoided if possible. Because these selective ventilation tubes are larger and more irritating to the bronchi, postoperative inflammation occurs. Postoperative inflammation and swelling result in increased morbidity owing to retained secretions and atelectasis.

■ Injury to the thoracic duct should be considered with every thoracic spinal intervention. Any pooling of lymphatic fluid at the end of the surgical procedure necessitates careful inspection and closure of the leak. If significant lymph is evident without a clear source, passage of a nasogastric tube and instillation of cream into the stomach should promptly demonstrate the area of damage to the thoracic duct. Repair of the duct or ligation of the duct at the level of the diaphragm should be performed.

■ Neurologic dysfunction is usually seen in reoperations when segmental vessels have already been ligated.
■ Chylothorax can occur from injury to the thoracic duct.
■ Persistent air leaks and/or bronchopleural fistulae can occur if lung parenchyma has been injured.
■ Atelectasis can occur from mucous plugging with associated hypoxia.
■ Arrhythmias can occur, most commonly atrial fibrillation secondary to atelectasis.

Illustrative Case Presentation

CASE 1. A 15-Year-Old Female with Progressive Thoracic Scoliosis Treated by Selective Anterior Thoracoscopic Fusion with Instrumentation*

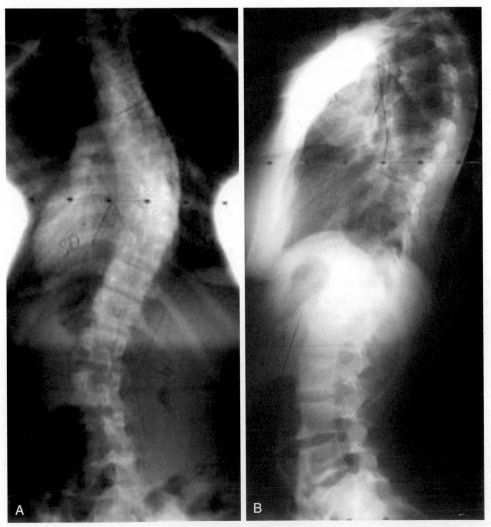

Figure 31-1. A and **B,** Preoperative posteroanterior and lateral radiographs.

Case courtesy of Baron S. Lonner, MD.

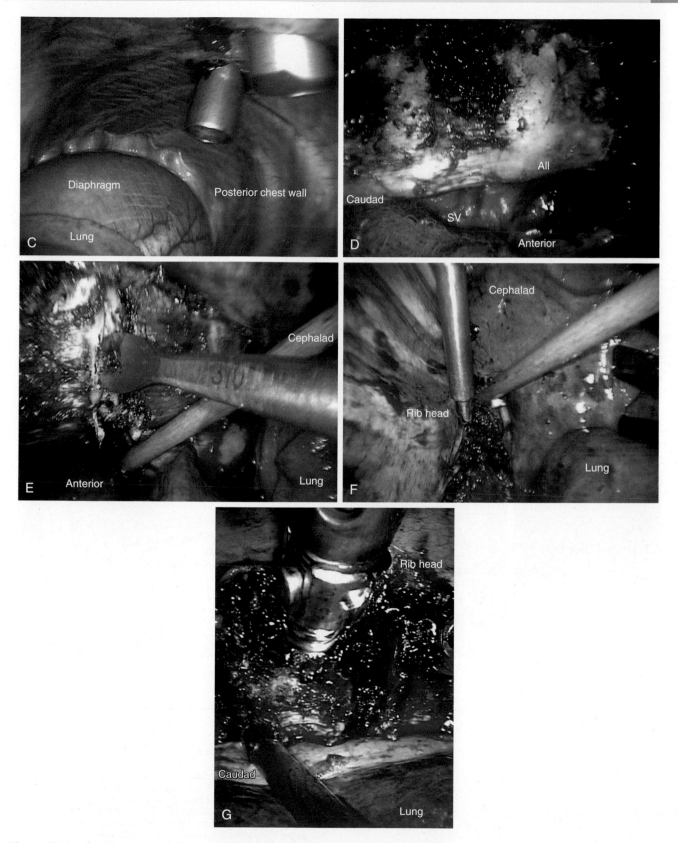

Figure 31-1, cont'd. C–G, Intraoperative images of the thoracoscopic technique. ALL, anterior longitudinal ligament; SV, segmental vessel.

Continued

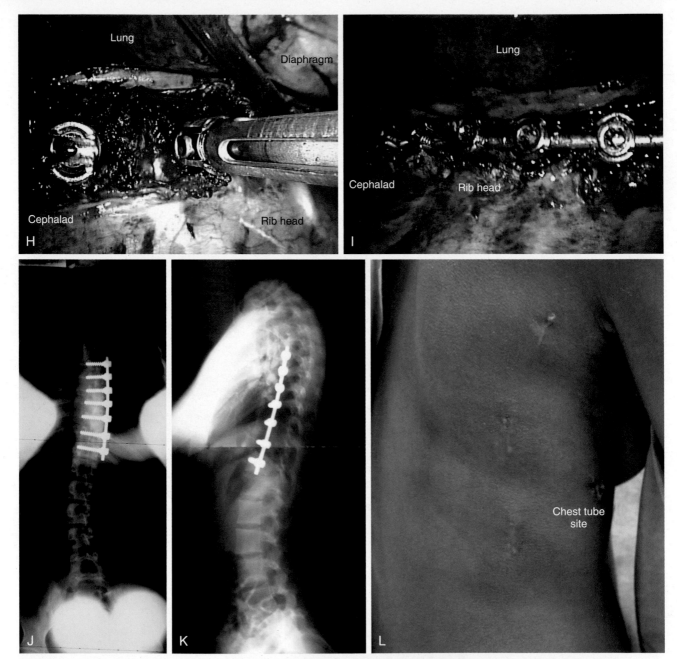

Figure 31-1, cont'd. H and **I,** Intraoperative images of the thorascopic technique. **J** and **K,** Postoperative posteroanterior and lateral radiographs. **L,** Postoperative image.

REFERENCES

Barone GW, Pait TG, Eidt JF, Howington JA: "General surgical pearls" for the anterior exposure of vertebral fractures. Am Surg 2001; 67:939–942.

Biglioti P, Spirito R, Roberto M, et al: The anterior spinal artery: The main arterial supply of the human spinal cord: A preliminary anatomic study. J Thorac Cardiovasc Surg 2000;119:376–379.

Cohen ZR, Fourney DR, Gokaslan ZL, et al: Anterior stabilization of the upper thoracic spine via an "interaortocaval subinnominate window": Case report and description of operative technique. J Spinal Disord Tech 2004;17:543–548.

Islam S, Hresko MT, Fishman SJ: Extrapleural thoracoscopic anterior spinal fusion: A modified video-assisted thoracoscopic surgery approach to the pediatric spine. J Soc Laparoendosc Surg 2001;5: 187–189.

Krbec M, Stulik J: Treatment of thoracolumbar spinal fractures using internal fixators. Acta Chir Orthop Traumatol Cech 2001;68:77–84.

Le Huec JC, Lesprit E, Guibaud JP, et al: Minimally invasive endoscopic approach to the cervicothoracic junction for vertebral metastases: Report of two cases. Eur Spine J 2001;10:421–426.

Niemeyer T, Freeman BJ, Grevitt MP, Webb JK: Anterior thoracoscopic surgery followed by posterior instrumentation and fusion in spinal deformity. Eur Spine J 2000;9:499–504.

Rubino F, Deutsch H, Pamoukian V, et al: Minimally invasive spine surgery: An animal model for endoscopic approach to the anterior cervical and upper thoracic spine. J Laparoendosc Adv Surg Tech A 2000;10:309–313.

Schwab FJ, Smith V, Farcy JP: Endoscopic thoracoplasty and anterior spinal release in scoliotic deformity. Bull Hosp Jt Dis 2000; 59:27–32.

SUGGESTED READINGS

Beisse R, Muckley T, Schmidt MH, et al: Surgical technique and results of endoscopic anterior spinal canal decompression. J Neurosurg Spine 2005;2:128–136.

The authors describe the endoscopic technique of anterior spinal canal decompression in the thoracolumbar spine. The morbidities associated with an open procedure were avoided, and excellent spinal canal clearance was accomplished, as was associated neurologic improvement.

Deutsch L, Testiauti M, Borman T: Simultaneous anterior-posterior thoracolumbar spine surgery. J Spinal Disord 2001;14:378–384.

The purpose of this study is to report the authors' experience with simultaneous anterior and posterior approach spine surgery.

Fraser JF, Diwan AD, Peterson M, et al: Preoperative magnetic resonance imaging screening for a surgical decision regarding the approach for anterior spine fusion at the cervicothoracic junction. Spine 2002;27:675–681.

This study demonstrates reliable and reproducible anatomic measurements that can aid spine surgeons in selecting surgical approaches for anterior spine fusion in the cervicothoracic region.

Holt RT, Majd ME, Vadhva M, Castro FP: The efficacy of anterior spine exposure by an orthopedic surgeon. J Spinal Disord Tech 2003; 16:477–486.

This retrospective study was designed to document the incidence and types of perioperative complications that occurred with anterior spinal fusion surgery performed solely by an orthopedic spine surgeon.

Huang EY, Acosta JM, Gardocki RJ, et al: Thoracoscopic anterior spinal release and fusion: Evolution of a faster, improved approach. J Pediatr Surg 2002;37:1732–1735.

The aim of this study was to compare the perioperative parameters and outcomes of video-assisted thoracoscopic surgery with open thoracotomy for anterior release and fusion in the treatment of pediatric spinal deformities.

Jin D, Qu D, Chen J, Zhang H: One-stage anterior interbody autografting and instrumentation in primary surgical management of thoracolumbar spinal tuberculosis. Eur Spine J 2004;13:114–121.

This study reports 23 cases of active thoracolumbar spinal tuberculosis treated by one-stage anterior interbody autografting and instrumentation.

Khoo LT, Beisse R, Potulski M: Thoracoscopic-assisted treatment of thoracic and lumbar fractures: A series of 371 consecutive cases. Neurosurgery 2002;51(5, suppl):S104–S117.

This retrospective study concludes that a complete anterior thoracoscopically assisted reconstruction of thoracic and thoracolumbar fractures can be safely and effectively accomplished, thereby reducing the pain and morbidity associated with conventional thoracotomy and thoracolumbar approaches.

Kim M, Nolan P, Finkelstein JA: Evaluation of 11th rib extrapleural-retroperitoneal approach to the thoracolumbar junction: Technical note. J Neurosurg 2000;93(1, suppl):168–174.

This study concludes that the 11th rib extrapleural-retroperitoneal approach was successfully used to treat patients with a variety of lesions in the thoracolumbar junction and was associated with little morbidity. The authors believe that previous criticism suggesting that this approach provides only limited access is unsubstantiated.

Knoller SM, Brethner L: Surgical treatment of the spine at the cervicothoracic junction: An illustrated review of a modified sternotomy approach with the description of tricks and pitfalls. Arch Orthop Trauma Surg 2002;122:365–368.

In this investigation, the anatomy and exposure of the cervicothoracic junction by means of a sternotomy are described. An illustrated review of the sternotomy approach to the cervicothoracic junction with a description of tricks and pitfalls is provided.

Levin R, Matusz D, Hasharoni A, et al: Mini-open thoracoscopically-assisted thoracotomy versus video-assisted thoracoscopic surgery for anterior release in thoracic scoliosis and kyphosis: A comparison of operative and radiographic results. Spine J 2005;5:632–638.

This retrospective study compares a mini open thoracoscopically assisted thoracotomy with a video-assisted thoracoscopic surgery for anterior release in thoracic scoliosis and kyphosis.

Lowry KJ, Tobias J, Kittle D, et al: Postoperative pain control using epidural catheters after anterior spinal fusion for adolescent scoliosis. Spine 2001;26:1290–1293.

This is a prospective review of patients undergoing epidural catheter placement after anterior spinal fusion and instrumentation for adolescent scoliosis. It concludes that epidural catheters can be used safely and effectively to control postoperative pain after anterior instrumentation and spinal fusion.

Perez-Cruet MJ, Kim BS, Sandhu F, et al: Thoracic microendoscopic discectomy. J Neurosurg Spine 2004;1:58–63.

The authors describe a retrospective study based on a novel posterolateral, minimally invasive thoracic microendoscopic discectomy technique that provides an approach to the thoracic spine which is associated with less morbidity.

Xu R, Grabow R, Ebraheim NA, et al: Anatomic considerations of a modified anterior approach to the cervicothoracic junction. Am J Orthop 2000;29:37–40.

This is an anatomic study on 30 human spines. It concludes that an adequate exposure of the low cervical spine to the upper thoracic spine can be obtained with this specific approach.

SECTION V

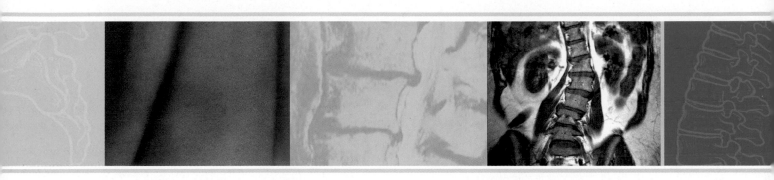

The Future of Spinal Deformity Surgery

CHAPTER 32

Future Developments in Spinal Deformity Surgery

PETER O. NEWTON

Idiopathic scoliosis remains a great challenge for those who are involved in spinal deformity care. The etiology eludes us, and the treatment for severe cases remains a radical procedure: fusion of an extensive portion of the spinal column. Our ability to perform such a correction and fusion procedure has advanced technologically since the introduction of the Harrington rod roughly 40 years ago, yet the desired outcome remains the same: a solid spinal arthrodesis. Posterior instrumentation systems are being developed at breakneck speed, whereas the early evolution from Harrington's rod to Cotrel and Dubousset's system took nearly 20 years. The past decade seems to have been devoted to the power of the thoracic pedicle screw. Undoubtedly, the correction of scoliosis has been greatly improved, particularly if one uses the somewhat flawed comparisons of the percent reduction of the Cobb angle—approximately 40% to 50% in the 1970s compared to 70% to 90% currently (Fig. 32-1). Great strides have also been made with anterior instrumentation methods. Problems with implant failures and the sagittal plane that plagued the early Dwyer and Zielke systems have largely been addressed with modern systems. The approach-related morbidity has been mitigated to some degree by the thoracoscopic method, but this has not been widely accepted into practice. Thus, in the 40 years of spinal instrumentation, we have become more successful at both achieving a solid arthrodesis of the spine and getting better spinal deformity correction in the process.

This, in my opinion, has been progress; however, we must remain cognizant of the fact that our procedures are designed to limit motion of substantial lengths of the spine. As we look to the future treatment of scoliosis, we must strive to make spinal mobility a priority. Granted, the vast majority of our patients seem to tolerate spinal fusion very well, but the lifelong effects of scoliosis instrumentation are not yet fully known. The first teenage scoliosis patients of Harrington are just now approaching their 60s. The next 20 years of evaluation will be critical and telling. It is unclear how the long-term status of the unfused segments

will fare over a lifetime. Lumbar degenerative disease is so prevalent that many fused and unfused scoliosis patients will face the symptoms associated with lumbar degeneration. One of the great unknowns is what degree of scoliosis the lumbar spine can tolerate with regard to late degeneration risk.

Recognizing the accomplishments in advancing scoliosis treatment along with the significant limitations that remain, we look to the future. What needs to be done to make "real" changes in the outcomes of scoliosis treatment? I think this can be summarized with two main objectives: (1) gaining a better understanding of the nature of the condition, diagnosis, and disease we call idiopathic scoliosis and (2) using this knowledge to design methods of redirecting or controlling spinal growth once a small curve has been detected, with the goal of reducing the need for spinal arthrodesis in adolescence.

We are beginning to home in on some of the genetic code that could be responsible for the generation of idiopathic scoliosis. It is undoubtedly a complex genetic disorder, and it is likely that there is more than one possible pathway for the development of abnormal adolescent spinal growth. Research in this area is critical if we are to have a chance at getting beyond spinal fusion procedures. With very few hard facts, theories as to the etiology of idiopathic scoliosis abound. These theories must be tested, and interrelationships between them must be sought. This puzzle, like many before, will be solved; the question is only "when."

In the meantime, there is much that can be done to understand if not the etiology, then the three-dimensional nature of this spinal deformity. Scoliosis is a complex deformity of a structure that, even in normalcy, has a complex sagittal plane geometry. The patterns of spinal deformity, although recognizable to some degree in the frontal plane, become much more challenging to categorize in the sagittal plane and particularly in the transverse plane. Our current imaging techniques do not allow a full appreciation of the three-dimensional nature of these

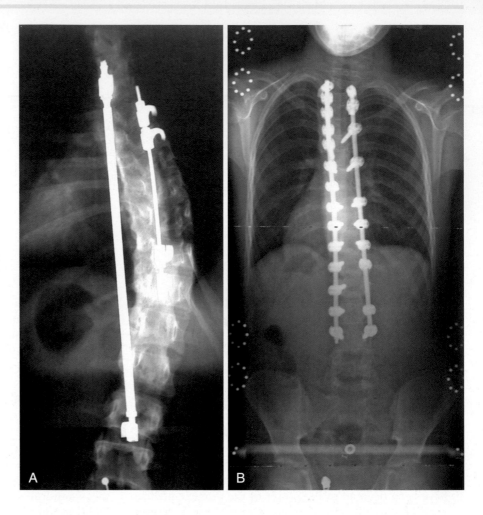

Figure 32-1. A, Example of Harrington rod instrumentation. **B,** Modern segmental thoracic pedicle screw instrumentation.

highly varied curve patterns. Just as we have realized the importance of the sagittal plane, we realize the value of understanding the transverse or axial plane, yet this dimension is much more challenging to image and analyze. I believe that as we master how to recognize what the transverse plane has to tell us, we will become better at correcting scoliosis in general as well as at designing a corrective procedure for each individual case. Although we tend to be more comfortable when we classify curve patterns into specific subtypes, the variation of scoliotic curves is so great that individual treatment approaches are needed if we seek better correction for each patient. To do this, however, requires a clear definition of all three planes of deformity.

What does "better correction" really mean? We would all agree in general that straighter is better and that a shorter fusion is better. Shorter and straighter are often conflicting goals, and global balance trumps both of these factors. The ultimate short fusion is none at all, and the ultimate straight spine could include a fusion of the entire thoracic and lumbar spine. Although each of these extremes might be the "best" choice for a given patient, we are often seeking a compromise between correction and length of fusion. Selective thoracic fusion promoted by Moe in the

Harrington era continues to ring true; we should spare the lumbar spine from fusion whenever possible. This often requires a balance between residual deformity and residual lumbar motion (Fig. 32-2). The deformity-flexibility quotient allows a quantification of the outcome of this compromise. The deformity-flexibility quotient is a ratio of the residual lumbar deformity as measured by the Cobb angle of the lumbar curve—fused or unfused, divided by the lumbar flexibility expressed as the number of unfused lumbar motion segments. A lower deformity-flexibility quotient value implies a smaller lumbar curve and greater lumbar flexibility—both theoretically "better." Long-term outcomes and three-dimensional analysis will ultimately be required to truly identify what "better correction" means.

The second major objective for the future is to develop effective means of controlling spinal growth. Our current best attempts use external braces in an attempt to mechanically influence spinal growth. Some clinicians remain skeptical of bracing efficacy, and even the "believers" would acknowledge serious limitations—at best curve stabilization rather than correction, as well as comfort and compliance issues. Internal mechanical methods designed to influence growth have been applied in the form of "growing rods." This is a misnomer, of course, since the rods do not

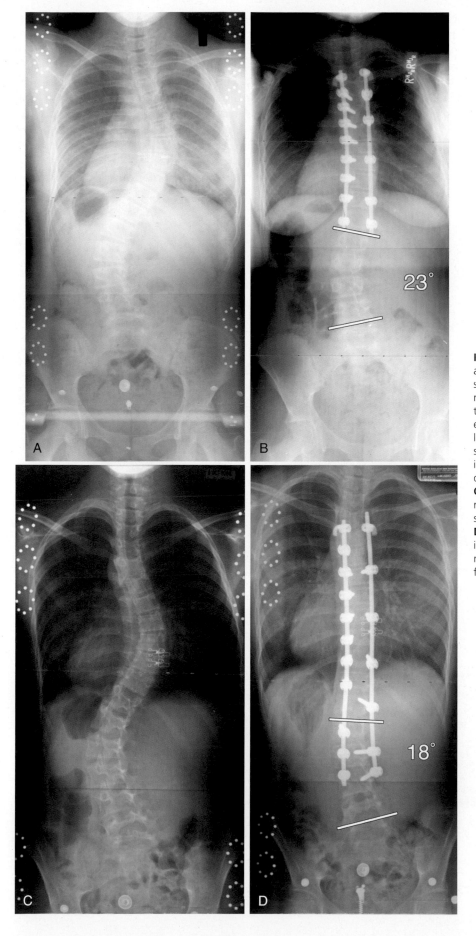

Figure 32-2. A, Right thoracic, left lumbar adolescent idiopathic scoliosis treated with selective thoracic fusion. **B,** This posteroanterior radiograph demonstrates the improvement in the thoracic deformity with instrumentation ending distally at T12. A 23-degree residual lumbar deformity remains; however, there are six discs that have not been fused distal to the instrumentation segment. This results in a deformity flexibility quotient of 23/6 = 3.8. **C,** Posteroanterior radiograph of a patient with right thoracic left lumbar scoliosis in which a selective thoracic fusion was not performed. **D,** Postoperative radiographs demonstrate instrumentation to L3 distally with an 18-degree residual lumbar deformity. The deformity flexibility quotient is 18/3 = 6.

grow; they can, however, be lengthened surgically at intervals to keep up with growth and, ideally, promote a normalization of spinal growth. This is one of our best options for early-onset scoliosis; however, it is merely a technique for delaying the eventual spinal fusion. The ideal solution would allow spinal growth to normalize the deformity and eliminate the need for later fusion, thus preserving all normal spinal motion and function.

The currently ongoing research involving techniques to slow convex anterior spinal growth might achieve these lofty aspirations of correction without loss of motion.

Present strategies include some form of a staple or tethering element placed across the disc space in an attempt to modulate or asymmetrically influence longitudinal vertebral growth. This is similar to the logic used by Blount when he introduced his staple to correct angular deformity in the lower extremities decades ago. There is one critical difference, however, and this is the disc. Because the vertebrae do not have an epiphysis, as in the long bones of the lower extremities, mechanical spinal growth modulation has necessarily crossed the disc space. What effect these devices will have on spinal motion and the condition

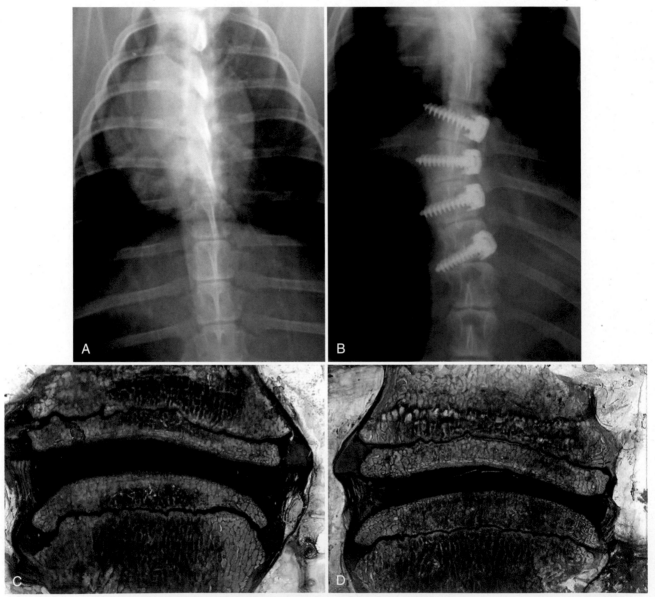

Figure 32-3. A, This posteroanterior radiograph represents the thoracic spine of a miniature pig prior to surgical implantation of a tethering element. **B,** In this experimental model, the miniature pig has been instrumented with an ultra-high-molecular weight polyethylene cable between the screws for 10 months. The resulting deformity is visible with wedging of the vertebral bodies due to mechanical modulation of spinal growth. **C,** A histologic specimen of a calf thoracic spine that has not undergone mechanical tethering. **D,** A corresponding thoracic disc space that has undergone 6 months of mechanical tethering. The physes remain intact; however, there is narrowing of the disc space. These specimens were also associated with vertebral wedging when analyzed by CT scan. These histologic images emphasize the need to monitor closely the effects on the disc space by mechanical tethering methods.

of the intervertebral disc remain to be proven. It does appear, however, that in experimental models, spinal growth can be mechanically manipulated (Fig. 32-3). This offers the potential for a means of correcting scoliosis as long as growth remains. How much correction and at what functional cost remain to be seen.

Mechanical growth modulation will likely come into clinical use in the relatively near future and could be the ideal option for the smaller progressive curves of juvenile and adolescent onset. This will be a welcome change from either bracing (motion without correction) or fusion (correction without motion). The greater challenge of early-onset scoliosis in children younger than 5 years of age will almost certainly require a more sophisticated approach. In these cases, we must be thinking long term about biologic solutions. This will obviously require greater knowledge of the etiology of scoliosis in this age group. This is a daunting task, given our current understanding of what controls spinal growth in scoliosis. I can only hope that we have the opportunity to reflect in 20 years and cringe at the solutions that we were able to offer this group of patients. There is great room for improvement in the treatment of scoliosis, and we must continue to aggressively seek the elusive answers we need to make these improvements.

REFERENCES

Alden KJ, Marosy B, Nzegwu N, et al: Idiopathic scoliosis: Identification of candidate regions on chromosome 19p13. Spine 2006;31:1815–1819.

Bashiardes S, Veile R, Allen M, et al: SNTG1, the gene encoding gamma1-syntrophin: A candidate gene for idiopathic scoliosis. Hum Genet 2004;115:81–89.

Bauer R, Mostegl A, Eichenauer M: An analysis of the results of Dwyer and Zielke instrumentations in the treatment of scoliosis. Arch Orthop Trauma Surg 1986;105:302–309.

Betz RR, et al: Vertebral body stapling procedure for the treatment of scoliosis in the growing child. Clin Orthop Relat Res 2005;434:55–60.

Blount WP, Clarke GR: The classic: Control of bone growth by epiphyseal stapling: A preliminary report: Journal of Bone and Joint Surgery, July, 1949. Clin Orthop Relat Res 1971;77:4–17.

Braun JT, Hoffman M, Akyuz E, et al: Mechanical modulation of vertebral growth in the fusionless treatment of progressive scoliosis in an experimental model. Spine 2006;31:1314–1320.

Burwell RG: Aetiology of idiopathic scoliosis: Current concepts. Pediatr Rehabil 2003;6:137–170.

Cotrel Y, Dubousset J: [A new technique for segmental spinal osteosynthesis using the posterior approach]. Rev Chir Orthop Reparatrice Appar Mot 1984;70:489–494.

Dickson RA, Weinstein SL: Bracing (and screening): Yes or no? J Bone Joint Surg Br 1999;81:193–198.

Dong L, Cheriet F, Labelle H: Three-dimensional classification of spinal deformities using fuzzy clustering. Spine 2006;31:923–930.

Faro FD, Marks MC, Newton PO, et al: Perioperative changes in pulmonary function after anterior scoliosis instrumentation: Thoracoscopic versus open approaches. Spine 2005;30:1058–1063.

Giampietro PF, Blank RD, Raggio CL, et al: Congenital and idiopathic scoliosis: Clinical and genetic aspects. Clin Med Res 2003;1:125–136.

Harrington PR: Treatment of scoliosis: Correction and internal fixation by spine instrumentation. J Bone Joint Surg Am 1962;44:591–610.

Helfenstein A, Lankes M, Ohlert K, et al: The objective determination of compliance in treatment of adolescent idiopathic scoliosis with spinal orthoses. Spine 2006;31:339–344.

Humke T, Grob D, Scheier H, Siegrist H: Cotrel–Dubousset and Harrington instrumentation in idiopathic scoliosis: A comparison of long-term results. Eur Spine J 1995;4:280–283.

Kaneda K, Shono Y, Satoh S, Abumi K: New anterior instrumentation for the management of thoracolumbar and lumbar scoliosis: Application of the Kaneda two-rod system. Spine 1996;21:1250–1261; discussion 1261–1262.

Kim YJ, Lenke LG, Kim J, et al: Comparative analysis of pedicle screw versus hybrid instrumentation in posterior spinal fusion of adolescent idiopathic scoliosis. Spine 2006;31:291–298.

King HA, Moe JH, Bradford DS, Winter RB: The selection of fusion levels in thoracic idiopathic scoliosis. J Bone Joint Surg Am 1983;65:1302–1313.

Lenke L: Debate: Resolved, a 55 degree right thoracic adolescent idiopathic scoliotic curve should be treated by posterior spinal fusion and segmental instrumentation using thoracic pedicle screws: Pro: Thoracic pedicle screws should be used to treat a 55 degree right thoracic adolescent idiopathic scoliosis. J Pediatr Orthop 2004;24:329–334.

Liljenqvist UR, Halm HF, Link TM: Pedicle screw instrumentation of the thoracic spine in idiopathic scoliosis. Spine 1997;22:2239–2245.

Mariconda M, Galasso O, Barca P, Milano C: Minimum 20-year follow-up results of Harrington rod fusion for idiopathic scoliosis. Eur Spine J 2005;14:854–861.

Miller NH, Justice CM, Marosy B, et al: Identification of candidate regions for familial idiopathic scoliosis. Spine 2005;30:1181–1187.

Moe JH: Modern concepts of treatment of spinal deformities in children and adults. Clin Orthop 1980;150:137–153.

Morcuende JA, Minhas R, Dolan L, et al: Allelic variants of human melatonin 1A receptor in patients with familial adolescent idiopathic scoliosis. Spine 2003;28:2025–2028; discussion 2029.

Picetti GD 3rd, Ertl JP, Bueff HU: Endoscopic instrumentation, correction, and fusion of idiopathic scoliosis. Spine J 2001;1:190–197.

Suk SI, Lee CK, Kim WJ, et al: Segmental pedicle screw fixation in the treatment of thoracic idiopathic scoliosis. Spine 1995;20:1399–1405.

Thompson GH, Akbarnia BA, Kostial P, et al: Comparison of single and dual growing rod techniques followed through definitive surgery: A preliminary study. Spine 2005;30:2039–2044.

Ugwonali OF, Lomas G, Choe JC, et al: Effect of bracing on the quality of life of adolescents with idiopathic scoliosis. Spine J 2004;4:254–260.

Wall EJ, Bylski-Austrow DI, Kolata RJ, Crawford AH: Endoscopic mechanical spinal hemiepiphysiodesis modifies spine growth. Spine 2005;30:1148–1153.

Wu J, Qiu Y, Zhang L, et al: Association of estrogen receptor gene polymorphisms with susceptibility to adolescent idiopathic scoliosis. Spine 2006;31:1131–1136.

SUGGESTED READINGS

Akbarnia BA, Marks DS, Boachie-Adjei O, et al: Dual growing rod technique for the treatment of progressive early-onset scoliosis: A multicenter study. Spine 2005;30(17, suppl):S46–S57.

The study aims to determine the safety and effectiveness of the previously described dual growing rod technique in achieving and maintaining scoliosis correction while allowing spinal growth. It concludes that the dual growing rod technique is safe and effective. The technique maintains correction obtained at initial surgery while allowing spinal growth to continue. It provides adequate stability, increases the duration of treatment period, and has an acceptable rate of complication in compaison with previous reports using the single-rod technique.

Braun JT, Hines JL, Akyuz E, et al: Relative versus absolute modulation of growth in the fusionless treatment of experimental scoliosis. Spine 2006;31:1776–1782.

The objective of this study is to differentiate relative and absolute changes in growth on the concavity and convexity of an experimental scoliosis treated with anterior vertebral stapling. Data in this study show the ability to modulate relative and absolute growth, according to the Hueter-Volkmann Law, at the apical spinal segment of a progressive experimental scoliosis. However, anterior vertebral stapling, though able to control progressive wedging and scoliosis at the apical spinal segment, was not able to reverse fully the Hueter-Volkmann effect.

Helenius I, Remes V, Yrjönen T, et al: Harrington and Cotrel-Dubousset instrumentation in adolescent idiopathic scoliosis: Long-term functional and radiographic outcomes. J Bone Joint Surg Am 2003; 85-A:2303–2309.

This study compares Cotrel-Dubouset instrumentation with Harrington instrumentation and concludes that Cotrel-Dubousset instrumentation yielded better long-term functional and radiographic outcomes in patients with adolescent idiopathic scoliosis than did Harrington instrumentation. However, complications were more common in the Cotrel-Dubousset instrumentation group.

Lee SM, Suk SI, Chung ER: Direct vertebral rotation: A new technique of three-dimensional deformity correction with segmental pedicle screw fixation in adolescent idiopathic scoliosis. Spine 2004;29: 343–349.

This is a new technique described by Dr. Suk; the authors concluded that segmental pedicle screw fixation with "direct vertebral rotation" showed better rotational and coronal correction than did "simple rod derotation."

Lenke LG, Betz RR, Harms J, et al: Adolescent idiopathic scoliosis: A new classification to determine extent of spinal arthrodesis. J Bone Joint Surg Am 2001;83-A:1169–1181.

This new two-dimensional classification of adolescent idiopathic scoliosis, as tested by two groups of surgeons, was shown to be much more reliable than the King system. It concludes that additional studies are necessary to determine the versatility, reliability, and accuracy of the classification for defining the vertebrae to be included in an arthrodesis.

Lonner BS, Scharf C, Antonacci D, et al: The learning curve associated with thoracoscopic spinal instrumentation. Spine 2005;30:2835–2840.

This study concludes that the learning curve associated with thoracoscopic spinal instrumentation appears to be acceptable. Significant differences were noted in operating time and percent curve correction after 28 cases, and the complication rates remained stable throughout the surgeon's experience.

Newton PO, Faro FD, Farnsworth CL, et al: Multilevel spinal growth modulation with an anterolateral flexible tether in an immature bovine model. Spine 2005;30:2608–2813.

This study aims to evaluate the radiographic changes in a growing spine with a multilevel anterolateral tether. It concludes that given adequate bony fixation, a flexible lateral spinal tether can affect growth modulation. This technique of growth modulation could serve as a future fusionless method of correction in a growing patient with scoliosis.

Newton PO, Marks M, Faro F, et al: Use of video-assisted thoracoscopic surgery to reduce perioperative morbidity in scoliosis surgery. Spine 2003;28:S249–S254.

This study evaluates the morbidity associated with thoracoscopic instrumentation compared to the open approach for thoracic scoliosis. It concludes that the thoracoscopic approach for instrumentation of scoliosis has advantages of reduced chest wall morbidity compared with the open thoracotomy method but allows comparable curve correction.

Newton PO, Parent S, Marks M, Pawelek J: Prospective evaluation of 50 consecutive scoliosis patients surgically treated with thoracoscopic anterior instrumentation. Spine 2005;30(17, suppl):S100–S109.

This study confirms that thoracoscopic anterior instrumentation for adolescent idiopathic scoliosis is a viable surgical option. The outcomes of this consecutive series of patients are comparable to prior open and endoscopic series presented in the literature. The technical challenges of this operation are evident in the learning curve effect, which has been demonstrated.

Ogilvie JW, Braun J, Argyle V, et al: The search for idiopathic scoliosis genes. Spine 2006;31:679–681.

This study aims to quantify the genetic effect in adolescent idiopathic scoliosis, determine the expressivity and penetrance of adolescent idiopathic scoliosis in large family groupings, and examine larger scoliosis pedigrees for evidence of multiple genes. It concludes that nearly all (97%) cases of adolescent idiopathic scoliosis have familial origins. There appears to be at least one major gene, and the differences in penetrance and expressivity in two large unconnected pedigrees might suggest the presence of more than one gene.

Suk SI, Lee CK, Min HJ, et al: Comparison of Cotrel-Dubousset pedicle screws and hooks in the treatment of idiopathic scoliosis. Int Orthop 1994;18:341–346.

This article compares Cotrel-Dubousset pedicle screws and hooks in the treatment of idiopathic scoliosis and concludes that screw fixation can be used in the thoracic spine without neurological complications. The screws provided immediate stability with rigid fixation, together with better correction of frontal, sagittal, and rotational deformity. There is less loss of correction, a shorter fusion, and less risk of neurologic complications because of the placement outside the spinal canal and the rigid fixation in derotation. The technique was simpler and the operating time shorter than with the other methods.

Sweet FA, Lenke LG, Bridwell KH, et al: Prospective radiographic and clinical outcomes and complications of single solid rod instrumented anterior spinal fusion in adolescent idiopathic scoliosis. Spine 2001;26:1956–1965.

This study concludes that anterior instrumented fusions for adolescent idiopathic scoliosis using a single solid rod had good radiographic and clinical outcomes. Consideration should be given to alternative techniques in larger adolescents (>70 kg) with thoracic hyperkyphosis (>40 degrees), and smoking should be avoided. Poor radiographic outcomes did not correlate with final Scoliosis Research Society scores.

Wise CA, Bennett LB, Pascual V, et al: Localization of susceptibility to familial idiopathic scoliosis. Spine 2000;25:2372–2380.

This study focuses on the genetic etiology of adolescent idiopathic scoliosis, with the objective of identifying chromosomal loci encoding genes that are involved in susceptibility to idiopathic scoliosis by positional cloning. It concludes that according to the study's data, there are a limited number of genetic loci predisposing to idiopathic scoliosis.

Note: Page numbers followed by b indicate boxes; those followed by f indicate figures; and those followed by t indicate tables.